MEDICAL RADIOLOGY

Diagnostic Imaging and Radiation Oncology

Springer
Berlin
Heidelberg
New York
Barcelona
Hong Kong
London
Milan
Paris
Singapore
Tokyo

A. L. Baert (Ed.)

G. Delorme and L. Van Hoe (Co-Eds.)

Radiology of the Pancreas

2nd Revised Edition

With Contributions by

A. L. Baert · P. H. Bernard · J. C. Brichaux · J.-M. Bruel · M. Brun · P. Brys · J. F. Chateil
B. Claikens · F. Diard · B. Dousset · C. Douws · J. Drouillard · P. M. Dubois · J.-F. Flejou
R. Függer · F. Grabenwöger · P. Grelet · J. Grellet · N. Grenier · A. M. Herneth
G. Klöppel · F. Laurent · R. Lecesne · G. Lechner · P. Legmann · G. Marchal · D. Mathieu
E. Ponette · A. Rahmouni · J. W. A. J. Reeders · H. Rigauts · A. Roche · E. Schlüter
N. J. Smith · P. Taourel · E. Thérasse · H. Trillaud · O. M. Van Delden · L. Van Hoe
W. Van Steenbergen · O. Vignaux · V. Vilgrain

Foreword by

F. H. W. Heuck

With 386 Figures in 690 Separate Illustrations, 18 in Color

Springer

Albert L. Baert, MD
Professor
Department of Radiology, University Hospital K.U.L.
Herestraat 49, B-3000 Leuven
Belgium

Guy Delorme, MD
Professor
Centre Hospitalier, Régional de Bordeaux, Hôpital Pellegrin
Place Amélie-Raba-Léon, F-33076 Bordeaux Cédex
France

Lieven Van Hoe, MD, PhD
Assistant Professor
Department of Radiology, University Hospital K.U.L.
Herestraat 49, B-3000 Leuven
Belgium

MEDICAL RADIOLOGY · Diagnostic Imaging and Radiation Oncology

Continuation of
Handbuch der medizinischen Radiologie
Encyclopedia of Medical Radiology

ISBN 3-540-63479-7 Springer-Verlag Berlin Heidelberg New York

Library of Congress Cataloging-in-Publication Data. Radiology of the pancreas / (ed) A. L. Baert ; co-edited by G. Delorme and L. Van Hoe ; with contributions by A. L. Baert ... [et al.]. -- 2nd rev ed. p. cm. -- (Medical radiology) Includes bibliographical references and index. 1. Pancreas--Radiography. I. Baert, A. L. (Albert L.), 1931- . Delorme, G. (Guy) III. Hoe, L. van, 1963- . IV. Series. [DNLM: 1. Pancreatic Diseases--diagnosis. 2. Pancreas--pathology. 3. Diagnostic Imaging--methods. WI 800 R129 1999] RC857.5.R33 1999 616.3'70754--dc21 DNLM/DLC for Library of Congresws 98-50337 CIP

Printed in Germany

Typesetting: Verlagsservice Teichmann, Mauer

SPIN: 10561016 21/3135 – 5 4 3 2 1 0 – Printed on acid-free paper

Foreword

The rapid developments in new imaging modalities as applied to the diagnostic work-up of pancreatic diseases have made a new edition of *Radiology of the Pancreas* necessary. The first edition of this important book by Albert Baert and a number of other renowned specialists covered the whole spectrum of normal and pathological imaging findings of the pancreas. Very soon this excellent volume was sold out. Because of the rapid methodological advances in spiral CT, MRI and sonography it has been necessary to revise the chapters on pancreatitis as well as those on primary and secondary tumors of the pancreas. The results of MR cholangiopancreatography have been introduced and special attention has been paid to the newly written chapters on normal radiological anatomy and variants of the pancreas. More detailed information on pathomorphological findings as seen by high-resolution spiral CT, sonography with color and power Doppler, and MRI with subsecond "snap-shot" sequences and specific contrast media is provided. Accordingly, a number of new illustrations have been included. The chapters on "Pancreatic Diseases in Childhood", "The Postoperative Pancreas" and "Pancreatic Transplantation" deserve attention.

The authors gathered by Albert Baert are all outstanding radiologists experienced in this special field. I am convinced this book will be of great value to all radiologists and other medical specialists who treat patients with pancreatic disease, as well as to physicians in training and students.

I wish this important second edition of Radiology of the Pancreas the same remarkable popularity and success as the first edition.

Stuttgart FRIEDRICH HEUCK

Preface

During the 5 years that have elapsed since the first edition of "Radiology of the Pancreas", published in 1994, further technical developments have taken place in three diagnostic modalities that play a key role in the diagnosis and management of pancreatic diseases. I refer to computed tomography (CT), with further technical advances in spiral CT, to sonography, with the clinical diffusion of color and power Doppler, and, even more importantly, to magnetic resonance imaging (MRI), with the introduction of "snap-shot", subsecond sequences, of projective and cross-sectional MR cholangiopancreaticography (MRCP) and of specific MR contrast media. The amount of new data available and the success of the first edition prompted us to prepare a second revised version of our book, the short time interval since publication of the first edition notwithstanding.

In comparison with the first edition, numerous new illustrations have been introduced in order to provide a maximum of state-of-the-art high-resolution CT figures. The chapter on radiological anatomy has been completely rewritten and considerably expanded. The possibilities and clinical applications of MRCP are introduced where needed and the new possibilities of the rapid sequences in MRI for the diagnosis of benign and malignant tumors are illustrated appropriately.

I would hereby like to thank my co-editors, Guy Delorme and Lieven Van Hoe, for their enthusiastic and efficient support. I express my great appreciation to the authors, all internationally known experts in their field of interest, for their overwhelmingly positive response to the preparation of a revised version, as well as for the timely delivery of their excellent and up-to-date chapters.

Lieven Van Hoe has been particularly helpful in assuming a lot of editorial tasks, which allowed us to reduce the production time of this book to an absolute minimum.

Special thanks go also to the staff of Springer-Verlag involved in the preparation of this volume, and particularly to Ursula Davis, for their very professional and efficient support in order to ensure optimal technical publishing quality and extremely rapid publication of this volume.

Leuven — Albert L. Baert

Acknowledgements

The editors acknowledge the excellent technical support from the photographers responsible for the preparation of the illustrations as well as the superb secretarial help from Mrs. Monika Philips.

Contents

1 The Exocrine and Endocrine Pancreas: Embryology and Histology

P. M. Dubois

CONTENTS

1.1 Introduction

The pancreas is both an exocrine and an endocrine gland. The exocrine part is arranged in *acini.* The exocrine secretion products are collected and delivered by a duct system which is drained by the pancreatic ducts. The endocrine component is composed of small clumps of cells, named the *islets of Langerhans,* which are scattered throughout the exocrine glandular tissue. The history of the endocrine pancreas has been recently reviewed (Samols 1991).

1.2 Gross Anatomy

The pancreas is a large gland located retroperitoneally at the level of L1–L3. On its right side it lies in the concavity of the duodenum, while on the left it extends to the hilus of the kidney, touching the spleen anteriorly. It is divided grossly into several parts: the head and uncinate process resting in the concavity of the duodenum, the body, and the tail extending to the left. All of these regions are drained horizontally by the main pancreatic duct, the duct of Wirsung, which enters the duodenum through the ampulla of Vater. Sometimes, an accessory pancreatic duct, the duct of Santorini, found in about 10% of individuals, enters the duodenum rostral to the ampulla; this duct derives from the embryonic dorsal pancreas and drains the head of the gland.

The *blood supply* is derived from the celiac and superior mesenteric arteries within the gland. The intralobular arteries contribute one or more arterioles either to acini or to islets. The pancreatic parenchyma is supplied by an extensive capillary network. However, several capillaries radiate from the islets to supply the periacinar capillary network. Thus an islet-acinar blood portal system exists in the pancreas (Fujita 1973) and a large part of the blood first supplies the islets. Consequently, islet hormones may be distributed to the acinar tissue and interact with acinar cells.

The pancreas is *innervated* by both parasympathetic fibers from the vagus nerve and sympathetic fibers from the celiac, the superior mesenteric, and the hepatic plexus. Nerve fibers are essentially distributed along the blood vessels, around ducts, and in the stromal, acinar, and insular compartments. Besides cholinergic, adrenergic, and gabaergic nerve fibers, numerous peptide-containing neurons have been demonstrated in the pancreas, with some differences in the density and pattern of fiber distribution (De Giorgio et al. 1992); the peptides in question are vasoactive intestinal peptide, substance P, cholecystokinin, enkephalins, gastrin-releasing peptide, bombesin, neuropeptide Y, neurotensin, calcitonin gene-related peptide (CGRP), and galanin.

P. M. Dubois, Professeur, CNRS-URA 1454, Université Claude Bernard, Faculté de Médicine Lyon-Sud, Laboratoire d'Histologie et d'Embryologie, BP 12, F-96900 Oullins, France

1.3 Embryology

1.3.1 Organogenesis

The pancreas develops from two separate evaginations of the foregut arising at about the third and fourth weeks of gestation in humans. These evaginations appear as a pair of blind-ended tubes.

The dorsal pancreas is first located at the dosral wall of the duodenum opposite to the hepatic diverticulum (Fig. 1.1). The ventral bud arises a little later, in the angle below the hepatic anlage. (Fig. 1.1). Each of these buds rapidly grows by branching. The duodenum undergoes a rotation so that its ventral surface is directed to the right. At this time, the ventral pancreas, which is connected to the duodenum by the duct of Wirsung, lies caudal to the dorsal pancreas. It is separated from the dorsal pancreas by the left vitelline vein, which becomes the portal vein. The dorsal pancreas is connected to the duodenum by the duct of Santorini. At the seventh week, the two pancreatic primordia fuse to form a simple organ. The upper part of the head, the body, and the tail derive from the dorsal bud, and the uncinate process from the ventral bud. At the time of fusion of the primordia, the ducts of each bud also fuse: the duct of Wirsung is formed distally by the duct of the dorsal pancreas and proximally by that of the ventral pancreas.

1.3.2 Development of the Exocrine Pancreas

By the time of fusion of the two oancreatic buds, hollow branchings from the endoderm outgrowth have appeared. These increase in length and invade surrounding mesenchyma. These blindended tubes are lined by undifferentiated simple columnar epithelial cells. From their blind ends epithelial sprouts arise which become canalized to form the collecting ducts. The acini arise by sprouting from the tips of the latter. The ducts continue to elongate and produce numerous branches of decreasing caliber. Acini, lobules, and lobes begin to organize into mesenchymal tissue.

During the development, the epithelial cells come into contact with a blanket of mesenchymal tissue, which, it has been suggested, plays a role in the morphogenesis of the pancreas. These adult characteristics are first discernible at the third or fourth month of gestation. The exocrine pancreas grows by the in situ proliferation of acinar cells as confirmed by the observation in mouse chimaeras of large patches of exocrine pancreas cells with a aingle genotype (Dewey and Mintz 1978). In the human fetus, the exocrine pancreas may be functional from the 5th or 6th month.

1.3.3 Development of the Endocrine Pancreas

1.3.3.1 Histogenesis of Islets

It has been generally accepted that the endocrine cells of islets develop from the pancreatic duct system. Clumps of cells fail to develop a lumen, become completely detached from the duct system, and form truly isolated islets of Langerhans. This phenomenon is probably due to a change in the axis of cell division, allowing the escape from the ductule lumen of one of the daughter cells (Pictet and

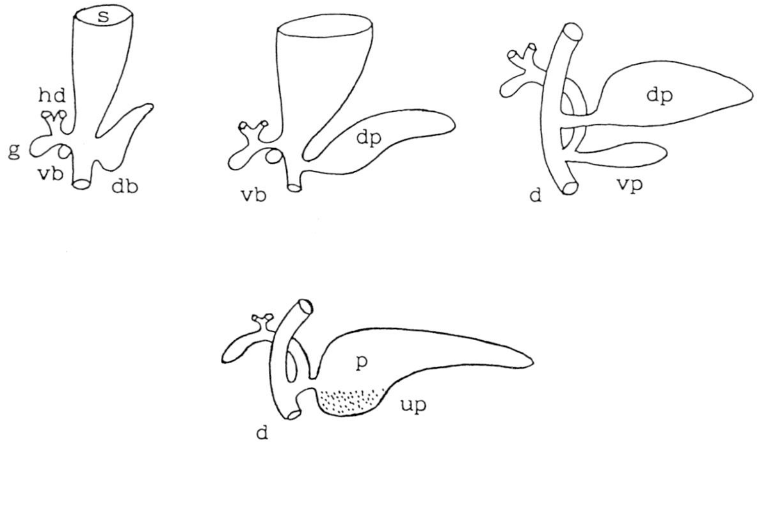

Fig. 1.1. Schematic drawings showing the development of pancreatic buds. Dorsal and ventral buds are shown before (*top*) and after (*bottom*) their fusion. The *dotted region* is the uncinate process which derives from the ventral bud. *d*, Duodenum; *db* , dorsal bud; *dp*, dorsal pancreas; *g*, gallbladder; *hd*, hepatic ducts; *p*, pancreas; *s*, stomach; *up*, uncinate process; *vb*, ventral bud; *vp*, ventral pancreas

Rutter 1972). Thus the endocrine cells arise by differentiating from progenitor cells within the ductular epithelium. Different endocrine pancreatic cells have been observed in the wall of the pancreatic duct in various species (Dubois 1989) and particularly in the pancreas of mouse chimaeras (Deltour et al. 1991).

1.3.3.2
Origin of Islet Cells

The results of cytochemical and ultrastructural studies on the endocrine cells of the pancreas, and more generally on the endocrine cells associated with endomesodermal structures, and advances in our knowledge of the peptides produced by these cells, led Pearse (1969) to develop the concept of an APUD system. The common ability of all these cells to concentrate amines, to take up their precursors, and to decarboxylate them support this concept. Pancreatic A and B endocrine cells are included in this APUD system, together with pituitary corticotrophs, thyroid C cells, gastrointestinal argyrophil or argentaffin cells, and adrenal medullary cells. The cytochemical and ultrastructural similarities of these cells are realted to their origin from a common ancestor. It has been postulated that all of these hormoneproducing cells, but especially the endocrine pancreatic cells, originate from the neural crest. More recently, the neuroectoderm has been proposed as the embryologic ancestor. This hypthesis has been reinforced by the transient production of thyrosine hydroxylase, the first enzyme in the catecholamine biosynthetic pathway, by all pancreatic islet cell. However, experimental data have shown that the endocrine pancreatic cell do not originate from the neuroectoderm but rather are derived from the endoderm (Le Douarin 1988).

1.3.3.3
Differentiation of Islet Cells

In the human fetus, glucagon-like material has been found in the pancreas at about the 6th week of gestation (Assan and Boillot 1973). Insulin has been detected at the 80-mm stage by radioimmunoassay (Schaeffer et al. 1973). Somatostatin has been identified at an early stage (Dubois et al. 1975), and later another peptide, the pancreatic polypeptide (PP), appears, but it is essentially localized in the uncinate process, derived from the ventral and (Paulin and Dubois 1976).

There is still little information on the processes that induce endocrine commitment and on the factors that control differentiation of the various pancreatic hormone-producing cells. However, some factors have been suggested: the tridimensional matrix of collagen (Montesano et al. 1983), glucagon (Pictet et al. 1975), nutritional conditions, and glucocorticoids (Pictet et al. 1975).

1.3.3.4
Islet Growth

In the human fetus, as well as in other mammals, the first differentiated cells are isolated in the pancreatic parenchyma. As gestation progresses, the endocrine cells form small clusters. At the end of the third month of gestation, these clusters resemble pancreatic islets. Two generations of islets may appear.

The mechanisms of islet growth are still unclear. Several processes have been suggested. Unlike in the case of the exocrine pancreas, in situ cell divisions do not account significantly for islet growth, and there are more DNA-synthesizing cells around the growing fetal islets than in the islets themselves. Moreover, analysis of the B cell population in several mouse chimaeras suggests a polyclonal origin of pancreatic islets (Deltour et al 1991).

1.3.4
Histologic Features and Hormonal Content of the Islets of Langerhans

The morphologic characteristics of fetal islets are identical to those described in adults. The distribution of different cell types is frequently of the mantle type: most insulin-containing cells form a central core surrounded by glucagon- and somatostatin-containing cells that form a discontinous ring.

The number of islets is greater in the tail than in the head (Goldman et al. 1982). The volume density of the total endocrine cell population decreases from 15% in neonates to 2% in adults (Rahier et al. 1981). The number of endocrine cells varies throughout life (Orci et al. 1979; Rahier et al. 1981). In the uncinate process, the percentage of PP-containing cells increases from about 40% during fetal life to 60% in adults, while the insulin-containing cells remain stable at 30%. In the upper part of the head and in the body and tail, the percentage of glucagon-containing cells remains stable at about 20%, while that of insulin-containing cells increases from fetal (30%) to adult (70%) life. The percentage of somatostatin-containing cells decreases from 20% to 10% in all regions of the pancreas.

Some other peptides have been located in islets of Langerhans in the human fetus. Thyroliberin (TRH) is present very early; the highest concentrations have been detected at between 6 and 8 weeks of gestation (1588.5 ± 382.3 pg/ml wet weight), after which they decline and remain low (LEDUQUE et al. 1986). TRH is synthesized in insulin-producing cells (THEODOROPOULOS and ZOLMAN 1985). Histidyl-proline diketopiperazine has been detected in glucagon-producing cells in the human fetus (LEDUQUE et al. 1987). Insulin-like growth factors I and II have also been reported in the fetal pancreas (BRYSON et al. 1989; HILL et al. 1987).

1.3.5 Malformations

The various congenital malformations were reviewed by WARKANY in 1971. One of them, complete aplasia, occurs in monstrous fetuses that lack the portion of the foregut from which the liver and pancreas are derived. Some malformations concern the exocrine pancreas only, e.g., congenital hypoplasia. Pancreatic hyperplasia is associated with hyperplasia of other organs (Beckwith-Wiedemann syndrome). Ectopic pancreas can be found in different regions of the intestine, lung, and spleen. Annular pancreas usually manifests late in life. Mucoviscidosis is essentially a disease of postnatal life, but it can begin early in fetal life, and some pathologic changes are then present at birth.

1.4 Histology

The main exocrine functional unit, responsible for synthesizing and secreting enzymes and proenzymes, is the acinus. Acinar (i.e., exocrine) cells occupy about 80% of the pancreatic volume, the ducts about 4%, and blood vessels and extracellular space about 14%. The endocrine part (islet cells) forms about 2% of the total gland. In this section, the morphologic characteristics of the pancreas will be briefly reviewed; more details have been given elsewhere (BAUER 1988; GORELICK and JAMIESON 1987; LACY and GREIDER 1979).

1.4.1 Histologic Organization of the Exocrine Pancreas

A remarkably thin capsule of connective tissue separates the pancreas from adjacent structures. This capsule is covered with peritoneum. From the capsule, very thin septa of connective tissue extend to divide the pancreas into several lobules. Connective tissue is often condensed around the main duct and its more immediate branches. The connective tissue matrix continues with basal lamina or basement membrane surrounding each acinus. Its basal lamina consists of type IV and V collagen, laminin, and heparan sulfate proteoglycan, and it is produced by epithelial cells themselves.

1.4.1.1 Acini and Acinar Cells

Each acinus is composed of several acinar cells surrounding the centroacinar lumen (Fig. 1.2). At the light microscopic level, acinar cells often appear as pyramidal in shape and are highly polarized. The basal zone contains basophilic elements termed ergastoplasm, corresponding to the rough endoplasmic reticulum (RER). The central median region is paler and corresponds to elements of the Golgi complex. The nucleus is basally located in this area. The apical region contains acidophilic zymogen granules.

At the electron microscopic level, the same cell polarity is observed. The basal lobe is packed with abundant parallel cisternae of RER with numerous mitochondria between the cisternae. The RER occu-

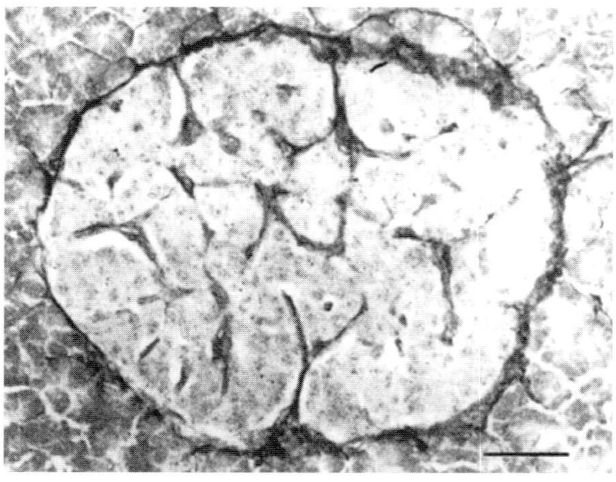

Fig. 1.2. Photomicrograph showing the pancreatic parenchyma. An islet of Langerhans is present in the acinar tissue. (Courtesy od Dr. P. Leduque) H&E; *scale bar*; 40μm

pies approximately 20% of the cytoplasmic volume and its membranes account for about 60% of the total membrane area of the acinar cells. The Golgi complex consists of some cisternae of smooth membranes whose *trans* side faces the apical pole of the cell, condensing vacuoles budding from the *trans* side and numerous small vesicles between the RER and the *cis* side of Golgi cisternae (Fig. 1.3). The membranes of the Golgi zone occupy about 8% of the cytoplasmic volume and about 10% of the membrane area of the cell. The apical cytoplasm is occupied by numerous zymogen granules which have a homogenous electron-opaque content. These granules account for about 20% of the cytoplasmic volume and about 7% of the total cell membranes. In addition to these different compartments, mitochondria, microfilaments (actin and intermediate filaments), and microtubules are found in the cytoplasmic matrix. The apical plasma membrane has numerous microvilli which project into the centroacinar lumen. The apical plasma membrane is segregated from the basolateral plasma membrane by junctional complexes: tight junctions, zonulae adherens, and desmosomes. Gap junctions located in the lateral plasma membrane are responsible for metabolic coupling of acinar cells.

The acinar cell has served as a paradigm for the study of protein synthesis (see ALBERTS et al. 1989). It has the morphologic and biochemical machinery which permits to it to perform the synthesis, transport, storage, and release of different constituents of the pancreatic juice (cf. Chap. 2). The regulation of pancreatic secretion is complex because various factors act at several levels of the glandular components.

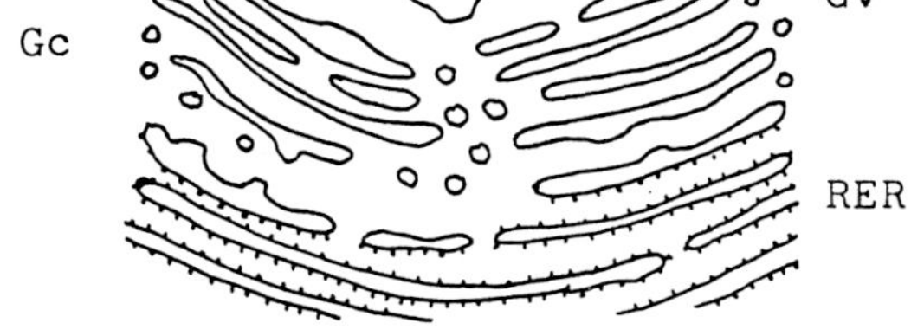

Fig. 1.3. Schematic drawing of opical pole of a polarized acinar cell. Proteins are synthesized by the RER and carried in the Golgi complex, where they are modified, concentrated, and stored in the secretory granules or zymogen granules. The release of proteins in the acinar lumen is achieved by exocytosis of secretory granules. *am*, Apical plasma membrane; *blm*, basolateral plasma membrane; *Gc*, Golgi complex; *Gv*, Golgi vesicles; *L*, acinar lumen; *RER*, rough endoplasmic reticulum; *sg*, secretory granules

The centroacinar cells are seen in the central part of acini. They are smaller than acinar cells, and their cytoplasm is devoid of zymogen granules. Their histochemical characteristics suggest that centroacinar cells may be specialized in electrolyte secretion.

1.4.1.2
Ducts

Small ducts emerge from acini. They are called intercalated ducts because they are inserted between the secretory units and the intralobular ducts proper. Their epithelium is flattened. This epithelium becomes cuboidal in the intralobular ducts, and sometimes it is low columnar, as in the interlobular ducts. The duct of Wirsung has a large lumen lined by columnar epithelium. Goblet cells may be interspersed between the columnar cells.

1.4.2
Islet Cell Morphology

In the adult human, as in other mammals, islets of Langerhans account for up to 2% of the pancreas volume. Recent evidence indicates that, in the adult human, the pancreas contains approximately 500 000 to one million islets. Most of them are between 100 an 200 μm in diameter. Each islet is demarcated from the surrounding acini by a delicate investment of reticular fibers. Islet cells are polyhedral and are arranged in irregular cords that follow the course of the capillary bed.

Several cell types have been reported. Here, the main ones will be described, and the existence of the other cell types only briefly mentioned.

1.4.2.1
Glucagon-Secreting Cells or A Cells

Histologically, A cells are identified by their argyrophylia using the Grimelius technique. They constitute approximately 15%-20% of the islet cell population (Fig. 1.4b) but there are regional variations in their distribution within the pancreas; thus islets in the uncinate process have few or no A cells.

The ultrastructural appearance of their secretory granules makes A cells easy to identify. The diame-

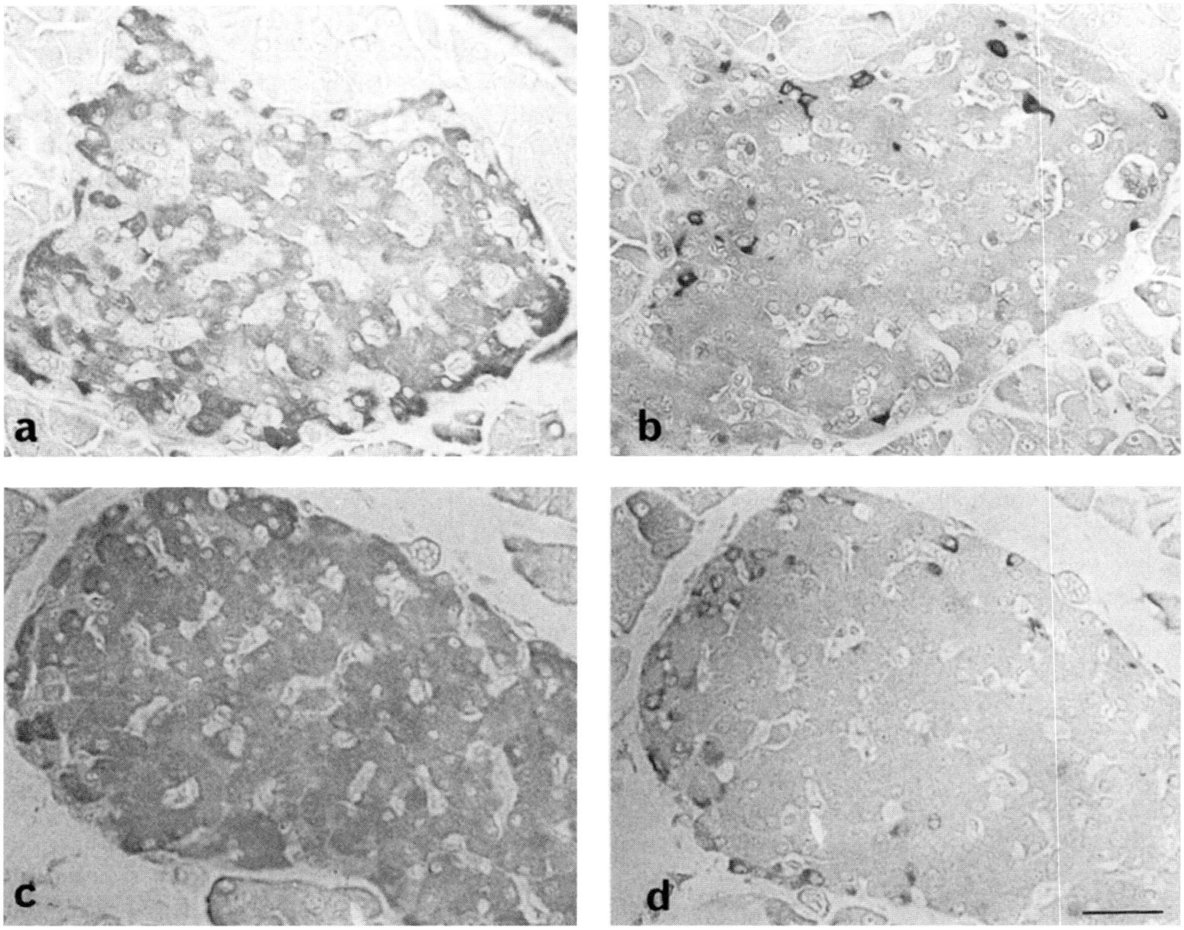

Fig. 1.4a–d. Distribution of endocrine cells in the islet of Langerhans. Immunocytochemical study with an anti-insulin serum (**a**, **c**), an anti-glucagon serum (**b**), and an antisomatostatin serum (**d**). (Courtesy of Dr. P. Leduque) Indirect immunoperoxidase method; *scale bar*: 80µm

ter of the granules (250nm) is generally uniform. In man, A cell granules are round with a closely applied membrane. The center of the granule is extremely electron dense with a less dense area surrounding it. Filamentous mitochondria, a small Golgi apparatus, and the RER are evident.

Immunocytologic studies (Fig. 1.4) have shown that glucagon is stored in the dense core granule. However, recent studies suggest that in the adult, the A cell may produce other peptides such as cholecystokinin and corticoliberin.

1.4.2.2 Insulin-Secreting Cells or B Cells

B cells can be identified with stains such as aldehyde fuchsin or aldehyde thionin, which are believed to react with the sulfhydryl group within insulin. They are the most numerous of the islet cells and usually constitute 70% of the total endocrine cell population. In man, they occupy the central core of the islet (Fig. 1.4a,b).

Ultrastructurally, the B cell is characterized by numerous secretory granules that vary remarkably in appearance between species. In man, the granules, about 300nm in diameter, have a rhomboid or polygonal profile, with a crystalline matrix containing lines of repeating periodicity of approximately 5 nm that are believed to represent insoluble insulin. A finer granular material fills the space between the core and the limiting unit membrane of the secretory granule. The different steps of insulin synthesis have been analyzed (Fig. 1.5). Some secretory granules contain a homogenous spherical core exhibiting no subunit structure and surrounded by a clathrin coat. These vesicles derive from the Golgi complex and are believed to be an intermediate stage in the maturation of insulin secretory granules (Orci 1982).

Immunocytologic studies have confirmed that insulin is synthesized by B cells by the way of a polypeptide named preproinsulin. In the lumen of RER the initial portion of this peptide (about 25 amino acids) is removed. The resulting polypeptide, proinsulin, is carried in the Golgi complex, where the connecting peptide (C peptide), which extends between A and B chains, is cleaved. The C peptide is stored in the secretory granules in a concentration equimolecular to insulin (Fig.1.5). The microtubules and microfilaments act synergeistically on the migration of the secretory granules from the Golgi zone to the plasma membrane. The release of insulin, C peptide, and also a small amount of proinsulin by exocytosis of secretory granules is regulated by various stimuli.

Other peptides, such as CGRP, prolactin, and chromogranins have been detected in B cells by immunocytochemistry.

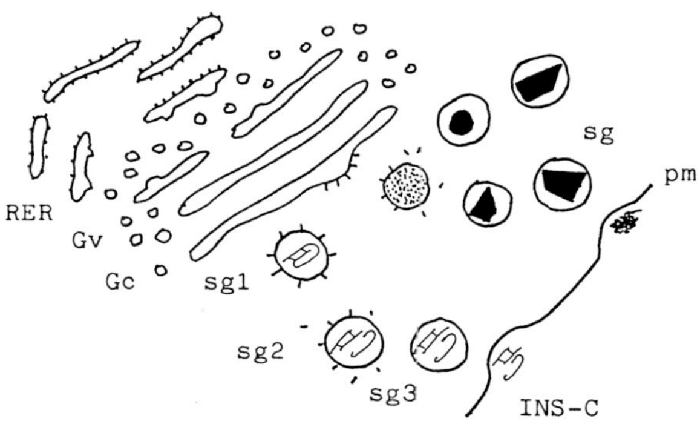

Fig. 1.5. Schematic representation of insulin synthesis in B cells. Proinsulin is synthesized in the RER and carried in the Golgi complex. Proinsulin is deaved in insulin (A and B chains) and C peptide in clathrin-coated vesicles located at the *trans* face of the Golgi complex. These vesicles subsequently shed clathrin. Insulin and C peptide are stored in the secretory granules. Both insulin and C peptide are released by exocytosis of secretory granules. *Gc*, Golgi complex; *Gv*, Golgi vesicles; *INS-C*, insulin and C peptide (schematic release); *pm*, plasma membrane; *RER*, rough endoplasmic reticulum; *sg*, secretory granules; *sg1,2,3*, schematic representation of maturation process of insulin molecule

1.4.2.3
Somatostatin-Secreting or D Cells

The D cells or delta cells are identified using the Mallory-Heidenhain stain, but they have also been identified by silver stains. They are less numerous than other cell types, accounting for about 5% -10% of the endocrine cells (Fig. 1.4d). They are usually located in the vicinity of A cells.

The ultrastructural appearance of their secretory granules is characteristic, with a pale matrix of variable electron density which almost fills the vesicles. Their diameter is about 300-350nm. Somatostatin has been localized in the secretory granules by immunocytochemistry. CGRP has also been found.

1.4.2.4
Pancreatic Polypeptide-Secreting or PP Cells or F Cells

PP cells are known under this name because they have been identified as reacting immunocytologically with anti-pancreatic polypeptide serum. They are mainly located in the uncinate process. Ultrastructurally they are identified by small-diameter (140-200nm) secretory granules with a homogenous core. Somatoliberin and peptide YY have also been detected in these cells.

1.4.2.5
Other Cell Types

Enterochromaffin cells or EC cells have been identified. They are argentaffinic and have pleomorphic vesicles (about 175-400nm in diameter).

Some other cell types have been cescribed under different names. Some of them are also observed in gastrointestinal mucosa or sometimes in one species. This diversity exists because precise criteria for their description have not always been applied, and the nature of their peptidic content is still discussed.

The different endocrine cells in an islet of Langerhans are interlinked by junctional complexes such as tight and gap junctions and desmosomes. The gap junctions enable chemical information to be quickly transmitted from one cell to another. The existence of a complex vascular relationship within the islets and between islets and acini and the presence of gap junctions between acinar cells make the pancreas a highly integrated organ.

References

Alberts B, Bray D, Lewis J, Raff M, Roberts K, Watson JD (1989) Molecular biology of the cell, 2nd edn. Garland, New York

Assan R, Boillot J (1973) Pancreatic glucagon and glucagon-like material in tissues and plasma from human fetuses 6–26 weeks old. Pathol Biol 21:149–155

Bauer GE (1988) Islets of Langerhans. In: Weiss L (ed) A textbook of histology, 6th edn. Urban and Schwarzenberg, Baltimore, pp 738-749

Bryson JM, Tuch BE , Baxter RC (1989) Production of insulin-like growth factor-II by human fetal pancreas in culture. J Endocrinol 121:367–373

De Giorgio R, Sternini C, Brecha NC, Widdison AL, Karanjia ND, Reber HA, Go VLW (1992) Pattern of innervation of vasoactive intestinal polypeptide, neuropeptide Y, and gastrin-releasing peptide immunoreactive nerves in the feline pancreas. Pancreas 7:376–384

Deltour L, Leduque P, Paldi A , Ripoche MA, Dubois P, Jami J (1991) Polyclonal origin of pancreatic islets in aggregation mouse chimaeras. Development 112:1115–1121

Dewey MJ, Mintz B (1978) Genetic control of cell-type-specific levels of mouse β-galactosidase. Dev Biol 66:550–559

Dubois P (1989) Ontogeny of the pancreas. Horm Res 32:53-60

Dubois P. Paulin C, Assan R, Dubois MP (1975) Evidence for immunoreactive somatostatin in the endocrine cells of human fetal pancreas. Nature 256:731–732

Fujita T (1973) Insulo-acinar portal system in the horse pancreas. Arch Histol Jap 35:161–171

Goldman H, Wong J, Patel JC (1982) A study of the structural and biochemical development of human fetal islets of Langerhans. Diabetes 31:897–902

Gorelick FS, Jamieson JD (1987) Structure-function relationship of the pancreas. In: Johnson LR (ed) Physiology of the gastrointestinal tract, 2nd edn. Raven, New York, pp 1089–1108

Hill DJ, Frazer A, Swenne I, Wridnam PK, Milner RDG (1987) Somatomedin-C in human fetal pancreas. Cellular localization and release during organ culture. Diabetes 36:465–471

Lacy PE, Greider MH (1979) Anatomy and ultrastructural organization of pancreatic islets. In: Cahill GF Jr, Odell WD, Martini L, Pott JT Jr, Nelon DH, Steinberger E, Winegrad AI (eds) Endocrinology. Grune and Stratton, New York, pp 907–919

Le Douarin NM (1988) On the origin of pancreatic endocrine cells. Cell 53:169–171

Leduque P, Aratan-Spire S, Czernichow P, Dubois PM (1986) Ontogenesis of thyrotropin-releasing hormone in the human fetal pancreas. A combined radioimmunological and immunocytological study. J Clin Invest 78:1028–1034

Leduque P, Jackson IMD, Kervran A, Aratan-Spire S, Czernichow P, Dubois PM (1987) Histidyl-proline diketopiperazine (His-Pro DKP) immunoreactivity is present in the glucagon-containing cells in the human fetal pancreas. J Clin Invest 79:875–880

Montesano R, Mouron P, Amherdt M, Orci L (1983) Collagen matrix provokes reorganization of pancreatic endocrine cell monolayer into islet-like organoid. J Cell Biol 97:935–939

Orci L (1982) Banting lecture (1981). Macro- and microdomains in the endocrine pancreas. Diabetes 31:538–572

Orci L, Stefan Y, Malaisse-Lagae F, Perrelet A (1979) Instability of pancreatic endocrine cell population throughout life. Lancet 1:615–616

Paulin C, Dubois PM (1978) Immunohistochemical identification and localization of pancreatic polypeptide cells in the pancreas and gastrointestinal tract of the human fetus and adult man. Cell Tissue Res 188:251–257

Pearse AGE (1969) The cytochemistry and ultrastructure of polypeptide hormone-producing cells of the APUD series and the embryologic, physiologic and pathologic implications of the concept. J Histochem Cytochem 17:303–313

reintel L, (eds) Handbook of physiology, vol I. Williams and Wilkins, Baltimore, pp 25–66

Pictet RL, Rall L, De Gasparo M, Rutter WJ (1975) Regulation of differentation of endocrine cells during pancreatic development in vitro. In: Camerini-Davalos RA, Cole HS (eds) Early diabetes in early life. Academic, New York, pp 25–39

Rahier J, Wallon J, Henquin JC (1981) Cell populations in the endocrine pancreas in human neonates and infants. Diabetologia 20:540-546

Samols E (1991) The history of the endocrine pancreas. In: Salmols E (ed) The endocrine pancreas. Raven, New York, pp 1–12

Schaeffer LD, Wilder ML, Williams RH (1973) Secretion and content of insulin and glucagon in human fetal pancreas slices in vitro. Proc Soc Exp Biol Med 143:314–319

Theodoropoulos TJ, Zolman JC (1985) Thyrotropin-releasing hormone biosynthesis in neonatal pancreas. Endocrinol Exp 19.77–82

Warkany J (1971) Congenital malformations. Notes and documents. Year Book Medical, Chicago

2 Physiology of the Exocrine Pancreas

P. H. BERNARD

CONTENTS

2.1 Introduction

The pancreas is an organ with both exocrine and endocrine functions. The exocrine pancreas plays an essential role in the digestion and absorption of nutrients through the secretion into the proximal duodenum of digestive enzymes and bicarbonates. The endocrine pancreas, on the other hand, releases hormones that regulate metabolism and the distribution of the breakdown products of food within the body. These combined exocrine and endocrine functions make the pancreas one of the most important organs involved in the assimilation of food.

2.2 Structure of Exocrine Pancreas

The major structural components of the exocrine pancreas are the acini and a duct system composed of intralobular and interlobular duct cells. The acinus is a grapelike cluster of six to eight pyramid-shaped acinar cells which represent about 90% of the total pancreatic population. From each acinus emerges a small ductule termed an intercalated duct. A lobule is composed of several acini. Inside this lobule, intercalated ducts are drained by an intralobular duct. Each lobule is linked by interlobular ducts to the main duct, which finally enters the duodenum.

P. H. BERNARD, MD, Practicien Hospitalier, Service des Maladies de l'Appareil, Digestif (Pr Quinton), Centre Hôspitalier et Universitaire, Hôpital Saint-André, 1, Rue Jean Burguet, F-33075 Bordeaux Cédex, France

2.3 Formation and Composition of Pancreatic Juice

The composition of normal human pancreatic juice has been extensively analyzed since it has become possible to avoid duodenal juice contamination of samples by cannulation of the pancreatic ducts. The human pancreas secretes approximately 0.2–0.3 ml/min of a clear colorless liquid during the interdigestive phase; this rate increases after a meal to reach a maximal flow rate of 4 ml/min in response to the exogenous release of secretin. Recent reviews have been provided by SCHULZ (1987), RINDERKNECHT (1986), ZIMMERMAN and JONOWITZ (1986), and OWYANG and WILLIAMS (1991).

2.3.1 Water and Electrolytes

Pancreatic juice and plasma are isotonic. The major cations are sodium (Na^+) and potassium (K^+); both are secreted at concentrations slightly greater than their plasma concentrations. The major anions in pancreatic juice are bicarbonate (HCO_3^-) and chloride (Cl^-). If concentrations of both cations – sodium and potassium – are constant and independent of secretory rates (160 mmol/l and 5 mmol/l respectively), chloride an bicarbonate concentrations vary with the rate of secretion of pancreatic juice (Fig. 2.1). At a low rate of fluid secretion, bicarbonate concentration is about 30 mmol/l and chloride concentration about 130 mml/l. As the flow rate increase, bicarbonate concentration rises, approaching a maximal plateau value which is species dependent (130–140 mmol/l in humans). The concentration of chloride falls reciprocally as the secretory rate increases, so that the sum of the two anions remains constant and approximately equal to the sum of sodium and potassium at all secretory rates. In humans and other mammals, pancreatic juice also contains calcium (1.7 mmol/l) and traces of magnesium, zinc, sulfates, and phosphates, the latter four always being associated with enzymatic proteins.

2.3.2 Enzymes

Pancreatic juice is the main source of digestive enzymes and contains protein at a concentration that varies from 1 to 10g/l (6–20g per day) depending on the level of hormonal stimulation. Enzymes constitute more than 85% of this protein; the remainder is composed of plasma proteins, trypsin inhibitors, and mucoproteins. The four major enzyme groups are proteolytic, lipolytic, amylolytic, and nucleolytic (Rinderknecht 1986). Table 2.1 lists the major pancreatic enzymes and proteins.

2.3.2.1 Proteolytic Enzymes

The proteolytic enzymes, which include trypsinogen, chymotrypsinogen, proelastase, and procar-

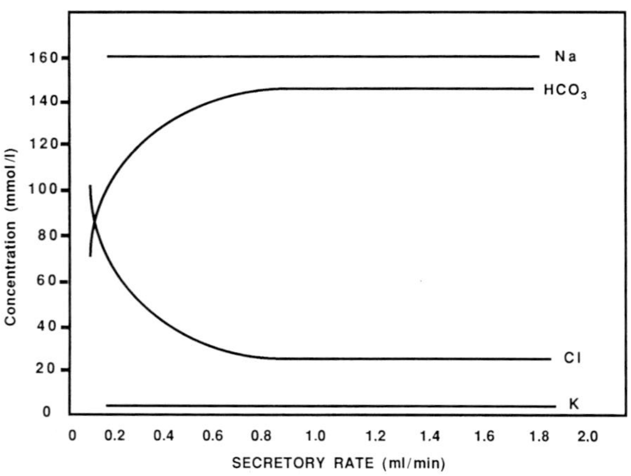

Fig. 2.1. Relationship of secretory rate of the electrolyte composition of pancreatic juice

Table 2.1. Human pancreatic juice proteins

Proteolytic enzymes	Amylolytic enzymes
Endopeptidases	α-Amylase
Trypsinogens 1 and 2	Nucleolytic enzymes
Chymotrypsinogen A and B	Ribonuclease
Proelastase	Desoxyribonuclease
Prekallikrein	Trypsin inhibitor
Exopeptidases	Lactoferrin
Procarboxy peptidase A	Serum proteins
Procarboxy peptidase B	Lysosomal enzymes
Lipolytic enzymes	
Lipase	
Procolipase	
Phospholipase A	

boxypeptidase and account for the majority of enzymatic proteins, are released as inactive precursors packaged into zymogen granules. The pancreas is thus protected from autodigestion. There are, however, cases for which the mechanisms are not entirely clear, where pancreatic enzymes can become active in the pancreatic parenchyma, digesting the pancreatic tissue and precipitating a cascade of events that leads to acute pancreatitis. In the small intestine, pancreatic proteolytic enzymes continue the digestion of proteins that has been begun in the stomach by pepsin and acid. The enzymes that hydrolyze proteins can be classified as endopeptidases and exopeptidases. Endopeptidases attack peptide bonds near the center of the molecule; exopeptidases hydrolyze amino-terminal or carboxy-terminal peptides.

Endopeptidases include trypsin, chymotrypsin, elastase, and kallikrein. Trypsinogen represents about 20% of the total protein content of pancreatic juice. Enterokinase, a specific enteropeptidase secreted by the duodenal mucosa, converts inactive trypsinogen into active trypsin. At a certain concentration, trypsin stimulates the autoactivation of more trypsinogen to trypsin and converts chymotrypsinogen and all other pancreatic zymogens into their active forms (Fig. 2.2). Trypsin specifically hydrolyzes the peptide bonds next to the basic amino acids, lysine and arginine. Chymotrypsin hydrolyzes the peptide bonds next to aromatic amino acids such as tryptophan, phenylalanine, and tyrosine. Its action, however, is relatively unspecific. Two proelastases have also been identified. When activated by trypsin, these elastases hydrolyze specific bonds involving the carboxyl groups of the neutral aliphatic amino acids. Kallikrein is also present as a zymogen in pancreatic secretion, but its physiologic significance is, as yet, unknown. In plasma, kallikrein

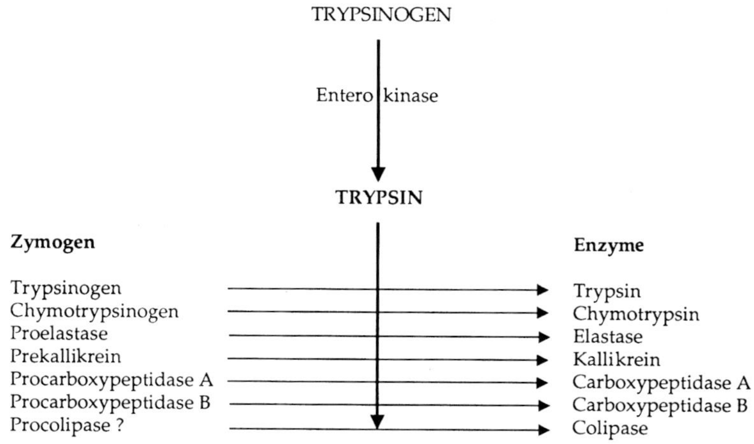

Fig. 2.2 Transformation of pancreatic zymogens

possesses highly specific functions of which the most important appears to be the release of kinins from kininogens. Kinins play an important role in the circulatory disturbances that occur in pancreatitis.

Exopeptidases are proteolytic enzymes that hydrolyze the first or last bond in the peptide chain, liberating amino acids one by one. There are two of these enzymes, both of which contain zinc ions. Carboxypeptidase A is specific for carboxy terminal aromatic and neutral aliphatic amino acids, and carboxypeptidase B for basic residues.

Trypsin inhibitors are polypeptides that inactivate trypsin in a 1:1 ratio. The presence of trypsin inhibitors in the pancreas is thought to protect the organ from autodigestion by the small amounts of trypsin present in the nonstimulated pancreas. The concentration of this inhibitor, however, would seem too low to offer efficient protection against trypsinogen activation.

Using the dual techniques of two-dimensional isoelectric focusing and sodium dodecylsulfate gel electrophoresis, Scheele et al. (1981) defined 19 different exocrine proteins in normal human pancreatic juice. Some proteolytic enzymes can exist in the form of isoenzymes, which catalyze the same types of reaction but have a slightly different amino acid composition. For example, enzymes such as trypsinogen and chymotrypsinogen can be found in two forms termed, respectively, trypsinogen A and B. On the other hand, the two elastocytic enzymes, protease E and elastase, are not isoenzymes because they do not hydrolyze the same substrate.

Protein synthesis: According to the classic Palade model (Palade 1975), amino acids are actively transported into the acinar cells and protein synthesis occurs in the ribosomes (Scheele 1986). Pancreatic enzymes are synthesized in the ribosomes bound to the cytoplasmic surface of the rough endoplasmic reticulum within acinar cells, progress through the Golgi apparatus, and are packaged into zymogen granules (Palade 1975; Scheele 1986; Kelly 1985). These secretory proteins are transported from the base of the cell to the apex through a series of membrane-enclosed compartments. The fact that enzymes are transported inside zymogen granules means that they are protected from contact with the cell cytoplasm, which avoids damage to the cell. The zymogen granuls are then discharged into the pancreatic duct by exocytosis. The entire process from synthesis to the point at which enzymes are ready to be secreted into the lumen requires approximately 50 min.

In contrast to the proteolytic enzymes, amylase, lipase, and ribonucleases are secreted by acinar cells in an active form.

2.3.2.2 Lipolytic Enzymes

Lipase is a pancreatic enzyme that hydrolyzes two external bonds of triglycerides to yield two free fatty acids and a monoglyceride. It acts on hydrophobic phases but cannot act alone on hydrophilic substrates. Unlike the proteolytic enzymes, lipase is not secreted as a proenzyme. Lipase activity is enhanced when fats, through the action of bile salts, are in fine emulsion with a large interface area. For this hydrolytic effect, lipase requires a protein cofactor, colipase, which is also secreted by the pancreas as a proenzyme and so needs trypsin activation. Pancreatic juice also contains colipase, a low-molecular-weight peptide, which is essential for optimal lipolysis. Although bile salts stabilize the lipid-water interface, they inhibit lipolysis. This is restored by colipase, which binds with bile salt-lipid surfaces to increase the interaction of lipase with tryglyceride (Borgstrom and Donner 1975; Borgstrom 1975). The marked increase in serum liapse that occurs in acute pancreatitis has long been used as one of the main criteria for diagnosis of this disease.

Phospholipase is secreted as a proenzyme and therefore requires trypsin activation. Phospholipase hydrolyzes dietary phospholipids to generate one molecule of free fatty acids and one molecule of lysolecithin. Like lipase, phospholipase is active only at the lipid-water interface and thus acts on substrates present as micelles or molecular dispersed solutions or monomolecular surface films. Elevated levels of serum phospholipase have been observed in acute pancreatitis, and serum concentrations correlate with the severity of the disease and mortality.

2.3.2.3 Amylolytic Enzymes

Pancreatic α-amylase has similar properties to salivary amylase, but is the only endoenzyme capable of hydrolyzing the α-1,4 linkages of starch substrates to short-chain polysaccharides termed dextrins. The final products of amylase hydrolysis are two disaccharides – maltose and maltotriose – and amylopectin, a polysaccharide with α-1,4 and α-1,6 bonds, a branched structure which prevents digestion by α-amylase.

2.3.2.4 Nucleases

Nucleases hydrolyze the phosphodiester bonds that bind the monoclueotides in nucleic acids. Ribonuclease acts on ribonucleic acid, desoxyribonucleases on desoxyribonucleic acid.

2.3.2.5 Lysosomal Enzymes

Several lysosomal enzymes have been identified in human pancreatic juice, among them galactosaminidase, fucosidase, mannosidase, glucosidase, and glucuronidase. The function of lysosomal enzymes remains unclear but they would seem to play an important role in modifying or inactivating ligands or hormones that stimulate the secretion of digestive enzymes.

2.3.3 Other Constituents of Pancreatic Juice

Lactoferrin is an iron-binding protein normally found at a very low concentration (less than 0.02% of total protien content). Levels rise markedly in patients with chronic calcifying pancreatitis.

Serum proteins are thought to be migrants from blood plasma which have filtered through the intracellular space. More than 60% are albumin, with small quantities of IgA, IgG, and IgM.

Other constituents are enzymes such as γ-glutamyltransferases, alanine transaminases, and alkaline phosphatase, and nonenzymatic substances such as carcinoembryonic antigen. The physiologic role of these substances in pancreatic juice has yet to be elucidated.

2.4 Regulation of Pancreatic Secretion

Pancreatic secretion is regulated by both neural and humoral mechanisms. Mediation of postprandial pancreatic secretion was for a long time ascribed mainly to the hormones secretin and cholecystokinin (CCK) and to vagovagal reflexes that activate cholinergic postganglionic neurons in the pancreas. Recent studies, however, indicate that other regulatory peptide hormones and neurotransmitters are also involved (Table 2.2) (Chey 1986; Holst 1986).

Table 2.2. Hormones or peptides that influence exocrine pancreatic secretion

Stimulation	Inhibition
Secretin	Glucagon
Cholecystokinin-pancreozymin (CCK-PZ)	Pancreatic polypeptide (PP)
Gastrin	Somatostatin
Bombesin	Opiate peptides
Vasoactive intestinal peptide (VIP)	Pancreatone
Neurotensin	Thyrotropin-releasing hormone (TRH)

2.4.1 Stimulation of Pancreatic Secretion

2.4.1.1 Hormonal Control

Secretin

Secretin is a strong stimulant of a pancreatic fluid rich in bicarbonate and with a low enzyme concentration. Duodenal pH is the major regulator of secretin release, with a threshold value of 4.5 (FAHRENKRUG et al. 1978). At a lower pH, pancreatic bicarbonate output is related to the total amount of titratable acid presented to the duodenum. The technique of radioimmunoassay has enabled precise evaluation of postprandial secretin levels and shown that the increase is, in fact, very slight (SCHAFFALIZKY DE MUCKADELL et al. 1981; SCHAFFALIZKY DE MUCKADELL and FAHRENKRUG 1978) because of the buffering of an appreciable amount of acid produced in the stomach by food and the neutralization of the remaining acid entering the duodenum by pancreaticobiliary secretion. Exogenous secretin given intravenously in a dose range that mimics postprandial plasma secretin levels can stimulate pancreatic secretion of water and bicarbonate (SCHAFFALIZKY DE MUCKADELL et al. 1981); there is a linear correlation between the increases in secretin levels and the bicarbonate secretion (SCHAFFALIZKY DE MUCKADELL et al. 1978). It has been shown, in dogs, that the administration of secretin antiserum reduces pancreatic bicarbonate response to a meal. In humans, elevation of postprandial secretin levels can be inhibited with antacids (SCHAFFALIZKY DE MUCKADELL and FAHRENKRUG 1978). Although acidification remains the most potent stimulant, nonacid factors may also play a role in the postprandial release of secretin, such as fatty acids (oleic acid and other digestive fat products) and bile salt in the upper small intestine (WATANABE et al. 1986; HANSSEN 1980). Although the release of secretin after duodenal acidification would not seem to be affected by cholinergic stimulation, the stimulating action of secretin in a physiologic dose range is significantly reduced by atropine or vagotomy (YOU et al. 1982; CHEY et al. 1979).

Secretin is a polypeptide hormone composed of 27 amino acids released from the duodenum and upper jejunal mucosa, which acts on pancreatic centroacinar and ductal epitheolial cells. It shares structural similarities with glucagon, gastric inhibitory polypeptide, and vasoactive intestinal polypeptide (VIP). Secretin is released by endocrine cells (S cells) present in large numbers in the duodenal bulb and decreasing towards the jejunum.

Cholecystokinin

Cholecystokinin is the other gut hormone that plays an important role in pancreatic secretion. In contrast to secretin, CCK is a potent stimulant of enzyme or protein secretion, but a weak stimulant of volume and bicarbonate (DEBAS and GROSSMAN 1973). It is released by various hydrolytic products of digestion such as amino acids and fatty acids. Undigested fat or proteins are ineffective stimulants: thus, pancreatic secretion itself plays a prominent role in the release of CCK due to its hydrolytic action on nutrients. Products of lipolysis such as fatty acids are the most potent stimulants of CCK release (WALSH et al. 1982): their chain length, degree of saturation, concentration, and total load are factors that influence CCK response. Under fasting conditions, plasma CCK levels are very low: a protein- and fat-rich meal results in a five- to ten-fold increases in CCK concentrations within 10–30 min, followed by a gradual decline to basal levels during the ensuing 3 h (WALSH et al. 1982; OWYANG et al. 1986). Reproduction of meal-stimulated plasma CCK levels by exogenous infusion of CCK produces the same levels of pancreatic enzyme secretion as during postprandial secretion, suggesting that endogenous CCK release is a major regulator of meal-induced pancreatic secretion (BEGLINGER et al 1985). In addition to this stimulating effect on the secretion of a pancreatic fluid rich in enzymes, CCK also exercises a trophic effect on the pancreas, causing increases in pancreatic weight, DNA protein content, and the functional capacity of the gland.

Cholecystokinin is a 33-amino acid polypeptide hormone which acts on acinar cells. Several biologically active variants of this molecule, such as CCK 8, CCK 39, and CCK 58, have been identified in the blood. Additional intermediate froms, including CCK 33, can be detected postprandially. CCK 8 has the same physiologic properties as CCK 33 but is more active in its effects on pancreatic secretion. There is a structural similarity between CCK and gastrin but CCK is a more potent stimulant of pancreatic enzyme secretion, particularly because CCK potentiates the action of secretin on the pancreas.

Other Regulatory Factors

Many other peptides are involved in postprandial pancreatic secretion but their physiologic role in the regulation of this secretion appears to be relatively minor.

Gastrin has the same carboxy-terminal structure as CCK and acts in a similar way on pancreatic secretion. It is, however, only one-third as effective as CCK. Most recent experiences show that gastrin does not play any significant role in postprandial pancreatic response.

Bombesin [or gastrin-releasing peptide (GRP) in mammals] acts directly on pancreatic acinar cells and has been shown to stimulate the secretion of pancreatic fluid that contains small amounts of bicarbonates and high concentration of enzymes (Basso et al. 1975). In addition it has been shown in dogs that the intraventricular administration of bombesin inhibits interprandial pancreatic secretion, which proves the existence of central specific receptors involved in the modulation of pancreatic stimulation.

Vasointestinal peptide although similar in structure to secretin, is a very weak stimulant of pancreatic secretion of water and bicarbonate in humans. Recent immunocytochemical studies have revealed the presence of several peptides in nerve cell bodies: those containing VIP are the most abundant. Vagal stimulation after administration of atropine increases pancreatic venous outflow of VIP as well as pancreatic bicarbonate secretion; these effects are blocked by somatostatin.

Neurotensin, a peptide mainly found in the distal small intestine and released by intestinal fatty acids, stimulates bicarbonate secretion but decreases enzyme secretion stimulated by secretin and cerulein (a CCK analog) in humans (Baca et al. 1983; Fletcher et al. 1981). Neurotensin, like VIP, is present in nerves and may function as a peptidergic neurotransmitter.

2.4.1.2 Neural Control

In common with most parts of the gastrointestinal system, the pancreas has a dual extrinsic innervation: parasympathetic, principally through the vagus nerve, and sympathetic through splanchnic nerves. Vagal efferent fibers emerge from the dorsal vagal nucleus, enter the abdomen as the anterior and posterior vagi, and extend to the pancreas where they synapse with cell bodies within pancreatic parenchyma. Additional cholinergic fibers reach the pancreas with splanchnic nerves. Vagal pathways to the pancreas may be either cholinergic or noncholinergic. Although most vagal stimulatory effects on pancreatic secretion are mediated by acetylcholine acting on muscarinic receptors, there is evidence for noncholinergic transmission, for example through peptides. On reaching the abdomen, sympathetic nerves from the splanchnic system synapse at the celiac, superior mesenteric, or gastroduodenal plexus. Adrenergic innervation of the pancreas is mainly through the splanchnic nerves. The majority of these fibers are distributed to the blood vessels and very few pass to the acini or ducts.

Parsympathetic Nervous System
In anesthetized animals, stimulation of the vagus nerve elicits an increase in the secretion of protein and bicarbonate equivalent to 40% of the response to secretin, and a protein output similar to that observed after administration of CCK (Chariot et al. 1982). The functional response to vagal stimulation varies greatly among species due to differences in the liberation of noncholinergic mediators. In humans, insulin-induced hypoglycemia, which is presumed to stimulate the vagus, augments secretin-stimulated pancreatic protein output (Rosenberg et al. 1976). Vagotomy reduces the bicarbonate secretory response to exogenous hormones as well as pancreatic enzymes responses to a meal (MacGregor et al. 1977) or to intraintestinal stimulants (Malagelada et al. 1974). Stimulation of volume and osmoreceptors present in the duodenum elicits a pancreatic enzyme response mediated by way of cholinergic neurons (Owyang et al. 1986b). It has also been shown that the gastric distention (Andrews et al. 1980) and intestinal perfusion with HCl (Andrews and Andrews 1971) induce increased firing rates in peripheral afferent vagal neurons and in central sites. Acetalcholine released by intrapancreatic postganglionic neurons during the gastric and intestinal phases may act directly on acinar cells or potentiate the action of secretin on bicarbonate secretion from duct cells. The interaction between acetylcholine and CCK is additive.

Sympathetic Nervous System
Adrenergic nerves appear to affect exocrine pancreatic secretion mainly by modulating pancreatic blood flow. The splanchnic nerves are inhibitory for exocrine and endocrine secretion as shown by the fact that stimulation of the nerves usually decreases the response to pancreatic stimulation whereas splanchnicectomy increases these response. The pancreatic inhibitory effect of splanchnic nerve stimulation appears to be synchronous with, and dependent on, intense vasoconstriction caused by stimulation of α-adrenergic receptors on the blood vessels.

2.4.1.3
Intracellular Control of Pancreatic Secretion

The two major effector enzymes in acinar cell membranes are the polyphosphoinositide-specificphospholipase C, which cleaves phosphatidylinositol-4,5-biphosphate, producing 1,4,5-inositol triphosphate (IP_3) and 1,2-diacylglycerol (DAG), and adenylate cyclase, which converts ATP to cyclic AMP (cAMP) (Hootman and Williams 1987). Among the major intracellular messenger involved in the regulation of pancreatic secretion, IP3, Ca2+, and DAG are predominant in acinar cells and increase after the activation of phosphoinositide-specific phospholipase C by CCK, acetylcholine, and gastrin, while cAMP is the predominant messenger in duct cells and is activated by secretin or VIP. CA2+ is released from stores in the cytosol or plasma membranes.

2.4.2
Inhibition of Pancreatic Secretion

The regulation of pancreatic secretion depends on a balance between inhibitory and stimulatory influences on the gland, which are exerted through hormones and the autonomic nervous system. While much has been written about pancreatic stimulation, less is known about the inhibitory influences on the pancreas.

2.4.2.1
Inhibitory Phase of Pancreatic Secretion

It is indicative of the importance of inhibitory mechanisms that studies have shown that pancreatic response to a meal is less than the maximal response induced by exogenous hormonal stimulation (via CCK and secretin). Three main inhibitory hormones have been clearly identified: glucagon, pancreatic polypeptide (PP), and somatostatin. A hormonal inhibitory substance which has not yet been identified has been termed pancreotone.

Glucagon: Both pancreatic glucagon released by pancreatic endocrine cells and enteroglucagon, identified in the gastrointestinal tract, inhibit pancreatic secretion that has been stimulated by either secretin or CCK or both, or by ingestion of a test meal (Dyck et al. 1970). This postprandial level of glucagon may be sufficient to inhibit secretin- or CCK stimulated pancreatic secretion.

Pancreatic polypeptide is produced almost exclusively in the islets of Langerhans in the cephalic pancreas. A significant increase in the plasma concentration of PP occurs after ingestion of a meal and inhibits secretion of both bicarbonate and pancreatic enzymes. PP is also released by exogenous CCK-PZ, gastrin, secretin, and bombesin. The effects of these peptides appear to depend on cholinergic influence, since atropine or truncal vagotomy abolished the cephalic phase of pancreatic secretion. Because secretion is under cholinergic control, PP plays a key role in the modulation of pancreatic secretion stimulated by the cholinergic enteropancreatic reflex (Schwartz 1983). After ingestion of a meal, the enteropancreatic reflex is activated to stimulate pancreatic enzyme secretion and PP release. PP, in turn, inhibits cholinergic transmission and reduces pancreatic enzyme secretion.

Somatostatin is a strong inhibitor of CCK-stimulated pancreatic enzyme secretion and a modest inhibitor of secretin-stimulated bicarbonate secretion (Dollinger et al. 1976). It also inhibits endocrine pancreatic secretion of insulin, glucagon, and PP.

Pancreotone is an inhibitory substance extracted from the colonic mucosa. This humoral agent, known to be a polypeptide, inhibits the action of secretin and CCK on the pancreas and gallbladder (Harper et al. 1979).

2.4.2.2
Feedback Regulation of Pancreatic Secretion

Some observations suggest that the intraluminal action of pancreatic proteases plays an important role in the regulation of pancreatic enzyme secretion. It has been demonstrated that, in rats, diversion of pancreatic juice from the duodenum stimulates CCK release and thereby pancreatic enzyme secretion while the intraduodenal administration of trypsin or chymotrypsin inhibits the release of CCK and pancreatic enzymes (Louie et al. 1986). The increase in plasma CCK levels and pancreatic secretion after diversion of pancreatic juice appears to be mediated by a trypsin-sensitive substance secreted by the proximal small intestine: the "CCK-releasing factor" (CCK-RF) (Lu et al. 1989). This peptide, cleaved and inactivated when trypsin is present, may act as a mediator of pancreatic enzyme secretion in response to dietary protein intake. In humans, intestinal administration of trypsin or chymotrypsin suppresses CCK release and partially blocks the pancreatic response to intestinal administration of amino acids or oral ingestions of a test meal (Owyang et al. 1986a). On the other hand, inhibitor of chymotrypsin and elastase infused intraduodenally markedly stimulates pancreatic enzyme secretion. These observations suggest that not only trypsin but also other proteases such as chymotrypsin and elastase should be removed to envoke pancreatic enzyme secretion in humans.

As noted above, postprandial pancreatic secretion is under both hormonal and neural control. Distention or administration of hyperosmolar solutions into the duodenum elicits pancreatic enzyme secretion without raising plasma CCK levels; moreover, this stimulatory effect is inhibited by atropine. In contrast to amino acid-stimulated pancreatic enzyme secretion, pancreatic responses to stimulation by volume or osmolality in the duodenum are not suppressed by trypsin. This indicates that feedback regulation of pancreatic secretion by trypsin is stimulus specific and is mediated by inhibiting the release of CCK (Owyang et al. 1986b).

The existence of feedback regulation of pancreatic enzyme secretion in humans may have important clinical implications. It is conceivable that in patients with chronic pancreatitis, decreased pancreatic enzymes secretion may result in elevated CCK levels, reflecting a failure in the feedback modulation of CCK release. This, in turn, may cause hyperstimulation of the pancreas and produce pain.

2.5 Phases of Pancreatic Secretion

Ingestion of a meal stimulates pancreatic secretion by a variety of impulses that are mediated by integrated humoral and neural mechanisms. Stimulatory impulses may originate at different levels, for example cephalic, gastric, and intestinal. These levels or phases are not independent but interact and frequently overlap in response to a meal. In addition, there is evidence that between meals there is an interdigestive phase during which a small but discernible amount of pancreatic secretion is delivered to the intestine (Singer 1986).

2.5.1 Interdigestive Phase (Fasting)

Under basal conditions, pancreatic secretion occurs at very low rates, although a small amount of enzymes is always present in the pancreatic juice. A pattern of cyclic change in basal pancreatic secretion has been demonstrated in dogs and humans; this is characterized by brief increases in bicarbonate and enzyme secretion which recur every 60-120 min during the interdigestive period. These secretions show cyclic variations that are related to cyclic motor activity in the gastrointestinal tract. This cyclic activity is characterized by bursts of peristalsis that begin in the lower esophagus and progress distally through the stomach and the entire small intestine. The rate of secretion increases during phase II (irregular contractions) to reach a peak just before the onset of phase III (peristaltic and propulsive contractions). The relationship between these cyclic secretory and peristaltic patterns is not yet entirely clear, but it has been proposed that this cycle may represent a clearance process for residual food particles or cell debris in the gastrointestinal tract.

2.5.2 Digestive Phase (Feeding)

After ingestion of a meal, the exocrine pancreas is stimulated to secrete enzymes and bicarbonate. Total postprandial pancreatic output is approximately 60%-70% of the output attained in response to maximal stimulation with intravenous infusion of CCK (Beglinger et al. 1985). The stimulatory effect of a meal can be described by separating its components into cephalic, gastric, and intestinal phases (Table 2.3).

Table 2.3. Stimulatory phase of pancreatic enzyme secretion

Phase	Intermediate mechanisms	Chemical mediator to acinar cells
Cephalic	Sight, smell, taste, eating →	ACH VIP?
Gastric	Distension →	ACH
Intestinal	Digested proteins → Reflects →	ACH, CCK
	Fats → Reflects; Fats →	CCK, secretin
	Distension →	ACH
	Hyperosmolality →	ACH

2.5.2.1 Cephalic Phase

A cephalic phase of pancreatic secretion has been demonstrated in both animals and humans. The sight, smell, and/or taste of appetizing food stimulates the secretion of small amounts of proteinrich fluid (Sarles et al. 1968; Anasgnostides et al. 1984). In humans, the contribution of the cephalic phase to postprandial pancreatic enzyme secretion amounts approximately to 50% of the maximal response induced by exogenous CCK 8 (DeFillipi et al. 1982). The pancreatic response to sham feeding is abolished by vagotomy but only partially suppressed by atropine. These findings suggest that the vagus nerve is the main mediator of the cephalic phase and that it is not only the release of acetylcholine that expresses these impulses. It is possible that other peptidergic neurotransmitters, such as VIP, are involved in this mechanism and are responsible for the effects that are not abolished by atropine.

2.5.2.2 Gastric Phase

For many years it was considered that the pancreatic secretory response to a meal was entirely dependent on the passage of gastric contents from the stomach to the small intestine. It is now known that gastric distention stimulates pancreatic secretion in humans and that it affects enzyme output rather than the secretion of water and bicarbonates. Both vagotomy and atropine reduce or abolish the pancreatic response to gastric distention, suggesting that it is mainly mediated by vagal-cholinergic pathways (White et al. 1963). The presence of food in the stomach also releases antral hormones such as gastrin or GRP, which can stimulate secretion of both bicarbonate and enzymes. These vagovagal gastropancreatic reflexes may be counteracted by inhibitory factors, since the presence of food in the stomach results in the release of PP, which inhibits gallbladder contraction and pancreatic secretion.

2.5.2.3 Intestinal Phase

The intestinal phase represents the most important phase of postprandial pancreatic secretion. In this phase, secretin and CCK are the main hormonal mediators. It is also intestinal mucosa that processes receptors for important vagal cholinergic reflexes that regulate both pancreatic bicarbonate and enzyme secretion. Although duodenal pH is the major regulator of the release of secretin (itself the major stimulant of the production of pancreatic bicarbonate), fatty acid and bile present in the intestine may also participate. The hydrolytic products of digestion such as amino acids and fatty acids are potent releasers of CCK, a strong stimulant of pancreatic enzyme secretion. Studies carried out in humans demonstrate that the mechanism responsible for the pancreatic response to amino acids are confined to the duodenum and jejunum; these show that, when amino acids are perfused in the ileum, no reaction can be observed (DiMagno et al. 1973). Although secretin and CCK are both potent stimuli, only small amounts are released by the duodenum after a meal. The strong stimulatory effect is explained by the interaction of these two hormones, termed potentialization. The pancreatic response to these hormones is lower after a meal than after exogenous administration of an equivalent dose of these hormones. This is the result of inhibitory impulses elicted by the meal in the gastrointestinal tract, such as the release of PP or enteroglucagon, or a possible inhibition of the release of CCK by proteases (trypsin and chymotrypsin) in contact with the duodenal mucosa (feedback regulation).

References

Anasgnostides A, Chadwick V, Selden AC, Maton PN (1984) Sham feeding and pancreatic secretion. Gastroenterology 87:109–114

Andrews CJH, Andrews WHH (1971) Receptors activated by acid in the duodenal wall of rabbits. QJ Exp Physiol 56:221–230

Andrews PLR, Grundy D, Scratcherd T (1980) Vagal afferent discharge from mechanoreceptors in different regions of the ferret stomach. J Physio (Lond) 298:513–524

Baca I, Feurle GE, Hass M, Nernitz T (1983) Interaction of neurotensin, cholecystokinin and secretin in the stimulation of pancreas exocrine in the dog. Gastroenterology 84:556–561

Basso N, Gini S, Improta G. et al. (1975) External Pancreatic secretion after bombesin infusion in man. Gut 16:994–998

Beglinger C, Fried M, Whitehouse I, Jansen JB, Caners CB, Gyr K (1985) Pancreatic enzyme response to a liquid meal and to hormoral stimulation. Correlation with plasma secretion and cholecystokinin level. J Clin Invest 75:147–1476

Borgstrom B (1975) On the interactions between pancreatic lipase and colipase and the substrate and the importance of bile salts. J Lipid Res 16:411–417

Borgstrom B, Donner J (1975) Binding of bile salts to pancreatic colipase and lipase. J Lipid Res 16:287–292

Chariot J, Roze C, de la Tour J, Vaille C (1982) Stimulation vagale non cholinergique de la secretion pancreatique externe chez la rat. Gastroenterol Clin Biol 6:371–378

Chey WY (1986) Hormoral control of pancreatic exocrine secretion: In: Go VLW et al. (eds) The exocrine pancreas: biology, pathobiology and diseases. Raven, New York, pp 301–313

Chey WY, Kim MS, Lee KY (1979) Influence of the vagus nerve on the release and action of secretin in dog. J Physiol 293:435–446

Debas HT, Grossman MI (1973) Pure cholecystokinin: pancreatic protein and bicarbonate response. Digestion 6:469–481

DeFillipi C, Solomon TE, Valenzuela JE (1982) Pancreatic secretory response to sham feeding in humans. Digestion 23:217–223

DiMagno EP, Go VLW, Summerskill WHJ (1973) Intraluminal and post absorptive effects of amino acids on pancreatic enzyme secretion. J Lab Clin Med 82:241–248

Dollinger HC, Raptis S, Pfeiffer EF (1976) Effects of somatostatin on exocrine and endocrine function stimulated by intestinal hormones in man. Horm Metab Res 8:74–78

Dyck WP, Texter EC, Lasater JM, Hightower NC (1970) Influence of glucagon and pancreatic exocrine secretion in man. Gastroenterology 58:532–539

Fahrenkrug J, Schaffalizky de Muckadell OB, Rune SJ (1978) pH treshold for release of secretin in normal subjects and in patients with duodenal ulcer and patients with chronic pancreatitis. Scand J Gastroenterol 13:177–186

Fletcher DR, Blackburn AM, Adrian TE, Chadwick VS, Bloon SR (1981) Effects of neurotensin on pancreatic function in man. Life Sci 29:2157–2161

Hanssen LE (1980) Pure synthetic bile salts release immunoreactive secretin in man. Scand J Gastroenterol 15:461–463

Harper AA, Hood AJC, Mushens J, Smy JR (1979) Inhibition of external pancreatic secretion by intracolonic and intraileal infusion in the cat. J Physiol (Lond) 292:445–454

Holst JJ (1986) Neural regulation of pancreatic exocrine function. In: Go VLW et al. (eds) The exocrine pancreas: biology, pathobiology and diseases. Raven, New York, pp 287–300

Hootman SR, Williams JA (1987) Stimulus-secretion coupling in the pancreatic acinus. In: Johnson LR (ed) Physiology of the gasrointestinal tract, 2nd edn. Raven, New York, pp 1129–1145

Kelly RB (1985) Pathways of protein secretion in eukaryotes. Science 230:25–32

Louie DS, May D, Miller P, et al. (1986) Cholecystokinin mediates feedback regulation of pancreatic enzyme secretion in rats. Am J Physiol 250:G252–G259

Lu L, Louie D, Owyang C (1989) A cholecystokinin releasing peptide mediates feedback regulation of pancreatic secretion. Am J Physiol 256:G430–G435

MacGregor I, Parent J, Meyer JH (1977) Gastric emptying of liquid meals and pancreatic and biliary secretion after subtotal gastrectomy or truncal vagotomy and pyloroplasty in man. Gastroenterology 72:-195–198

Malagelada JR, Go VLW, Summerskill HJ (1974) Altered pancreatic and biliary function after vagatomy and pyroloplasty. Gastroenterology 66:22–27

Owyang C, Williams J (1991) Pancreatic secretion. In: Yamada T, Alters DH, Owyang S, Powell DW, Silverstein FE (eds) Textbook of gastroenterology. J.B. Lippincott, Philadelphia, 294–314

Owyang C, Louie DS, Tatum D (1986a) Feedback regulation of pancreatic enzyme secretion in man: suppression of cholecystokinin release by trypsin. J Clin Invest 77:2042–2047

Owyang C, May D, Louie DS (1986b) Trypsin suppression of pancreatic enzyme secretion. Gastroenterology 91:637–643

Palade GE (1975) Intracellular aspects of the process of protein synthesis. Science 189:347–358

Rinderknecht H (1986) Pancreatic secretory enzymes. In: GO VL et al. (eds) The exocrine pancreas: biology, pathobiology and diseases. Raven, New York, pp 163–183

Rosenberg IR, Zambrano VJ, Janowitch HD, Rudick J (1976) Parasympathetic innervation and pancreatic secretion: the role of the gastric antrum. Ann Surg 183:247–251

Sarles H, Dani R, Prezelin G, Souville C, Figarella C (1968) Cephalic phase of pancreatic secretion in man. Gut 9:214

Schaffalizky de Muckadell OB, Fahrenkrug J (1978) Secretion pattern of secretin in man. Regulation by gastric acid. Gut 19:812–818

Schaffalizky de Muckadell OB, Fahrenkrug J, Watt-Boolsen S, Worning H (1978) Pancreatic response and plasma secretin concentration during infusion of low dose secretin in man. Scand J Gastroenterol 13:305–311

Schaffalizky de Muckadell OB, Fahrenkrug J, Nielsen J, Westfall, Worning H (1981) Meal-stimulated secretin release in man: effect of acid and bile. Scand J Gastroenterol 16:981–988

Scheele G (1986) Cellular processing of proteins in the exocrine pancreas. In: Go VL et al. (eds) The exocrine pancreas: biology, pathobiology and diseases. Raven, New York, pp 69–85

Scheele G, Bartelt D, Bieger W (1981) Characterization of human exocrine pancreatic proteins by two-dimensional isoelectric focusing/sodium dodecyl sulfate gel electrophoresis. Gastroenterology 80:461–473

Schulz I (1987) Electrolyte and fluid secretion in the exocrine pancreas. In: Johnson LR (ed) Physiology of the gastrointestinal tract. Raven, New York, pp 1147–1171

Schwartz TW (1983) Pancreastic polypeptide: a hormone under vagal control. Gastroenterology 85:1411–1425

Singer MV (1986) Neurohormonal control of pancreatic enzyme secretion in animals. In: Go VLW et al. (eds) The exocrine pancreas: biology, pathobiology and diseases. Raven, New York, pp 315–331

Walsh JH, Laners CB, Valenzuela JE (1982) Cholecystectokinin-octapeptide-like immunoreactivity in human plasma. Gastroenterology 82:438–444

Watanbe S, Chey WY, Lee KY, Chang TM (1986) Secretin is released by digestive products of fat in dog. Gastroenterology 90:1008–1017

White TT, McAlexander RA, Magee DF (1963) The effects of gastric distension on duodenal aspirates in man. Gastroenterology 44:48–53

You CH, Rominger JM, Chey WY (1982) Effects of atropine on the action and release of secretin in humans. Am J Physiol 242:608–611

Zimmerman MJ, Jonowitz HD (1986) Water and electrolyte secretion in the human pancreas. In: Go VL et al. (eds) The exocrine pancreas: biology, pathobiology and diseases. Raven, New York, pp 275–281

3 The Pancreas: Normal Radiological Anatomy and Variants

L. Van Hoe and B. Claikens

CONTENTS

L. Van Hoe, MD, PhD Assistant Professor, Department of Radiology, University Hospitals K.U. Leuven, Herestraat 49, B-3000 Leuven, Belgium

B. Claikens, MD, Department of Radiology, University Hospitals K.U. Leuven, Herestraat 49, B-3000 Leuven, Belgium

3.1 Normal Development

The pancreas develops from two separate anlagen, which arise as diverticula off the caudal end of the foregut during the 4th week of development (Fig. 3.1). The dorsal anlage or dorsal bud is the most cranial one and arises between the leaves of the dorsal mesogastrium (Langman 1975). The ventral component arises at the basis of the hepatic diverticulum and is initially composed of separate right and left lobes. The left lobe usually regresses completely. During further development, the ventral pancreas rotates clockwise around the duodenum to come to lie to the right of the dorsal pancreas. During the 7th week, the two pancreatic components fuse. The dorsal pancreas becomes the tail, body, and portions of the head of the pancreas. The ventral pancreas becomes the remainder of the head. Classic descriptions state that the cephalad portion of the head of the pancreas is derived from the dorsal pancreas, while the caudal portion is derived from the ventral pancreas (Kleitsch 1955). However, this is a simplified description that does not necessarily correspond to the real situation in all patients. This is illustrated by the fact that the duct of Santorini, which is derived from the dorsal pancreas, often receives a branch from the caudal portion of the pancreatic head. This particular feature is occasionally observed at endoscopic retrograde cholangiopancre-

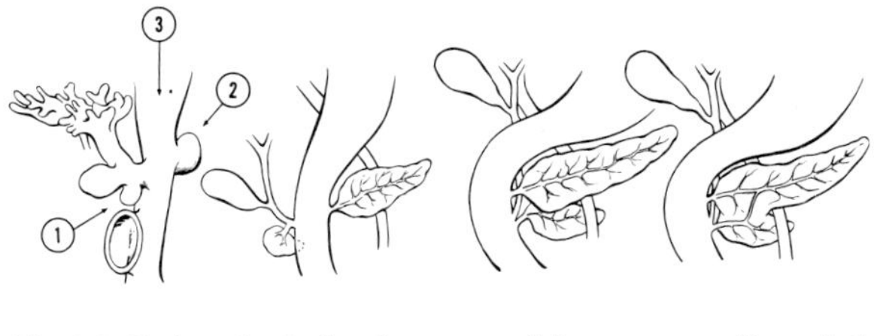

Fig. 3.1. Embryologic development of the pancreas (from *left* to *right*). Both the ventral pancreas (*1*) and dorsal pancreas (*2*) are buds off of the foregut (*3*). The ventral pancreas develops as a separate anlage and rotates posteriorly during maturation. Finally, fusion of the ventral and dorsal ductal system occurs. [Reprinted with permission from Stewart et al. (1977)]

atography (ERCP) or magnetic resonance cholangio pancreatography (MRCP). Furthermore, a caudally looping duct of Santorini may be observed. While both the dorsal and ventral anlagen may contribute to the upper and lower portion of the pancreatic head, their relationship with the anterior and posterior portions of the head is more constant: the ventral pancreas is located *posteriorly* and the *dorsal* pancreas anteriorly.

The ductal systems of the ventral and dorsal pancreatic anlagen fuse in the region of the neck. The duct of the dorsal pancreas becomes the main pancreatic duct, and, distal to the site of fusion, it becomes the accessory duct (duct of Santorini) which drains into the duodenum through the minor papilla. The duct of the ventral pancreas becomes the continuation of the main pancreatic duct and drains into the duodenum through the major papilla, which is located 1–3 cm caudal to the minor papilla.

There has been some confusion about terminology. As proposed by Schulte (1994), it is best to use "main pancreatic duct" to refer to the portion of the main duct in the body and tail, and to reserve the terms "duct of Santorini" and "duct of Wirsung" for the ducts distal to the site of fusion (Fig. 3.2).

As the fetus matures, the dorsal mesogastrium fuses with the posterior parietal layer of the peritoneum, except for its lateral portion, which persists as a ligament (splenorenal ligament) containing the pancreatic tail (Fig. 3.3). This fusion makes the pancreas a retroperitoneal organ. The fusion plane between the dorsal mesogastrium and the parietal layer of the peritoneum is a dissectable plane that constitutes a potential pathway for the spread of disease (see Sect. 3.2.2).

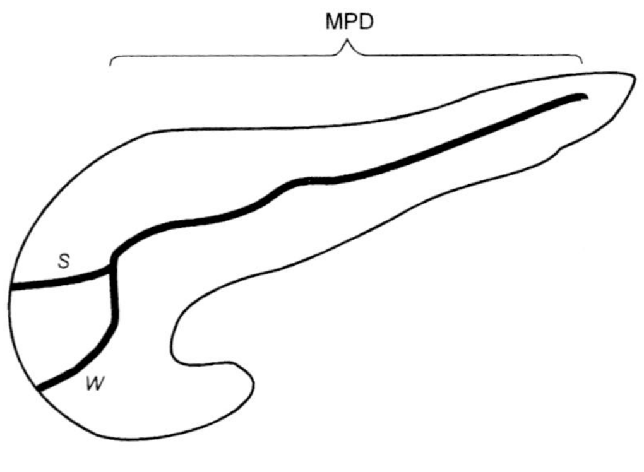

Fig. 3.2. Simplified representation of pancreatic ductal anatomy. The "main pancreatic duct" (*MPD*) is the portion of the main duct in the body and tail, while the terms "duct of Santorini" (*S*) and "duct of Wirsung" (*W*) are used for those portions distal to the site of fusion

3.2 General Anatomy

3.2.1 Historical Introduction

The pancreas has been called the "hidden organ" of the abdomen (Rhoades and Folin 1987). The name pancreas was given to this organ by the Greek Ruphos (*pan*, all; *kreas*, flesh). More than a millenium passed before anatomic descriptions were completed. In 1642, Johann Wirsung demonstrated the pancreatic duct. Santorini of Venice described the accessory duct in 1724. The papilla of Vater and the sphincter complex were described by Abraham Vater in 1720 and by Oddi in 1887. Langerhans revealed the histologic structure in 1869. Surgery for pancreatic disease was not popular until the pioneering work of Whipple in 1930. Nowadays, classic anatomical descriptions of the pancreas have been correlated or completed with observations made with ERCP, catheter angiography, computed tomography (CT), ultrasonography (US), and magnetic resonance imaging (MRI).

3.2.2 Peripancreatic Abdominal Compartments

The pancreas is localized deep in the epigastric region just ventral to the lumbar vertebrae, partially surrounded by the duodenum and behind the stomach. The head usually lies at the level of L1–2 and the body crosses the spine at L1. Most frequently, the pancreas is oriented slightly oblique to the left and cranially, resulting in a curved form against the lumbar spine. The long axis has an average angulation of 20° with respect to the transverse plane (Fig. 3.4).

The pancreas is usually divided into a head, neck, body, and tail with the mesenteric vessels as a reference point (see Sect. 3.2.3). The head, neck, and body are fixed in the retroperitoneal space. The last portion, the tail, is loosely developed in between the double peritoneal layer of the splenorenal ligament. Thus, the space behind the pancreatic tail is an extension of the peritoneal space. It is called the retropancreatic recess and forms a potential pathway for intraperitoneal spread of pancreatic disease (Fig. 3.5).

The retroperitoneal space is subdivided into three spaces by the anterior and posterior layers of the

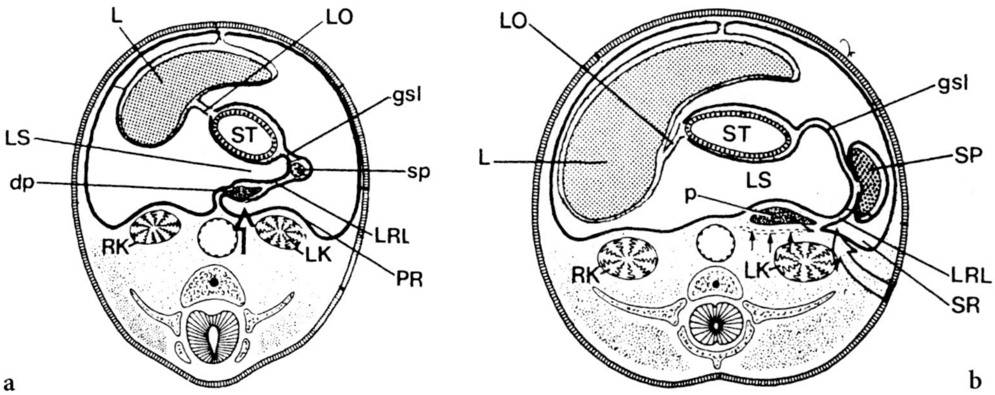

Fig. 3.3a,b. Developmental anatomy of the pancreas. **a** Schematic transverse section of a 7-week-old fetus. The dorsal pancreas (dp) lies within the leaves of the dorsal mesogastrium, between the lesser sac (*LS*) anteriorly and the retroperitoneal pancreatic recess (*open arrow*) posteriorly. The developing spleen (*SP*) lies more laterally within the dorsal mesogastrium, dividing into an anterior gastrosplenic ligament (*gsl*) and a posterior lienorenal ligament (*LRL*). *ST*, stomach; *LO*, lesser omentum; *L*, liver; *RK*, right kidney; *LK*, left kidney **b** Transverse section of a 4-month-old fetus. The spleen (*SP*) has moved laterally, and the lesser sac (*LS*) is deeper than in (**a**). The dorsal mesogastrium has fused (*closed arrows*) with the posterior parietal layer of the peritoneum, except for its lateral portion, which persists as the adult lienorenal ligament (*LRL*). Thus, the embryonic retropancreatic recess is obliterated, except laterally (*open arrow*) where it persists behind the lienorenal ligament in continuity with the splenorenal space (*SR*). If the line of fusion (*arrows*) is incomplete, the retropancreatic recess can extend behind the pancreas (*p*). *gsl*, Gastrosplenic ligament; *st*, stomach; *LO*, lesser omentum; *L*, liver; *RK*, right kidney; *LK*, left kidney. [Reprinted with permission from Rubinstein et al. (1985)]

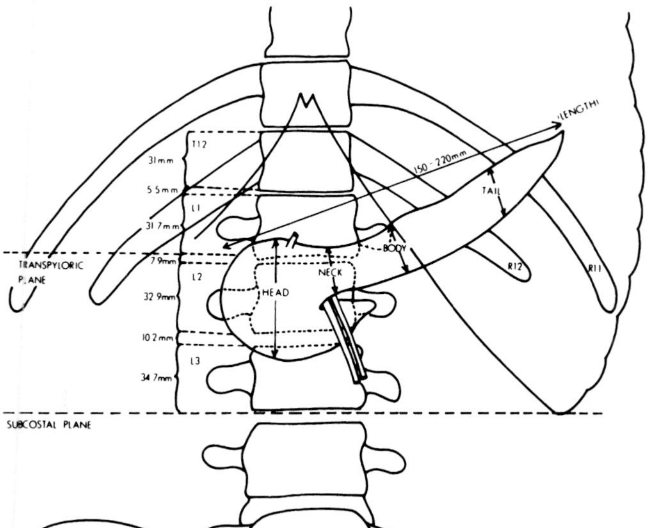

Fig. 3.4. Normal pancreatic orientation and dimensions. [Reprinted with permission from Zylak and Pallie (1981)]

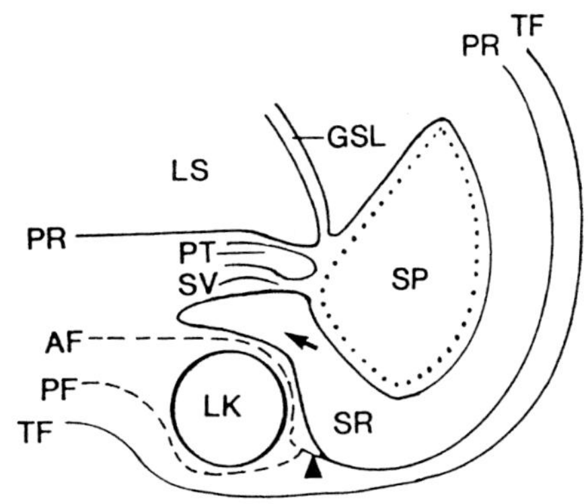

Fig. 3.5. The splenorenal space. The peritoneal compartments have been exaggerated. The splenorenal space (*SR*) extends posteriorly between the spleen (*SP*) and the left kidney (*LK*) to the level of the lateroconal fascia (*arrowhead*) and anteromedially (*arrow*) behind the pancreatic tail (*PT*). *SV*, splenic vein; *PR*, parietal layer of peritoneum; *AF*, anterior renal fascia; *PF*, posterior renal fascia; *TF*, transverse fascia; *LS*, lesser sac; *GSL*, gastrosplenic ligament. [Reprinted with permission from Rubinstein et al. (1985)]

renal fascia (Gerota's fascia): the anterior and posterior pararenal spaces and the perirenal spaces (Rubinstein et al. 1985; Meyers 1988; Molmenti et al. 1996) (Fig. 3.6).

The *anterior pararenal space* contains the pancreas and is bounded anteriorly by the posterior or parietal layer of the lesser sac, posteriorly by the anterior leaf of the Gerota's fascia, and at its lateral border by the lateroconal fascia. It is continuous with the contralateral side and also harbors the duodenum, descending and ascending colon, and the peripancreatic blood vessels. Importantly, it extends cra-

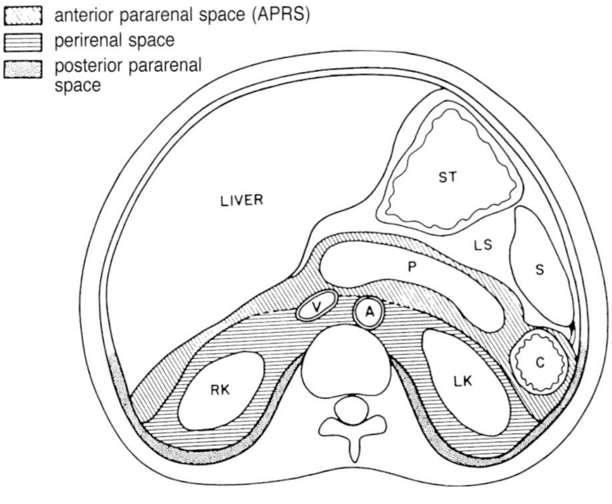

Fig. 3.6. Retroperitoneal compartments. The pancreas (*P*) lies in the anterior pararenal space (APRS), the borders of which are the posterior parietal peritoneum, the anterior renal (Gerota's) fascia dorsally, and the lateral conal fascia laterally. Other important structures in the APRS are the duodenal loop (not shown) and the ascending and descending colon (*C*). *A*, aorta; *LS*, lesser sac; *RK* and *LK*, right and left kidney; *S*, spleen; *ST*, stomach; *V*, vena cava. [Reprinted with permission from FEDERLE and GOLDBERG (1992)]

nially to the subdiaphragmatic area and caudally to the pelvis. Therefore, disease processes originating in the pancreas can extend far cranially and caudally. Extension into the peritoneal cavity is also possible because the posterior pariental peritoneum constitutes a relatively weak barrier. The anterior pararenal space is also connected with the transverse mesocolon and small bowel mesentery (Fig. 3.7). The parietal peritoneum forms the two leaves of the transverse mesocolon somewhat below the level of the pancreas. A nonperitonealized "bare area" results which is in close proximity to the pancreas. The root of the small bowel mesentery originates inferior to the pancreatic body and is continuous with the transverse mesocolon. Pancreatic processes may affect the small bowel loops and colon via the small bowel mesentery and transverse mesocolon, respectively (Meyers 1988).

The *perirenal space* contains the adrenal gland, the kidney, and the ureter. There is no direct connection between the pancreas and the perirenal space.

The *posterior pararenal space* is bounded ventrally by the posterior leaf of the Gerota's fascia and dorsally by the transversalis facia and back muscles. It is continous with the properitoneal space and therefore with the other side. The posterior pararenal space contains no organs.

This compartmental model for describing the anatomy of the retroperitoneal spaces was originally proposed by MEYERS (1988) and has recently been refined. MOLMENTI and coworkers (1996) have suggested that previously described lines of fusion (e.g., between the mesentery of the descending colon and the left renal fascia) are dissectable planes, and that fluid collections that accumulate due to pathologic processes extend easily into these planes (Fig. 3.8). Clinical observations support this hypothesis. Fluid collections observed at CT in patients with pancreatitis, for instance, do not conform to the classically determined boundaries of the anterior pararenal space. In some patients, the fluid appears to extend *into* the perirenal and/or lateroconal fascia (Fig. 3.9) (KOROBKIN et al. 1992). This observation is now explained by the presence of an "interfascial space", also called "plane of fusion" of "fusion fascia" (KURODA and NAGAI 1998). This concept also nicely explains: (a) the observation that pancreatic exsudates may extend to the psoas muscle, and (b) the relatively caudal position of the flank discoloration that composes the "Gray Turner sign" in pancreatitis (MOLMENTI et al. 1996).

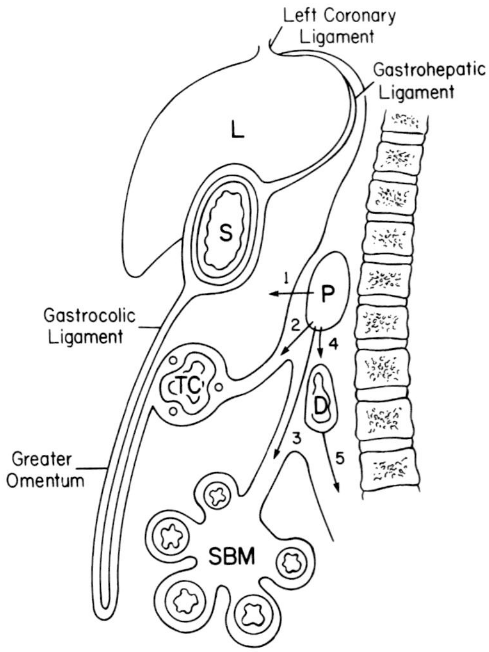

Fig. 3.7. The mesenteric, omental, retroperitoneal, and subperitoneal relationships of the pancreas (*P*): sagittal perspective. Pancreatic disease may spread into the lesser sac (*1*), transverse mesocolon (*TC*) (*2*), root of the small bowel mesentery (*SBM*) (*3*), duodenum (*D*) (*4*), and anterior pararenal space (*5*). *L*, liver; *S*, spleen. [Reprinted with permission from GORE et al. (1994)]

a b
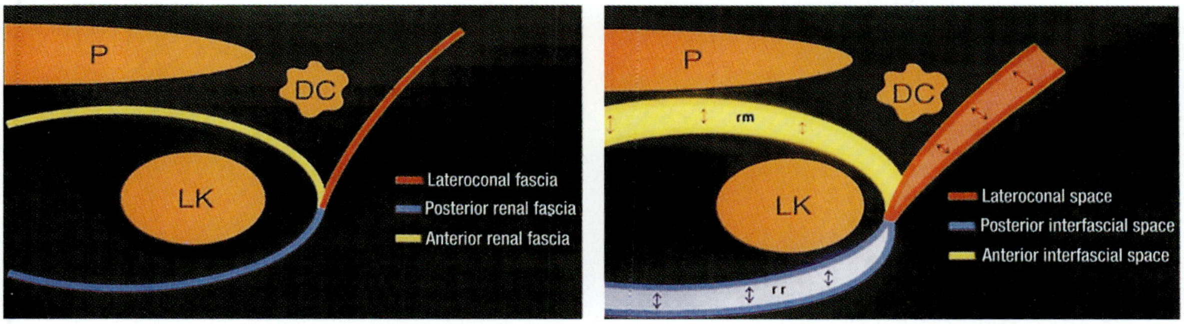

Fig. 3.8a,b. Proposed position of retromesenteric and retrorenal planes. **a** Standard retroperitoneal anatomy at the level of the upper left renal pole. The pancreas (*P*) and descending colon (*DC*) lie in the anterior pararenal space and are separated from the left kidney (*LK*) and surrounding perirenal fat by the anterior renal fascia (*yellow*), and from the posterior pararenal fat (not shown) by the lateroconal fascia (*red*). The posterior renal fascia (*blue*) divides the perirenal space from the posterior pararenal space. **b** Proposed position of pathologic fluid collections. Expandable planes lie in place of the fascial boundaries illustrated in (**a**). The retromesenteric plane (*rm*) on the left side lies anterior to the perirenal fat and posterior to the mesentery of the descending colon (*DC*) and, superiorly, to the pancreas (*P*). The retrorenal plane (*rr*) lies posterior to the perirenal fat. This theory proposes that rapidly accumulating fluid that originates within any of the three classically described retroperitoneal spaces can extend into one or more of these planes, from which further extension inferiorly to the pelvis or superiorly to the diaphragm is possible. *LK*, left kidney. [Reprinted with permission from MOLMENTI et al. (1996)]

a b
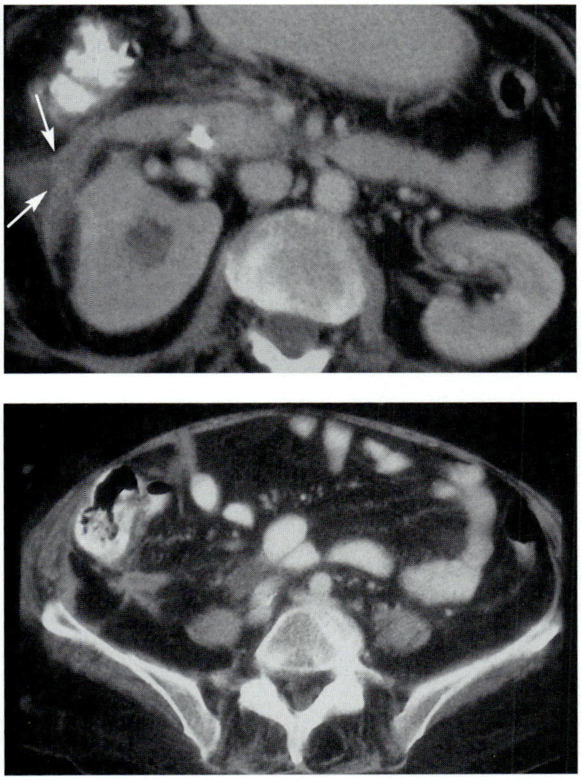

Fig. 3.9a,b. Distribution of pancreatic exsudate in lateroconal and anterior interfascial spaces (patient with acute pancreatitis). **a** Image obtained at caudal border of pancreatic head shows fluid in anterior interfascial space (*arrow*) with extension into the lateroconal space (*arrowheads*). **b** Image obtained 8 cm more caudally shows small tubular collection still located in the anterior (retromesenteric) interfascial space (*arrow*) and clearly separated from the ascending colon. Note limited extension into posterior interfascial space (*arrowheads*)

In the surgical literature, the fusion fascias behind the head and behind the body/tail are named after Treitz and Toldt, respectively.

3.2.3
The Pancreatic Gland

The pancreas is a soft, pale yellow, coarsely lobulated organ 12–20 cm long, 3–5 cm wide, and 1–3 cm thick, weighing 60–125 g in adults (QUINLAN 1991).

Macroscopically, the pancreas has a rose aspect, a hard consistence, and a granular surface. Its contour is smooth in about 80% and lobulated in 20%.

The pancreatic parenchyma is divided into acinar lobules by multiple fibrous septa containing arteries, veins, and variable amounts of fat. Fat-laden interlobular septa are more common in obese individuals, and in conditions with glandular atrophy.

The pancreas is divided in a head, neck, body, and tail, with the mesenteric vessels as a reference point (Fig. 3.10).

The head is the broad right end of the gland lying within the curve of the duodenum and is defined as the portion to the right of the superior mesenteric and portal vein (KURODA and NAGAI 1998).

The uncinate process is the polongation of the left and caudal borders of the head. It projects like a hook, dorsal to the superior mesenteric vein, and has a triangular appeance, with the tip oriented to the left. Its antero- and posteromedial borders are usually straight or concave. A convex appeance of the

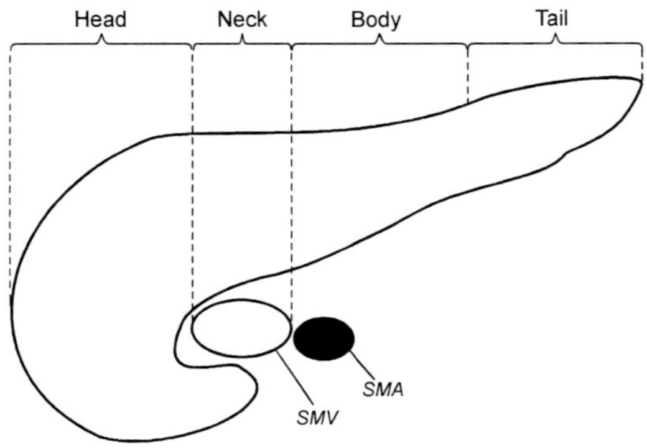

Fig. 3.10. Division of the pancreas into a head, neck, body, and tail. The head is defined as the portion to the right of the superior mesenteric vein (*SMV*). The neck is located to the left of the right border of the superior mesenteric vein and to the right of its left border. The portion of the gland left of the left border of the superior mesenteric vein is bisected into the body (the right half) and the tail (the left half). *SMA*, superior mesenteric artery

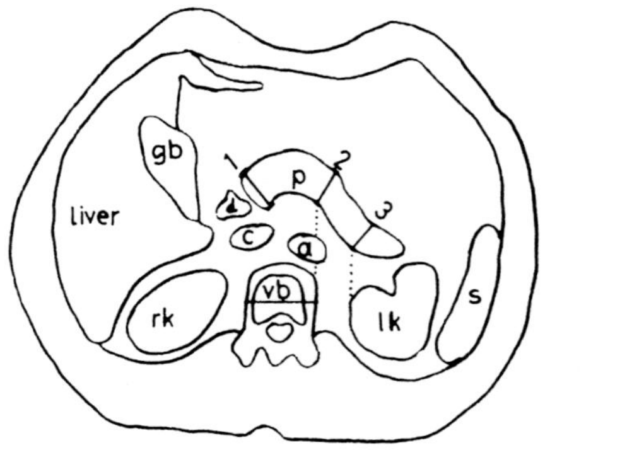

Fig. 3.11. Localization of measured diameters in the study by Heuck and colleagues. *1*, Head of pancreas; *2*, body; *3*, tail; *p*, pancreas; *a*, aorta; *c*, vena cava; *d*, duodenum; *gb*, gallbladder; *vb*, vertebral body; *s*, spleen; *rk*, right kidney; *lk*, left kidney. [Reprinted with permission from Heuck et al. (1987)]

borders should suggest the possibility of underlying disease.

The neck is the constricted portion to the left of the head, lying ventral to the superior mesenteric vessels (to the left of the right border of the superior mesenteric vein and to the right of the its left border).

The body lies behind the lesser sac (omental bursa) and stomach. The border between the body and tail is not clearly defined (Kuroda and Nagai 1998). According to the classification proposed by the Japanese Pancreas Society, the portion of the gland left to the left border of the superior mesenteric vein is bisected into the body (the right half) and the tail (the left half) (Japanese Pancreas Society 1996) (see Fig. 3.10). The body may be somewhat thinner than the head and tail.

The size of the pancreas shows some variation with age: a gradual decrease in size occurs in older patients (Heuck et al. 1987). Several studies have focused on the normal diameters of the different portions of the gland at CT. Kreel and collegues investigated patients in their fifth decade and found the following average normal values for anteroposterior diameter: head: 23–24 mm, neck 17 mm, body 20 mm, tail: 15 mm (Kreel et al. 1977). More recently, Heuck et al. investigated 360 patients with a 4.5-s scanner. Their results are given in Tables 3.1 and 3.2. Importantly, all the measurements were done at right angles to the long axis of the organ (Fig. 3.11).

3.2.4 Anatomical Landmarks

3.2.4.1 Great Vessels

3.2.4.1.1 Arteries (Fig. 3.12)

The pancreas maintains a more or less constant relationship with the major vessels and the loop of the

Table 3.1. Normal pancreas: anteroposterior diameters (mm) of the pancreas according to the patient's age

Age (years)	Head	Body	Tail
20–30	28.6 (±3.8)	19.1 (±2.1)	18.0 (±1.6)
31–40	26.0 (±3.4)	18.2 (±2.4)	16.5 (±1.8)
41–50	25.2 (±3.6)	17.8 (±2.2)	15.8 (±1.7)
51–60	24.0 (±3.6)	16.0 (±2.0)	15.1 (±1.9)
61–70	23.4 (±3.5)	15.8 (±2.4)	14.7 (±1.8)
71–80	21.2 (±4.3)	14.4 (±2.7)	13.0 (±2.1)

Table 3.2. Vertebral body/pancreas ratio (%) in different age groups. [Reprinted with permission from Heuck et al. (1987)]

Age (years)	Head	Body	Tail
20–30	68.2 (±8.5)	47.0 (±5.6)	45.1 (±4.4)
31–40	62.1 (±9.3)	43.2 (±6.0)	38.9 (±5.9)
41–50	58.0 (±7.8)	41.6 (±6.0)	36.1 (±4.3)
51–60	55.0 (±9.7)	37.2 (±6.4)	35.6 (±5.7)
61–70	53.4 (±7.8)	36.1 (±6.2)	33.6 (±4.7)
71–80	48.2 (±12.2)	32.4 (±6.1)	29.4 (±5.1)

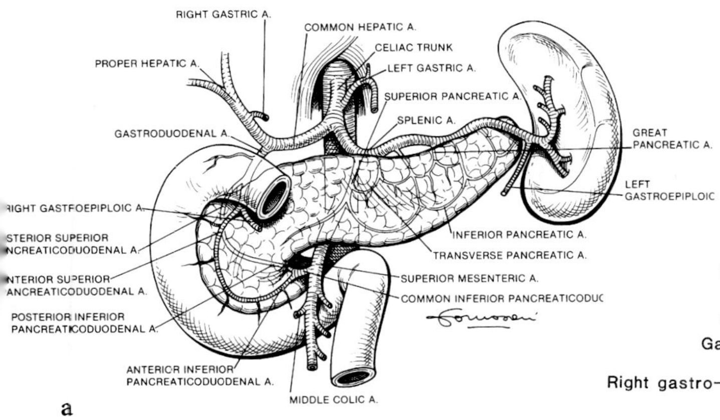

a

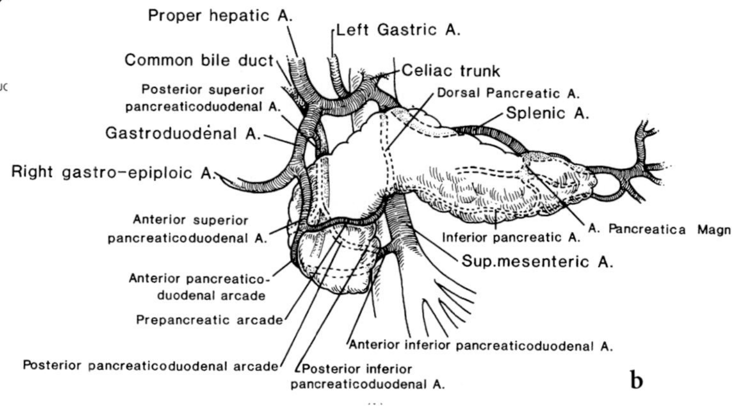

b

Fig. 3.12a,b. The arterial anatomy of the pancreas. [Reprinted with permission from Tersingni and Toledo-Pereyra (1985)]

duodenum. It is located ventral to the abdominal aorta and inferior vena cava. The celiac axis, which is the first branch of the abdominal aorta, is located at the superior margin of the pancreatic neck. The splenic artery, which is a major branch of the celiac trunk, is usually located in a groove along the posterior and superior border of the pancreas. However, this relationship is rather inconstant as the splenic artery may be very tortuous. The hepatic artery, which is the second major branch of the celiac trunk, courses cranially to the pancreatic head and gives rise to the gastroduodenal artery, which runs caudally along the anterolateral border of the pancreatic head. The superior mesenteric artery arises from the aorta 1–2 cm inferior to the celiac artery and courses inferiorly beneath the pancreatic neck.

3.2.4.1.2 Veins (Fig. 3.13)

The splenic vein is perhaps the most important anatomical landmark because of its consistent location in a groove along the posterior margin of the pancreas. Unlike the splenic artery, it has a rather straight course.

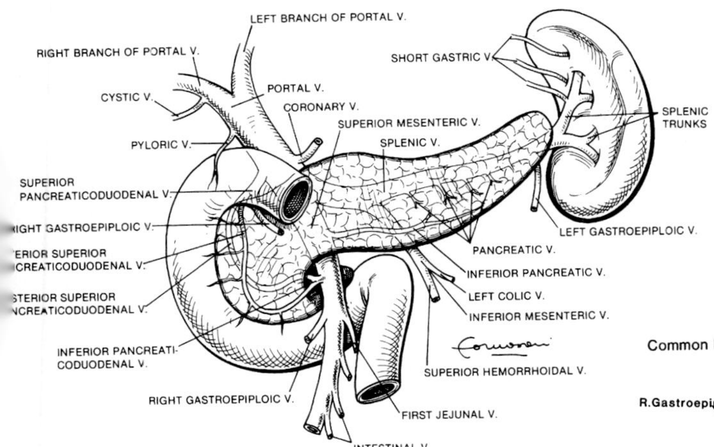

a

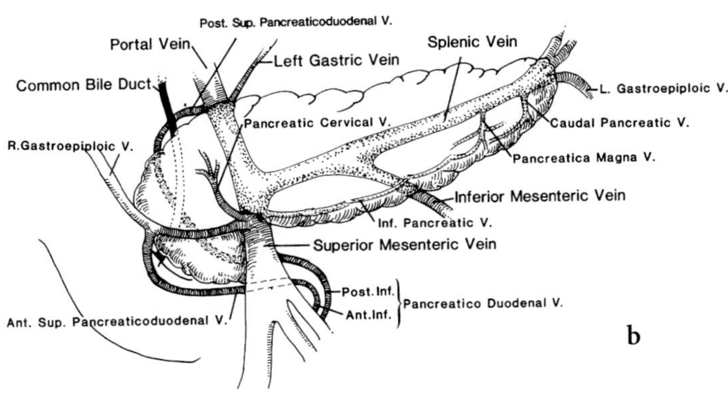

b

Fig. 3.13a,b. The venous anatomy of the pancreas. [Reprinted with permission from Tersingni and Toledo-Pereyra (1985)]

The superior mesenteric vein parallels the superior mesenteric artery and, importantly, lies to the right of it. The junction of the splenic and superior mesenteric veins ("venous confluence") is located immediately dorsal to the cranial portion of the pancreatic head and neck, and continues superiorly and laterally towards the porta hepatis as the portal vein. The common bile duct and hepatic artery are located close to the portal vein. The left renal vein is located somewhat caudal to the portovenous confluence and drains into the inferior caval vein dorsally to the pancreatic head. The inferior caval vein is located close to the pancreatic head.

3.2.4.2 Pancreatic Head

The head of the pancreas is in intimate relationship to the duodenum (Figs. 3.12, 3.13). The first part of the duodenum is completely surrounded by peritoneum and is located above and anterior to the pancreatic head. The portal vein and common bile duct are posterior to it. The second, descending, part of the duodenum has a retroperitoneal location and is immediately contiguous to the lateral border of the pancreatic head. The third part is in contact with the inferior margin of the pancreatic head and uncinate process. The gallbladder is positioned ventral to the pancreatic head. Anteriorly, the head is covered by the pylorus above and the transverse colon below. The posterior surface of the head faces the hilum of the right kidney, the inferior vena cava, the left renal vein, and aorta.

The uncinate process extends dorsal to the superior mesenteric vein, in the space between the aorta and the mesenteric vessels (see Fig. 3.4).

3.2.4.3 Pancreatic Neck

The posterior surface of the neck is grooved by the portal vein, which is formed by the confluence of the superior mesenteric vein and the splenic vein (Fig. 3.14a). Anteriorly, the neck is covered by the pylorus and the lesser sac, and superiorly it is related to the celiac trunk. The pylorus is located ventral to the pancreatic neck.

3.2.4.4 Pancreatic Body

The dorsal boundary of the body faces the abdominal aorta, the left diaphragmatic pillar, the left adrenal gland, and the left kidney (Fig. 3.14b). The upper part of the pancreatic body is in close contact with the celiac trunk and the solar plexus. The gastric body and antrum lie anterior to the body of the pancreas. The transverse mesocolon attaches to the inferior aspect of the body and tail. Inferiorly, the body lies adjacent to the fourth portion of the duodenum and the ligament of Treitz.

a b

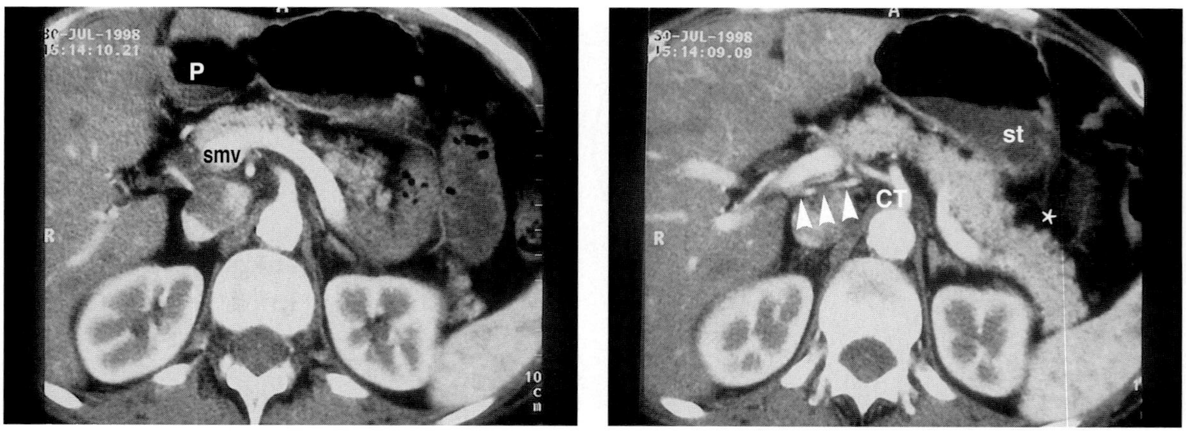

Fig. 3.14a,b. Topographic relationships. **a** Computed tomography (*CT*) image obtained at level of pancreatic neck. The neck is bounded dorsally by the superior mesenteric vein (*smv*). Anteriorly, it is covered by the lesser sac (not seen in physiologic state) and pylorus (*P*). **b** CT image obtained at level of pancreatic body. The upper part of the pancreatic body is in close contact with the celiac trunk (*CT*). Anteriorly, the body and tail are bordered by the stomach (*st*) and transverse mesocolon (*asterisk*). The tail may or may not reach the hilum of the spleen. Note the presenece of an anatomic variant in this patient: a replaced right hepatic artery (*arrowheads*)

3.2.4.5
Pancreatic Tail

The pancreatic tail is completely covered by the peritoneum and relatively mobile.

The most proximal portion – which has a variable length – is usually oriented to the splenic hilum. The anterior surface of the tail lies closely to the posterior part of the lesser sac. The posterior surface is in close contact with the left kidney. The spleen lies along the lateral and superior aspect of the pancreatic tail.

3.2.5
Ductal Anatomy

The main pancreatic duct begins in the tail and has a gradually enlarging caliber as it courses from the tail to the ampulla. Its length ranges from 9.5 cm to over 25 cm (average 16 cm). Based on measurements obtained with ERCP, the average caliber is 3.5 mm in the head, 2.5 mm in the body, and 1.5 mm in the tail (Sivak and Sillivan 1976). A large variability in caliber exists and diameters up to 7 mm may be seen in normal patients free of pancreatic disease. The pancreatic duct gently arches in an anterior direction and then passes in a posterior direction to enter the head. In the head, the duct inclines further dorsally and caudally and passes to the left caudal side of the common bile duct. It runs midway between the superior and inferior surfaces through the body and closer to the posterior surface at the neck.

By describing the course of the pancreatic duct in the head, body, and tail as either descending, horizontal, or ascending, 27 possible ductal configurations can be defined. According to Varley and coworkers, the sigmoid configuration (ascending-horizontal-ascending) and the pistol pattern (ascending-horizontal-horizontal) are the most common types (40% and 30%, respectively) (Varley et al. 1976) (Fig. 3.15). Other groups have reported slightly different results (Classen et al. 1973; Kasugai et al. 1972). From a practical point of view, it should be stressed that variations in the course of the pancreatic duct are so numerous that nearly every configuration can be normal.

The main pancreatic duct drains 20–30 collateral canals (side branches) (Silvis et al. 1995). The side branches in the body and tail have an average caliber of 0.2 mm (!) and generally enter the duct at right angles.

The main pancreatic duct usually bifurcates into the duct of Wirsung (duct of ventral pancreas) and the duct of Santorini (see Fig. 3.2). At the entrance of the duodenum, the duct of Wirsung unites with the distal common bile duct and drains in the duodenum at the papilla major, which is a small, mucosa-covered, protuberance in the medial wall of the duodenum. The location, size, and shape of the papilla major are variable. According to Schwartz and coworkers, it is located in the middle third of the descending duodenum in 74% of cases. Other possible locations are at the junction of the second and third portions of the duodenum (18%) and in the third portion (8%) (Schwartz and Birnbaum 1962). The average size of the papilla is 14.7 mm. It may be flat, hemispheric, or papillary. The orifices of the pancreatic duct and common bile duct are usually located at the tip of the papilla.

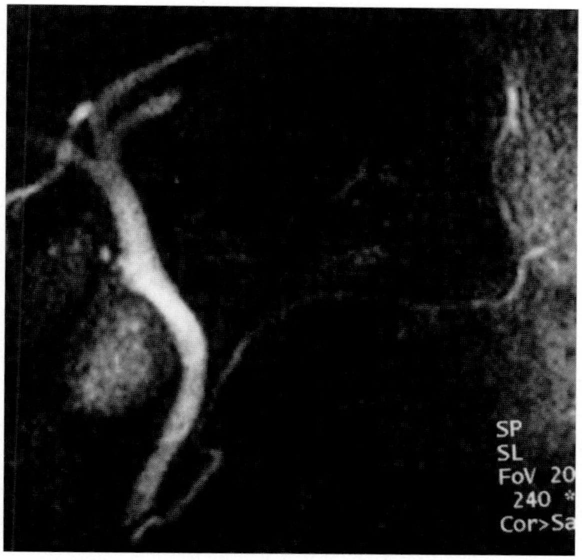

Fig. 3.15. Magnetic resonance image showing normal pancreatic duct with sigmoid configuration. [Reprinted with permission from Van Hoe et al. (1998b)]

As the distal bile duct and pancreatic duct approach the duodenal wall, they become invested by smooth muscle fibers. This muscle is referred to as the Vaterian sphincter, or Oddi's sphincter, and has an average length of 14 mm (range 10–15 mm) (Fig. 3.16) (Stewart et al. 1977). The terminal portions of the common bile duct and pancreatic duct course obliquely in a latero-caudal direction. Importantly, the diameter of the intramuscular portions of both ducts is only a few millimeters. In 60%–80% of patients, the pancreatic and bile ducts unite to form *a common channel* [length 2–15 mm, average 5 mm (Misra and Dwivedi 1990)]. The slightly dilated distal segment of the common channel is also called the ampulla (Sterling 1954). The anatomical rela-

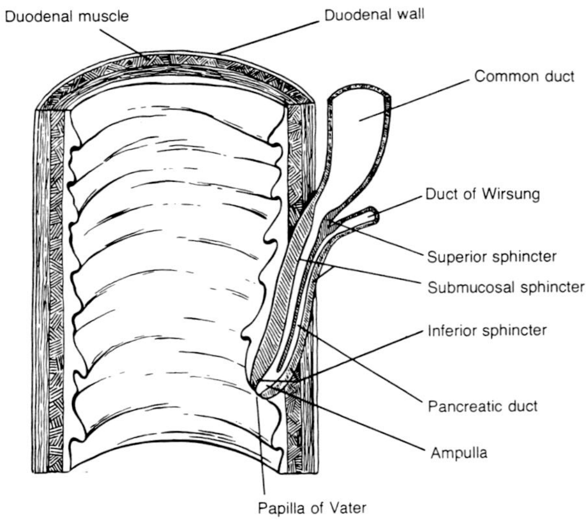

Fig. 3.16. The Vaterian sphincter complex. The most distal portions of the pancreatic duct and bile duct become invested with smooth muscle fibers as they approach the duodenal wall. [Reprinted with permission from STEWART et al. (1977)]

tionship of both ducts has been termed V-, U-, or Y-shaped (TAYLOR and BOHORFOUSH 1997).

The functional complex consisting of the papilla, the ampulla (if present), and the distal portions of both ducts with their muscular and fibrous coverings has been called the Vaterian system or Vaterian sphincter complex (VSC) (STEWART et al. 1977). This sphincter complex consists of separate muscle groups including the sphincter choledochus, the sphincter pancreaticus (present in 33% of patients only), and the ampullary sphincter. It regulates the passage of bile and pancreatic juice into the duodenum. Manometric studies have shown that the physiological function of the Vaterian sphincter is characterized by phasic contractions superimposed on a baseline pressure. While the basal pressure measures 15 ± 5 mmHg, phasic wave contractions usually measure 150 ± 16 mmHg. These phasic waves occur at a mean frequency of four/min and last 4.3 ± 0.5 s (STARITZ 1988).

The accessory duct of Santorini drains the anteroir and superior portion of the head of the pancreas, usually as a separate duct terminating at the papilla minor. This smaller papilla is located 1–2 cm proximal to the major papilla.

The exact location of the common bile duct with respect to the pancreatic head also deserves some attention, since it may determine morphologic changes seen in pancreatic disease. The common bile duct enters the head of the pancreas after it passes posterior to the first part of the duodenum in the hepatoduodenal ligament. It passes inferiorly and dorsally to join the Wirsung duct. There are three major patterns of the relationships between common bile duct and head of pancreas: (1) partial coverage of the duct by pancreatic tissue from behind (51.5%), (2) total coverage (30%), and (3) the duct running externally in a groove on the posterior aspect of the gland (16.5%) (SMANIO 1954) (Fig. 3.17). Occasionally, the common bile duct courses lateral to the pancreatic head, within the peripancreatic fat medial to the descending duodenum.

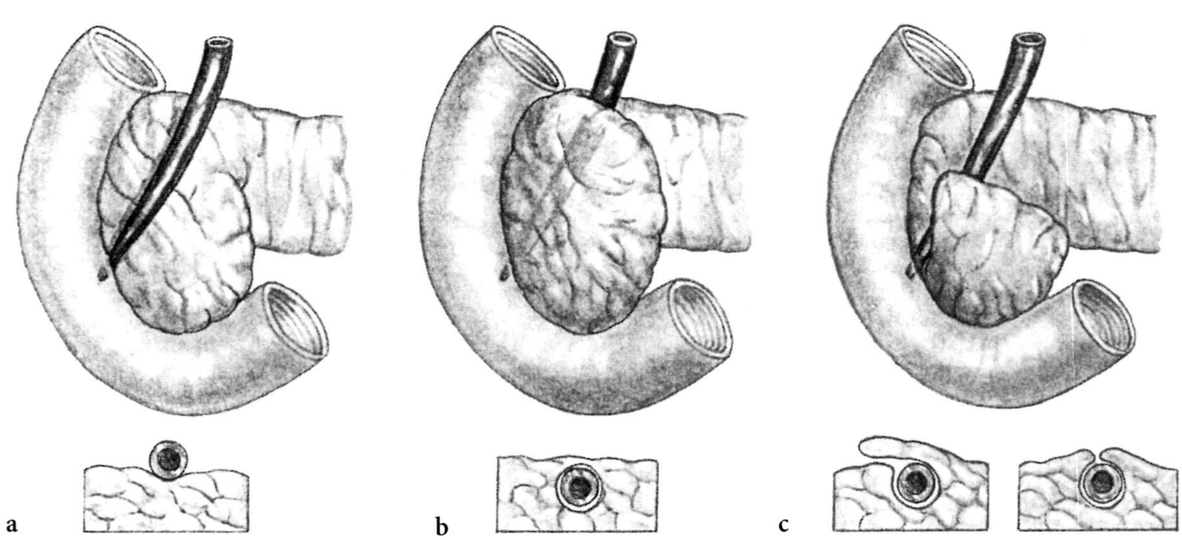

Fig. 3.17a–c. Relationships of the common bile duct to the posterior aspect of the pancreatic head. **a** Partially covered; **b** completely covered; **c** uncovered. [Reprinted with permission from KURODA and NAGAI (1998)]

3.2.6
Arterial Anatomy (see Fig. 3.12)

A detailed knowledge of the arterial anatomy of the pancreas is required for those performing superselective arteriography. Nowadays, many of these vessels are also visible on cross-sectional images obtained with thin-section CT.

3.2.6.1
Major Vessels

The arterial blood supply of the pancreas arises from the celiac trunk and the superior mesenteric artery (Freeny and Lawson 1982).

The *celiac artery* arises from the anterior aspect of the aorta at the level of T12-L1, above the neck of the pancreas. Its primary branches are the common hepatic, splenic, and left gastric arteries. It may also give rise to the dorsal pancreatic artery.

The *common hepatic artery* divides into the proper hepatic artery and the gastroduodenal artery (see Sect. 3.2.6.2).

The *splenic artery* directly gives rise to several important vessels which represent the major vascular supply to the tail of the pancreas including the dorsal pancreatic artery, the pancreatic magna artery, and the caudal pancreatic artery.

The *superior mesenteric artery* arises from the anterior aspect of the aorta 1–2 cm below the origin of the celiac artery. It forms an acute or open angle with the aorta, courses posterior to the pancreas, crosses the small tip of the uncinate process anteriorly, and emerges ventral to the third portion of the duodenum to enter the mesentery (Michels 1955). It usually gives rise to the inferior pancreaticoduodenal artery.

3.2.6.2
Distal Branches

The *gastroduodenal artery* represents the primary source of vascular supply to the head of the pancreas. It gives a first branch, the *posterior superior pancreaticoduodenal artery* (PSPDA), and then crosses the first portion of the duodenum. Together with a posterior branch of the the inferior pancreaticoduodenal artery, which originates from the superior mesenteric artery, the PSPDA froms an anastomotic network that is called the *posterior arcade* (Rouviere and Delmas 1985; Kadir 1991).

At the anterior surface of the pancreas, the gastroduodenal artery bifurcates into the *anterior superior pancreaticoduodenal artery* (ASPDA) and the right gastro-epiploic artery. An *anterior arcade* is formed by anastomoses between the ASPDA and an anterior branch of the inferior pancreaticoduodenal artery.

The *dorsal pancreatic artery* usually provides a significant contribution to the head and neck and, therefore, is one of the most important arteries for superselective pancreatic angiography. It most commonly (40%) arises from the proximal suprapancreatic segment of the splenic artery and is located at the dorsal surface of the neck of the gland. It may also arise from the celiac (22%), superior mesenteric (14%), and common hepatic (12%) arteries. It runs downward to the lower border of the pancreas and typically has four main branches: two "head branches" that may anastomose with the pancreatic arcades described above, a third descending branch communicating with the superior mesenteric artery or one of its branches, and a fourth left branch that is called the *transverse pancreatic artery*. This artery courses along the inferior surface of the gland.

The *pancreatic magna artery* is the largest constant branch of the splenic artery and arises from its midportion (usually around the border between body and tail). It courses along the superior margin of the body and tail and divides into left and right branches to anastomose with the transverse pancreatic, dorsal pancreatic, and caudal pancreatic arteries. It forms a major source of blood supply for the body and tail.

The *caudal pancreatic artery* arises from the third or fourth portion of the splenic artery and may be represented by several small, independent branches.

The *inferior pancreaticoduodenal artery* arises from the right side of the superior mesenteric artery or from the first or second jejunal branch. It divides into anterior and posterior branches on the surface of the pancreatic head. These branches communicate with the corresponding anterior and posterior superior arcade vessels. The inferior pancreaticoduodenal artery thus contributes to the blood supply of the pancreatic head, including the uncinate process.

3.2.7
Venous Anatomy (see Fig. 3.13)

Knowledge of the venous anatomy is important for at least three reasons. Firstly, as described above, some veins constitute major anatomical landmarks for localization of the pancreas. Secondly, subtle venous abnormalities may indicate extrapancreatic extension of a pancreatic tumor on CT or MR images, a finding which may be of critical importance for therapy planning. Finally, venous sampling may be the last diagnostic step in patients with suspected endocrine pancreatic tumors. This technique, of course, requires thorough knowledge of the anatomy. This point is extensively discussed in Chap. 10.

Those peripancreatic veins that are important as anatomical landmarks are described above (Sect. 3.2.4.1.2). Here, a short overview is given of the venous drainage of the different parts of the pancreas.

The head of the pancreas is drained by the pancreaticoduodenal veins. These are referred to as the anterior and posterior superior and inferior veins, corresponding to the arterial arcades. The *posterior superior pancreaticoduodenal vein* (PSPDV) terminates directly in the right posterior wall of the portal vein (Fig. 3.18). Its course is more or less parallel to the common bile duct (it may even be confused with the common bile duct (see Sect. 3.5.3). The *anterior superior pancreaticoduodenal vein* (ASPDV) joins the gastrocolic trunk before it drains into the superior mesenteric vein (Figs. 3.18, 3.19). The gastrocolic trunk is present in 72%–100% of patients and formed by the confluence of the right gastroepiploic and right colic veins. Alternatively, the ASPDV may join the right gastroepiploic vein before its entry into the superior mesenteric vein, with the right superior colic vein having a separate insertion site into the superior mesenteric vein.

The drainage of the venous blood of the body and tail is ensured by 3–13 small corporal veins that drain directly into the splenic vein (KADIR 1991). As a general rule, the veins tend to follow the corresponding arteries.

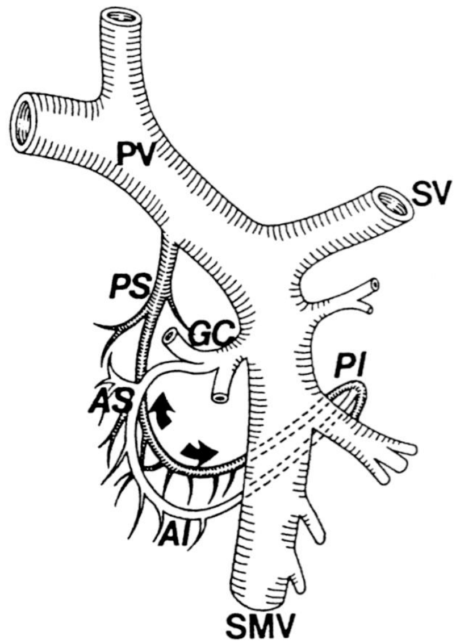

Fig. 3.18. Anatomy of the anterior superior pancreaticoduodenal vein (ASPDV) and posterior superior pancreatocoduodenal vein (PSPDV). *PV*, portal vein; *SV*, splenic vein; *PS*, PSPDV; *PI*, posterior inferior pancreaticoduodenal vein; *AS*, ASPDV; *AI*, anterior inferior pancreaticoduodenal vein; *GC*, gastrocolic trunk. *Arrows* indicate direction of venous drainage. [Reprinted with permission from MORI et al. (1991)]

3.2.8 Lymphatic System

The intralobular tissue of the pancreas is devoid of lymphatics, and lymph capillaries of the gland arise in the interlobular tissue. Lymph capillaries are collected by anastomosing networks to form large lymph ducts that reach the surface of the pancreas, usually along blood vessels. The main lymphatic flow of the pancreas reaches the anterior and posterior pancreaticoduodenal nodes (Fig. 3.20). Some lymphatics from the head skip this pathway to flow directly to the inferior head, juxta-aortic, or para-aortic nodes. These para-aortic nodes are located on the lateral and anterior aspects of the aorta, from the celiac axis to the origin of the inferior mesenteric

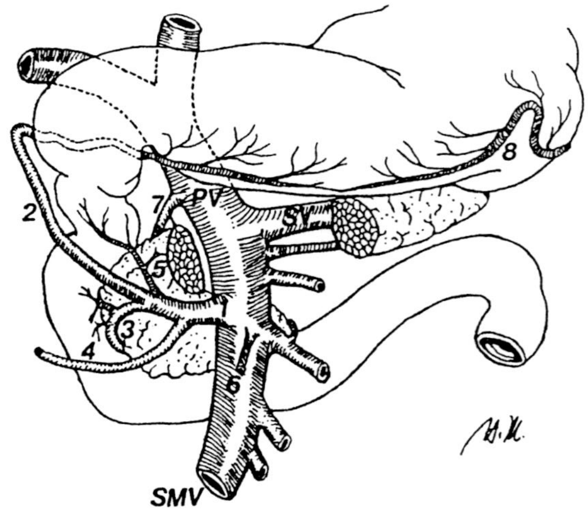

Fig. 3.19. Anatomy of gastrocolic trunk and its tributaries (frontal veiw). *PV*, portal vein; *SV*, splenic vein; *SMV*, superior mesenteric vein; *1*, gastrocolic trunk; *2*, right gastroepiploic vein; *3*, anterior superior pancreaticoduodenal vein; *4*, right colic vein; *5*, subpyloric vein; *6*, middle colic vein; *7*, posterior superior pancreaticoduodenal vein; *8*, left gastroepiploic vein. [Reprinted with permission from MORI et al. (1992)]

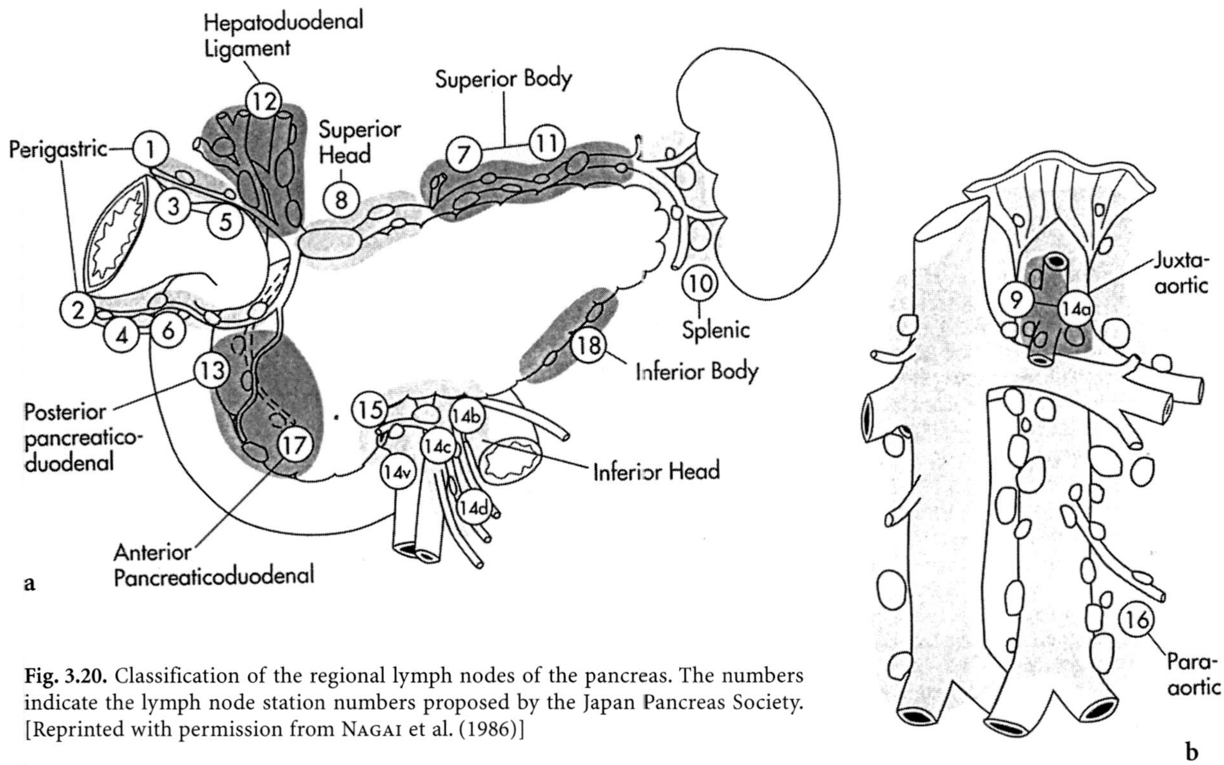

Fig. 3.20. Classification of the regional lymph nodes of the pancreas. The numbers indicate the lymph node station numbers proposed by the Japan Pancreas Society. [Reprinted with permission from NAGAI et al. (1986)]

artery. Some lymphatics flow directly into the cisterna chyli or thoracic duct.

Most lymphatics of the body and tail empty into the splenic and superior body nodes. They further drain to the juxta- and para-aortic nodes. Connections with the inferior head and inferior body nodes also exist.

The nodes of the splenic hilum and gastropancreatic fold receive the drainage of the pancreatic tail. The porta hepatis drains some of the pancreatic head and proximal body (WILLIAMS and WARWICK 1980).

Particular features of the lymphatic drainage of the pancreas are: (a) the presence of many connections between the different peripancreatic nodal systems, and (b) presence of several direct connections to para-aortic groups. These anatomical features could, together with the absence of a true pancreatic capsula, explain why tumor recurrence is so common after partial pancreatectomy for cancer.

3.2.9 Nerve Supply

The pancreas recieves sympathetic and parasympathic innervation. The sympathetic nerves carry the pain fibers. These pierce the diaphragm to enter the celiac plexus and celiac ganglion that are located close to the celiac trunk. The superior mesenteric ganglia and plexus surround the superior mesenteric artery. Interruption of afferent pain fibers ("celiac nerve block") can be obtained by injection of a chemical agent between the superior mesenteric and celiac arteries, either antecrurally or retrocrurally (HAAGA 1984). This technique may be of great clinical value in patients with severe pain resulting from pancreatic carcinoma or chronic pancreatitis.

3.3 Anatomical Variants and Developmental Anomalies

3.3.1 Variations in Position, Size, Shape, and Composition

3.3.1.1 Variations in Position

The entire pancreas may be displaced in patients who have undergone right or left nephrectomy. Alternatively, after right or left nephrectomy, the head or tail of the pancreas may fall back to occupy the space vacated by the kidney, while the remainder of the gland remains in an almost unchanged location. Interestingly, the pancreatic head almost invariably maintains a fixed relationship to the second portion of the duodenum and to the root of the superior mesenteric vessels.

While the splenic vein is located closely to the dorsal border of the pancreas in nearly all patients, the distal tip of the pancreatic tail may occasionally curve dorsal to the vein and lie adjacent to the left adrenal gland. The importance of this variant resides in the fact that, in these patients, the normal pancreatic tail may be confused with an adrenal mass on imaging studies.

3.3.1.2 Ectopic Pancreas

Ectopic pancreas (also called aberrant or accessory pancreas) is defined as pancreatic tissue located outside the normal confines of the pancreas, and lacking any anatomic or vascular connection with it. Presumably, heterotopic pancreas is a result of an error in embryological development, and it must be analogous to the multiple pancreatic nodules normally found in animals (MONTGOMERY 1965). Its reported incidence ranges from 0.6% to 13.7% (BARBOSA et al. 1946; LAI and TOMPKINS 1986; KONDI-PAPHITI et al. 1997). Most cases of ectopic pancreas have involved the stomach (26%–38%), duodenum (28%–36%), and jejunum (16%), with Meckel's diverticula and the ileum being the next most common sites (FREENY and STEVENSON 1994). Other locations have been described, including the gallbladder, bile duct and cystic duct, the liver, spleen, colon, omentum, mediastinum, and lung. Above the diaphragm it is sometimes observed in association with a duplication of the esophagus.

Ectopic pancreatic tissue is most commonly located within the submucosal layer, with an intact overlying mucosa. The nodules are usually single and vary from 0.5 to 2 cm in diameter. A rudimentary duct system often exists and opens into the gut lumen, thereby producing a central umbilication. Ectopic pancreas is usually clinically silent. However, like orthotopic pancreatic tissue, they may be affected by inflammatory and neoplastic disease (FÉKÉTÉ et al. 1996).

3.3.1.3 Agenesis and Hypoplasia

Complete agenesis of both the dorsal and ventral components of the pancreas is an extremely rare anomaly and is associated with stillbirth or early neonatal death. Partial agenesis of the pancreas may involve either the ventral or dorsal component (LECHNER and READ 1966). While both entities are rare, agenesis or hypoplasia of the dorsal pancreas is certainly much more common than agenesis of its ventral counterpart (WANG et al. 1990). Patients may suffer from diabetes and recurrent abdominal pain. Based on ERCP observations, it is reasonable to state that a spectrum exists ranging from complete agenesis to mild hypoplasia. Indeed, filling of the duct of Santorini could be obtained in some cases, indicating that only portions of the dorsal pancreas did not develop (GILINSKI et al. 1985).

Isolated hypoplasia of the uncinate process has also been described. In persons with normal intestinal rotation it is relatively rare (3%) (INOUE and NAKAMURA 1997). In patients with intestinal nonrotation, the uncinate process is commonly hypoplastic or even aplastic. This association can be explained by the fact that development of the pancreas is intimately related to rotation of the duodenojejunal loop in the embryo. Abnormal rotation of the intestine may interrupt the normal rotation of the pancreatic primordia, with malpositioning of the pancreatic buds. Malposition of the ventral bud may result in abnormal morphology of the uncinate process (ADDA et al. 1984).

3.3.1.4 Duplication Anomalies

While partial duplication of the pancreatic duct is relatively common, partial duplication of the parenchyma is rare, with only a few cases reported. KIKUCHI and collegues reported on a case of duplication of the pancreatic tail (KIKUCHI et al. 1983). In their case, the "aberrant" (duplicated) tail presented as a gastric submucosal tumor. Communication of the duct of the duplicated tail with duplications of the stomach or intestine has also been described (HALPERT et al. 1990; HOFFMAN et al. 1987). Finally, Agha described a case of a duplex ventral pancreas (AGHA 1987).

3.3.1.5 Variations in Migration: Annular Pancreas

In annular pancreas, pancreatic tissue partially or completely encircles the duodenum, usually in its second portion, while remaining continuous with the remainder of the gland. According to recent series, its incidence is 4/8000 (YOGI et al. 1987). The annular tissue may consist of a fibrous band or of glandular pancreatic tissue. The etiology of annular pancreas is not entirely clear, but is most likely related to failure of normal migration. The most widely accepted theory is that adherence of the tip of the ventral pancreatic anlage to the duodenum before rotation results in formation of the annulus (LECCO 1910) (Fig. 3.21). An alternative explanation is that failure of the left lobe of the ventral bud to involute results in the ring of pancreatic tissue around the descending duodenum (Fig. 3.21) (BALDWIN 1910). The duct within the annulus usually passes dorsally to the right and enters the duct of Wirsung. This type of anatomy has been identified in 69% of cases (ENGLAND et al. 1995). It may occasionally connect to the duct of Santorini or have its own orifice into the duodenum (ITOH et al. 1989; CLIFFORD 1980).

Interestingly, a coexisting pancreas divisum occurs in up to 36% of cases ["annular pancreas divisum" (LEHMAN and O'CONNOR 1985)]. This is not surprising since migration of the ventral pancreas and fusion of the ductal systems occurs at approximately the same time in intrauterine life. In case of annular pancreas divisum, the annular duct communicates with the ventral duct system.

Annular pancreas may remain asymptomatic, may present in the neonatal period with duodenal obstruction, or may present in adulthood with signs suggesting complicated duodenal stasis (e.g., ulcers, 26%–48% of patients), or complicated obstruction of the pancreatic duct (acute or chronic pancreatitis, 13%–50%) (LLOYD-JONES et al. 1972; ITOH et al. 1989).

3.3.1.6 Other Variations in Shape

There may be a normal focal enlargement of the gland in the body or tail just to the left of the midline. Marked tortuosity of the pancreatic duct and gland in the body or tail may be observed and may appear as a "pseudomass" on cross-sectional imaging studies.

Minor variations in the lateral contour of the head and neck of the pancreas have recently been described at CT (see Sect. 3.6.3). They probably represent a spectrum of fusion patterns of the dorsal and ventral analogues and have no other significance than that they may mimic a pancreatic mass.

The uncinate process may rarely extend over the left margin of the superior mesenteric artery or even encircle the mesenteric vessels (KURODA and NAGAI 1998).

3.3.1.7 Variations in Composition

The posterior and inferior portion of the pancreatic head may contain less fat than the remainder of the pancreatic head. This has been attributed to the increased content of densely packed, polypeptide-rich acinar lobules, and the greater content of interlobular fibrous tissue within this portion of the pancreatic head, which originates from the ventral pancreatic anlage (JACOBS et al. 1994). Similarly, uneven lipomatosis may be observed in other portions of the gland. According to Matsumoto and coworkers, it can be detected at CT in approximately 3% of patients (MATSUMOTO et al. 1995) (see Sect. 3.6.3).

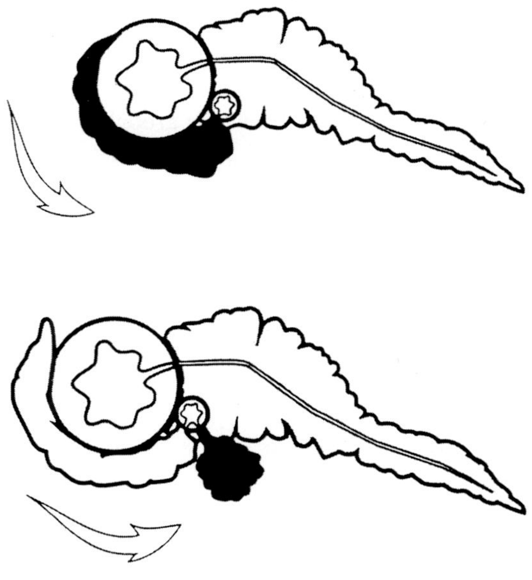
a

b

Fig. 3.21. Theories of the development of annular pancreas. **a** LECCO proposes that the tip of the right ventral bud (black) adheres to the duodenum before it undergoes rotation, while the left bud atrophies. **b** BALDWIN proposes that failure of the left bud (*white*) to involute results in the annulus. The right bud rotates in the usual fashion. [Reprinted with permission from ENGLAND et al. (1995)]

3.3.2
Variations in Ductal Anatomy

There is considerable variation in the anatomy of the pancreatic duct stystem (Rienhoff and Pickrell 1945; Dawson and Langman 1961). Some of these variations have a clear clinical significance. It should be noted that conditions where variations in ductal anatomy coexist with variations in parenchymal shape (annular pancreas, duplication) have been discussed above.

3.3.2.1
Variable Types of Communication Between the Dorsal and Ventral Ducts

In approximately 60% of the population, the dorsal and ventral ducts have fused, which results in communicating dual drainage of the main pancreatic duct ("bifid configuration") (Fig. 3.22a). Rarely (1% of patients), the duct of Santorini is larger than the duct of Wirsung ("dominant duct of Santorini"). In approximately 30%, the dorsal and ventral ducts have also fused, but the main pancreatic duct only drains through the duct of Wirsung (Fig. 3.22b). In these cases, the duct of Santorini is rudimentary. Finally, in 5%–10% of cases, the dorsal and ventral ducts have not fused. This anatomic variant is called pancreas divisum (see below). Dawson and Langman have described a caudally looping communication between the ducts of Santorini and Wirsung, which they called "ansa pancreatica" (Fig. 3.23) (Dawson and Langman 1961). It probably develops from an inferior branch of the ventral duct that communicates with the distal part of the accessory duct. Although this ansa pancreatica connects the main duct to the minor papilla, its entrance into the duodenum was patent in only one third of cases. Besides these major categories of fusion patterns, many other variants exist. These are illustrated in Fig. 3.24.

3.3.2.2
Absence of Communication Between the Dorsal and Ventral Ducts: Pancreas Divisum

Pancreas divisum originates from a failure of complete fusion of the dorsal and ventral pancreas: the common bile duct and ventral pancreatic duct drain into the duodenum through the major papilla, and the dorsal pancreatic duct drains through the minor papilla (see Fig. 3.22). It occurs in 5%–10% of patients undergoing ERCP (Taylor and Bohorfoush 1997).

The ventral ducts vary in size, ranging from barely visible to several centimeters long (Belber and Bill 1977). The ducts usually arborize and gradually decrease in diameter.

Chronic as well as acute pancreatitis have been reported to be associated with pancreas divisum (Warshaw et al. 1990).

A variant of pancreas divisum, called incomplete pancreas divisum, is much rarer than complete pancreas divisum. It is characterized by the presence of a small-caliber duct connecting the dorsal and ventral pancreatic ductal system (Farkas 1982).

3.3.2.3
Fusion Narrowing and Other Variations in Caliber

There may be focal narrowing of the main pancreatic duct at its junction with the accessory duct, the site where the ventral and dorsal ducts fuse (Belber and Bill 1977; Fink et al. 1986). Fusion narrowing is characterized mainly by the typical location, but also by the

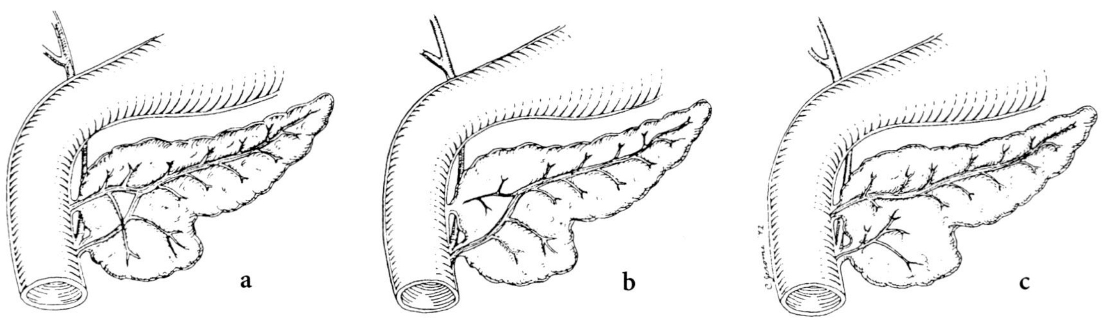

Fig. 3.22a–c. Main categories of pancreatic duct drainage. **a** Communicating dual-duct drainage. The dorsal and ventral ducts have fused, and there is dual drainage into the duodenum. **b** Single-duct drainage. The dorsal and ventral ducts have fused, but the accessory duct of Santorini is rudimentary and does not communicate with the duodenum at the minor papilla. **c** Pancreas divisum. The dorsal and ventral ducts have not fused. The entire dorsal pancreas drains at the minor papilla and the ventral pancreas at the major papilla. [Reprinted with permission from Schulte (1994)]

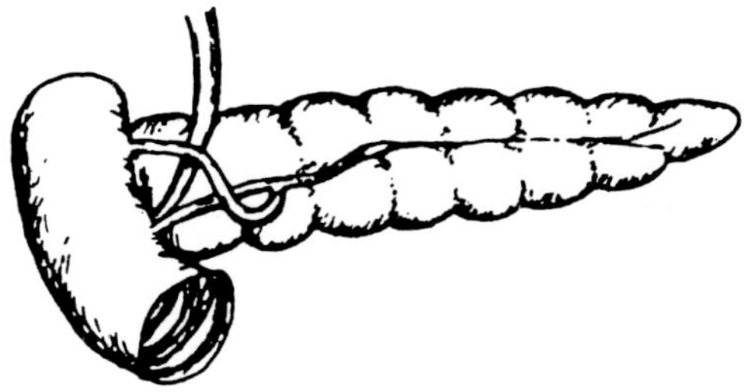

Fig. 3.23. Ansa pancreatica. [Reprinted with permission from GOODMAN et al. (1991)]

relatively short length and by the absence of obstructive dilation of the proximal ductal system (Fig. 3.25). It is thought to represent another variant related to fusion of the two embryological portions of the head.

Focal ductal narrowing may also occur at the pancreatic isthmus, i.e., in the part of the gland that lies anterior to the superior mesenteric artery (OGOSHI et al. 1973).

Slight fusiform dilatation of the duct of Wirsung is not uncommonly seen just proximal to the papillary orifice (Fig. 3.26).

3.3.2.4 Anomalous Junction of Common Bile Duct and Pancreatic Duct

In less than 0.2% of patients, the common bile duct and pancreatic ducts have separate orificia. This variant is clinically silent. An anomalous junction of the pancreatico-biliary ductal system, on the other hand, is clinically important because it may predispose to intrabiliary reflux of pancreatic juice and formation of a choledochal cyst (KOCHHAR et al. 1989). It is defined as a union of the common bile duct and pancreatic duct occurring outside the duodenum and beyond the influence of the sphincter. It is diagnosed if the length of the common channel of both ducts is more than 15 mm (Fig. 3.27). Other types of anomalous junction include insertion of the common bile duct into the pancreatic duct or an accessory duct, or a more complex union of the ducts (GOODMAN et al. 1991).

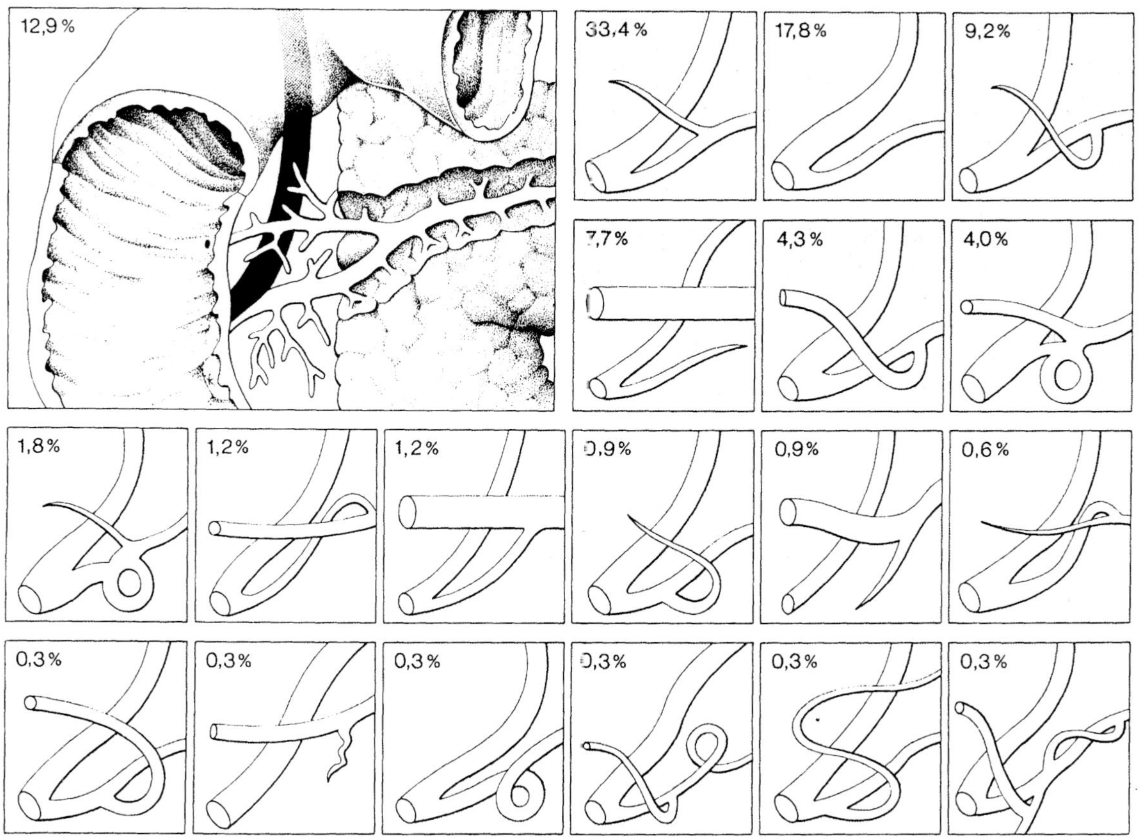

Fig. 3.24. Variations in pancreatic duct anatomy. [Reprinted with permission from DEMLING et al. (1979)]

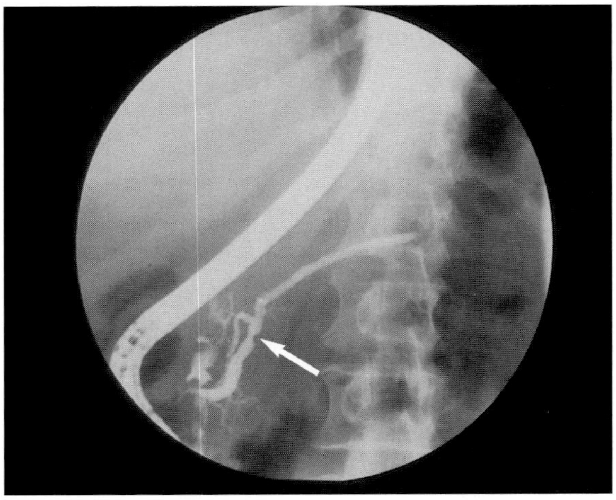

Fig. 3.25. Fusion narrowing. Retrograde cholangiopancreatography image shows narrowing at junction of the two embryologic parts of the pancreatic duct (*arrow*). No associated pancreatic abnormalities were found

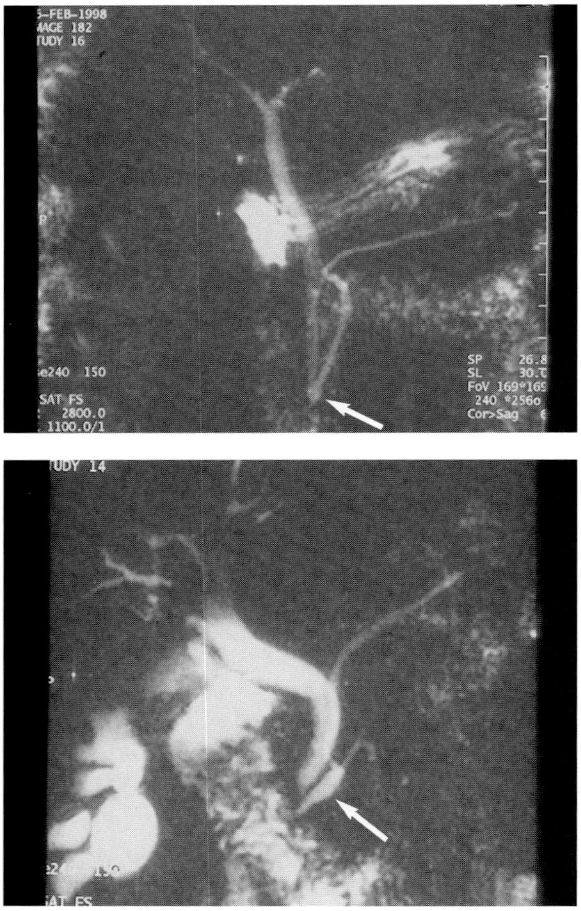

a

b

Fig. 3.26a,b. Fusiform dilatation of the duct of Wirsung in the pancreatic head. Magnetic resonance cholangiopancreatography images showing fusiform dilatation of the distal portion of the duct of Wirsung (*arrows*)

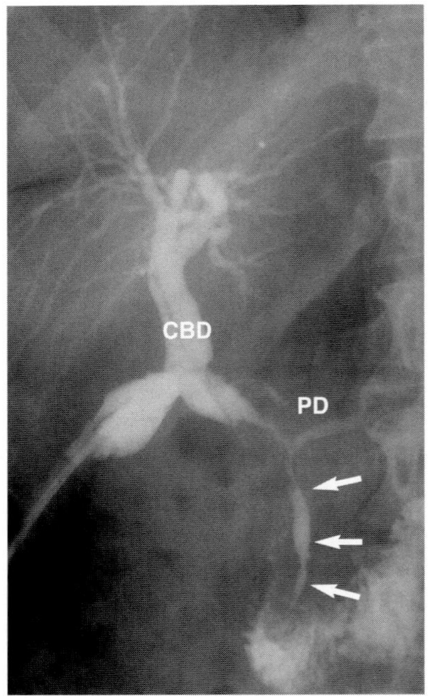

Fig. 3.27. Anomalous junction of common bile duct and pancreatic duct. Image obtained after injection of contrast material via Kehr-drain shows long common channel (*arrows*) of common bile duct (*CBD*) and pancreatic duct (*PD*)

3.3.2.5
Ducts Draining in Duodenal Diverticulum (Fig. 3.28)

The incidence of duodenal diverticula is 5%–10%. Occasionally, the papilla may be located on the rim of a diverticulum or even in the diverticulum (Shemesh et al. 1987). This variant may be the cause of a failed examination with ERCP. Furthermore, an increased incidence of pancreatitis has been suggested in these patients (Osnes et al. 1981).

3.3.2.6
Senescent Changes

Small cystic dilatations at the tips of the side branches of the main pancreatic duct have been described in elderly patients. They appear to be without any clinical significance (Kreel and Sandin 1973). The ductal diameter also appears to increase with increasing patient age. Kreel and Sandin noted an average increase of 8% per decade. An important feature of a "normal" aging pancreas is that the pancreatic duct should maintain its gradual increase in diameter towards the ampulla (Kreel and Sandin 1973).

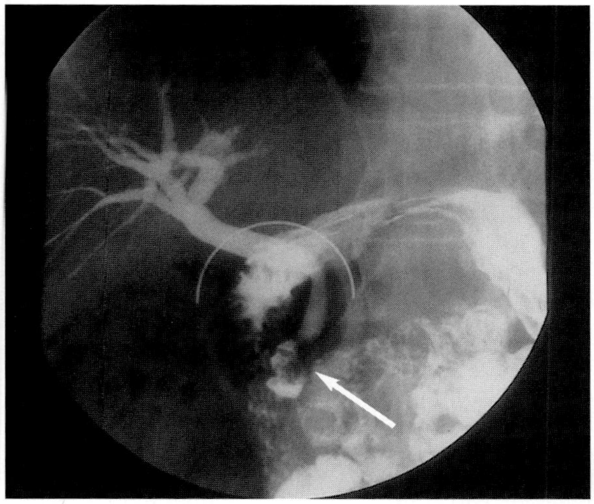

Fig. 3.28. Ducts draining in duodenal diverticulum. Image obtained during a barium follow-through shows retrograde filling of a duodenal diverticulum (*arrow*) and of the common bile duct with contrast medium, pointing to an incompetent sphincter mechanism

3.3.3
Variations in Vascular Anatomy

The multiple variations of the celiac and superior mesenteric arteries and their branches are nicely explained by several authors (Michels 1955; Nebasar et al. 1969; Freeny and Lawson 1982). A detailed description of these variants is beyond the scope of this text. The discussion will be limited to those variants that may be of importance in clinical radiological practice, either because they have surgical relevance (see Sect. 3.3.3.1) or because they may cause difficulties in the interpretation of imaging studies (see Sects. 3.3.3.2 and 3.3.3.3)

3.3.3.1
Celiac Trunk and Hepatic Artery

The "classic" anatomy of the celiac trunk is found in 55%–65% of patients only. In this configuration, the common hepatic artery, splenic artery, and left gastric artery arise separately from the celiac trunk. In anoter configuration, the left and right hepatic arteries have separate origins. In this case, the gastroduodenal artery is usually a branch of the left hepatic artery.

An aberrant common or right hepatic artery arising from the superior mesenteric artery ("replaced hepatic artery") occurs in 4.5% and 25% of subjects, respectively (Trede 1993). These variations are relevant for the surgeon considering duodenum-preserving pancreatic head resection. Both of these anomalous vessels usually run just behind the pancreatic head and uncinate process. Importantly, they may give off one or two large inferior pancreaticoduodenal arteries that anastomose with the anterior and posterior pancreatic arcades (see Figs. 3.14b, 3.29)

3.3.3.2
Pancreatic Arteries

The *gastroduodenal artery* may have a variety of origins. It typically arises from the common hepatic

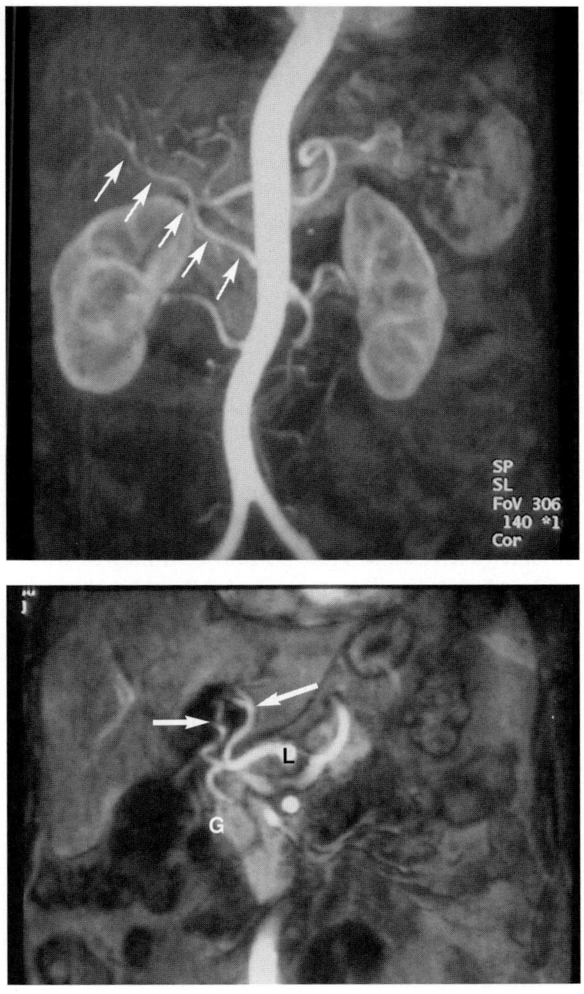

a

b

Fig. 3.29. Replaced right hepatic artery. **a** Maximum-intensity projection image obtained after postprocessing of magnetic resonance (MR) angiographic images obtained in the coronal plane shows right hepatic artery arising from the superior mesenteric artery (*arrows*). **b** Native MR angiographic image better showing the anatomy of the left hepatic branches. The main left hepatic artery (*L*) arises from the celiac trunk and divides into two branches (*arrows*). The gastroduodenal artery (*G*) is a third branch that courses in a caudal direction artery (75%), but may also arise from either the right (3.5%) or left (1%) hepatic arteries, or arise directly from the celiac artery, splenic artery, or superior mesenteric artery (2.5%). In the case of a replaced hepatic artery, it may arise from the left (11%), right (7%), middle (1%), or main (3.5%) hepatic artery.

The *dorsal pancreatic artery* may arise from the splenic (40%), celiac (22%), or superior mesenteric (14%) arteries (Nebasar et al. 1969). Rarely, it takes origin from a right hepatic artery replaced to the superior mesenteric artery (7%), from the gastroduodenal artery, or from the gastroepiploic (2%). It may also be represented by two separate vessels.

The *transverse pancreatic artery* usually arises from the dorsal pancreatic artery (90%). It may also take origin from the right gastroepiploic (3%), gastroduodenal (3%), or posterior superior pancreaticoduodenal arteries (1%).

3.3.3.3 Veins

The inferior mesenteric vein may occasionally be confused with other peripancreatic veins on imaging studies. In one third of the population, the inferior mesenteric vein enters at the splenomesenteric confluence, in another third it joins the splenic vein close to the junction, and in the remainder it drains into the superior mesenteric vein.

At the level of the neck, an inconstant vein may drain into the splenomesenteric confluence or into the left gastric vein. This isthmic vein may be anastomosed to veins of pancreatic body or head.

Another inconstant vein, the inferior pancreatic vein, may drain a major portion of the pancreatic body. This vein usually empties into the final portion of the inferior mesenteric vein (Kadir 1991; Crabo et al. 1993).

3.4 Gastrointestinal Contrast Studies

3.4.1 Technical Remarks

Gastrointestinal contrast studies that may provide useful indirect information about pancreatic disease are conventional barium radiography, tube-assisted duodenography, and double contrast duodenography.

The *conventional barium examination* is the simplest but also the least informative technique. Following ingestion of 150–200 ml of barium suspension, the patient is positioned in a prone left posterior oblique position in order to facilitate filling of the bulbus. Spot films are obtained in different positions.

Tube-assisted duodenography involves passage of a tube into the duodenum. Duodenal atony is obtained by IV injection of an antiperistaltic drug (e.g., glucagon 0.25–1 mg). With this technique, excellent distention of the duodenum can be obtained (Benedict et al. 1970).

Tubeless double contrast hypotonic duodendography is a modification of the conventional barium examination and has replaced tube-assisted duodenography for most indications (Laufer 1975). It relies on the administration of a high-density barium preparation, followed by an effervescent agent. Films showing the medial wall of the duodenum can be obtained in double contrast by turning the patient in a prone or prone-oblique position.

3.4.2 Normal Findings and Variants

The normal features of the papilla have been discussed in Sect. 3.2.5. The papillary complex is characterized by a triad of features: (1) the superior papillary fold, which may form a "hood" over the papilla, (2) the papilla itself, and (3) the distal longitudinal fold (Ferrucci et al. 1970). The normal papilla is usually well visualized with conventional double contrast studies (Fig. 3.30). An unusually large but

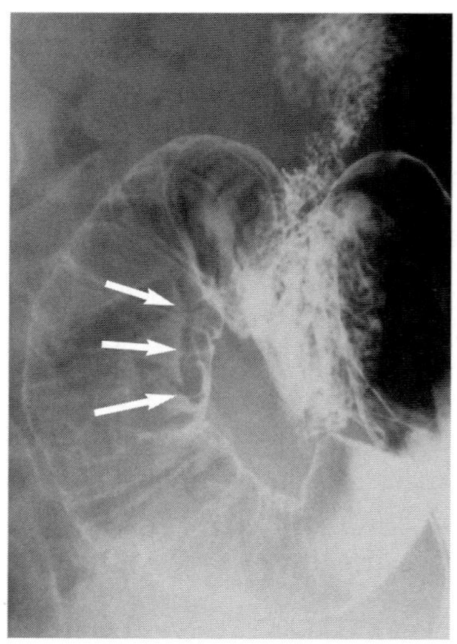

Fig. 3.30. Papilla of Vater: localization with gastrointestinal contrast studies. Image obtained with tubeless double contrast hypotonic duodendography shows distal longitudinal fold

normal papilla may be difficult to differentiate from a papilla enlarged by tumor or inflammation.

Ectopic pancreas appears as a broad-based and smooth lesion in the stomach or duodenum that sometimes resembles a gastric polyp. Often, a central niche is seen, correspondining to the orifice of the rudimentary ductal system. When filled with barium, this short ductal structure gives a very characteristic appearance (see Fig. 5.4).

Annular pancreas may be suggested if there is stenosis of the duodenum.

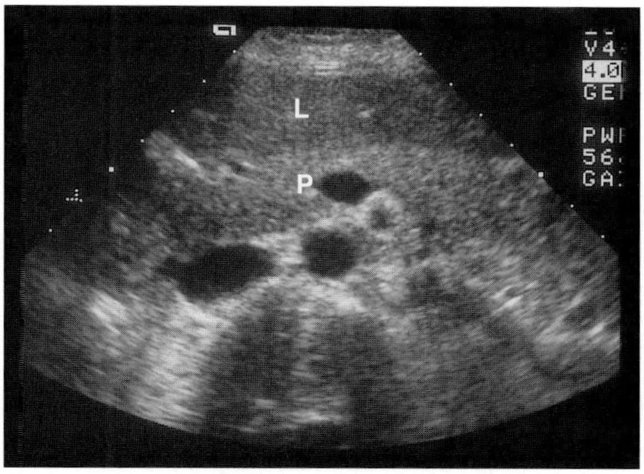

Fig. 3.31. Sonography of the pancreas: use of the liver as acoustic window. Ultrasonography image shows pancreas (*P*) that is well seen behind the left liver lobe (*L*)

3.5 Ultrasonography

3.5.1 Technical Remarks

3.5.1.1 Transabdominal Ultrasonography

This noninvasive, safe, and real-time examination should be performed in a fasting patient and started with the patient supine. Real-time US is preferentially performed with a sectorial or linear transducer. Frequencies of 3–5 MHz are suitable dependig upon the patent habitus. Because the acoustic window may be very small, it may be preferred to use a sectorial transducer with a small contact surface.

Anterior epigastric access in combination with a left and/or right intercostal access is necessary for optimal visualization of the whole pancreas. Transverse scans utilize the left liver lobe as an acoustic window (Fig. 3.31). Sagittal scanning begins in the midline and procedes to the right and left until the right kidney and spleen are seen.

The pancreatic tail is usually difficult to visualize over its complete length with a ventral approach. This may be true, in particular, in patients with excessive retroperitoneal fat and/or bowel distention. On the other hand, the tail is usually well seen in between the left kidney and the spleen on sagittal sonograms obtained with a dorsolateral approach (Fig. 3.32).

In general, superposition of air is the major drawback of the US examination. Positional changes may partially overcome this limitation. Increasing intra-abdominal pressure (Vasalva maneuver) can move the pancreas more ventrally to the abdominal wall and lead to a better sonographic visualization (Taylor et al. 1981). Another helpful approach is to examine the patient in an upright position (Op den Orth 1987). In addition, oral administration of 250–500 cc water may replace gas in the stomach and provide an improved acoustic window (Fig. 3.33). Intravenous administration of glucagon is also useful in this respect. Placing the patient in a right lateral decubitus position following water ingestion may well fill the second portion of the duodenum with fluid and provide excellent visualization of the contour of the head of the pancreas.

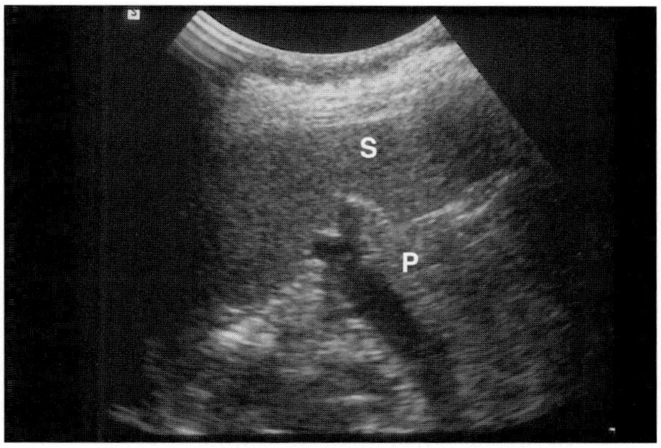

Fig. 3.32. Use of spleen as acoustic window. Ultrasonography image shows pancreatic tail (*P*) that is well seen using the spleen (*S*) as an acoustic window

US may also play a role in a more functional evalution of the pancreatic and biliary ductal systems. Warshaw et al. studied 100 patients with pancreas divisum or related disorders suffering from episodic acute pancreatitis or "pancreatic pain". They mon-

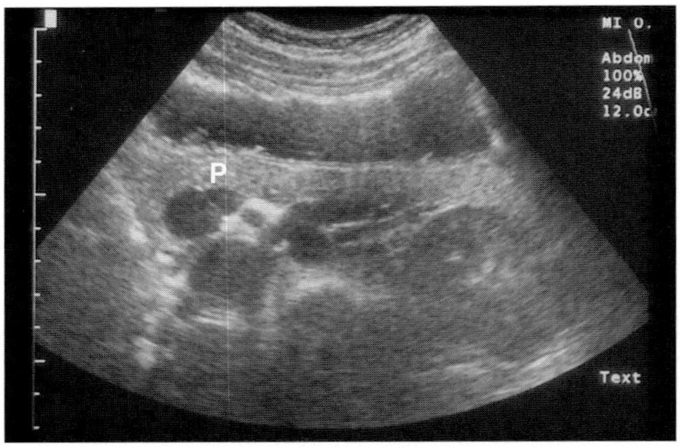

Fig. 3.33. Use of water as oral contrast medium. Ultrasonography image obtained after oral intake of water nicely shows the pancreatic neck (*P*). Note the presence of air in the gastric lumen with reverberations causing suboptimal visualization of part of the pancreatic body. This problem can usually be overcome by changing the position of the patient

itored the size of the pancreatic duct before and after administration of IV secretin. Prolonged (15–30 min) dilation of the pancreatic duct was nearly exclusively found in patients with stenosis of the accessory papilla (Warshaw et al. 1990). Similarly, oral administration of a fatty meal may be useful in the evaluation of the distal common bile duct and sphincter complex. After administration of a fatty meal, cholecystokinin is released, which leads to increased production of bile, and relaxation of the sphincter of Oddi. An enlarged duct that decreases in size after ingestion of a fatty meal is almost certainly not obstructed (Simeone et al. 1982).

Color Doppler US is nowadays an essential part of a transabdominal US examination of the pancreas. It facilitates the identification of vascular anatomical landmarks and, in case of doubt, allows the differentiation of vessels from other tubular structures.

3.5.1.2
Endoscopic, Laparoscopic, and Intraoperative Ultrasonography

Endoscopic US (EUS) has several advantages over transabdominal US (Rösch 1998). Besides eliminating the problems with bowel gas, a better spatial resolution can be obtained with the use of high frequency transducers (7.5–12 MHz) (Fig. 3.34). This technique is mainly used in the evaluation of patients with suspected (periampullary) malignancy (see Chap. 8) and for preoperative localization of endocrine tumors (see Chap. 10).

In laparoscopic and intraoperative US, the transducer can be applied directly to the surface of organs, and no tissues intervene to attenuate sound transmission (Pietrabissa et al. 1993). As in EUS, high-frequencey transducers can be used, providing images with high spatial resolution. In order to visualize lesions and structures located superficially within the organ, some stand-off is needed (Bandia and Makuuchi 1998). This can be obtained by applying gel or by submerging the pancreas in warm saline. A more detailed description of the technique of laparoscopic US is given in Chap. 8.

3.5.2
Normal Findings

3.5.2.1
Anatomical Landmarks

US is not as well suited as CT to demonstrate the exact topographic localization of the pancreas within the retroperitoneal space. The reason is that the different subcompartments of this space can usually not be distinguished. On the other hand, US exquisitely allows analysis of the major peripancreatic and retroperitoneal blood vessels. Identification of these vessels is of major help in the sonographic localization and subsequent analysis of the pancreas. Localization is not always straightforward; since the pancreas lacks a well-defined capsule, strong specular reflections do not return from the contours of the gland. Vascular structures that can be used to localize the pancreas with US are the aorta, the portal vein, the inferior vena cava, the splenic artery and vein, the superior mesenteric artery and vein, and the hepatic and gastroduodenal arteries.

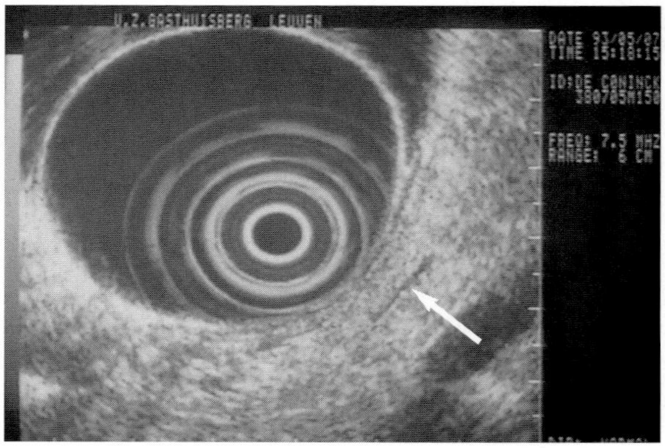

Fig. 3.34. Endoscopic Ultrasonography (EUS) image of the normal pancreas. EUS image shows echo pattern of normal pancreas. The pancreatic duct is also nicely displayed (*arrow*). (Courtesy of M. Hiele, MD, PhD)

After initial localization of the aorta and the inferior caval vein, the superior mesenteric artery is well visible as a vascular structure displaying an oblique craniocaudal and (slightly) posteroanterior course. The left renal vein can be identified as the vessel running in the axial plane within the aorto-mesenteric space. The splenic vein is visible more ventrally at the same anatomic level or somewhat more cranially. This vein is the most important anatomical landmark for sonographic identification of the pancreatic body. It is nearly invariably located at a dorsal groove within the pancreatic parenchyma. It joins the superior mesenteric vein slightly to the right of the midline to form the portal vein. This confluence is a landmark for the neck of the pancreas (Fig. 3.35). The pancreatic head is usually easily visualized because of its typical position at the right of the superior mesenteric vein. The uncinate process extends more caudally and medially, and is located dorsal to the vein (Fig. 3.36). Secondary landmarks for identification of the pancreatic head include the distal common bile duct and the gastroduodenal artery. On transverse sections, the common bile duct is seen as a rounded sonolucent structure. Its location usually corresponds to the dorsal boundary of the head. In case of doubt, the duct can be traced towards the liver hilum where it is located immediately ventral and lateral to the hepatic artery, and ventral and medial to the portal vein. The gastroduodenal artery has a similar appearance and is located on the ventral or ventrolateral surface. It is easily identified with use of color Doppler.

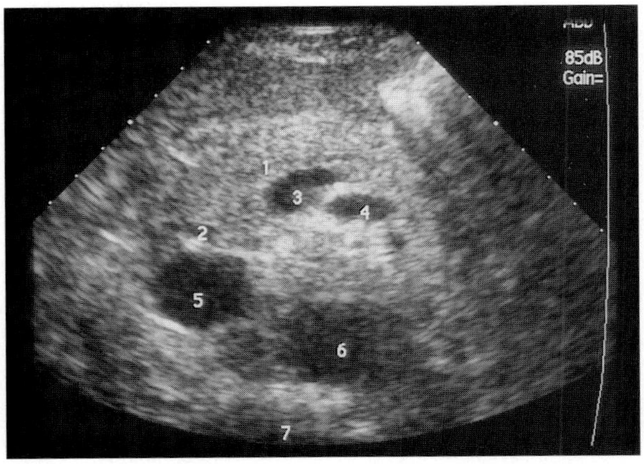

Fig. 3.35. Major sonographic landmarks. Ultrasonography image shows normal pancreas (*1*), distal common bile duct (*2*), confluence of splenic vein and superior mesenteric vein (*3*), superior mesenteric artery (*4*), inferior caval vein (*5*), and aorta (*6*). *7*, vertebra

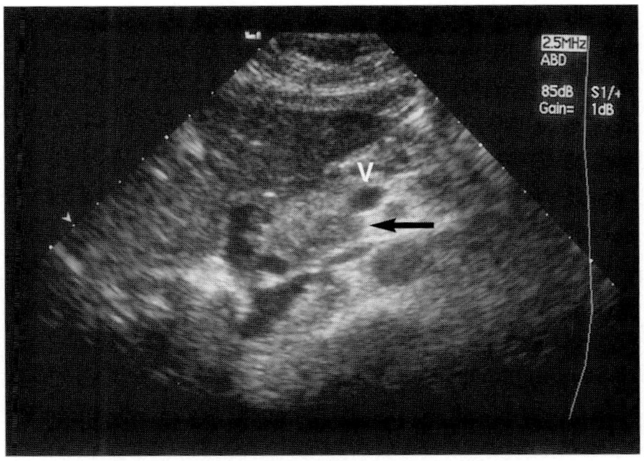

Fig. 3.36. Uncinate process. Ultrasonography image shows normal appearance of pancreatic head. Note the position of the uncinate process (*arrow*) dorsolaterally to the superior mesenteric vein (*V*). In this patient, the uncinate process had a hypoechoic appearance, which was caused by uneven lipomatosis

3.5.2.2
The Pancreatic Gland

The echo texture of the pancreas is homogeneous, consisting of thin and dense echoes. The discrete nodular contour, easily detected with computed tomography, especially at the ventral surface, is visualized only rarely at US.

The echogenicity of the pancreas varies with age (Fig. 3.37). In the infant it may be relatively hypoechoic, due to the predominance of glandular tissue and relative paucity of both fat and fibrous elements. In a study by Siegel et al., the pancreas was found to be less echogenic than the liver in 10% of 300 healthy children, aged between newborn and 18 years (Siegel et al. 1987). In adults, the pancreas is iso- or (usually) hyperechoic when compared to the liver (Weill 1987). In order to assess whether the echogenicity of the liver can be used as a normal internal standard, one may: (a) evaluate the definition of the collagen and fat in the portal triads, or (b) compare the echo pattern of the liver with that of the adjacent kidney.

The pancreas is normally slightly hypoechogenic with respect to the surrounding retroperitoneal fat. An increased echogenicity of the pancreas may be seen in obese or elderly patients and corresponds to lipomatous infiltration of the gland. Increased reflectivity usually does not have pathologic significance and, as an isolated finding, should not be mentioned in radiological reports. In patients with lipomatosis, the pancreatic parenchyma may be isoechoic to

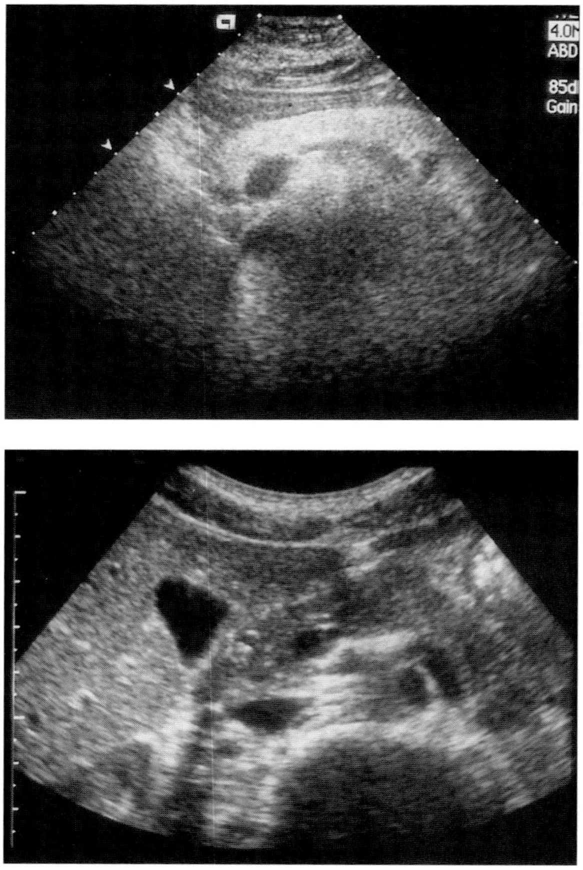

a

b

Fig. 3.37a,b. Echotexture of normal pancreas. Ultrasonography images obtained in a 67-year-old man (a) and a 16-year-old-girl (b), both free of pancreatic disease, illustrating the variability in normal echotexture: when compared to the liver, the pancreas is hyperechoic in (a), while it is hypoechoic in (b)

retroperitoneal fat, and it may be impossible to define the contours of the pancreas.

While various authors have cited the normal dimensions for individual segments of the pancreas at US, it is now accepted that diameter measurements per se do not have much diagnostic value. A maximal transverse diameter of 3.5 cm of the head and tail is normal with the body somewhat smaller (Johnson and Mack 1978). It should be remembered that the pancreas is proportionally larger in young people; it decreases in relative size with age (Niederau et al. 1983).

3.5.2.3 The Ductal System

The pancreatic duct is frequently seen in pancreatic body and neck, mostly over short distances. The visualization of the duct depends on its orientation with respect to the sound beam; the walls act as sound reflectors primarily if the duct is oriented perpendicular to the beam. This explains why it is more difficult to visualize the duct in the pancreatic head with use of a standard ventral approach (Bryan 1982; Hadidi 1983). Depending on the equipment used and on patient-related factors, the duct may be seen as two small parallel hyperechoic lines, corresponding to both walls of the duct (Fig. 3.38), or, less commonly, as one small hyperechoic line (Bryan 1982) . The internal diameter of the normal pancreatic duct in the body usually measures less than 2–2.5 mm (Lawson et al. 1982).

3.5.3 Variants and Pitfalls

The posterior wall of the stomach may assume a similar appearance as a dilated pancreatic duct. This pitfall is easily avoided in real-time US. The splenic vein may also be mistaken for a dilated pancreatic duct. In case of doubt, color Doppler allows for an easy differentiation. A circular or ovoid lucency similar to the gastroduodenal artery may occasionally be seen in the distal body or tail of the pancreas. This presents a turn of the normally tortuous splenic artery which may mimic a cyst within the pancreas.

The PSPDV may be seen in close proximity to the common bile duct. Wachsberg has demonstrated that this vein enters the posterior (82%) or anterior (18%) aspect of the portal vein. In the case of an anterior insertion, this vein may mimic the common bile duct on sagittal sonograms (Wachsberg 1993).

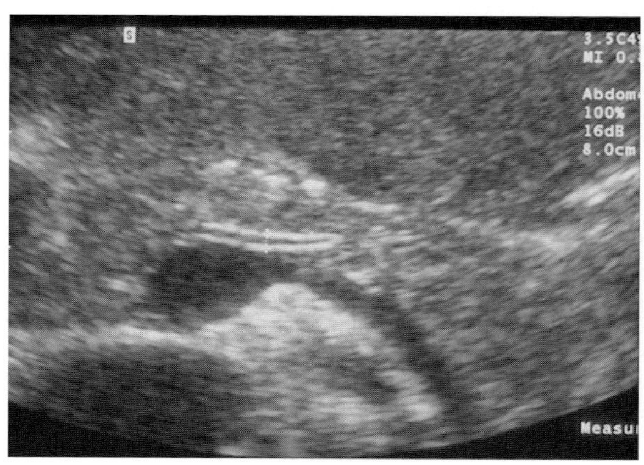

Fig. 3.38. Pancreatic duct: normal Ultrasonography (US) appearance. US images showing the normal pancreatic duct as a double line

Uneven lipomatosis is an important potential pitfall in pancreatic US, because it may appear as a hypoechoic area in the head and may simulate a pancreatic mass (Marchal et al. 1989; Donald et al. 1990). The hypoechoic area is usually located posteriorly (posterolateral, posteromedial) in the head and typically shows a straight and clear demarcation (Fig. 3.39).

Other congenital variants are more difficult to diagnose by real-time US and Doppler techniques. Annular pancreas may occasionally present with a pseudotumoral sonographic aspect. Enlargement of the pancreatic head may also be observed in patients with pancreas divisum.

3.6 Computed Tomography

3.6.1 Technical Remarks

CT is well suited for visualization of the pancreas. Meticulous technique should be followed in order to obtain optimal results in clinical practice. Thin-section helical CT is mandatory for adequate visualization of small anatomical and pathological structures. With this technique, the entire gland can be imaged during the optimal phase of contrast uptake and overlapping slices can be calculated a posteriori. A more detailed description of the optimal CT technique is given in Chap. 8. A few technical points concerning the CT visualization of normal anatomical structures deserve to be stressed here. Firstly, the use of a collimation of 3 mm or less is required for visualization of small peripancreatic veins (Ibikuro et al. 1996). Secondly, cine-display viewing of overlapping sections at the computer console affords a much better appreciation of the vascular and ductal anatomy than film-based viewing (Bonaldi et al. 1998). Finally, CT can be used to calculate arteriograms or venograms quite similar to those obtained with catheter angiography. The method relies on thin-section scanning, fast injection of contrast medium (4 ml/s), optimization of the scan delay, and calculation of three-dimensional images (either surface shaded displays, maximum intensity projections, or volume renderings) (Graf et al. 1997). Selective display of venous anatomy requires image editing ("removal" of bone and major arteries).

3.6.2 Normal Findings

3.6.2.1 Anatomical Landmarks

CT is the best imaging modality to depict the exact location of the pancreas within the retroperitoneal space. The different compartments of this space and the intervening fascias are usually well seen, except in very thin patients. The fascias are seen as thin, delicate stripes that have soft tissue density (Fig. 3.40).

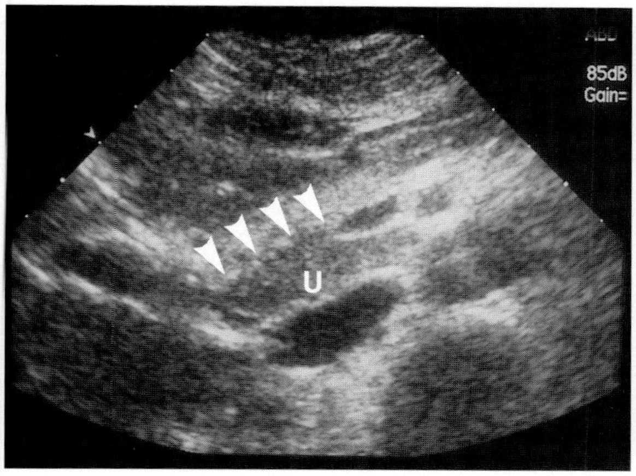

Fig. 3.39. Uneven lipomatosis. Ultrasonography image shows uncinate process (*U*) as a hypoechoic area. Note sharp demarcation line between ventral and dorsal portions of pancreatic head (*arrowheads*)

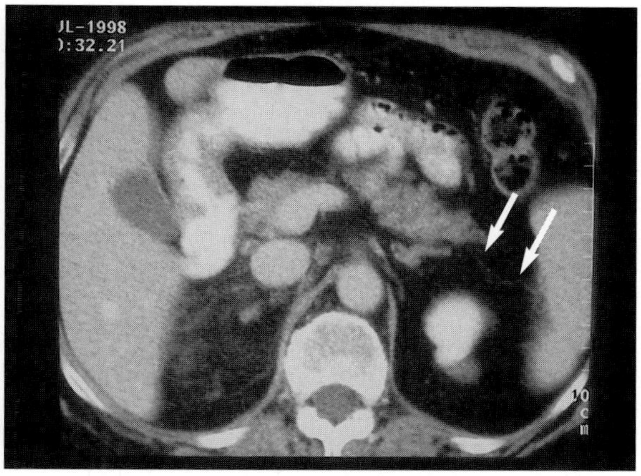

Fig. 3.40. Peripancreatic retroperitoneal compartments: computed tomography (CT) appearance. CT image shows left renal fascia (*arrows*) separating the anterior pararenal and perirenal spaces. The *asterisk* indicates the retropancreatic fat plane. Note increased density of fat in perirenal space on the right (patient with pyelonephritis)

A thin retropancreatic fat plane is identified in almost all patients. Absence of retropancreatic fat may be a sign of inflammatory or neoplastic disease. Identification of the fat plane around the superior mesenteric artery is also important. Obliteration of this fat plane is usually seen in pancreatic carcinomas with direct extrapancreatic extension, but has also been observed in inflammatory disease.

For a more detailed anatomical description, the reader is referred to Sects. 3.2.2 and 3.2.4. The CT appearance of the (peri-) pancreatic vessels is discussed in Sect. 3.6.2.4.

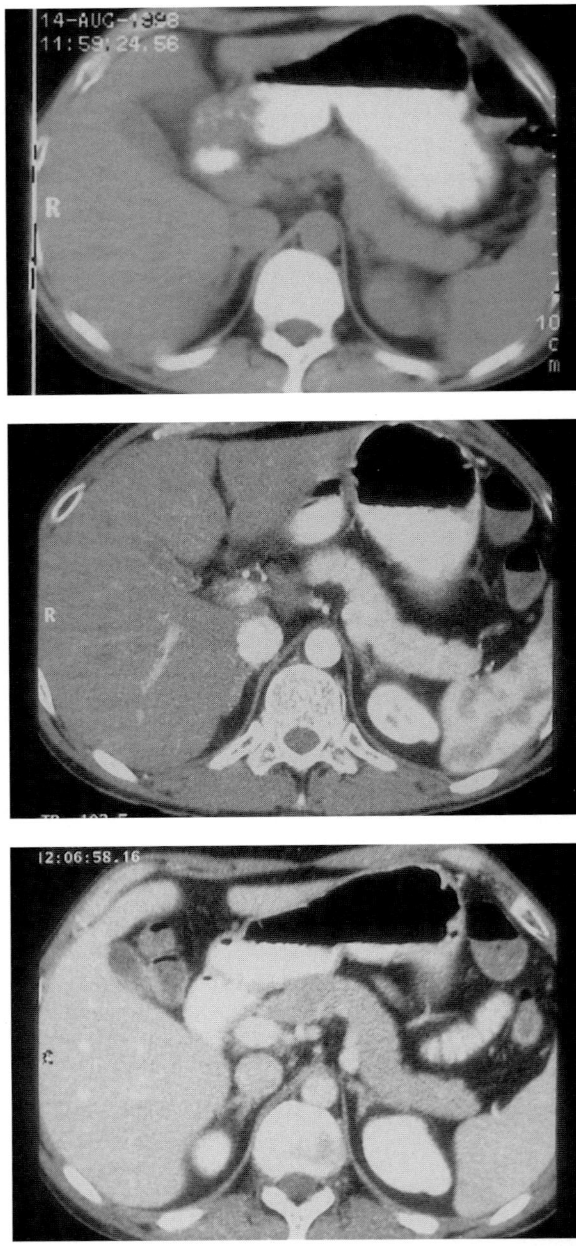

a b c

Fig. 3.41a–c. Normal pancreas: pattern of contrast uptake. **a** Non-contrast-enhanced image shows pancreas to be isodense to the liver. **b** Contrast-enhanced image obtained in pancreatic phase shows marked enhancement of the pancreatic parenchyma. **c** Contrast-enhanced image obtained in hepatic phase shows the pancreas to be less well enhanced when compared to (**b**)

3.6.2.2
The Pancreatic Gland

The pancreatic gland may have a smooth CT appearance with a homogeneous density. Alternatively, it may appear lobulated and inhomogeneous. The aspect is determined by the amount of fat present in the intralobular septa which separate the acinar lobules of the gland. Nodularity of the gland is usually most evident along the ventral surface. On unenhanced CT images, the pancreatic parenchyma usually shows a density of 40–50 Hounsfield units (HU). The variability among individuals mainly reflects the degree of lipomatous infiltration of the pancreas. The normal pancreas enhances rapidly after IV injection of iodinated contrast media. The time to peak enhancement depends on factors such as injection rate and cardiac function. From a practical point of view, it is important to note that peak pancreatic enhancement occurs earlier than peak hepatic enhancement. An optimized CT protocol scans the upper abdomen both in the pancreatic and hepatic phases of perfusion ("dual-phase scanning", see Chap. 8) (Fig. 3.41)

3.6.2.3
The Ductal System

The normal pancreatic duct is commonly seen on CT scans, even with use of conventional (non-helical) technology (Berland et al. 1981). Bonaldi et al. used 5-mm collimation helical CT and reported visualization of the normal pancreatic duct in the tail, body, and head in 48%, 73%, and 65%, respectively (Bonaldi et al. 1998). It is likely that these results may be improved with the use of thinner sections. The normal duct is identified as a thin, linear area of low density (Fig. 3.42). It may be seen in the center of the gland or may apparently be located close to the ventral or dorsal border. In the region of the body it may have a straight appearance or may show a ventral convexity as it arches over the spine and great vessels. In the neck and head, the more distal portions of the duct can be traced on more caudal sections, thereby progressively assuming a more lateral position with respect to the midline. In the pancre-

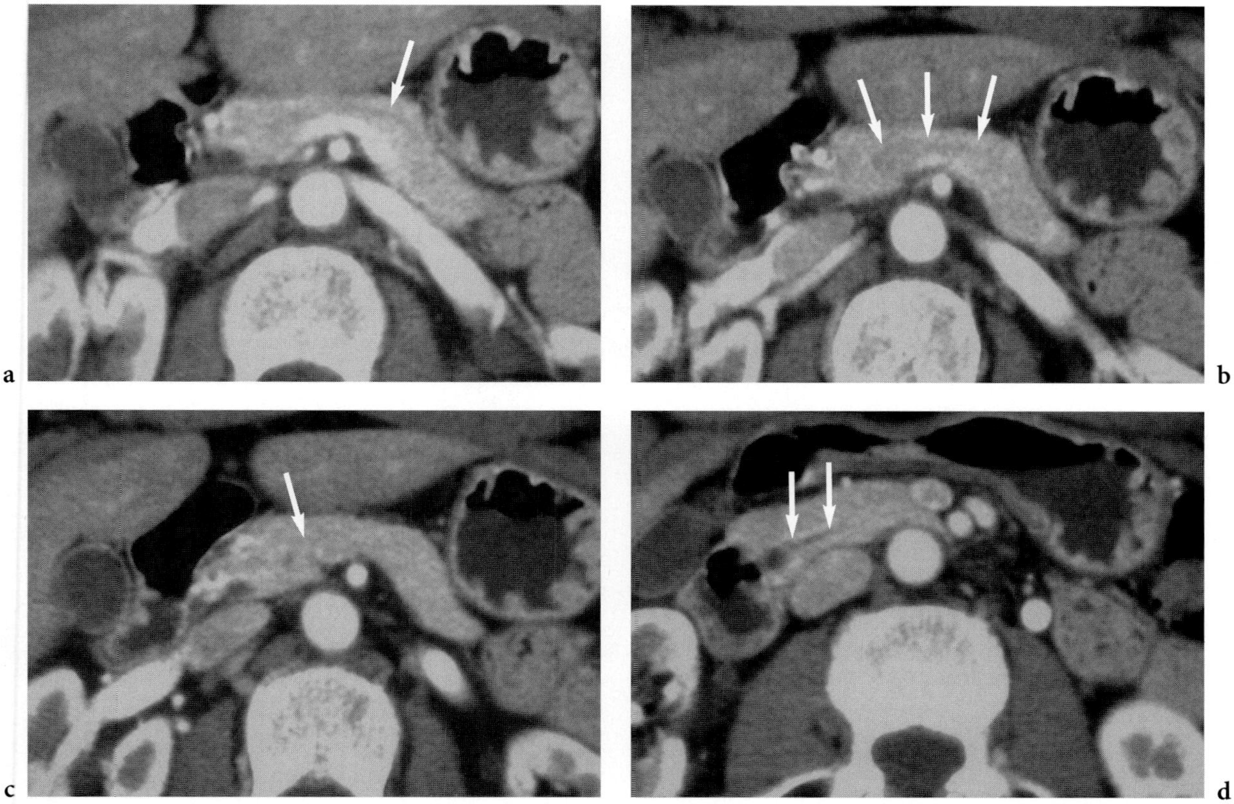

Fig. 3.42a–d. Computed tomography appearance of pancreatic duct. **a–d** Images obtained at four different anatomical levels, from cranial to caudal, show the typical course of the normal pancreatic duct (*arrows*)

atic head, the common bile duct and pancreatic duct are commonly seen as two adjacent hypodense structures. On CT, the normal pancreatic duct usually measures 2–4 mm or less.

3.6.2.4
Blood Vessels

The larger peripancreatic vessels (splenic artery, superior mesenteric artery and vein, splenic vein, venous confluence, gastroduodenal artery) are nearly invariably seen at thin-section (helical) CT images. The identification of small peripancreatic vessels with CT has recently been described (Figs. 3.43–3.46) (Chong et al. 1998).

At the level of the *cranial portion of the head*, the gastroduodenal artery is located in the retropyloric space at the anterolateral surface and can be seen in almost every patient (Figs. 3.43, 3.45). The PSPDA and PSPDV can be identified along the posterolateral surface accompanying the bile duct in 72%–88% of CT scans (*Mori* et al. 1991, 1992; *Crabo* et al. 1993; *Ibukuro* et al. 1996). The PSPDV is identified as a vertically oriented vessel within the sulcus of the common bile duct (and posterior to the duct itself), coursing cranially to drain into the posterolateral aspect of the undersurface of the portal vein, just cephalad to the venous confluence (Fig. 3.47) (Mori et al. 1991, 1992; Crabo et al. 1993; Vedantham et al. 1998). The following criteria aid in distinguishing the PSPDV from the accompanying artery: (a) the different course (the PSPDA originates from the gastroduodenal artery), and (b) the larger diameter of the vein (mean 3.5 mm, range 2–5.2 mm) (Mori et al. 1991).

Behind the pancreatic neck, the superior mesenteric vein is routinely seen. On occasion, a branch of the dorsal pancreatic artery to the head of the pancreas may be seen (Figs. 3.43, 3.44). The inferior mesenteric vein can be seen draining into the left side of the superior mesenteric vein in this location in 50%–70% of cases (Ibukuro et al. 1996).

At the *midlevel of the head*, the ASPDV runs horizontally across the anterior surface of the pancreatic head, coursing leftward to drain into the gastrocolic trunk. The gastrocolic trunk has a normal size

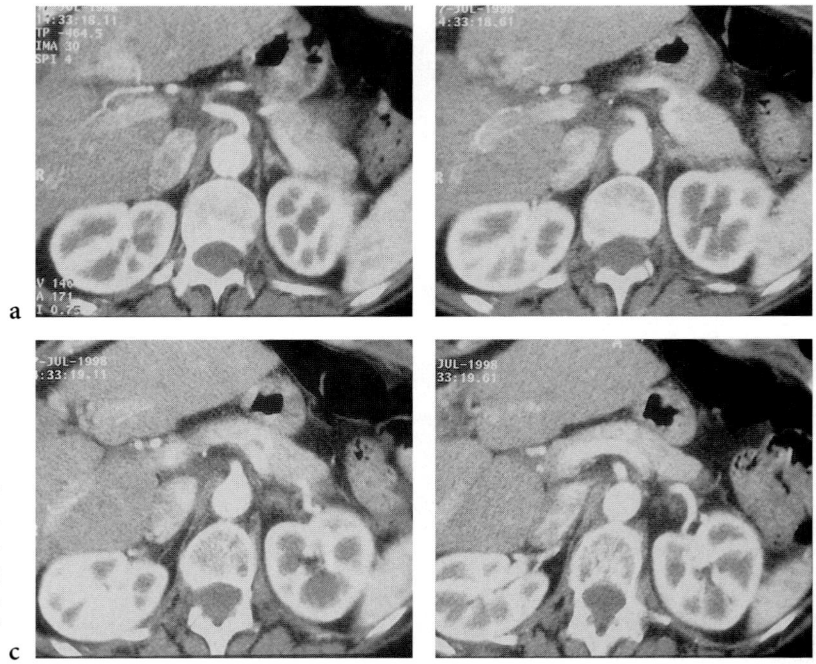

Fig. 3.43a–d. Computed tomography (CT) appearance of pancreatic arteries. **a–d** CT images obtained at 5-mm intervals, from cranial to caudal, showing the gastroduodenal artery (*arrow*) in (**d**) and the dorsal pancreatic artery (*arrowheads*) in (**b**) and (**c**)

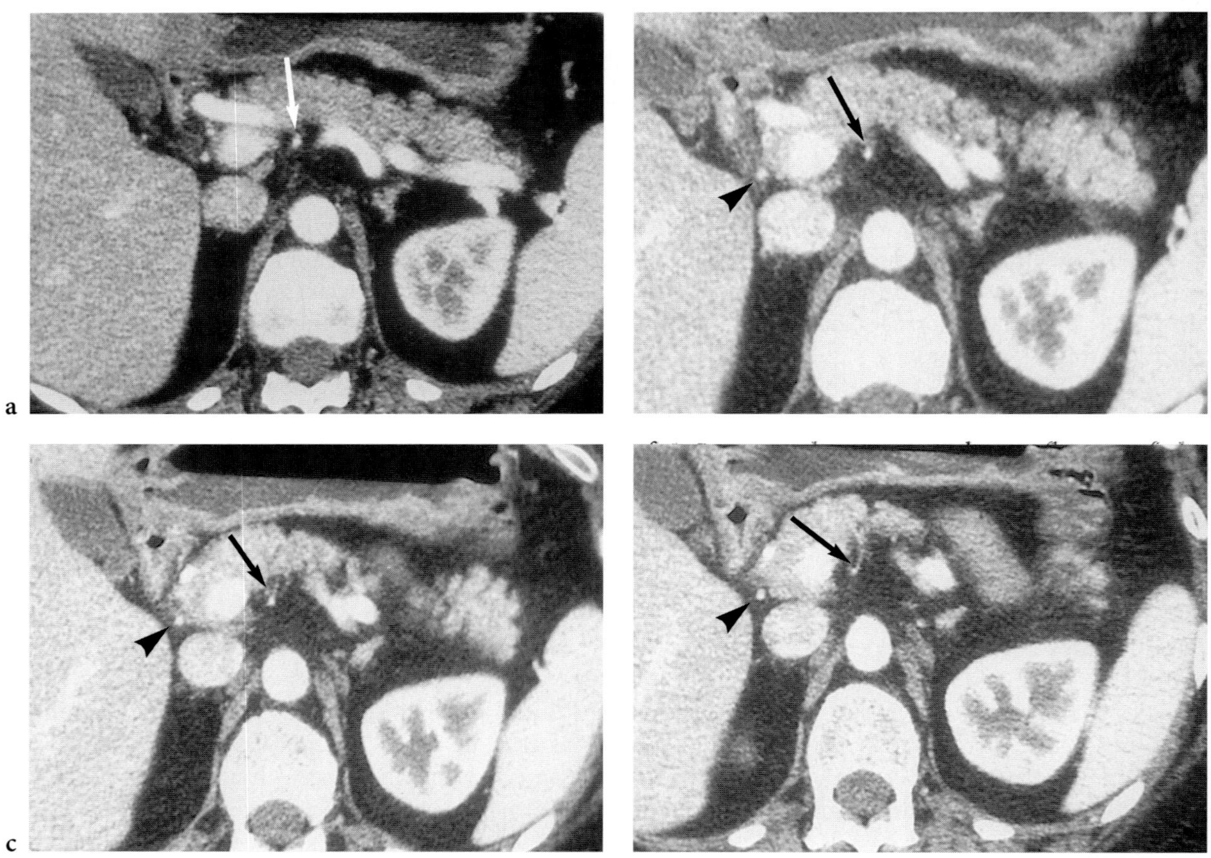

Fig. 3.44a–d. Computed tomography (CT) appearance of pancreatic arteries (different patient). CT images showing the dorsal pancreatic artery directly arising from the celiac trunk (*arrows* in **a–c**), coursing in the retropancreatic fat, and dividing in a small right branch and a larger left branch representing the transverse pancreatic artery (*arrow* in **d**). Also note visualization of the posterior superior pancreaticoduodenal vein (*arrowheads*)

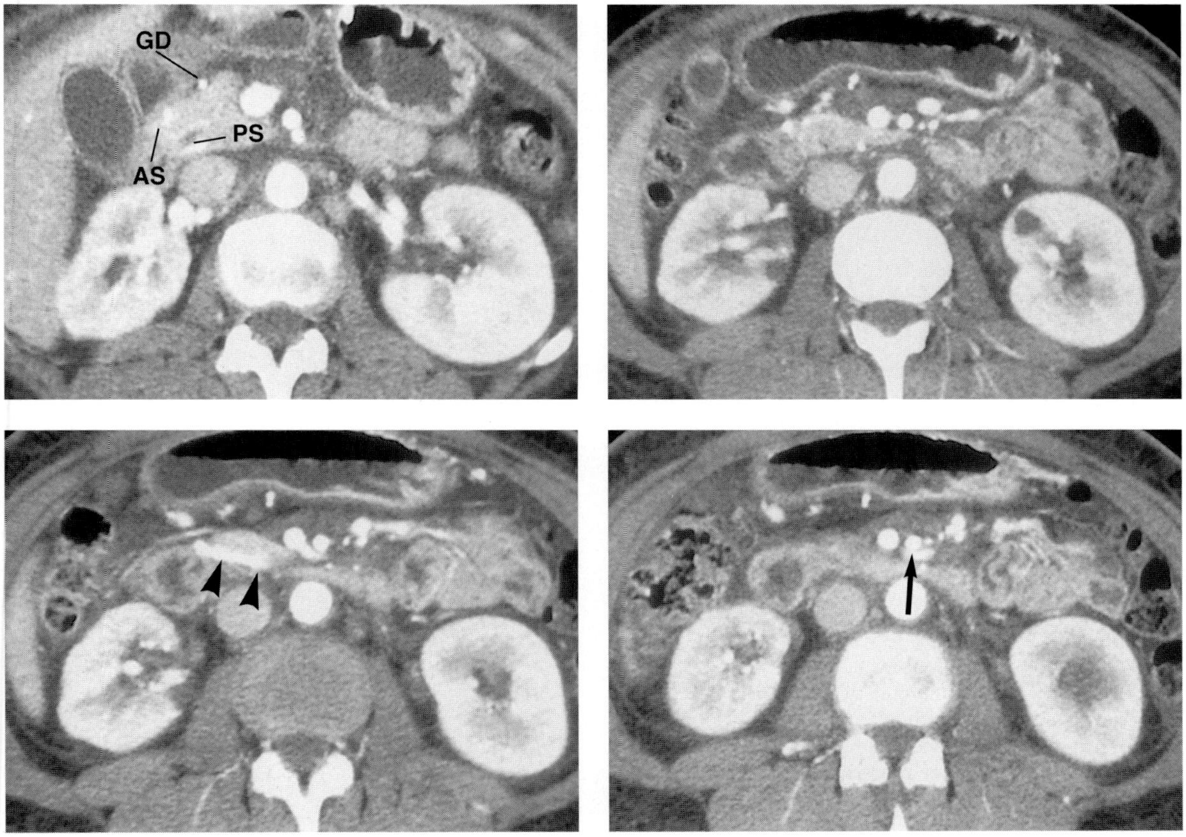

Fig. 3.45a–d. Computed tomography (CT) appearance of pancreatic arteries. **a** CT image obtained at level of mid portion of pancreatic head shows gastroduodenal artery (*GD*), anterior superior pancreaticoduodenal artery (*AS*), and posterior superior pancreaticoduodenal artery (*PS*) **b–d** CT images obtained at level of caudal portion of pancreatic head showing the anastomosis between inferior portion of the ventral pancreatic arcade (*arrow*) and a branch of the inferior pancreaticoduodenal artery (*arrowheads*). Also note first jejunal vein draining into the superior mesenteric vein in (**c**) and (**d**) (*arrow* in **d**)

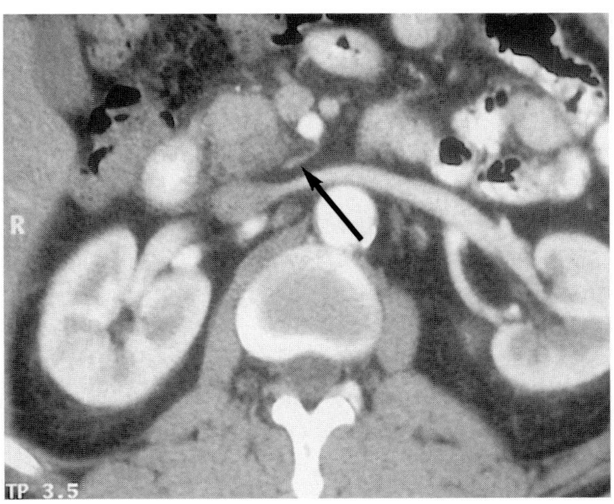

Fig. 3.46. Computed tomography (CT) appearance of inferior pancreaticoduodenal artery. CT image obtained at level of caudal portion of pancreatic head showing the inferior pancreaticoduodenal artery (*arrow*) arising from the posterior wall of the superior mesenteric artery

duct at the posterior surface of the head (see Fig. 3.47). At this same level, the branches of the inferior pancreaticoduodenal vein may be identified on the posterior surface of the head as it forms a network with the PSPDV. The anterior and posterior inferior pancreaticoduodenal veins are less than 5 mm in diameter.

At the level of the *caudal portion of the head*, the inferior pancreaticoduodenal vein can be identified medial to the head as it connects with the first jejunal vein before entering the posterior wall of the superior mesenteric vein. This type of anatomy is seen in 66%–90%; the first jejunal vein can be seen in 96%.

Other peripancreatic veins that may be seen at thin-section helical CT are the middle colic vein (72%), right superior colic vein (64%), inferior mesenteric vein (88%), left gastric vein (80%), and right gastroepiploic vein (100%) (Ibukuro et al. 1996). The left and right gastroepiploic veins form an

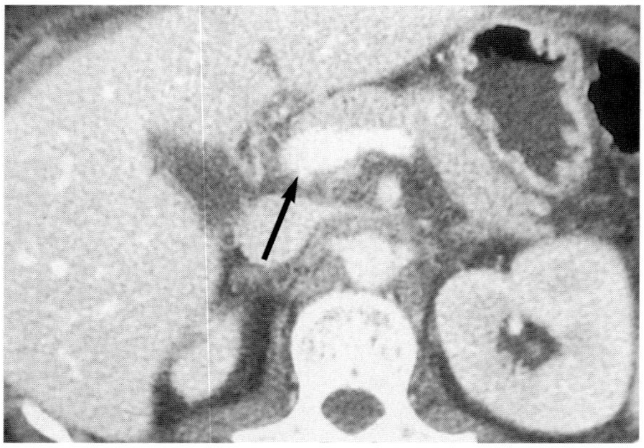
a

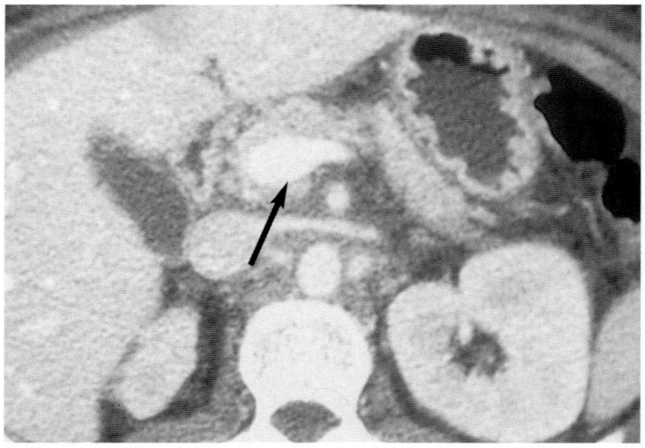
b

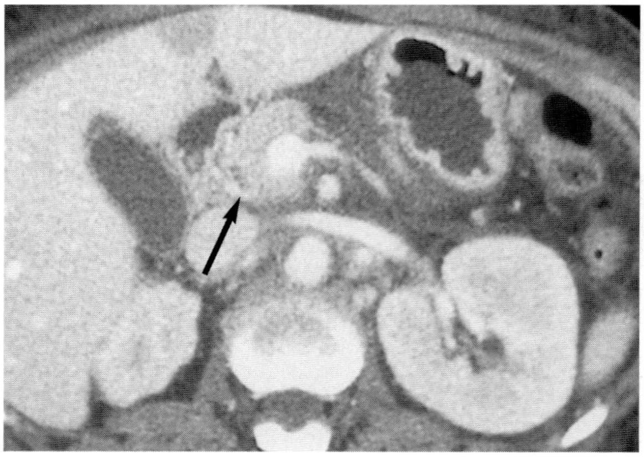
c

Fig. 3.47a–c. Computed tomography (CT) appearance of posterior superior pancreaticoduodenal vein. *a–c* CT images at level of pancreatic neck and head (from cranial to caudal) showing typical location of posterior superior pancreaticoduodenal vein at the posterolateral surface of the pancreatic head (*arrows*)

important collateral pathway to the portal vein in case of superior mesenteric vein or splenic vein obstruction.

The branching pattern of the inferior pancreaticoduodenal artery and the jejunal artery is very similar to that of the veins. This vessel usually arises from the posterior wall of the superior mesenteric artery (Fig. 3.46).

3.6.3 Variants and Pitfalls

3.6.3.1 Pitfalls Related to Changes in Position

Congenital or surgical absence of the left kidney alters the retroperitoneal compartments, and the pancreatic tail may be displaced into the empty renal fossa, simulating recurrent tumor or a primary retroperitoneal lesion. Positional variants may also be limited to a portion of the gland. A classical example is a retro-venous (posterior to the splenic vein) location of the pancreatic tail (Fig. 3.49).

3.6.3.2 Pitfalls Related to an Unusual Distribution or Amount of Fat

Several potential pitfalls are relatad to an unusual distribution or amount of fat.

Extension of infrapancreatic fat within the pancreatic gland is occasionally observed and could be mistaken for a lipomatous pancreatic tumor (see Chap. 8, Fig. 8.48).

Extreme lipomatosis is occasionally observed in diabetics, very obese patients, and elderly patients. On rare occasions, the pancreas may have a negative density on unenhanced scans similar to the density of the retroperitoneal fat. The only feature that allows differentiation with agenesis is the visualization of the ductal system and (sometimes) thin septa (Fig. 3.50).

As in sonography, *uneven fatty replacement* of the pancreas may mimic the appearance of a mass at CT.

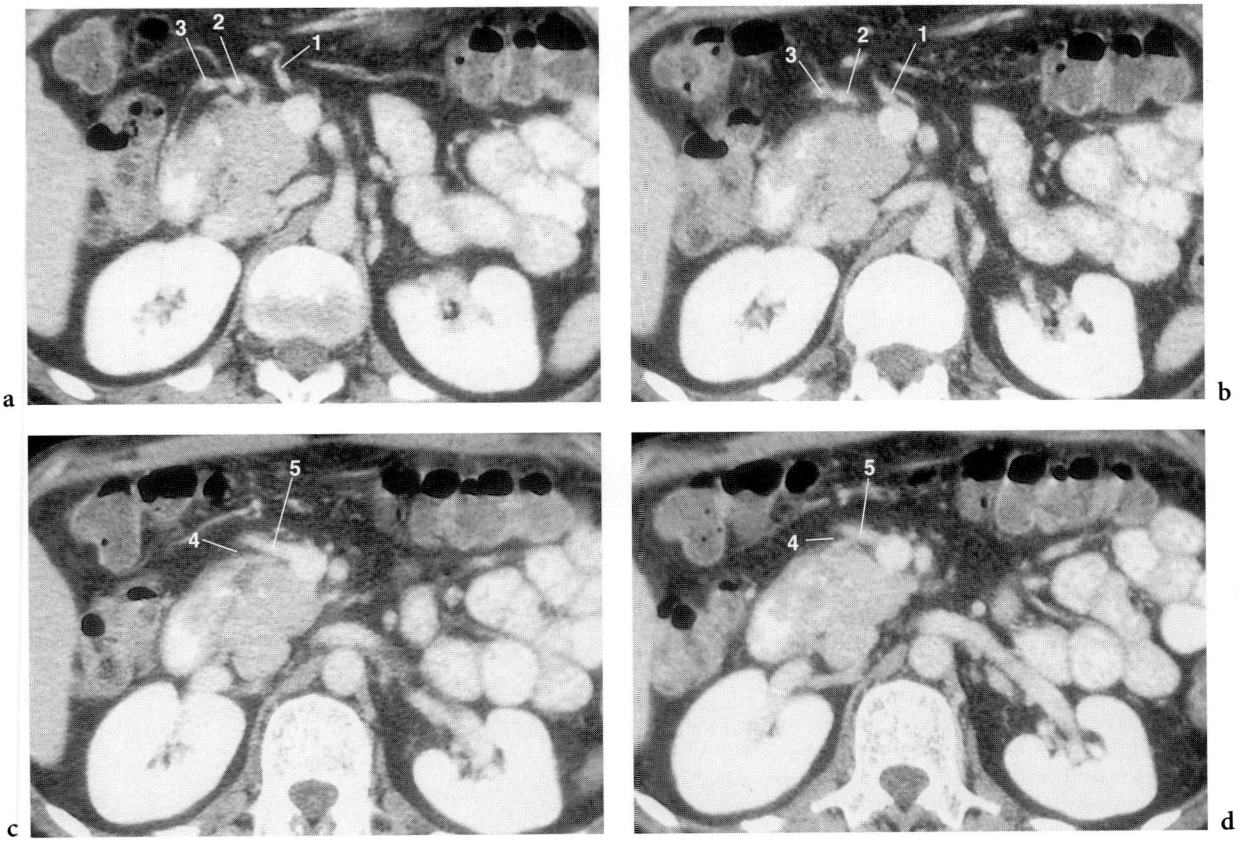

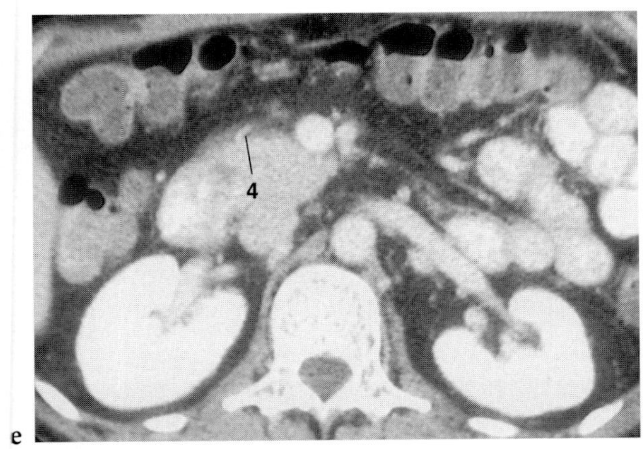

Fig. 3.48a–e. Computed tomography (CT) appearance of anterior superior pancreaticoduodenal vein. **a–e** CT images at level of pancreatic head (from cranial to caudal) showing middle colic vein (*1*) draining into superior mesenteric vein in (**a**) and (**b**) and junction of right gastroepiploic vein (*2*) and right colic vein (*3*) in (**a**) and (**b**). The anterior superior pancreaticoduodenal vein (*4*) is seen as a small vein draining into the gastrocolic trunk (*5*) in (**c–e**)

Since the early work of Marchal and coworkers (1989), it is well understood that the embryologic dorsal and ventral parts of the gland may have a different histologic composition. At CT, this may result in a higher density of the dorsal portion of the head when compared to the remainder of the gland, usually with a straight demarcation line. Matsumoto et al. described two additional features sometimes observed at CT: (1) the area of focal sparing may be limited to the peribiliary region, and (2) the anterior portion of the head may be the only part of the gland having fatty replacement. Based on these observations, two morphologic types and two subtypes were described (Fig. 3.51). In type 1, the posterior aspect of the head and uncinate process are spared from intense fatty replacement (Fig. 3.52). In type 2, the focal area around the common bile duct is spared (Fig. 3.53). Each type was subdivided on the basis of whether the body and tail had intense fatty replacement: subclass a, negative for fatty replace-

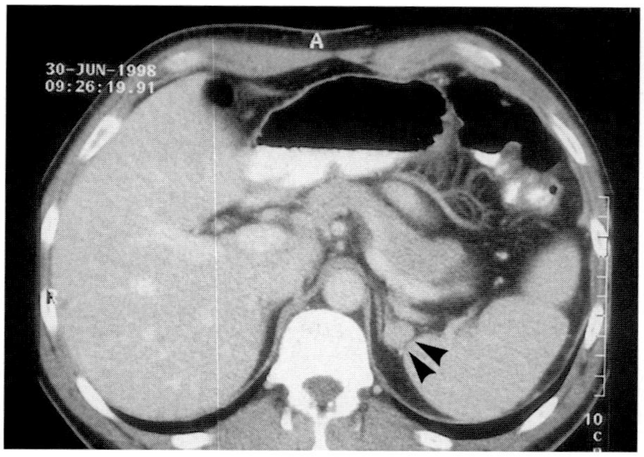

a

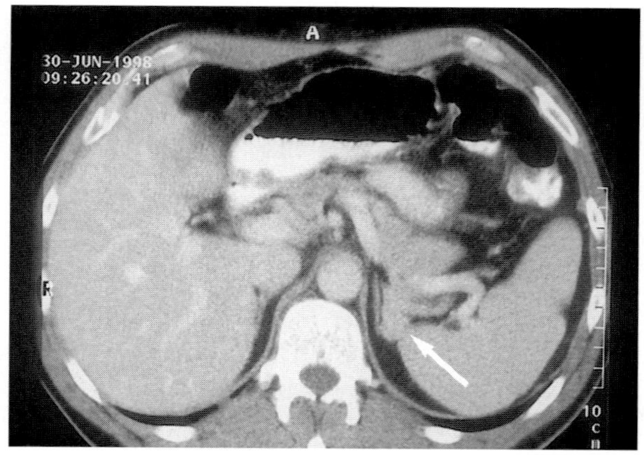

b

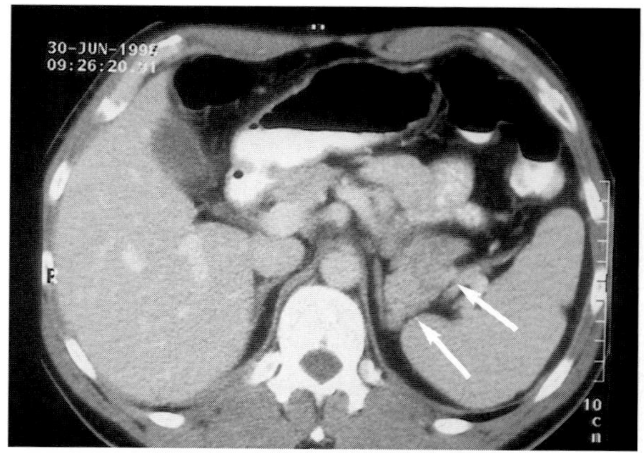

c

Fig. 3.49a–c. Retrovenous location of splenic vein (positional variant). a–c Computed tomography images obtained at 5-mm intervals (from cranial to caudal) showing pancreatic tail that is partially located posterior to the splenic vein (*arrows*). Also note accessory spleen (*arrowheads*)

ment; subclass b, positive. Matsumoto et al. reported the following relative frequencies: type 1a, 35%; type 1b, 36%; type 2a, 11%; type 2b, 18% (Matsumoto et al. 1995).

Ectopic pancreas is usually not seen at CT. On rare occasions, it may appear as focal thickening of the duodenal wall and thus simulate a tumor (Fig. 3.54). In the case of cystic dystrophia secondary to obstruction, a partially cystic enhancing mass may be seen, usually in the wall of the duodenum (Fékété et al. 1996).

Pancreas annulare may show as a well defined ring of pancreatic tissue that encircles the duodenum. However, the annulus may also appear as non-specific duodenal wall thickening (Inamoto et al. 1983; Novetsky et al. 1984). Other associated find-

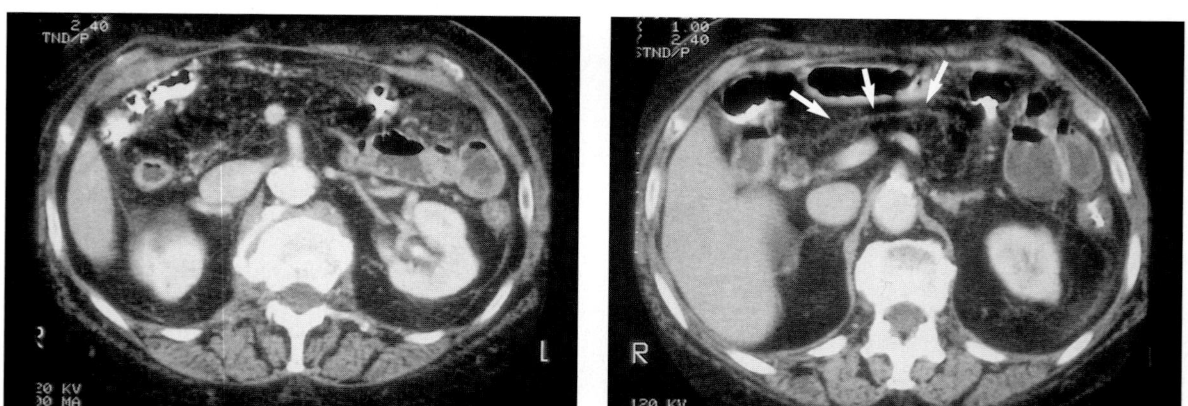

a b

Fig. 3.50a,b. Diffuse fatty replacement of the pancreas. a,b Computed tomography images showing pancreas that is isodense to retroperitoneal fat. Note that the main pancreatic duct and its branches are seen as hyperdense structures (*arrows*)

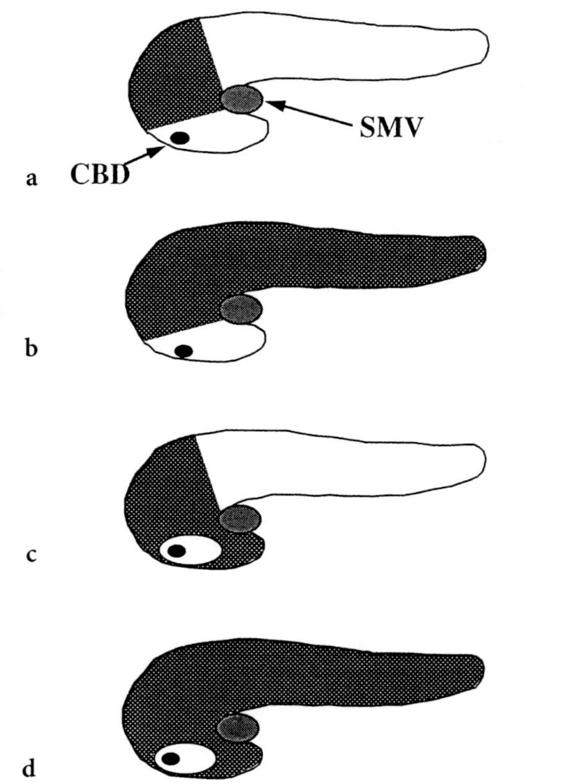

Fig. 3.51. Uneven lipomatosis of the pancreas: classification. From top to bottom, type 1a, 1b, 2a, and 2b fatty replacement of the pancreas. *Darkly shaded* areas represent an area of fatty replacement. *CBD*, common bile duct; *SMV*, superior mesenteric vein. [Reprinted with permission from MATSUMOTO et al. (1995)]

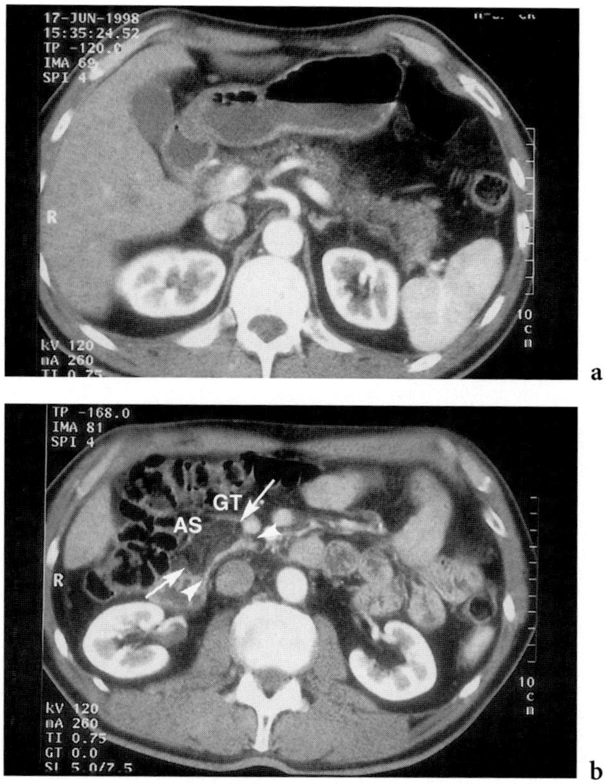

Fig. 3.52a,b. Uneven lipomatosis type 1. **a** Computed tomography (CT) image obtained at level of pancreatic body shows heterogenous and relatively low density of pancreatic parenchyma. **b** CT image obtained at level of pancreatic head shows marked lipomatosis of anterior portion of pancreatic head (*arrows*) with sparing of posterior portion (*arrowheads*). Note normal anterior superior pancreaticoduodenal vein (*AS*) and gastrocolic trunk (*GT*)

ings at CT may be dilation of the proximal duodenum, stenosis of the duodenal lumen, and presence of pancreatic calcifications (chronic pancreatitis).

Pancreas divisum may be diagnosed with CT using thin slices if the pancreatic duct within the body does not continue laterally and dorsally into the dorsal portion of the head on consecutive thin sections. The diagnosis can be confirmed if a direct lateral extension of this duct into the duodenum can be visualized.

While direct tracing of the course of the ducts constitutes the most reliable diagnostic approach, it is feasible only if the duct is clearly seen during cine-display evaluation of overlapping thin-section images obtained with helical CT. Other, more indirect CT signs of pancreas divisum have also been described, including: (a) a relative enlargement of the pancreatic head, (b) presence of two distinct moieties separated by a fat cleft or showing a clear difference in fat content, (c) prominent lobulation of the pancreatic head with presence of a marked lateral indentation (ZEMAN et al. 1988; BURDENY and KROEKER 1988; LINDSTORM and IHSE 1989). Another interesting feature is the presence of a prominent main pancreatic duct. Dilatation of the main pancreatic duct may occur secondary to a "functional" stenosis of the minor papilla (which must drain all secretions coming from the ventral head, body, and tail). As with US, secretin stimulation may be used to confirm the presence of a functional stenosis (LINDSTORM and IHSE 1990).

Pitfalls related to the presence of pancreas divisum are usually caused by a different fat content of the "ventral" and "dorsal" portions of the pancreas and may include: (a) erroneous interpretation of the non-lipomatous portion of the head as a (hyperdense) "mass" (SILVERMAN et al. 1989), and (b) erroneous interpretation of the lipomatous portion of the head as a hypoenhancing mass.

Agenesis or hypoplasia of the dorsal pancreas is

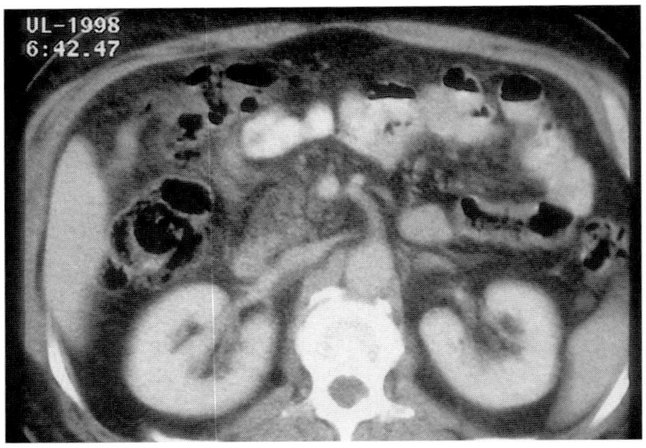

Fig. 3.53. Uneven lipomatosis type 2. Computed tomography image obtained at level of pancreatic head shows lipomatosis with sparing of the focal area around the common bile duct

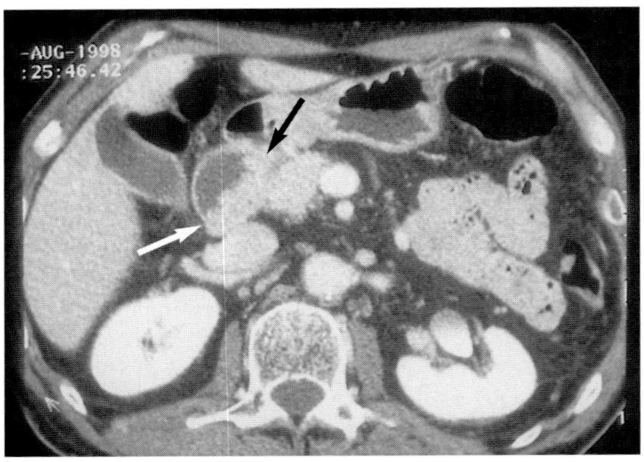

Fig. 3.54. Ectopic pancreas. Computed tomography image shows thickening of the medial wall of the duodenum (*arrows*), which was proved to represent ectopic pancreatic tissue. [Reprinted with permission from Van Hoe et al. (1998b)]

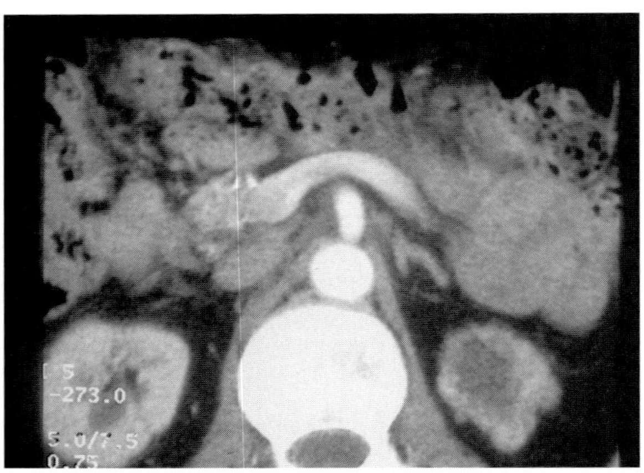

Fig. 3.55. Agenesis of dorsal pancreas. Computed tomography image shows absence of dorsal pancreas. The vacant space is now occupied by small bowel and transverse colon. Also note small size of pancreatic head and presence of tiny calcifications: the patient had chronic pancreatitis

seen as an absence of the tail and part or all of the body. Of course, this condition should be differentiated from extreme atrophy and extreme lipomatosis. This is always possible by a careful inspection of the tissue located in front of the splenic vein (Fig. 3.55).

3.6.3.3
Pseudomasses

Duplications as well as angulations of the pancreatic duct may present as a pseudomass on CT images (Churchill et al. 1978). Since the main pancreatic duct not uncommonly has a somewhat tortuous course, the presence of such a pseudomass on single CT sections is a common finding. Anterior protrusions of the pancreatic body towards the lesser sac have been called "omental tuberosity" (Choi et al. 1997). Similar protrusions may also, although more rarely, be observed in the pancreatic head (Fig. 3.56). Misinterpretation is easily avoided by assessing images obtained at adjacent anatomical levels. Another potential pitfall is represented by focal enlargement of the pancreatic tail (Fig. 3.57).

3.6.3.4
Variations in Lateral Contour of Pancreatic Head and Neck

Ross et al. used dual-phase helical CT to analyze contour variations of the head and neck. They found discrete lobulations of pancreatic tissue greater than 1 cm lateral to the gastroduodenal artery or ASPDA in 34% of patients. These contour variants were categorized as three main types: Type I, presence of a lobule with anterior orientation; type II, lobule oriented posteriorly; type III, lobule oriented horizontally (Figs. 3.58, 3.59). The relative incidence was: type I, 10%; type II, 19%; type III, 5%. Interestingly, these lobules were isodense to the remainder of the pancreas on all phases of perfusion. In other words, they should not be confused with a pancreatic neoplasm if an adequate CT technique is used (Ross et al. 1996).

3.6.3.5
Vessels

While the detection of subtle variations in vascular anatomy requires dedicated angiographic studies, CT may visualize variant anatomy of the larger vessels.

While the "normal" hepatic artery courses in the hepatoduodenal ligament anterior to the portal vein

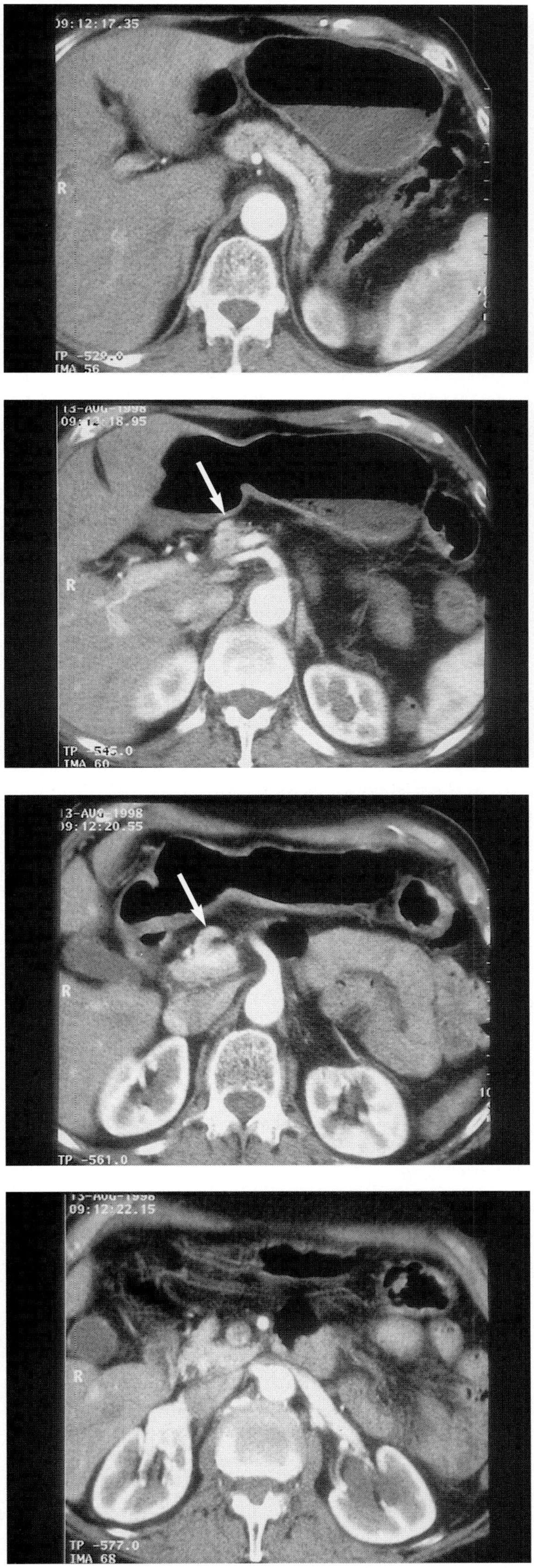

a

b

c

d

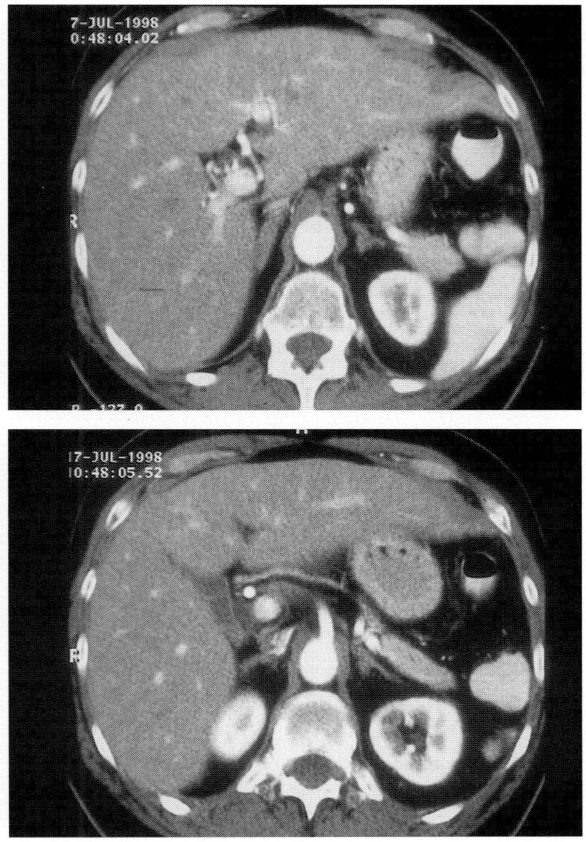

a

b

Fig. 3.57a,b. Focal thickening of pancreatic tail. **a,b** Images obtained at level of pancreatic tail (**a**) and body (**b**). There is marked focal thickening of the tail

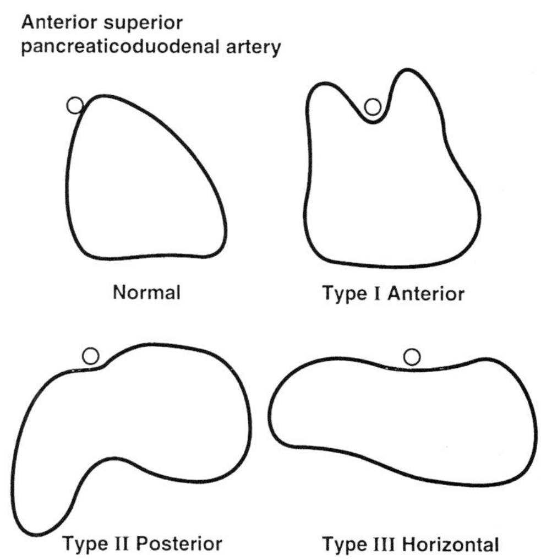

Fig. 3.58. Normal head of pancreas and variants. [Reprinted with permission from Ross et al. (1996)]

Fig. 3.56a–d. Lobulation of pancreatic head/neck. **a–d** Computed tomography images obtained at 15-mm intervals show normal pancreatic body and head. A focal protrusion is seen ventrally in the pancreatic head (*arrow*)

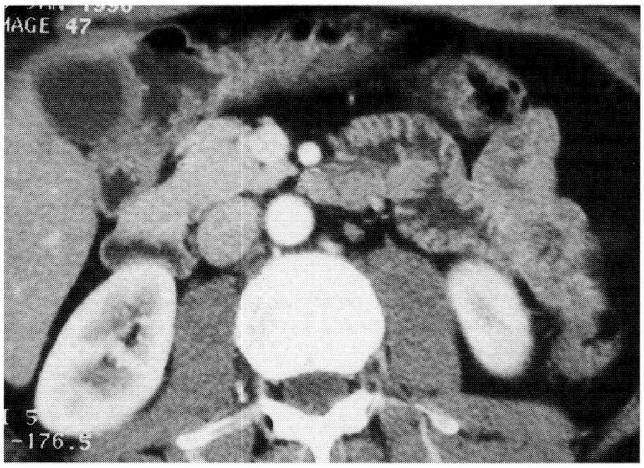

Fig. 3.59. Type II pancreatic lobule. Computed tomography scan shows pancreatic lobule oriented posteriorly and abutting the duodenum (*arrows*)

and medial to the common bile duct, a replaced right hepatic artery courses behind the portal vein and usually runs posterolateral to the bile duct. At the level of the head of the pancreas, it may be seen posterior to the pancreatic head, like the PSPDV. These vessels can be differentiated by tracing the vessel caudally or cranially (the PSPDV drains into the portal vein, a replaced hepatic artery arises from the superior mesenteric artery) (Fig. 3.60). Moreover, the PSPDV has a larger diameter (Mori et al. 1992; Crabo et al. 1993; Vedantham et al. 1998).

In a study on the anatomy of the mesenteric veins with helical CT venography, Graf and collegues found that the superior mesenteric vein was seen as a single common trunk formed by its chief tributaries (ileocolic, gastrocolic, right colic, and middle colic veins) in 87% of patients only. In 13%, the main trunk of the superior mesenteric vein (SMV) was not present and a large left and right mesenteric branch merged separately with the splenic vein. This variant has previously not been described in CT studies, which could be related to the fact that the left mesenteric branch, which drains separately into the splenic vein, may have been interpreted as the inferior mesenteric vein (Graf et al. 1997).

3.7 Magnetic Resonance Imaging

3.7.1 Technical Remarks

Due to the advances in scanner and sequence technology, pancreatic MRI has improved considerably over the past 10 years, providing a valuable alternative to CT.

The most important technical evolution in pancreatic MRI is the introduction of magnetic resonance cholangiopancreatography (MRCP), a technique capable of depicting fluid-containing structures or lesions within a relatively short imaging time and without administration of any contrast medium. Other simultaneous developments have been the introduction of breath-hold MR angiography (MRA), breath-hold dynamic contrast-enhanced MRI, and ultrafast "snapshot" T1- and T2-weighted MRI (Helmberger and Gryspeerdt 1998; Van Hoe et al. 1998b).

It is clear that these ongoing developments will change the place of MRI in the evaluation of patients with suspected pancreatic disease. Importantly, an interactive "staged" MRI examination of the pancreas is now possible. Since the value of the technique resides in the fact that it offers so many different pieces of information (signal intensity, ductal anatomy, vascular anatomy, glandular perfusion, etc.), the term "all-in-one" MRI (including "conventional" MRI, MRCP, and MRA) appears to be well chosen (Gaa et al. 1997). An extensive discussion of state-of-the-art MRI techniques used in the evaluation of pancreatic disease is given in Chap. 8.

3.7.2 Normal Findings

3.7.2.1 Anatomical Landmarks

CT remains the modality of choice for detailed anatomical evaluation of the retroperitoneum. Nevertheless, most peripancreatic structures and organs can also be displayed with MRI, particularly if non-fat-suppressed snapshot T2-weighted images are used (Fig. 3.61).

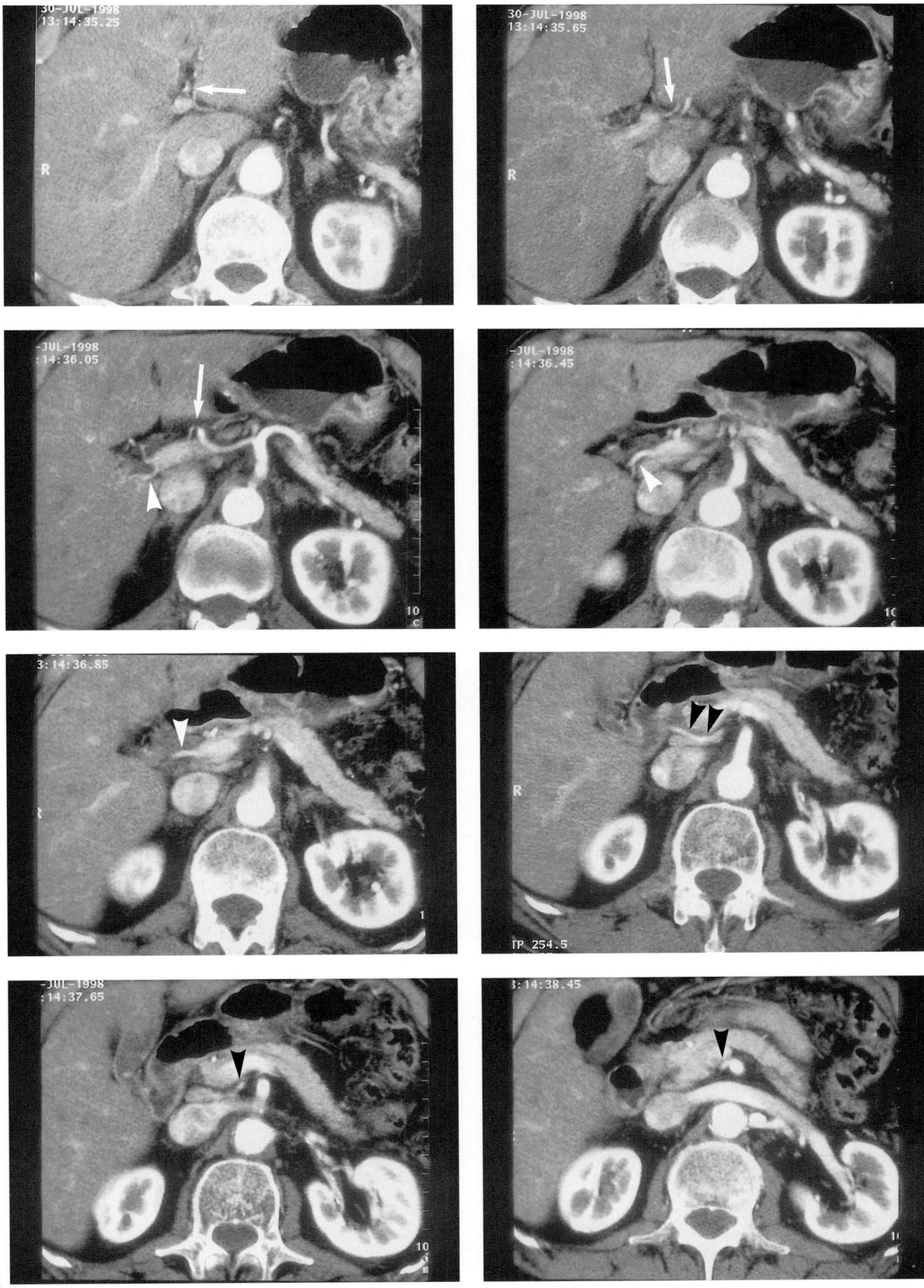

a b c d e f g h

Fig. 3.60a–h. Replaced right hepatic artery. **a–h** Computed tomography images obtained from cranial to caudal showing left hepatic artery arising from celiac trunk (*arrows*) and right hepatic artery arising from the superior mesenteric artery (*arrowheads*). Note typical course of right hepatic artery behind the portal vein

3.7.2.2
The Pancreatic Gland (Fig. 3.62)

The pancreas shows a relatively similar signal intensity to that of the liver on T1-weighted images (SEMELKA and ASCHER 1993). On T2-weighted images the normal pancreas appears isointense to the liver parenchyma and hypointense to the spleen and the kidneys. The contrast between fat and pancreas is maximal on fat-suppressed T1-weighted images (WINSTON et al. 1995). The high signal intensity of the pancreatic gland on these images is related to the presence of aqueous protein in the acini. The pattern of contrast uptake after IV administration of aspecific contrast media (usually a gadolinium compound) is similar to what is know from CT studies (Fig. 3.63). Since the total injection time is shorter in MRI (only 15–20 ml is injected instead of 100–150 ml), peak enhancement may be expected to occur somewhat earlier than in CT.

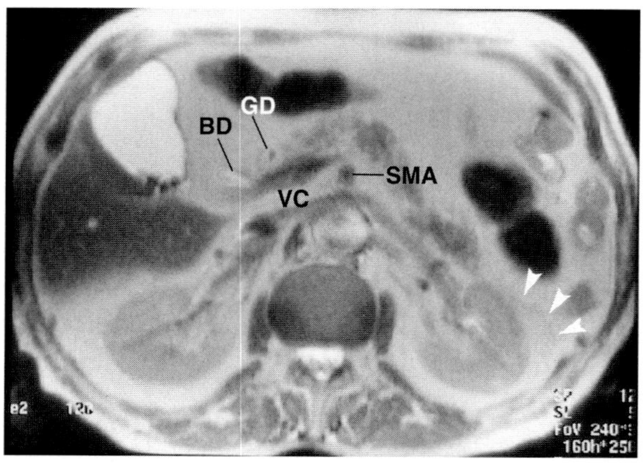

Fig. 3.61. Anatomical landmarks: magnetic resonance imaging (MRI). T2-weighted snapshot MR image (obtained with HASTE sequence) showing pancreatic neck, body, and tail, and gastroduodenal artery (*GD*), extrahepatic bile duct (*BD*), superior mesenteric artery (*SMA*), portomesenteric venous confluence (*VC*), left renal vein, inferior caval vein, etc. Also note visibility of left renal fascia (*arrowheads*)

3.7.2.3
The Ductal System

The rate of successful visualization of the pancreatic duct critically depends on the technique used. It approaches 100% using optimized rapid acquisition relation-enhanced (RARE) and half-Fourier single-shot turbo spin echo (HASTE) sequences during breath-holding (LAUBENBERGER et al. 1995; REUTHER et al. 1996) (Fig. 3.64). In other words, if a portion of the duct is not visualized on these images, pathology should be suggested. Importantly, normal side branches are not routinely depicted. This may also be an advantage: visualization of side branches at MRCP usually allows us to suggest underlying disease (usually chronic pancreatitis or obstruction).

It has recently been shown that dynamic (repetitive) single-shot MRCP has the ability to show the anatomy and contractility of the Vaterian sphincter complex in 95% of "normal" patients. During contraction of the sphincter, the terminal portions of both ducts are usually not seen. During relaxation, they are seen as very thin linear, hyperintense structures (Fig. 3.65) (VAN HOE et al. 1998a).

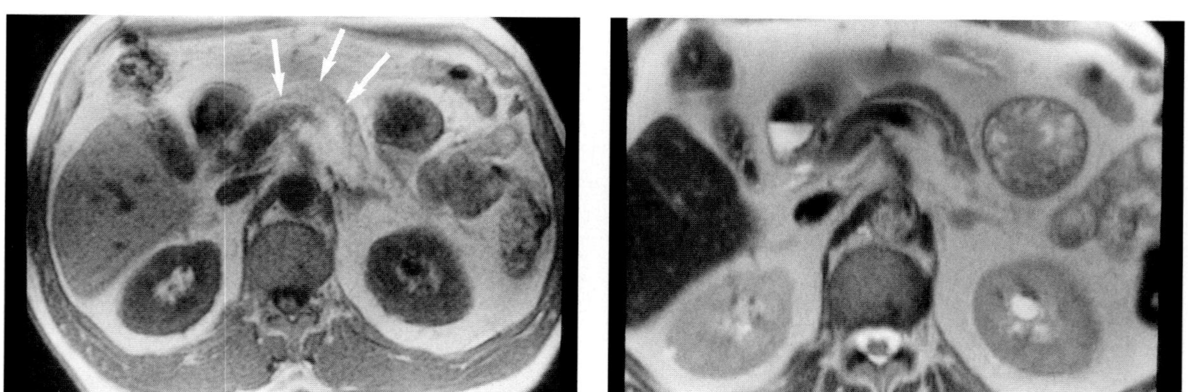

a b

Fig. 3.62a,b. Normal pancreas: signal intensity. **a** T1-weighted magnetic resonance (MR) image showing the pancreas to be relatively hyperintense (approximately isointense to fat) (*arrows*). **b** T2-weighted MR image showing the pancreas to be relatively hypointense. A more hyperintense aspect of the pancreas may be a sign of lipomatosis or pancreatic disease (e.g., acute pancreatitis)

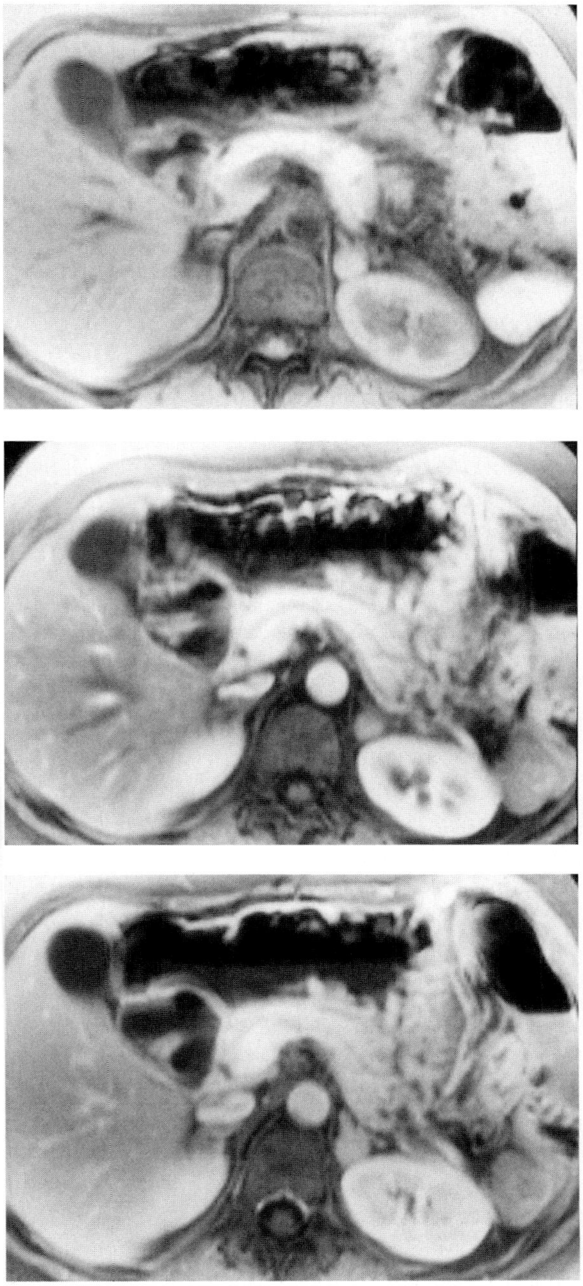

a

b

c

Fig. 3.63a–c. Pancreas: appearance on contrast-enhanced magnetic resonance (MR) images. Fat-suppressed images before (**a**) and 30 s (**b**) and 60 s (**c**) after contrast injection. The pancreas is markedly hyperintense in (**a**). In MRI, the rich vascular blood supply of the pancreas is not reflected by a dramatic increase in signal intensity after IV injection of contrast media [compare (**b**) and (**c**) to (**a**)], which is related to the high 'baseline' intensity. When comparing (**b**) to (**c**), it is clear that early-phase images have to be preferred

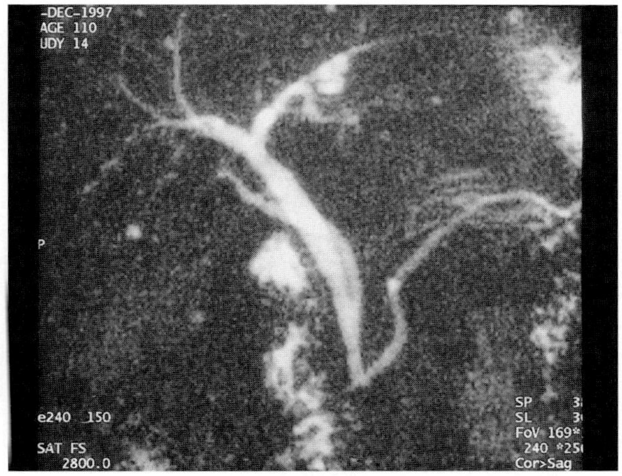

Fig. 3.64. Normal pancreas: ductal anatomy. Projective magnetic resonance image showing normal pancreatic duct, gradually tapering towards the tail. Also note low insertion of cystic duct

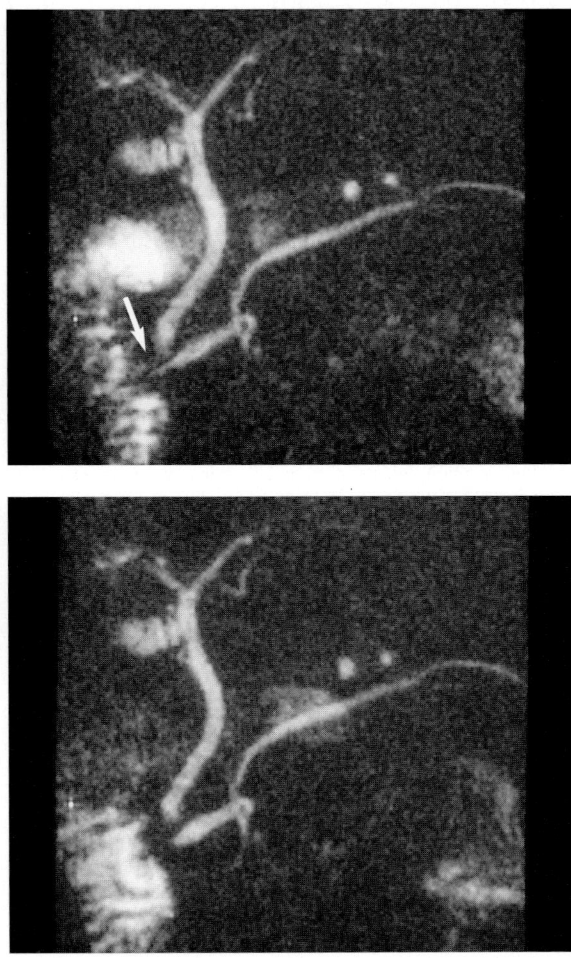

a

b

Fig. 3.65a,b. Dynamic magnetic resonance imaging for evaluation of contractile function of sphincter of Oddi. Image obtained during relaxation (**a**) and during contraction (**b**) of the sphincter. The intramural portions of the common bile duct and pancreatic duct are seen in (**a**) only (*arrows*)

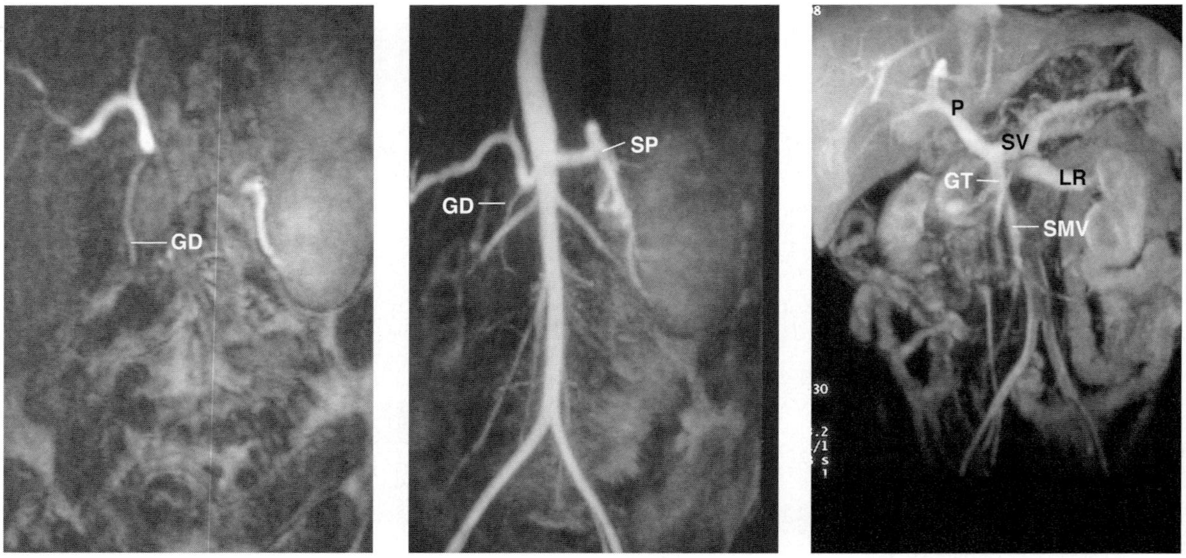

a,b c

Fig. 3.66a–c. Peripancreatic blood vessels: magnetic resonance (MR) angiography. **a** Contrast-enhanced MR image shows gastroduodenal artery (*GD*) arising from common hepatic artery. More cranially, the common hepatic artery bifurcates in a left and a right branch. **b** Same patient. Maximum-intensity projection (MIP) image shows gastroduodenal artery (*GD*) and splenic artery (*SP*). **c** Subtraction MR angiogram shows portal vein (*P*), superior mesenteric vein (SMV), splenic vein (*S*), and gastrocolic trunk (*GT*). Also shown is the left renal vein (*LR*). This image is a MIP of images obtained by subtraction (venous phase minus arterial phase)

3.7.2.4
Blood Vessels

Contrast-enhanced MRA can demonstrate the most important peri-pancreatic vessels (Fig. 3.66). Demonstration of small vessels such as the dorsal pancreatic artery is currently beyond the scope of this technique.

3.7.3
Variants and Pitfalls

The presence of motion artifacts was previously a major problem in abdominal MRI. This problem has largely been eliminated with the introduction of breath-hold and snapshot MRCP techniques. In comparison with ERCP, some specific problems and pitfalls may be encountered in MRI-MRCP. It is of critical importance to be aware of the fact that images obtained with MRCP are fundamentally different from those obtained with ERCP, not only because a different imaging technique is used, but also because the ducts are imaged in their physiologic state, i.e., ducts are not distended due to filling with contrast medium. As a consequence, ERCP and MRCP images should be interpreted differently. Unawareness of this concept all too often leads to the conclusion that an MRCP examination was "not accurate" because it did not show the same features as ERCP.

Pitfalls in pancreatic MRI-MRCP may be related to artifacts caused by surgical clips, metallic stents, and pneumobilia.

MRI-MRCP has the ability to demonstrate nearly all anatomic variants of the ductal system. The discussion is limited to a few examples.

In pancreas divisum, key cholangiographic findings include: (a) the visualization of a dorsal duct draining into the duodenum via the papilla minor, separated from the distal common bile duct, and (b) the absence of a connection between dorsal and ventral ductal system. The course of the main pancreatic duct and duct of Santorini should be assessed both on projective and on axial cross-sectional images (Figs. 3.67, 3.68). The ventral duct may be difficult to visualize at MRCP: according to Bret and coworkers, it may be either small (29%) or invisible (71%) (Bret et al. 1996).

Direct diagnosis of stenosis of the accessory ampulla, responsible for recurrent episodes of acute pancreatitis, is impossible with MRCP. Stenosis, however, results in a dilatation of pancreatic ducts, which can be diagnosed on MRCP.

Annular pancreas is well shown with MRCP by demonstrating an encirclement of the duodenum by the pancreatic duct (Fig. 3.69).

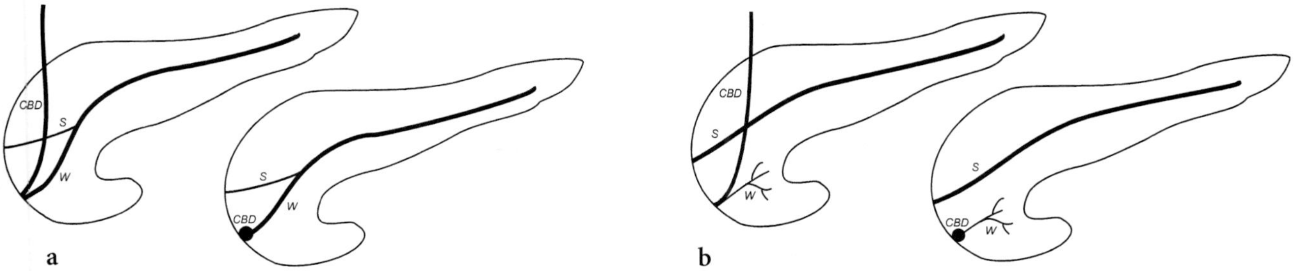

Fig. 3.67a,b. Ductal anatomy in pancreas divisum. **a** Classical ductal anatomy: posterior view (*left*) and cranial view (*right*). **b** Pancreas divisum: posterior view (*left*) and cranial view (*right*) *CBD*, common bile duct; *S* duct of Santorini, splenic vein; *W*, duct of Wirsung

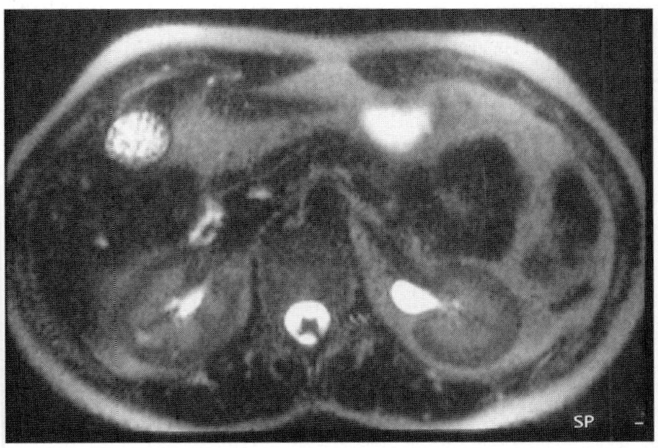

a

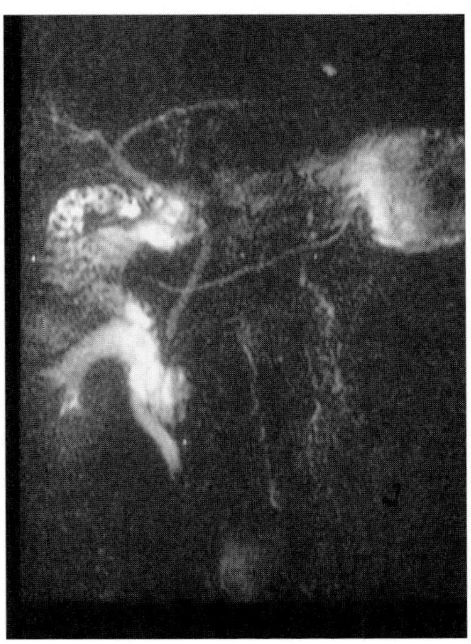

b

Fig. 3.68a,b. Pancreas divisum: magnetic resonance imaging (MRI). Cross-sectional (**a**) and projective (**b**) MR image showing typical features of pancreas divisum. [Reprinted with permission from Van Hoe et al. (1998b)]

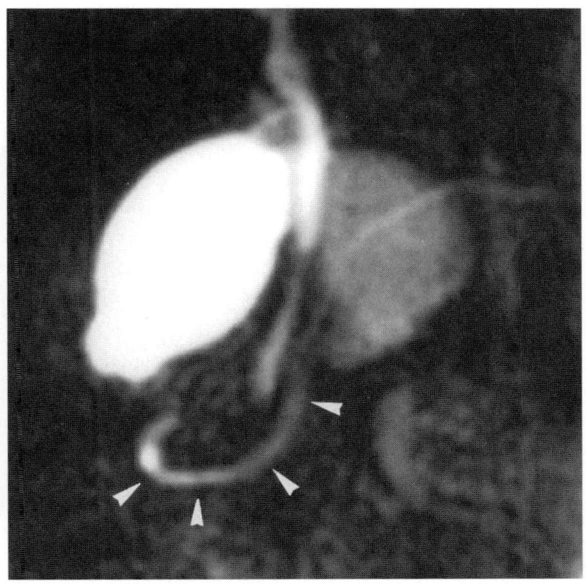

a

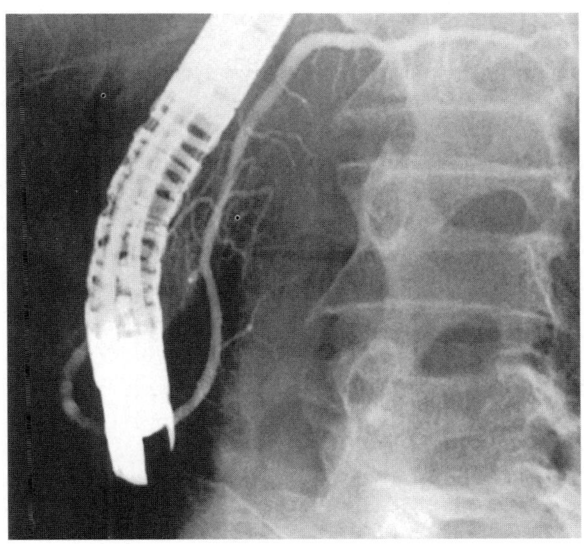

b

Fig. 3.69. Annular pancreas: magnetic resonance imaging (MRI). Projective MR image (**a**) and endoscopic retrograde cholangiopancreatography (**b**) show loop configuration of distal pancreatic duct (*arrowheads*). In (**b**), the duct encircles the endoscope. [Reprinted with permission from Van Hoe et al. (1998)]

Partial *duplication* of the pancreatic duct in the tail is a relatively common finding on MRCP studies. Parenchymal duplication is well seen by evaluating T1- or T2-weighted cross-sectional images.

Anomalous junction of the common bile duct and pancreatic duct. This anomaly can also be detected at MRCP. In particular, a long common channel can be appreciated on projective images (Fig. 3.70)

3.8 Endoscopic Retrograde Cholangiopancreatography

3.8.1 Technical Remarks

A complete overview of the technique, indications, imaging findings, results, potential problems, and complications in ERCP can be found in several excellent books devoted exclusively to this technique (Stewart et al. 1977; Silvis et al. 1995; Taylor and Bohorfoush 1997). Because of its superior spatial resolution, ERCP remains the most accurate technique for the visualization of small anatomical details of the pancreatic ducts.

A side-viewing fiber-duodenoscope is used to reach the papilla. The endoscope is passed into the duodenum with the patient in a left lateral decubitus position. Once the second portion of the duodenum has been entered, the patient is rotated into a right anterior oblique position on the fluoroscopic table. The ampulla is then identified and cannulated. Contrast medium is injected until side-branch filling is noted along the entire course of the main duct. Care must be taken not to acinarize into the pancreatic parenchyma. Filming in early stages is required to detect subtle intraluminal filling defects. The pancreatic duct must be filled out to the tail. Delayed films may be useful to detect papillary stenosis. The best position to promote drainage of the biliary tree is with the patient supine.

One point of concern in ERCP is the risk of procedure-related acute pancreatitis (0.5%–10%), which is believed to be related to overfilling of the pancreatic ducts. In order to avoid this complication in as many patients as possible, strict guidelines have been proposed by Bilbao and coworkers, including: (a) slow injection of contrast medium, (b) stopping the injection when side-branch filling is observed, (c) limiting the number of injections and delaying consecutive injections until the initially injected contrast medium has drained into the duodenum (Bilbao et al. 1976).

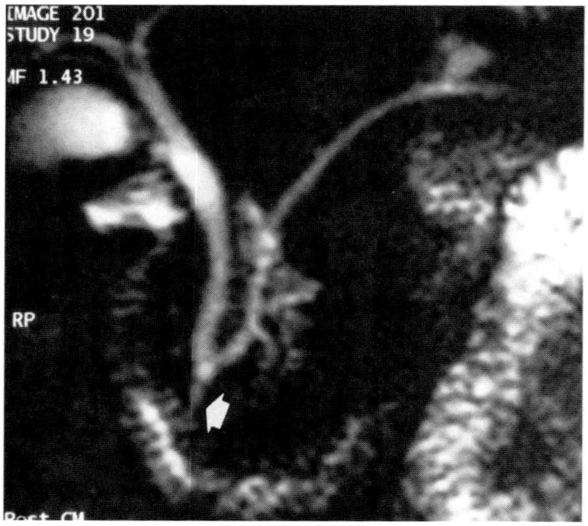

Fig. 3.70. Anomalous junction of the common bile duct and pancreatic duct. Projective image shows relatively long common channel (approximately 16 mm) (*arrow*). [Reprinted with permission from Van Hoe et al. (1998b)]

3.8.2 Normal Findings

As previously discussed (see Sect. 3.2.5), the normal duct should gradually taper towards the tail (Fig. 3.71). Reported normal values for the diameter of the main pancreatic duct exceed those obtained with US or CT, which is related to the distention caused by injection of contrast material. Average diameters of 3.5, 2.5, and 1.5 mm have been reported for the duct in the head, body, and tail, taking into account magnification at ERCP (Sivak and Sullivan 1976). The upper limits of normal are more generous – 6.5, 5, and 3 mm, respectively (Axon 1989). These dimensions may increase with age.

The normal emptying time of the pancreatic duct at ERCP is about 2–7 min. In older patients, it may be prolonged to 10 min (Kasugai et al. 1972). Note that the common bile duct is usually emptied at 15 min; if the gallbladder has been filled with contrast medium, complete emptying of the bile duct may require more time.

Quantifiable criteria for the side branches do not exist. More important than a definable number of side branches is the periodicity of the branch points.

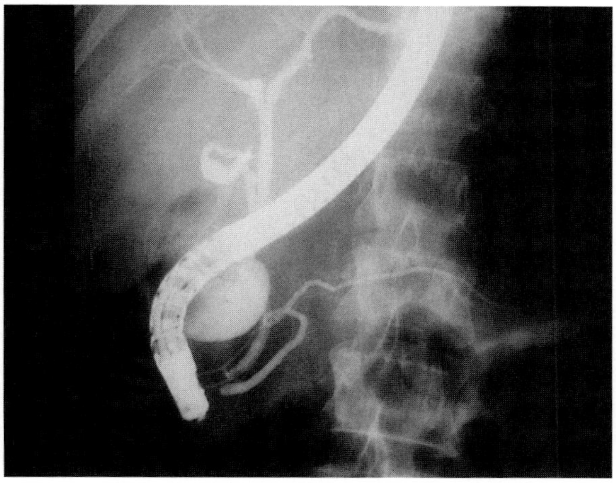

Fig. 3.71. Endoscopic retrograde cholangiopancreatography (ERCP) appearance of normal pancreatic duct

This regular interval is usually constant in the body and tail. The side branch itself should gently taper as it courses into the parenchyma. All the body and tail branches should appear uniform. However, the presence of one or two ectatic branches is usually considered normal (Axon 1989). Larger branches may be seen in the pancreatic head (Fig. 3.72). The uncinate process may be served by one single dominant branch. Alternatively, a set of smaller branches may be seen. As in MRCP, the contractility of the sphincter may be assessed (Fig. 3.73), although spasm caused by cannulation is probably a limiting factor in some patients.

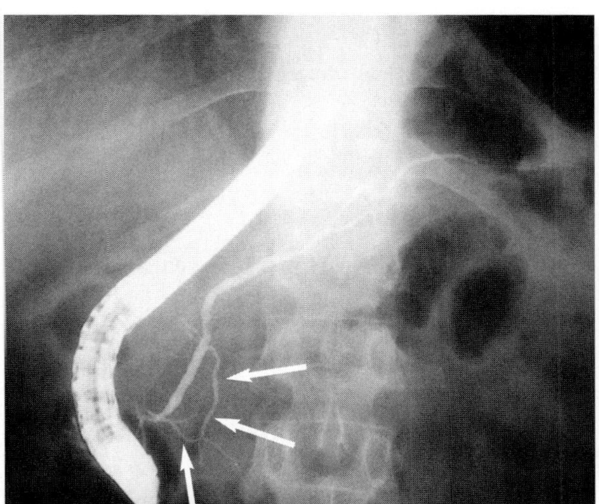

Fig. 3.72. Large side branches in pancreatic head. Endoscopic retrograde cholangiopancreatography image shows large side branches in pancreatic head (*arrows*)

3.8.3 Variants and Pitfalls

ERCP is the standard of reference for detection and evaluation of anatomical variants of the pancreatic ducts. However, it is not a perfect technique: injections at the major papilla often do not show extension into the duodenum via the minor papilla, even when the duct of Santorini is patent. If cannulation of the minor papilla is technically impossible, it may be difficult to get an exact idea of the precise anatomical situation. In this respect, ERCP and MRCP may be complementary.

The reader is referred to Sect. 3.3.2 for a discussion of the anatomical variants of the ducts. Here, only those features specific for ERCP are discussed.

Agenesis of the dorsal pancreas is seen as a sudden obstruction of the duct of Wirsung (or main

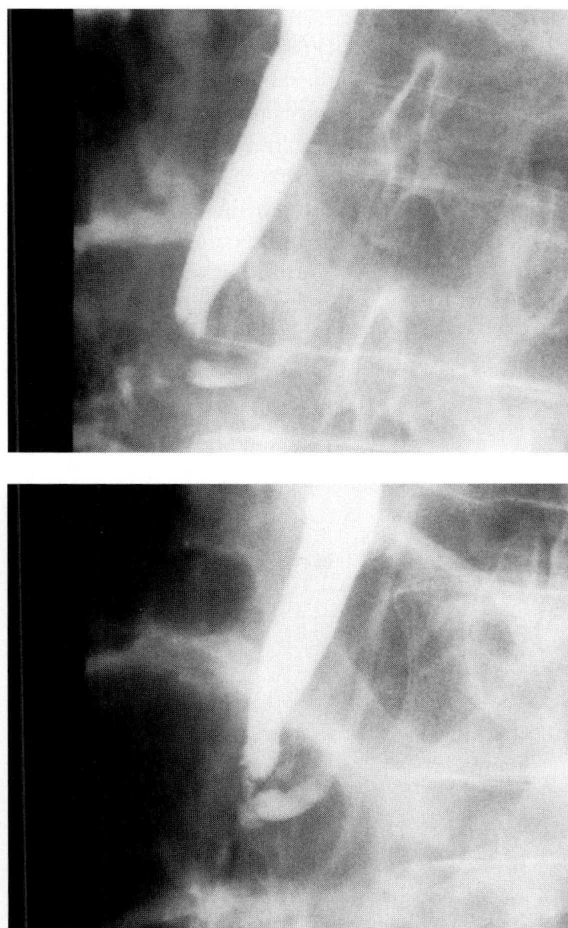

a

b

Fig. 3.73a,b. Contractility of the sphincter of Oddi: evaluation with endoscopic retrograde cholangiopancreatography (ERCP). **a,b** Two consecutively obtained ERCP images showing the sphincter area. The distal portion of the common bile duct is well seen in (**b**) while it is not seen in (**a**) pancreatic duct in the case of hypoplasia). It may be impossible to differentiate agenesis from obstruction.

Ectopic pancreas can be located in the duodenum. If injected during ERCP, a rudementary duct system may be identified, confirming the diagnosis.

Pancreas divisum is easily recognized when the ventral portion is completely opacified and the ventral duct is recognized by its smaller caliber and branching pattern (Fig. 3.74). In case of doubt, pancreas divisum can be confirmed by injecting contrast into the dorsal duct (GULLIVER et al. 1991). ERCP also nicely demonstrates the presence of a connection between the ventral and dorsal pancreatic ducts in patients with incomplete pancreas divisum (Fig. 3.75).

Bifid pancreatic ducts (usually in tail or body) (Fig. 3.76) and unusually tortuous pancreatic ducts generally do not cause diagnostic difficulty.

Many *other variants* have been described with ERCP (Figs. 3.77–3.80) (STEWART et al. 1977). Their importance resides in the fact that they may be interpreted as signs of disease. In case of doubt, correlation with cross-sectional imaging studies may be required.

In *elderly patients*, the main duct can be diffusely ectatic and present with mural contour changes. Side branches change in appearance with variations in number and size. Therefore, one should be careful with the diagnosis of chronic pancreatitis based on ERCP findings in this patient group.

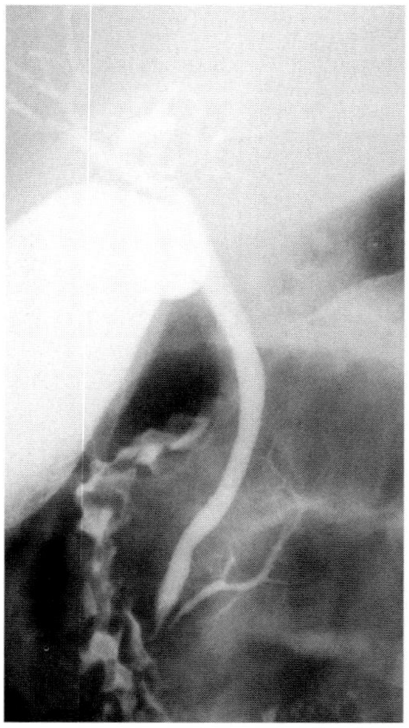

Fig. 3.74. Typical endoscopic retrograde cholangiopancreatography (ERCP) features in pancreas divisum. ERCP image obtained after cannulation of the major papilla shows typical branching pattern of ventral duct

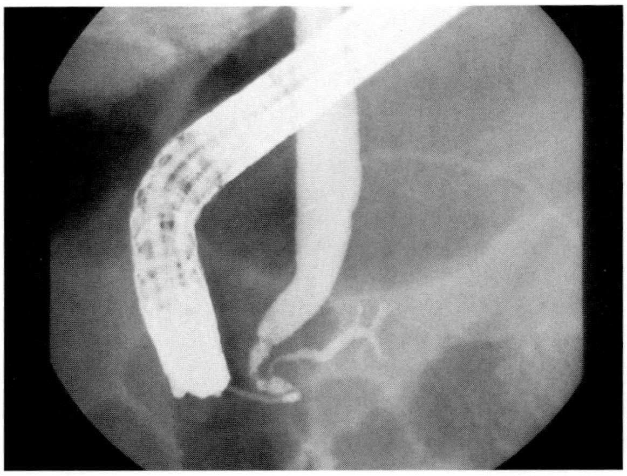

Fig. 3.75. Incomplete pancreas divisum. Endoscopic retrograde cholangiopancreatography image obtained after cannulation of the major papilla shows arborization of ventral pancreatic duct as typically seen in pancreas divisum. Moreover, there is some opacification of the main pancreatic duct, indicating the presence of a communication between the ventral and dorsal ductal system

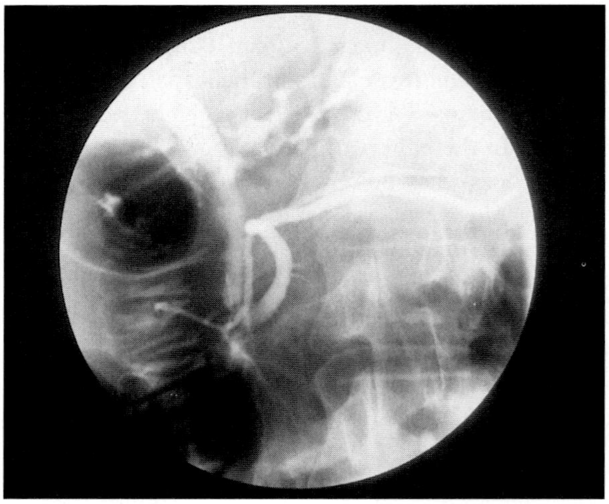

Fig. 3.76. Bifid pancreatic duct. Endoscopic retrograde cholangiopancreatography image shows bifurcation of pancreatic duct in neck/body

3.8.4 Potential Problems and Pitfalls

Failure to cannulate the ductal system occurs in 3%–9% of procedures (SILVIS et al. 1995). One of the causes may be an anatomical variant whereby the papilla is located on the rim of a duodenal diverticulum or in the diverticulum itself.

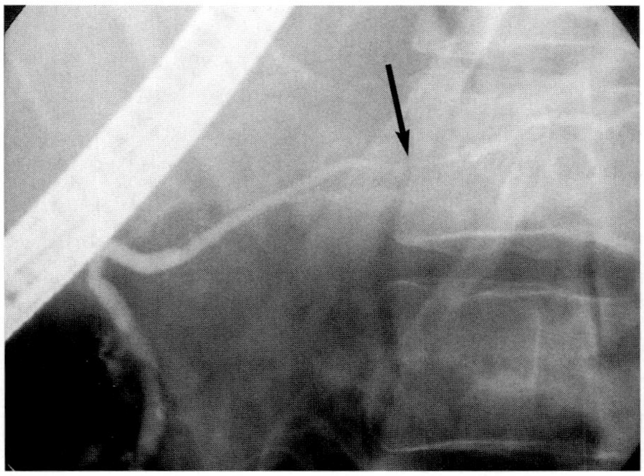

Fig. 3.77. Segmental narrowing of pancreatic duct (*arrow*). Further investigations and clinical follow-up revealed no underlying cause

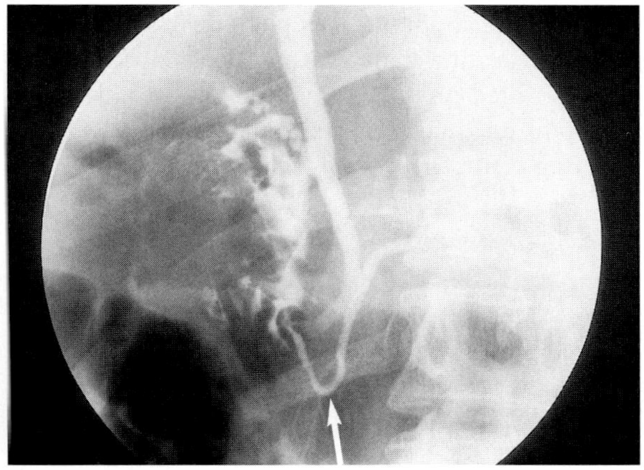

Fig. 3.78. Curved Wirsung. Endoscopic retrograde cholangiopancreatography image shows marked convexity of duct of Wirsung (*arrow*)

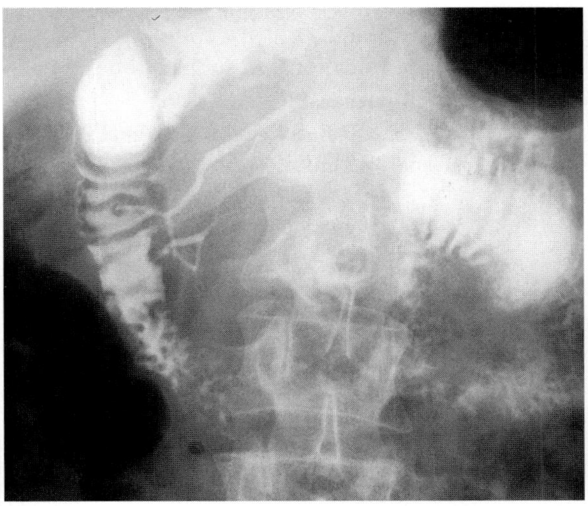

Fig. 3.79. Variant of fusion between ventral and dorsal ductal system (see also Fig. 3.24)

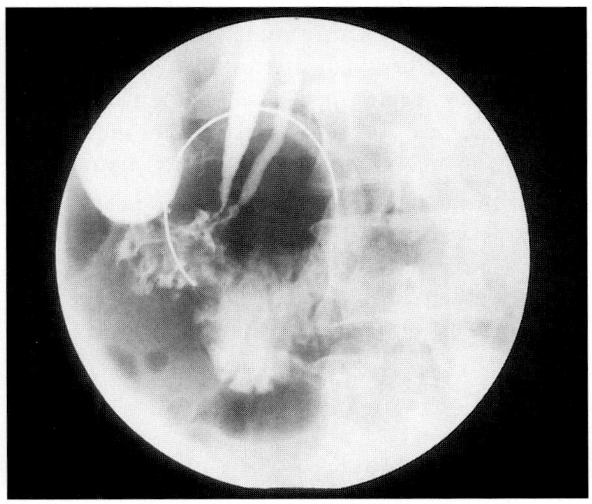

Fig. 3.80. Separate drainage of common bile duct and pancreatic duct into duodenum

Pancreatic duct underfilling is a potential cause of diagnostic inaccuracy. It may be particularly difficult to diagnose a stricture or obstruction in the tail if sufficient filling has not been obtained. Therefore, no diagnostic statement should be made concerning this area unless side-branch filling is observed, indicating that injection pressure has been sufficient.

Inadvertent injection of a small volume of air produces bubbles that are usually easily recognized. However, if a larger amount of air is injected before the contrast material, the duct in the tail may be filled with air, which may escape attention during fluoroscopy. During subsequent injection of contrast material, the abrupt transition between contrast material and air may be interpreted as a stricture (Gulliver et al. 1991).

A contracted sphincter may mimic a calculus in the distal bile duct ("pseudocalculus sign") (Ferrucci et al. 1976). A similar phenomenon may simultaneously be observed in the adjacent pancreatic duct.

Overfilling the ductal system potentially obscures small lesions, particularly intraluminal filling defects.

Initial deep cannulation of the duct can place the tip in a side branch, filling only this part of the duct and suggesting a pancreas divisum (Taylor and Bohorfous 1997). This may also lead to rupture of the side branch and contrast extravasation.

A calcified abdominal lymph node or renal calculus overlying the pancreas may be mistaken for a contrast-filled cavity. It may therefore be advocated to obtain an image of the upper abdomen before injecting contrast medium (Stewart et al. 1977).

3.9 Catheter Angiography

3.9.1 Technical Remarks

Under local anesthesia, the femoral artery is punctured in the groin, using the Seldinger technique (Seldinger 1953). Other routes of access, such as the axillary or brachial arteries, may also be used. The axillary route may facilitate superselective catheterization of the celiac and superior mesenteric branches in many patients because of a straighter access to these vessels. A 5–6.5-F simple curved catheter is passed into the aorta over a guidewire. Modern coaxial guidewire/catheter systems have facilitated superselective catheterization of small arterial branches (Freeny and Lawson 1982). For adequate opacification of the celiac and superior mesenteric territories, a total volume of 40–50 ml is injected at 8–10 ml/s. The portal venous system can be visualized by continuing the filming sequence for approximately 20 s.

If a diagnosis is possible on the basis of celiac and superior mesenteric injections, no further injections need to be performed. However, if the findings are equivocal or normal, superselective injections into the hepatic, dorsal pancreatic, gastroduodenal, or inferior pancreaticoduodenal vessels should be performed. The degree of demonstration of small intrapancreatic arteries is an index of the adequacy of pancreatic arteriography (Finlay and Herlinger 1977). Image magnification and subtraction is nowadays an essential part of the procedure.

The portal venous system may be visualized by several techniques, including indirect arterioportog-

a

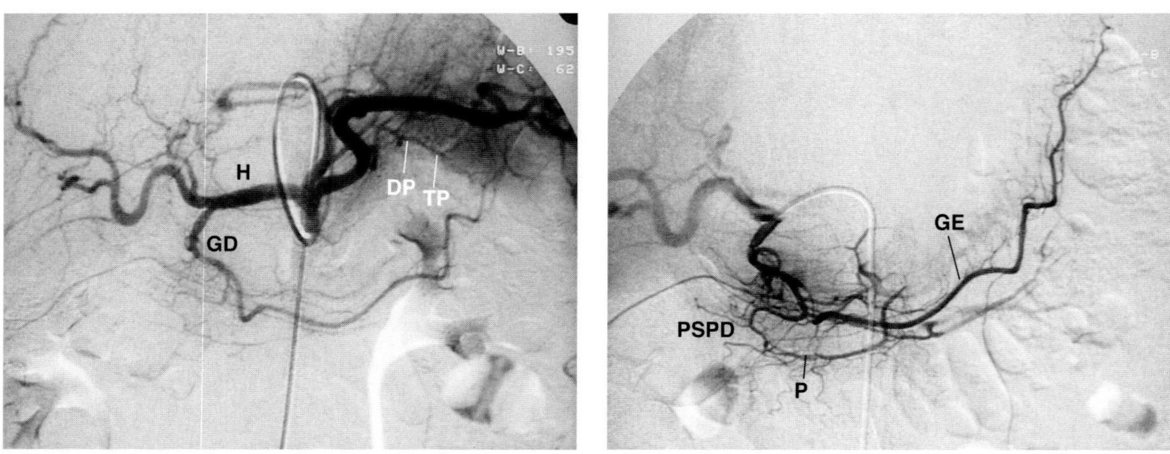

b

c

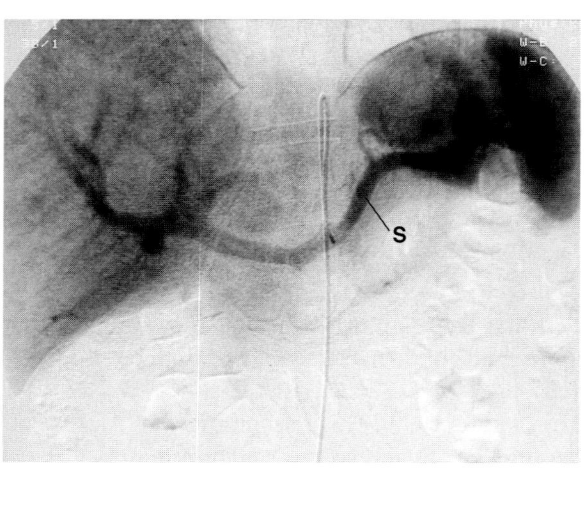

Fig. 3.81a–c. Pancreatic vascular anatomy: catheter angiography. **a,b** Images obtained after selective catheterization of the celiac trunk (**a**) and gastroduodenal artery (**b**) showing the common hepatic artery (*H*), gastroduodenal artery (*GD*), posterior superior pancreaticoduodenal artery (*PSPD*), posterior arcade (*P*), right gastroepiploic artery (*GE*), dorsal pancreatic artery (*DP*), and transverse pancreatic artery (*TP*). **c** Image obtained in a more delayed phase showing enhancement of splenic vein (*S*) and portal vein (*P*)

raphy and direct venography through a transhepatic, splenic, or transjugular approach (Rousselot et al. 1953). A more detailed discussion including specific techniques of localization of endocrine tumors is given in Chap. 10, Sects. 10.5, 10.6.

3.9.2 Findings

The normal arterial vascular supply of the pancreas and its normal variants has been described in Sect. 3.2.4.7 (Fig. 3.81). As stated above, the procedure should be continued until all major branches have been identified. In some patients, this may not be an easy task. The transverse pancreatic artery, for instance, usually arises from the dorsal pancreatic artery (90%), but may also take origin from the right gastroepiploic (3%), gastroduodenal (3%), or posterior superior pancreaticoduodenal arteries (1%). While it is usually best demonstrated by a selective dorsal pancreatic injection (87%), it may be filled with selective gastroduodenal (67%), hepatic (50%), inferior pancreaticoduodenal (58%), or splenic (84%) injections (Reuter 1969).

Catheter angiography remains the gold-standard technique for evaluation of congenital variants (Fig. 3.82).

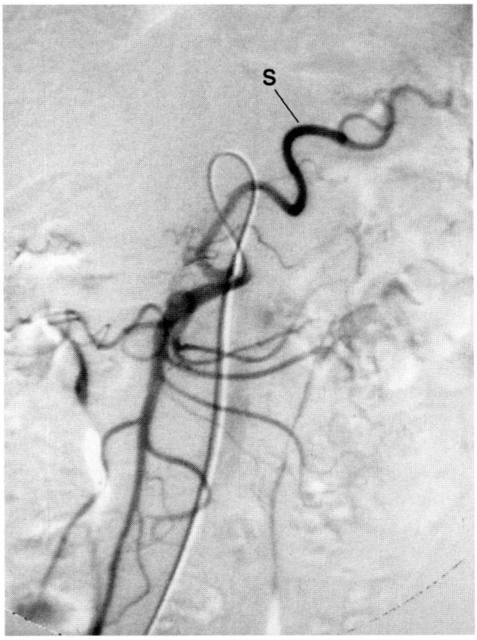

Fig. 3.82. Anatomical variant: splenic artery (S) arising from superior mesenteric artery

Acknowledgements. The authors wish to thank E. Ponette MD, PhD, for providing the following illustrations: Figs. 3.25, 3.27, 3.28, 3.71–3.78.

References

Adda G, Hannoun L, Loygue J (1984) Development of the human pancreas: variations and pathology – a tentative classification. Anat Clin 5:275–283

Agha FP (1987) Duplex ventral pancreas. Gastrointest Radiol 12:23–25

Axon AT (1989) Endoscopic retrograde cholangiopancreatography in chronic pancreatitis. Cambridge classification. Radiol Clin North Am 27:39–50

Baldwin WM (1910) A specimen of annular pancreas. Anat Rec 4:299–304

Bandia Y, Makuuchi M (1998) Intraoperative ultrasound. In: Howard J, Idezuki Y, Ihse I, Prinz R (eds) Surgical diseases of the pancreas. Williams and Wilkins, Baltimore, pp 1107–1110

Barbosa J, Dockerty MB, Waugh JM (1946) Pancreatic heterotopia. Surg Gynecol Obstet 82:527–542

Belber JP, Bill K (1977) Fusion anomalies of the pancreatic ductal system: differnetiation from pathologic states. Radiology 123:637–642

Benedict KT, Ferrucci JT, Eaton SB (1970) Hypotonic duodenography: current concepts in technique, interpretation, and clinical usefulness. Crit Rev Radiol Sci 1:567–578

Berland LL, Lawson TL, Dennis Foley W, Geenen JE, Stewart ET (1981) Computed tomography of the normal and abnormal pancreatic duct: correlation with pancreatic ductography. Radiology 141:715–724

Bilbao MK, Dotter CT, Lee TG, et al. (1976) Complications of endoscopic retrograde cholangiopancreatography. Gastroenterology 70:314–320

Bonaldi VM, Bret PM, Atri M, Reinhold C (1998) Helical CT of the pancreas : a comparison of cine display and film-based viewing. AJR 170:373–376

Bret PM, Reinhold C, Taourel P, Guibaud L, Atri M, Barkun AN (1996) Pancreas divisum: evaluation with MR cholangiopancreatography. Radiology 199:99–103

Bryan PJ (1982) Appearance of normal pancreatic duct: a study using real time ultrasound. J Clin Ultrasound 10:63–66

Burdeny DA, Kroeker MA (1988) CT appearance of the ventral pancreas. J Can Assoc Radiol 39:190–192

Choi YH, Rubenstein WA, Ramirez de Arellano E, Intriere L, Kazam E (1997) CT and US of the pancreas. Clin Imaging 21:414–440

Chong M, Freeny PC, Schmiedl UP (1998) Pancreatic arterial anatomy: depiction with dual-phase helical CT. Radiology 208:537–542

Churchill R, Reynes C, Love L (1978) Pancreatic pseudotumors: computed tomography. Gastrointest Radiol 3:251–256

Classen M, Hellwig H, Rösch W (1973) Anatomy of the pancreatic duct. A duodenoscopic-radiological study. Endoscopy 5:14–17

Clifford KM (1980) Annular pancreas diagnosed by endoscopic retrograde cholangio-pancreatography. Br J Radiol 53:593–595

Crabo LG, Conley DM, Granley O, Freeny PC (1993) Venous anatomy of the pancreatic head: normal CT appearence in cadavers and patients. AJR 160:1039–1045

Dawson W, Langman J (1961) An anatomical-radiological study on the pancreatic duct pattern in man. Anat Rec 139:59–68

Demling L, Koch H, Rösch W (1979) ERCP. Schattauer, Stuttgart

Donald JJ, Shorvon PJ, Lees WR (1990) A hypoechoic area within the head of the pancreas – a normal variant. Clin Radiol 41:337–338

England RE, Newcomer MK, Leung JW, Cotton PB (1995) Case report: annular pancreas divisum – a report of two cases and review of the litterature. Br J Radiol 68:324–328

Farkas IE (1982) Rare anomaly of the pancreatic duct: communication between the two ductal systems in pancreas divisum. Diagn Imag 51:284–287

Federle MP, Goldberg HI (1992) The pancreas. In: Moss A, Gamsu G, Genant H (eds) Computed tomography of the body. Saunders, Philadelphia, p 870

Fékété F, Noun R, Sauvanet A, Fléjou JF, Bernades P, Belghiti J (1996) Pseudotumor developing in heterotopic pancreas. World J Surg 20:295–298

Ferrucci JT, Benedict KT, Page DL, Fleischli DJ, Eaton SB (1970) Radiographic features of the normal hypotonic duodenogram. Radiology 96:401–408

Ferruci J, Wittenberg J, Stone L, Dreyfuss J (1976) Hypotonic cholangiography with glucagon. Radiology 118:466–467

Fink AS, Perez de Ayala V, Chapman M, Cotton PB (1986) Radiologic pitfalls in endoscopic retrograde cholangiopancreatography. Pancreas 1:180–187

Finlay DB, Herlinger H (1977) The intrapancreatic anatomy as an index of adequacy of pancreatic arteriography. Clin Radiol 28:595–599

Freeny PC, Lawson TL (1982) Radiology of the pancreas. Springer, Berlin Heidelberg New York

Freeny PC, Stevenson GW (1994) Margulis' and Burhennen alimentary tract radiology, 5th edn. Mosby, St. Louis

Gaa J, Georgi M, Trede M (1997) New concepts in MR imaging of pancreatic tumors. Imaging Decis MRI 1:2–7

Gilinski NH, Del Favero G, Cotton PB, Lees WR (1985) Congenital short pancreas: a report of two cases. Gut 26:304–307

Goodman P, Halpert RD, Rabassa AE (1991) Aberrant insertion of the common bile duct into an accessory pancreatic duct: cholangiographic demonstration. Am J Gastroenterol86:1268–1270

Gore RM, Levine MS, Laufer I (eds) (1994) Textbook of gastrointestinal radiology. Saunders, Philadelphia

Graf O, Boland GW, Kaufman JA, Warsghaw AL, Fernandez del Castillo C, Mueller PR (1997) Anatomic variations of the mesenteric veins: depiction with helical CT venography. AJR 168:1209–1213

Gulliver DJ, Cotton PB, Baillie J (1991) Anatomic variants and artifacts in ERCP interpretation. AJR 156:975–980

Haaga JR (1984) Improved CT technique for CT-guided celiac ganglia block. AJR 142:1201–1204

Hadidi A (1983) Pancreatic duct diameter: sonographic measurement in normal subjects. J Clin Ultrasound 11:17–22

Halpert RD, Shabot JM, Heare BR, Rogers RE (1990) The bifid pancreas: a rare anatomical variation. Gastrointest Endosc 36:60–62

Helmberger T, Gryspeerdt S (1998) Advanced MR imaging techniques for the pancreas, with emphasis on MR pancreatography. In: Heuck A, Reiser M (eds) Magnetic resonance imaging of the abdomen and pelvis. Springer, Berlin Heidelberg New York, pp 83–90

Heuck A, Maubach PA, Reiser M, et al. (1987) Age-related morphology of the normal pancreas on computed tomography. Gastrointest Radiol 12:18–22

Hoffman M, Sugerman HJ, Heuman D, Turner MA, Kisloff B (1987) Gastric duplication cyst communicating with aberrant pancreatic duct: a rare cause of recurrent acute pancreatitis. Surgery 101:369–372

Ibukuro K, Tsuikiyama T, Mori K, Inoue Y (1996) Peripancreatic veins on thin-section (3 mm) helical CT. AJR 167:1003–1008

Inamoto K, Ishikawa Y, Itoh N (1983) CT demonstration of annular pancreas: a case report. Gastrointest Radiol 8:143–145

Inoue Y, Nakamura H (1997) Aplasia or hypoplasia of the pancreatic uncinate process: comparison in patients with and patients without intestinal nonrotation. Radiology 205:531–533

Itoh Y, Hada T, Terano A, Itai Y, Harada T (1989) Pancreatitis in the annulus of annular pancreas demonstrated by the combined use of computed tomography and endoscopic retrograde cholangiopancreatography. Am J Gastroenterol 84:961–964

Jacobs JE, Coleman BG, Arger PH, Langer JE (1994) Pancreatic sparing of focal fatty infiltration. Radiology 190:437–439

Japanese Pancreas Society (1996) Japanese classification of pancreatic carcinoma, 1st English edn. Kanehara, Tokyo

Johnson ML, Mack LA (1978) Ultrasonographic evaluation of the pancreas. Gastrointest Radiol 3:257–266

Kadir S (1991) Atlas of normal and variant angiographic anatomy. Saunders, Philadelphia

Kasugai T, Kuno N, Kobayashi S, Hattori K (1972) Endoscopic pancreatocholangiography. The normal endoscopic pancreatocholangiogram. Gastroenterology 63:217–226

Kikuchi K, Nomiyama T, Miwa M, Harasawa S, Miwa T (1983) Bifid tail of the pancreas: a case presenting as a gastric submucosal tumor. Am J Gastroenterol 78:23–27

Kleitsch WP (1955) Anatomy of the pancreas. Arch Surg 71:795–803

Kochhar R, Nagi B, Chawla S, et al. (1989) The clinical spectrum of anomalous pancreatico-biliary junction. Surg Endoscop 3:83–86

Kondi-Paphiti A, Antoniou AG, Kotsis T, Polimeneas G (1997) Aberrant pancreas in the gallbladder wall. Eur Radiol 7:1064–1066

Korobkin M, Silverman PM, Quint L, Francis IR (1992) CT of the retroperitoneal space: normal anatomy and fluid collections. AJR 159:933–941

Kreel L, Sandin B (1973) Changes in pancreatic morphology associated with aging. Gut 14:486–494

Kreel L, Haertel M, Katz D (1977) Computed tomography of the normal pancreas. J Comput Assist Tomogr 1:290–299

Kuroda A, Nagai H (1998) Surgical anatomy of the pancreas. In: Howard J, Idezuki Y, Ihse I, Prinz R (eds) Surgical diseases of the pancreas. Williams and Wilkins, Baltimore, pp 11–21

Lai E, Tompkins R (1986) Heterotopic pancreas. Am J Surg 151:697–700

Langman J (1975) Medical embryology, 3rd edn. Williams and Wilkins, Baltimore

Laubenberger J, Büchert M, Schneider B, Blum B, Hennig J, Langer M (1995) Breath-hold projection magnetic reso-

nance cholangio-pancreaticography (MRCP): a new method for the examination of the bile and pancreatic ducts. Magn Reson Med 33:18–23
Laufer I (1975) A simple methd for routine double contrast study of the upper abdomen. Radiology 117:513–518
Lawson TL, Berland LL, Dennis Foley W, Stewart ET, Geenan JE, Hogan WJ (1982) Ultrasonic visualization of the pancreatic duct. Radiology 144:865–871
Lecco TM (1910) Zur Morphologie des Pancreas Annulare. Sitzungsber Wien Akad Wissen Math Naturw Kl 119:391–406
Lechner GW, Read RC (1966) Agensesis of the dorsal pancreas in an adult diabetic presenting with duodenal ileus. Ann Surg 163:311–313
Lehman GA, O'Connor KW (1985) Coexistence of annular pancreas and pancreas divisum – ERCP diagnosis. Gastrointest Endoscop 31:25–28
Lindstorm E, Ihse I (1989) Computed tomography findings in pancreas divisum. Acta Radiol 30:609–613
Lindstorm E, Ihse I (1990) Dynamic CT scanning of the pancreatic duct after secretin provocation in pancreas divisum. Dig Dis Sci 35:1371–1376
Lloyd-Jones W, Mountain JC, Warrent KW (1972) Annular pancreas in the adult. Ann Surg 176:163–170
Marchal G, Verbeken E, Van Steenbergen W, Baert AL (1989) Uneven lipomatosis: a pitfall in pancreatic sonography. Gastrointest Radiol 1989:233–237
MatsumotoS, Mori H, Miyake H, et al. (1995) Uneven fatty replacement of the pancreas: evaluation with CT. Radiology 194:453–458
Meyers MA (1988) Dynamic radiology of the abdomen. Springer, Berlin Heidelberg New York, pp 348–363
Michels N (1955) Blood supply and anatomy of the upper abdominal organs. Lippincott, Philadelphia
Misra SP, Dwivedi M (1990) Pancreaticobiliary ductal union. Gut 31:1144–1149
Molmenti EP, Balfe DM, Kanterman RY, Bennet HF (1996) Anatomy of the retroperitoneum: observations of the distribution of pathologic fluid collections. Radiology 200:95–103
Montgomery G (1965) Congenital and miscellaneous anomalies of the liver and pancreas. In: Montgomery G (ed) Textbook of pathology, vol 1. Churchill Livingstone, London
Mori H, Miyake H, Aikawa H, et al. (1991) Dilated posterior superior pancreaticoduodenal vein: recognition with CT and clinical significance in patients with pancreatobiliary carcinomas. Radiology 181:793–800
Mori H, McGrath FP, Malone DE, Stevenson GW (1992) The gastrocolic trunc and its tributaries: CT evaluation. Radiology 182:871–877
Nagai H, Kuroda A, Morioka T (1986) Lymphatic and local spread of T1 and T2 pancreatic cancer: a study of autopsy material. Ann Surg 204:65–71
Nebasar RA, Kornblith PL, Pollard JJ, et al. (1969) A correlation of angiograms and dissections. Little Brown, Boston
Niederau C, Sonnenberg A, Muller J, Erkenbrecht J, Scholten T, Fritsch W (1983) Sonographic measurements of the normal liver, spleen, pancreas and portal vein. Radiology 149:537–540
Novetsky GJ, Berlin L, Smith C, Epstein AJ (1984) CT diagnosis of annular pancreas. J Comp Assist Tomogr 8:1031–1034
Ogoshi K, Niwa M, Hara Y, Nebel OT (1973) Endoscopic pancreatocholangiography in the evaluation of pancreatic and biliary disease. Gastroenterology 64:210–216
Op den Orth JO (1987) Sonography of the pancreatic head aided by water and glucagon. Radiographics 1:85–100
Osnes M, Lootveit T, Larsen S, Aune S (1981) Diverticula and their relationship to age, sex, and biliary calculi. Scand J Gastroenterol 16:103–107
Pietrabissa A, Shimi S, Chschieri A (1993) Detection of occult insulinoma by laparoscopic infragastric pancreatic contact ultrasound scanning. Surg Oncol 2:83–86
Quinlan RM (1991) Anatomy and embryology of the pancreas. In: Zuidema GD (ed) Shackelford's surgery of the alimentary tract, vol III, 3rd edn. Saunders, Philadelphia, pp 3–18
Reuter SR (1969) Superselective pancreatic angiography. Radiology 92:74–85
Reuther G, Kiefer B, Tuchman A (1996) Cholangiography before biliary surgery: single-shot MR cholangiography versus intravenous cholangiography. Radiology 198:561–566
Rhoades JE, Folin LS (1987) The history of surgery of the pancreas. In: Howard JM, Jordan GL, Reber HA (eds) Surgical diseases of the pancreas. Lea and Febiger, Philadelphia, pp 3–10
Rienhoff WF, Pickrell KL (1945) Pancreatitis: an anatomic study of the pancreatic and extrahepatic biliary systems. Arch Surg 51:205–210
Rösch T (1998) Endoscopic ultrasonography. In: Howard J, Idezuki Y, Ihse I, Prinz R (eds) Surgical diseases of the pancreas. Williams and Wilkins, Baltimore, pp 185–192
Ross BA, Brooke Jeffrey R, Mindelzun RE (1996) Normal variations in the lateral contour of the head of the pancreas mimicking neoplasm: evaluation with dual-phase helical CT. AJR 166:799–801
Rousselot LM, Ruzicka FF, Doehner GA (1953) Portal venography via the portal and percutaneous splenic routes. Surgery 34:557–569
Rouviere H, Delmas A (1985) Pancréas. Anatomie humaine Tome 2, 12th edn. Masson, Paris, pp 459–468
Rubenstein WA, Auh YH, Zirinsky K, Kneeland B, Whalen JP, Kazam E (1985) Posterior intraperitoneal recesses. Assessment using CT. Radiology 156:461–468
Schulte SJ (1994) Embryology, normal variation, and congenital anomalies of the pancreas. In: Freeny PC, Stevenson GW (eds) Margulis' and Burhenne's alimentary tract radiology, 5th edn. Mosby, St. Louis, pp 1039–1051
Schwartz A, Birnbaum D (1962. Roentgenologic study of the topography of the choledocho-duodenal junction. AJR 87:772–776
Seldinger SI (1953) Catheter placement of the needle in percutaneous arteriography: a new technique. Acta Radiol 39:368–376
Semelka RC, Ascher SM (1993) MR imaging of the pancreas. Radiology 188:593–602
Shemesh E, Friedman E, Czesniak A, Bat L (1987) The association of biliary and pancreatic anomalies with periampullary duodenal diverticula. Correlation with clinical presentations. Arch Surg 122:1055–1057
Siegel MJ, Martin KW, Worthington JL (1987) Normal and abnormal pancreas in children: US studies. Radiology 165:15–18
Silverman PM, McVay L, Zeman RK, Garra BS, Grant EG, Jaffe MH (1989) Pancreatic pseudotumor in pancreas divisum: CT characteristics. J Comput Assist Tomogr 13:140–141

Silvis S, Rohrmann C, Ansel H (eds) (1995) Endoscopic retrograde cholangiopancreatography. Igaku-Shoin, New York, pp 446–469

Simeone JF, Mueller PR, Ferrucci JT, et al. (1982) Sonography of the bile ducts after a fatty meal: an aid in the detection of obstruction. Radiology 143:211–215

Sivak MV, Sillivan BH (1976) Endoscopic retrograde pancreatography: analysis of the normal pancreatogram. Am J Dig Dis 21:263–269

Smanio T (1954) Varying relations of the common bile duct with the posterior face of the pancreatic head in Negroes and white persons. J Int Coll Surg 22:150–172

Staritz M (1988) Pharmacology of the sphincter of Oddi. Endoscopy 20:171–4

Sterling JA (1954) The common channel for bile and pancreatic ducts. Surg Gynecol Obstet 98:420–424

Stewart E, Vennes J, Geenen J (eds) (1977) Atlas of endoscopic retrograde cholangiopancreatography. Mosby, St. Louis

Taylor A, Bohorfoush A (eds) (1997) Interpretation of ERCP, Lippincott-Raven, Philadelphia

Taylor K, Buchin P, Viscomi G, Rosenfield A (1981) Ultrasonographic scanning of the pancreas. Radiology 138:211–213

Tersingni R, Toledo-Pereyra LH (1985) Surgical anatomy of the pancreas. In: Toledo-Pereyra LH (ed) The pancreas: principles of medical and surgical practice. Churchill Livingstone, New York

Trede M (1993) Embryology and surgical anatomy of the pancreas. In: Trede M, Carter DS (eds) Surgery of the pancreas. Churchill Livingstone, Edinburgh, pp 17–27

Van Hoe L, Gryspeerdt S, Vanbeckevoort D, et al. (1998a) Normal Vaterian sphincter complex: evaluation of morphology and contractility with dynamic single-shot MR cholangiography. AJR 170:1497–1500

Van Hoe L, Vanbeckevoort D, Van Steenbergen W (1998b) Atlas of cross-sectional and projective MR cholangio-pancreatography. Springer, Berlin Heidelberg New York

Varley PF, Rohrmann CA, Silvis SE, Vennes JA (1976) The normal endoscopic pancreatogram. Radiology 118:295–300

Vedantham S, Lu DS, Reber HA, Kadell B (1998) Small peripancreatic veins: improved assessment in pancreatic cancer patients using thin-section pancreatic-phase helical CT. AJR 170:377–383

Wachsberg RH (1993) Posterior superior pancreaticoduodenal vein: mimic of distal common bile duct at sonography AJR 160:1033–1037

Wang JT, Lin JT, Chuang CN, et al. (1990) Complete agenesis of the dorsal pancreas: a case report and review of the literature. Pancreas 5:493–497

Warshaw AL, Simeone JF, Schapiro RH, Flavin-Warshaw B (1990) Evaluation and treatment of the dominant dorsal duct syndrome (pancreas divisum redefined). Am J Surg 159:59–66

Weill F (1987) Ultrasonographie en pathologie digestive, Vigot, Paris

Williams PL, Warwick R (eds) (1980) The pancreas. In: Gray's anatomy, 36th British edn. Saunders, Philadelphia, pp 1368–1374

Winston CB, Mitchell DG, Outwater EK, Ehrlich SM (1995) Pancreatic signal intensity on T1-weighted fat saturation MR images: clinical correlation. JMRI 5:267–271

Yogi Y, Shibue T, Hashimoto S (1987) Annular pancreas detected in adult, diagnosed by endoscopic retrograde cholangiopancreatography: report of four cases. Gastroenterol Jpn 22:92–94

Zeman R, Vay L, Silverman P, et al. (1988) Pancreas divisum: thin section CT. Radiology 169:395–398

Zylak CJ, Pallie W (1981) Correlative anatomy and computed tomography: a module on the pancreas and posterior abdominal wall. Radiographics 1:61–84

4 Pathology of the Pancreas

G. KLÖPPEL and E. SCHLÜTER

CONTENTS

G. KLÖPPEL MD, PhD, Professor and Chairman, Klinikum der Christian-Albrechts-Universität zu Kiel, Department of Pathology, Michaelisstr. 11, D-24105 Kiel, Germany
E. SCHLÜTER, MD, PHD, Department of Pathology, Academic Hospital Jette, Free University of Brussels. Laarbeeklaan 101, B-1090 Brussels, Belgium

4.1 Congenital Anomalies

4.1.1 Agenesis and Hypoplasia

Complete absence of the pancreas is extremely rare and is usually associated with other malformations such as cardiac defects, diaphragmatic hernia, or gallbladder aplasia (WÖCKEL and SCHEIBNER 1977). Clinically, these patients present with diabetes mellitus, malabsorption, and severe fetal growth retardation. In partial agenesis, i.e., hypoplasia, which is likewise rare, either the body and tail or the head of the pancreas is absent, suggesting that the dorsal or the ventral anlage has failed to develop. Recently, it has been suggested that a mutation of the developmental protein IPF1 may be responsible for pancreatic agenesis, since a patient with complete absence of the pancreas was found to be homozygous for a point deletion in the IPF1 gene (STOFFERS et al. 1997).

4.1.2 Annular Pancreas

In annular pancreas, pancreatic tissue encircles and sometimes obstructs the descending part of the duodenum (Fig. 4.1). A total of 10% of the cases of duodenal stenosis in childhood are due to annular pancreas. The annulus represents the ventral part of the duodenal pancreas, which has remained fixed to the duodenum (MACLEAN 1979; STARCK 1965) as a result of retardation of rotation. A distinction is made between an extramural and an intramural type. In the extramural type, the annulus is drained by ducts running around the duodenum to join the main pancreatic duct. In the intramural type, pancreatic tissue is intermingled with muscle fibers in the duodenal wall and small ducts drain directly into the duodenum.

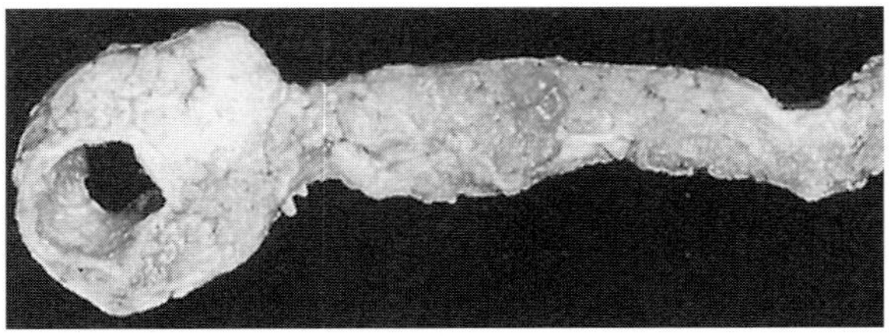

Fig. 4.1. Annular pancreas in a newborn: the duodenum is encircled by pancreatic tissue

4.1.3 Pancreas Divisum

Pancreas divisum is caused by an insufficient or incomplete fusion of the ventral and dorsal primordia of the pancreas. As a result, the dorsal duct of Santorini drains the majority of the gland (dorsal head, body, and tail), passing through the minor papilla, while the ventral duct of Wirsung drains the smaller ventral remnant. In unselected autopsy specimens, the incidence of pancreas divisum ranges from 4% to 10% (DELHAYE et al. 1985). In children, this malformation is usually silent. Adults may present with pancreatitis in the dorsal pancreas, probably because of intermittent relative obstruction at the minor papilla (GREGG 1977).

4.1.4 Abnormalities of the Pancreaticobiliary Junction

Marked variations in the anatomy of the ducts are seen at the pancreaticobiliary junction within the ampulla of Vater, with a complete separation of the orifices of the common bile duct and the major pancreatic duct at one end of the spectrum, and a long common channel at the other end.

4.1.5 Ectopic (Heterotopic) Pancreas

Ectopic pancreatic tissue has been noted in up to 15% of autopsy specimens (Feldman and Weinberg 1952). Most commonly, it is found in the stomach (25%–30%) and the duodenum (30%) (Fig. 4.2), followed by the jejunum, ileum, and Meckel's diverticulum (DOLAN et al. 1974). Uncommon localizations are the gallbladder (HORANYI and FÜSY 1963), liver (GADRAT et al. 1965), mesentery (KUBOTA 1955), spleen, and omentum. In trisomy 18, ectopic pancreatic tissue seems to be a frequent change (WARKANY et al. 1966).

In the bowel, ectopic pancreas presents as a small submucosal lump with a granular or ulcerated surface. Its diameter varies from some millimeters to several centimeters (2–4 cm). In more than 50% of cases it is located in the submucosa, in 25% in the muscular layer, and in 10% in the subserosal region (ELFRING and HÄSTBACKA 1965; Nicolesco and Velciu 1968). In at least one third of patients, the ectopic pancreas shows normal pancreatic tissue, while in the other cases it consists mainly of ducts intermingled with endocrine elements. Usually, one duct connects to the overlying mucosa through a nipple-like projection.

Ectopic pancreas usually remains asymptomatic, but occasionally it may result in stenosis, ulceration, bleeding, or invagination (JANSEN and ROTHEMUND 1965; MACKINNON and NASH 1957).

Pancreatic tissue with a normal exocrine and endocrine composition may be noted especially in mediastinal teratomas (HONICKY and de PAPP 1973; SCHLUMBERGER 1946; SUDA et al. 1984).

4.1.6 Congenital Cysts and Dysplastic Changes

Congenital cysts of the pancreas can be either single or multiple. Both types are uncommon, but, unlike solitary cysts (Fig. 4.3a), multiple cysts are usually associated with other congenital anomalies such as von Hippel-Lindau disease (CHENG et al. 1997; FISHMAN and BARTHOLOMEW 1979; NICOLESCO and VELCIU 1968; SEIFERT 1984) (Fig. 4.3b), or polycystic kidney disease. In these conditions, the cysts are of

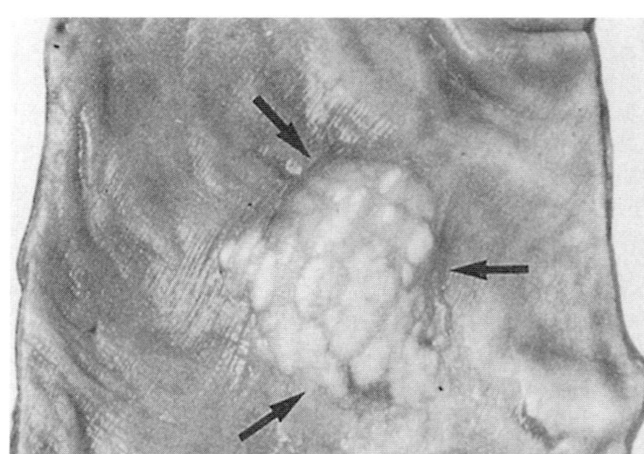

Fig. 4.2. Ectopic pancreas in the duodenum presenting as a submucosal nodule (*arrows*)

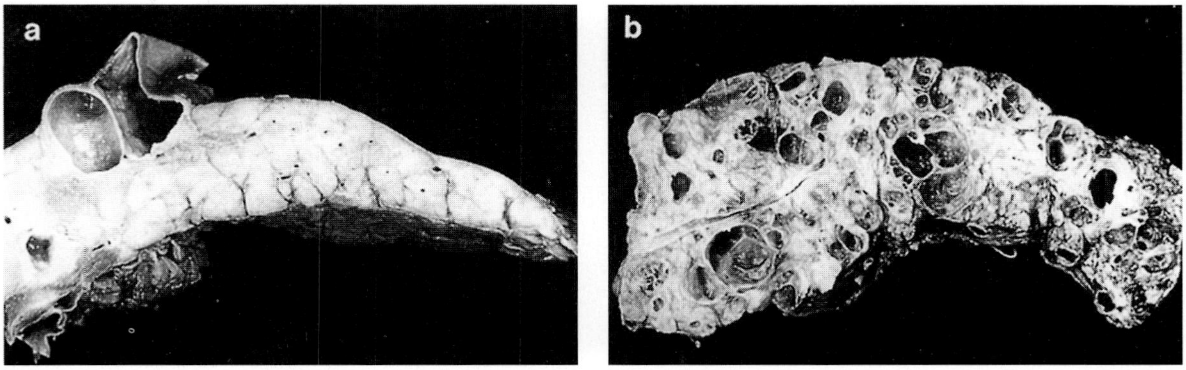

Fig. 4.3a,b. Congenital cysts of the pancreas. **a** Solitary cysts. **b** Multiple cysts in a left-sided resection specimen from a patient with von Hippel-Lindau disease

various sizes, filled with serous fluid and lined by cuboidal epithelium. Clinical symptoms or signs of exocrine pancreatic insufficiency are rare.

Polycystic dysplasia of the pancreas is seen in the Meckel-Gruber syndrome, Jeune's syndrome (JEUNE et al. 1955), Saldino-Noonan syndrome, and Ivemark's syndrome. Microcystic lesions, combined with multiple splenic islands in the pancreas, are a distinctive feature of trisomy 13 (HASHIDA et al. 1983).

Congenital enterogenous cysts are rare. These are gastrointestinal duplications, most often in the wall of the duodenum, but in rare cases they may lie in other parts of the pancreas.

4.2 Vascular and Traumatic Lesions

4.2.1 Vascular Lesions

4.2.1.1 Atherosclerosis

The severity of atherosclerosis in the pancreas correlates with that seen in the coronary arteries in about 85% of cases (POLLAK 1968). However, because of the extensive collateral circulation in the pancreas, atherosclerosis leads only in exceptional cases to ischemic changes in the pancreas.

4.2.1.2 Arteritis

Periarteritis nodosa almost always involves the pancreas (FROBOESE 1949), but ischemic pancreatic infarctions are uncommon. Arteritis of the pancreas may also be seen in other systemic diseases such as lupus erythematosus, scleroderma, and Wegener's granulomatosis.

4.2.2 Traumata

Penetrating injuries, blunt traumata, and operative complications should be differentiated. Penetrating shot or stab wounds frequently lead to rupture of the main pancreatic duct and/or the main vessels. Fistulae (50%), pseudocysts (10%), and hemorrhage are the usual complications (HESS 1976; THOMPSON and HINSHAW 1966; TORRANCE 1979).

Blunt traumata of the pancreas are based on the compression of the organ against the lumbar spine and lead to considerable destruction of the pancreatic tissue with bleeding or rupture of the main pancreatic duct (Fig. 4.4). In approximately 1%–2% of cases of blunt abdominal trauma the pancreas is involved (KÄUFER 1967). One third of cases concern children, with bicycle accidents being a particularly common cause (SCHEGA and DENNHARDT 1971). The mortality rate is about 40%. As late complications, fistulae, pseudocysts, abscesses, ileus, and thrombosis of the portal vein may develop.

Surgical damage to the pancreas occurs most commonly after gastrectomy, sphincterotomy, splenectomy, or biopsy of the pancreas. It results in acute pancreatitis with pseudocysts, hemorrhage, and/or fistulization.

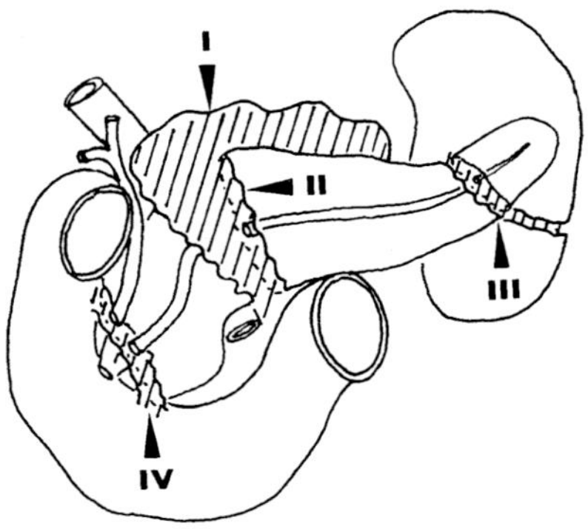

Fig. 4.4. Common types of injuries to the pancreas following blunt trauma. *I*, Retroperitoneal hematoma; *II*, prevertebral fracture of the body of the pancreas; *III*, blunt injury to the tail of the pancreas associated with rupture of the spleen; *IV*, disruption of duodenum with rupture of bile duct and pancreatic duct. [Adapted from Torrance (1979)]

4.3 Hereditary Diseases of the Pancreas

4.3.1 Cystic Fibrosis

Cystic fibrosis is the most common lethal autosomal recessive disease in Caucasians. The cystic fibrosis gene has been located at chromosome 7q31 and encodes the cystic fibrosis transmembrane conductance regulator (CFTR). This protein is involved in the regulation of secretory chloride channels (Stern 1997). Inadequate secretion of chloride is believed to cause insufficient hydration and increased viscosity of mucin in bronchi, pancreatic ducts, and other mucin-producing tissues. The high content of sodium, potassium, and chloride in the sweat, which is of diagnostic importance, is another sequela of a CFTR mutation.

Pathogenetically, all morphologic changes in cystic fibrosis, whether in the pancreas or elsewhere, are secondary to the high viscosity of the mucin (Klöppel 1983; Seifert and Klöppel 1984).

In the pancreas, the earliest microscopic lesions may be seen at birth. Gross changes, however, are not found until after 2–3 years of disease. The pancreas then reveals a more solid consistency and a more pronounced lobular appearance. Histologically, the pancreatic changes commence with ductular and acinar dilatations. These are followed by progressive fibrous and lipomatous atrophy of the parenchyma (Imrie et al. 1979) (Fig. 4.5). In late stages of the disease, which are reached by more than 80% of the patients today, the acinar tissue is largely replaced by fatty tissue and may contain some retention cysts of different sizes that are filled with white mucinous fluid (Seifert 1959; Stömmer 1980).

4.3.2 Lipomatous Atrophy (Shwachman-Diamond Syndrome)

Lipomatous hypertrophy with extensive atrophy of the exocrine acinar tissue and preservation of the islet system is found in Shwachman syndrome (Mack et al. 1996; Seifert 1984). The absence of acinar tissue leads to maldigestion and generalized growth retardation. These changes are associated with bone marrow dysfunction (neutropenia, anemia, and thrombocytopenia) and skeletal anomalies, such as metaphyseal dysostosis (Lebenthal and Shwachman 1977; Shwachman et al. 1964), and also occasionally with myelogenous leukemia (Caselitz et al. 1979). The syndrome is thought to be of genetic origin with autosomal recessive inheritance (Lebenthal and Shwachman 1977).

4.3.3 Hemochromatosis

Primary hemochromatosis is an inherited iron storage disease, while secondary hemochromatosis results from massive oral or parenteral iron uptake. The pancreas is involved in both conditions. In advanced stages of hemochromatosis, it shows a rusty color and increased consistency. Histological-

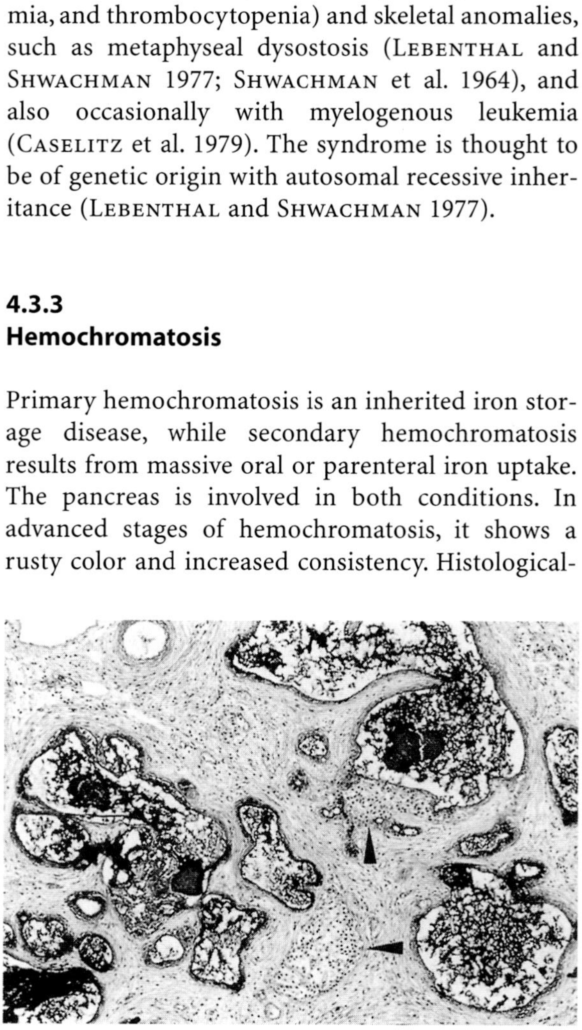

Fig. 4.5. Pancreas of a patient with end-stage cystic fibrosis of the pancreas: cystic dilatations of the pancreatic ducts by periodic acid–Schiff (PAS)-positive concretions. Acinar cells replaced by fibrosis. Islets are seen (*arrowheads*). PAS, ×125

ly, hemosiderin is found in the cytoplasm of the acinar and duct cells, but also in the b cells of the islets. The overload of ferritin molecules in the cells leads to atrophy of the acini and to inter- and intralobular fibrosis. In later stages of the disease, there is also b cell loss with concomitant development of diabetes. The most massive iron deposition in pancreatic acini is seen in neonatal hemochromatosis.

4.3.4 Hereditary Pancreatitis

Hereditary pancreatitis usually starts in childhood. It accounts for about 1%–2% of all cases of pancreatitis. The mode of inheritance is autosomal dominant with limited penetrance (80%) and no sex predilection. The genetic defect is located at 7q35 and concerns the trypsinogen gene. It is hypothesized that the mutated gene encodes a trypsin with an arginine to histidine substitution which, if prematurely activated in the pancreas, can no longer be inactivated by trypsin inhibitors. This defect leads to repeated episodes of acute pancreatitis, which eventually progress to chronic pancreatitis (Gorry et al. 1997; Whitcomb et al. 1996). Morphologically, hereditary pancreatitis is characterized in its late stage by parenchymal fibrosis, severe duct distortions and dilatations, and calcifications. An important point is that this type of pancreatitis is evidently complicated by the development of a pancreatic carcinoma in around 6% of patients.

4.4 Pancreatitis

4.4.1 Classification

The 1963 Marseilles classification differentiated pancreatitis on the basis of clinical features into: acute pancreatitis, relapsing acute pancreatitis, chronic relapsing pancreatitis, and chronic pancreatitis.

In 1984, again in Marseilles, this classification was revised and pancreatitis was differentiated according to its morphologic features into: (a) acute pancreatitis with mild or severe course, (b) chronic pancreatitis with diffuse or segmental fibrosis, with or without necrosis, and with or without calculi, and (c) obstructive pancreatitis (Gyr et al. 1984). However, this classification system was largely based on morphologic criteria, which in most instances cannot be assessed at the time of diagnosis. Consequently, a classification of pancreatitis was still needed that would consider both the clinical features and the morphologic findings. An important step towards this aim was taken during an expert meeting held in Atlanta in 1992. This conference succeeded in establishing a clinically based classification system for acute pancreatitis that also defines the morphologic basis of the disease (Bradley 1993). The classification distinguishes mild acute pancreatitis, i.e., acute pancreatitis with minimal organ dysfunction and an uneventful recovery, from severe acute pancreatitis, i.e., acute pancreatitis associated with organ failure and/or local complications, such as necrosis, abscess, or pseudocyst. The morphologic descriptions of acute pancreatitis given below will consider the definitions introduced by the Atlanta classification.

4.4.2 Acute Pancreatitis

4.4.2.1 Definition

Acute pancreatitis is an abruptly occurring necrotic and inflammatory process in and around the pancreas. The morphologic changes range from interstitial edema and minimal histologic evidence of necrosis (mild acute pancreatitis) to large confluent areas of necrosis and hemorrhage (severe acute pancreatitis). With the exception of infectious pancreatitis resulting from direct injury of the acinar cells by microorganisms, all types of acute pancreatitis, irrespective of their etiology, are due to autodigestion by pancreatic enzymes.

4.4.2.2 Epidemiology

The incidence of acute pancreatitis shows marked geographic variation. In Western countries, acute pancreatitis occurs in 5–15/100 000 inhabitants. The severe form accounts for approximately 20% of cases. In autopsy series, the frequency of fatal acute pancreatitis ranges from 0.18% to 1.65% (Dürr 1979; Höfler 1978). Over the past 20–30 years, the number of patients has doubled, probably due to increased alcohol consumption and the lower age at which people start drinking alcohol (Renner et al. 1985; Storck et al. 1976). Despite this increase, acute pancreatitis is still a rare disease, and in absolute numbers one can expect about 20–30 cases in 1000 autopsies.

Acute pancreatitis affects both sexes equally. In men, the maximum incidence is between the third and fifth decades, and in women in the fifth and sixth. This difference in the age distribution reflects the fact that the alcohol-related form is usually found in young men, whereas the gallstone-associated form predominates in women (Ammann 1976).

4.4.2.3 Etiology

The two most common causes of acute pancreatitis in Western countries are alcohol abuse and gallstone disease (Creutzfeldt and Schmidt 1976). Together they account for about 80% of cases. Rarer causes include shock, trauma, certain drugs, toxins, hypercalcemia, hyperlipidemia, pancreatic tumors, hereditary factors, and infections (mumps, Coxsackie B, cytomegalovirus, leptospirosis icterohemorrhagica, tuberculosis) (Capner et al. 1975; Imrie et al. 1985; Naficy et al. 1973; Witte and Schanzer 1968). In about 10% of patients, the cause remains unknown (idiopathic pancreatitis). Alcohol appears to cause acute pancreatitis only after continued abuse (Malagelada 1986), but the time of the damage cannot be predicted on the basis of the average amount of alcohol ingested over time. Nor is there a clear association between the severity of alcoholic liver disease and pancreatitis. In gallstone pancreatitis, initiation of the disease appears to result from gallstone migration from the gallbladder to the duodenum, with a temporary impaction at the ampulla of Vater (Acosta and Ledsma 1974).

If we try to relate the morphology of acute pancreatitis to its etiology, it seems that, except for infectious pancreatitis, all other causes lead to the same basic changes, i.e., primary autodigestive destruction of peripancreatic tissue and only later of pancreatic tissue. Only in infectious pancreatitis is primarily the pancreatic acinar tissue damaged. We therefore believe that infectious and noninfectious pancreatitis have a different pathogenesis.

4.4.2.4 Pathogenesis of Noninfectious Pancreatitis

It is not yet known how alcohol abuse and biliary disease, the most common causes of noninfectious pancreatitis, induce autodigestive tissue necrosis in and around the pancreas. The two most commonly discussed working hypotheses at present postulate either primary damage to the acinar cells or duct obstruction combined with reflux of bile (Steer 1989). A third hypothesis is based on a mutation of the trypsinogen gene, which has been discovered in hereditary pancreatitis (see Sect. 4.3.4).

The acinar cell damage theory focuses on a complex disturbance of acinar cell function culminating in deranged intracellular compartmentation and uncontrolled liberation of enzymes. These alterations could lead to intracellular enzyme activation by lysosomal hydrolases (Scheele et al. 1984; Steer 1989), and/or sudden effusion of enzymes into the interstitial space and adipose tissue (Klöppel et al. 1986). As these changes appear to occur predominantly in the peripheral acinar cells of a lobule, and as these cells are most remote from the artery supplying a lobule, it is conceivable that the effects of the different etiologic factors are mediated by microcirculatory changes.

The duct obstruction–bile reflux theory (based on Opie's common channel theory; Opie 1901) postulates that temporary obstruction of a common bile duct and the main pancreatic duct by a gallstone causes increased intraductal pressure and/or ampullary incontinence, with duodenopancreatic and bile reflux resulting in activation of pancreatic proenzymes and their leakage from small ducts into the interstitial space. Although there is no doubt that migration of gallstones is associated with the induction of pancreatitis, it has not been possible so far to obtain definite functional and morphologic proof that the pathogenesis of human acute pancreatitis is due to ductal obstruction.

Whatever the pathogenetic mechanisms that lead to autodigestion, the resulting damage pattern is the same for most (>95%) patients. The pancreatitis in these patients is usually associated with alcoholism and gallstone disease. The common damage pattern („type 1 necrosis pattern“) is characterized by interstitial fatty-tissue necrosis and its sequelae, i.e., necrosis of adjacent vessels (with hemorrhage), acinar cells, and ducts. Fatty tissue necrosis is probably caused by lipase (one of the few pancreatic enzymes that need no activation) after an abrupt effusion of zymogens from peripheral acinar cells into interstitial space (Klöppel et al. 1986; Schmitz-Moormann 1981). Whether fat necrosis depends on the action of lipase alone or the combined action of lipase and other enzymes, such as trypsin and phospholipase A2, is still uncertain, but it seems that proenzymes become activated during this process and may help to destroy the surrounding tissues.

Necrosis patterns that are distinct from the one described above are rare, but may occur. The „type 2 necrosis pattern“ seems to occur in patients with prolonged circulatory failure. It starts with ductal necrosis and proceeds to periductal inflammation (Foulis 1980). It is possible that this lesion is initiated by the activation of trypsinogen via autocatalyzation in precipitates of pancreatic secretions after impairment of all secretory processes in the exocrine pancreas due to a severe extrapancreatic disease.

4.4.2.5 Pathogenesis of Infectious Pancreatitis

The pathogenesis of infectious pancreatitis relates to the direct cytotoxic effect of microorganisms on the acinar cells. This leads to necrosis of these cells accompanied by an inflammatory response („type 3 necrosis pattern“).

4.4.2.6 Macroscopy

In mild pancreatitis with the type 1 necrosis pattern, the surface of the usually edematous gland shows spotty fatty tissue necrosis (Fig. 4.6a). Hemorrhage and intraparenchymal necrosis are absent. In severe acute pancreatitis, the chalky white fat necroses on the surface of the pancreas are large and confluent and alternate with hemorrhages (Fig. 4.6b). Disseminated foci of fat necrosis may also be present in the bursa omentalis, omentum, mesentery, and deep retroperitoneum. The peritoneal cavity contains turbid or hemorrhagic fluid. The cut surface of the pancreas usually displays only a few hemorrhagic foci associated with a network of fat necrosis between the lobuli. In the most severe cases, however, necrosis also involves parts of the lobular parenchyma, often transforming these areas into firm hemorrhagic-necrotic masses. Occasionally, necrosis may also affect the main pancreatic duct or the large tributaries, causing rupture. The pattern and distribution of necrosis differ from patient to patient, and in some patients necrosis may be present in only a portion of the gland.

The gross changes in a pancreas with the type 2 necrosis pattern do not seem to differ clearly from those seen in the usual acute pancreatitis described above. In infectious pancreatitis with the type 3 necrosis pattern, the gland may be swollen but lacks grossly visible autodigestive changes such as fat necrosis.

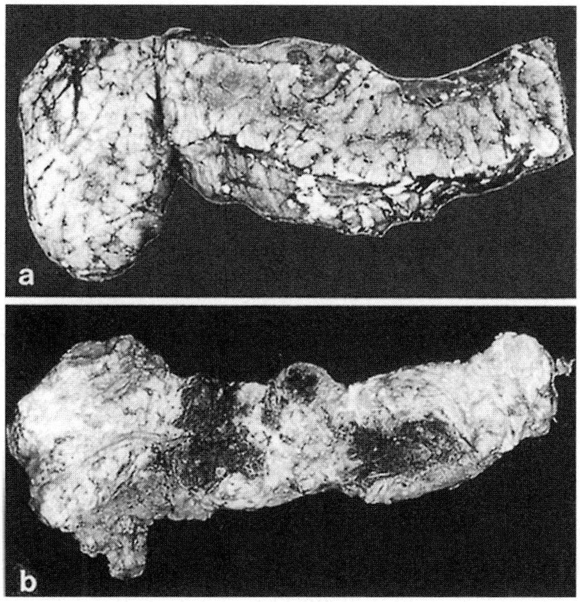

Fig. 4.6a,b. Acute pancreatitis. **a** Mild form with edema and spotty peripancreatic and intrapancreatic fatty tissue necrosis. **b** Severe form with disseminated intrapancreatic fat necrosis and hemorrhage

4.4.2.7 Microscopy

4.4.2.7.1 Type 1 Necrosis Pattern

In patients with mild pancreatitis, disseminated small peripancreatic fat necroses with or without interstitial edema are usually the only changes found (Klöppel et al. 1984). In severe pancreatitis, the peripancreatic tissue shows large fat necroses, while in the pancreatic parenchyma areas of necrosis alternate with unaffected regions, where only interstitial edema is present (Fig. 4.7). Intrapancreatic necrosis develops in the interlobular fatty tissue and may be so severe that the lobuli are embraced by confluent fat necrosis. Fat necrosis may also involve small veins and venules, leading to swelling of their walls, infiltration by granulocytes, thrombosis, and eventually necrosis, rupture, and hemorrhage. Arterial thrombosis is much less frequent, but may result in panlobular ischemic necrosis. Destruction of single interlobular ducts and peripheral acinar cells are further sequelae of expanding fat necrosis, but it is often striking how well preserved these structures are despite their proximity to fat necrosis. Intact acinar cells at the margin of fat necrosis usually form so-called tubular complexes, i.e., acini with widened lumina which may be filled with periodic acid–Schiff

(PAS)-positive secretions. Islets are only affected in lobuli with extensive necrotic changes. The necrotic areas are demarcated by granulocytes and macrophages.

4.4.2.7.2
Type 2 Necrosis Pattern

The type 2 necrosis pattern is characterized by disseminated ductal and periductal necroses which outnumber the foci of fat necrosis and, more importantly, may even be present without any fat necrosis (Foulis 1980; Kimura and Ohtsubo 1989). Ductal necrosis appears to start with a precipitation of eosinophilic secretions in small and medium-sized interlobular ducts, which then become infiltrated by granulocytes, although still lined by intact epithelium. The next step is necrosis of part of the duct epithelium with rupture of the duct wall (Fig. 4.8). This leads to periductal necrosis with an extensive acute inflammatory infiltrate extending through the interstitial spaces. In advanced periductal necrosis, the duct is replaced by necrotic material. Despite this heavy inflammatory process, the acinar tissue remains largely unaffected. Bacteria have so far not been identified in the lumina of the affected ducts. It seems, however, that these patients may easily develop purulent peritonitis (Kimura and Ohtsubo 1989).

4.4.2.7.3
Type 3 Necrosis Pattern

The type 3 necrosis pattern is characterized by scattered acinar cell necrosis without any concomitant fat necrosis or ductal necrosis. This type of necrosis signifies an infection either by certain viruses, such as mumps or Coxsackie B (Jenson et al. 1980; Silbert 1975), or by bacteria, as in the case of leptospirosis icterohemorrhagica or tuberculosis. The composition of the inflammatory infiltrate depends on the nature of the microorganism.

4.4.2.8 Immunocytochemical and Ultrastructural Findings

Immunostaining of the normal human pancreas for enzymes such as amylase, lipase, phospholipase A2, trypsin, and chymotrypsin strongly labels the acinar cells (Aho et al. 1983; Klöppel et al. 1986; Nevalainen et al. 1983; Willemer and Adler 1989; Willemer et al. 1989). In severe acute pancreatitis with the type 1 necrosis pattern, the staining intensity differs from cell to cell, with some acinar cells entirely negative for enzymes and others with a normal enzyme content (Fig. 4.9). Most enzyme-negative acinar cells are found at the periphery of lobuli adjoining fat necrosis (Klöppel et al. 1986). The acinar lumina lined by these cells may contain enzyme-positive secretions. Electron microscopically, the acinar cells adjacent to necrosis are small and severely degranulated (Bockman et al. 1987; Klöppel et al. 1986; Willemer and Adler 1989), with the remaining zymogen granules irregularly distributed in the cytoplasm and along the cell membrane. Some acinar cells display large autophagic vacuoles containing floccular material and remnants of membranes and zymogen granules (Willemer et al. 1989). Acinar lumina may be filled with fine fibrillar material, probably representing secreted pancreatic enzymes, and the same material may also be observed in interstitial spaces (Aho et al. 1982). Occasionally, the acinar lumina contain lethally damaged acinar cells and cellular debris. The epithe-

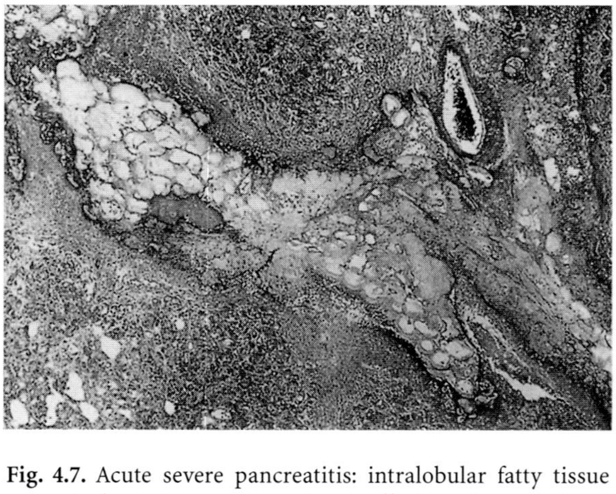

Fig. 4.7. Acute severe pancreatitis: intralobular fatty tissue necrosis (type 1 necrosis pattern) affecting the peripheral regions of the neighboring lobules. H&E, ×40

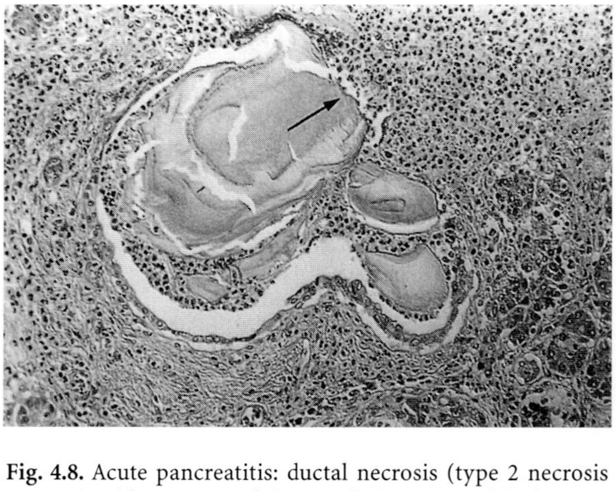

Fig. 4.8. Acute pancreatitis: ductal necrosis (type 2 necrosis pattern) with rupture of duct wall (*arrow*) and leukocytes infiltrating the interstitial space. H&E, ×125

lial lining of the duct system appears to be preserved, even in those regions where most of the acinar cells are damaged and infiltrated by granulocytes. Some of the duct cells display large lysosomes containing debris from membranes and zymogen granules.

4.4.2.9 Sequential Changes and Outcome

The resolution and outcome of fat necrosis depend on its localization and size (Fig. 4.10). Small foci of peripancreatic fat necrosis (<1 cm) resolve entirely. The necrotic material rich in lipids is phagocytosed by macrophages which are transformed to foam cells and later may be replaced by small foci of fibrotic tissue. The liquefied necrotic content of larger peripancreatic fat necroses exceeding 2–4 cm in diameter and often containing hemorrhagic material is demarcated by a rim of macrophages and also may be slowly reabsorbed by these cells. In those necrotic areas (>5 cm) that do not resolve spontaneously, the lining macrophages are replaced by a thin layer of granulation tissue within 10–20 days after the onset of the disease. After 20–30 days, the granulation tissue, rich in hemosiderin, forms a fibrotic capsule which gradually increases in thickness and forms a grossly visible wall (TRAPNELL 1971). The fully developed pseudocyst is round to ovoid and usually attached to the pancreas. The fact that many of the pseudocysts contain pancreatic juice suggests communications with the pancreatic duct system. This, in particular, may be the case in those pseudocysts which eventually increase in size, causing compression and/or perforation of structures such as the bile duct, duodenum, stomach, vessels, and peritoneum. Most pseudocysts occur in or around the head of the pancreas (SUGAWA and WALT 1979). If fat necrosis becomes infected with (mostly gut-derived) bacteria, infection usually takes place early in pseudocyst development, i.e., at the time (days 4–20) when the liquefied necrotic areas are only demarcated by a rim of macrophages or a thin layer of granulation tissue. Infection of the peritoneal cavity leads to purulent peritonitis.

Necrotic areas within the pancreas originating from interlobular fat necroses with hemorrhage usually resolve slowly and may induce interlobular fibrosis. If this process, which we term the necrosis-fibrosis sequence (KLÖPPEL and MAILLET 1992), takes place repeatedly, acute pancreatitis may evolve into chronic pancreatitis (KLÖPPEL and MAILLET 1991a, 1992).

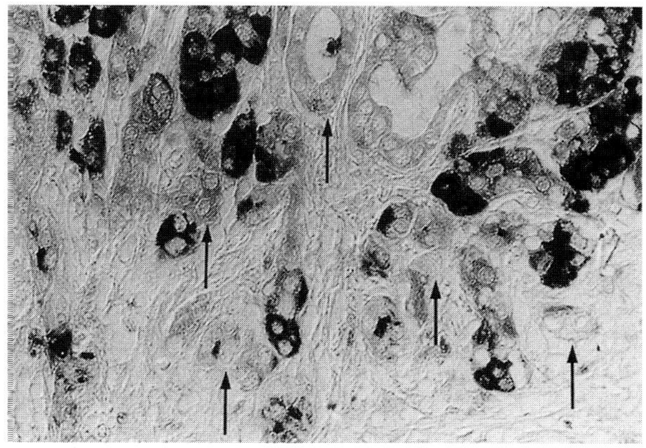

Fig. 4.9. Acute pancreatitis: pancreatic lobule adjacent to fat necrosis with severe degranulation (*arrows*) of numerous acinar cells. Immunostaining for trypsin. H&E, ×250

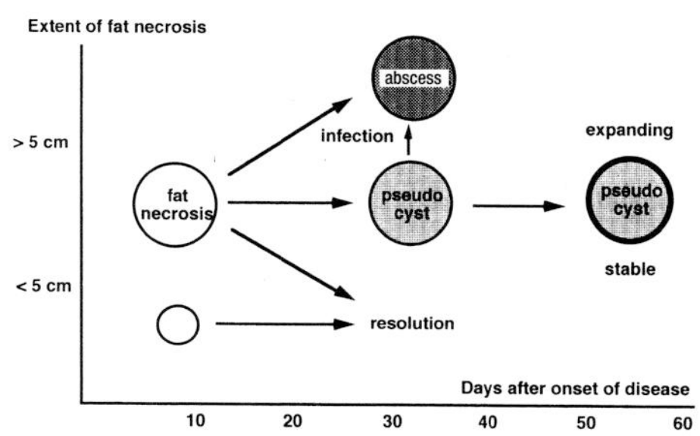

Fig. 4.10. Natural history of fat necrosis in acute pancreatitis

4.4.3 Chronic Pancreatitis

4.4.3.1 Definition

Chronic pancreatitis is an irreversible and irregular scarring of glandular parenchyma due to inflammatory processes involving the duct system. If progressive, it leads to loss of pancreatic exocrine and endocrine function.

4.4.3.2 Epidemiology

In Western countries, chronic pancreatitis affects predominantly young to middle-aged men (range 25–50 years). Chronic pancreatitis is an uncommon disease with an autopsy incidence between 0.18% and 2.8% (BECKER 1981; KLÖPPEL 1986; SARLES et al. 1976; UYS et al. 1973) and a clinical incidence of about 4/100 000 inhabitants (Worning 1990). Over the past 20 years, its incidence has been rising (Klöppel 1986).

4.4.3.3 Etiology

In Western countries, chronic alcohol abuse is the main cause of chronic pancreatitis (Marks 1990). Approximately 70%–80% of the patients presenting with chronic pancreatitis are young to middle-aged men who are heavy drinkers (Ammann et al. 1984; Durbec and Sarles 1978; Mössner 1993; Worning 1984). In approximately 25% of patients, no cause can be detected (idiopathic; Layer and Singer 1990). In rare cases, chronic pancreatitis is due to hyperparathyroidism or is of hereditary origin. In tropical countries, and especially in India, the development of chronic pancreatitis is probably related to nutritional factors (protein malnutrition, consumption of cassava or tapioca, etc.).

4.4.3.4 Pathogenesis of Alcoholic Chronic Pancreatitis

Several theories have been put forward to explain the pathogenesis of alcoholic chronic pancreatitis. The most popular hypothesis is that of Sarles, who suggested that chronic ethanol consumption increases the protein concentration in the pancreatic juice with subsequent precipitation of plug-forming secretions in the ducts, which later calcify (Sarles et al. 1976). More recently, Sarles' group (Multigner et al. 1985; Sarles et al. 1965, 1990) identified a protein in pancreatic juice that prevented $CaCO_3$ precipitation and was therefore called lithostatin (formerly pancreatic stone protein). It is thought that secretion of an abnormal lithostatin due to either an acquired or an inherited defect in its biosynthesis contributes to the calcification of protein plugs in the pancreatic ducts. The formation of stones leads in turn to duct obstruction and ulceration of duct epithelium, two mechanisms that cause acinar atrophy and fibrosis upstream of the obstruction, as well as periductular inflammation. Although this hypothesis is attractive, it has been criticized for several reasons. Firstly, the findings concerning altered lithostatin biosynthesis and function in chronic pancreatitis have not been universally confirmed (Hayakawa et al. 1995; Schmiegel 1993; Schmiegel et al. 1990). Secondly, the hypothesis only recognizes chronic pancreatitis as an alcohol-induced disease and neglects the fact that acute pancreatitis may also be caused by alcohol (Klöppel et al. 1986; Marks and Bornman 1994; Renner et al. 1985; Seligson et al. 1982). Thirdly, alcoholic acute and chronic pancreatitis have many features in common, such as clinical symptoms and the presence of pseudocysts. Fourthly, in alcoholic acute pancreatitis, no preexistent changes due to chronic pancreatitis have been found, whereas the pancreas of patients with chronic pancreatitis may show signs of acute pancreatitis, such as autodigestive tissue necrosis (Klöppel and Maillet 1991b; Uys et al. 1973). Finally, in its early stages, chronic pancreatitis lacks calcifications (Ammann et al. 1996). The questions that are not answered by the plug hypothesis have found special consideration in the concept of a necrosis-fibrosis sequence (Comfort et al. 1946; Klöppel and Maillet 1993). This theory postulates that alcoholic chronic pancreatitis is the result of relapsing severe acute pancreatitis (Ammann et al. 1996; Klöppel and Maillet 1993). The resorption of large areas of fat necrosis and hemorrhagic necrosis, which are the main events in severe acute (necrotizing) pancreatitis (Klöppel and Maillet 1992), induce fibrosis, possibly through the action of growth factors such as TGFα and TGFβ (Korc et al. 1994; van Laethem et al. 1995). The fibrosis develops primarily in the perilobular space, where fat necrosis and most of the hemorrhagic necrosis occur (Klöppel and Maillet 1992). Perilobular fibrosis in turn affects the structure of the interlobular ducts, gradually creating duct dilations and strictures. In these altered ducts, the flow of secretions is most likely impaired, a situation that may trigger the spontaneous precipitation of proteins with subsequent calcification. In addition, the impaired and eventually interrupted flow of pancreatic secretions leads to fibrotic replacement of the acinar cells upstream from the occluded duct, and finally results in intralobular fibrosis.

Although the necrosis-fibrosis sequence nicely explains the perilobular fibrosis pattern, the patchy distribution of fibrosis, and the late occurrence of calcifications in the pancreas of patients with alcoholic chronic pancreatitis, certain questions still need to be answered. Firstly, it is difficult to reconcile the fact that the necrosis-fibrosis sequence also holds true for the primary painless chronic pancreatitis that may be observed in 5%–10% of alcoholics (Bank 1986; DiMagno et al. 1993; Tabata et al. 1993). Secondly, biliary acute pancreatitis, which may occasionally be as severe as alcoholic pancreatitis, virtually never progresses to chronic pancreatitis.

A third hypothesis, called the „toxic-metabolic hypothesis", was put forth by Bordalo and colleagues (BORDALO et al. 1984; NORONHA et al. 1981). This hypothesis postulates that chronic alcohol consumption induces progressive acinar lipid deposition, with acinar atrophy and intrapancreatic fibrosis, by exerting direct toxic and metabolic effects on the acinar cells. Because the described pancreatic changes, particularly the fatty degeneration of acinar cells, have not been confirmed by others, the significance of this concept for the pathogenesis of alcoholic chronic pancreatitis seems to be minor.

The fourth hypothesis, the „oxidative stress hypothesis" (BRAGANZA 1983), postulates that oxidative stress in pancreatic acinar cells induced by excess free radicals causes a blockade of the intracellular pathway, fusion of lysosomal and zymogenic compartments, and membrane lipid oxidation. These events then lead to an inflammatory response. The hypothesis focuses on possible functional disturbances underlying acinar failure, but fails to explain the particular fibro-inflammatory process that characterizes chronic pancreatitis.

4.4.3.5 Pathogenesis of Nonalcoholic Chronic Pancreatitis

The pathogenesis of the various types of chronic pancreatitis summarized under the term nonalcoholic chronic pancreatitis is not known. In particular, we do not know the exact mechanisms leading to hereditary, idiopathic, autoimmune, or tropical pancreatitis. Interesting recent findings, however, have shed new light on the pathogenesis of chronic pancreatitis associated with a hereditary or autoimmune background (see Sects. 4.3.4 and 4.4.4.2).

4.4.3.6 Macroscopy

In early chronic pancreatitis, the gland is always unevenly affected. Grossly, the affected parts are usually enlarged and indurated. On the cut surface, these areas show coarse lobulation or nodular scarring. If the fibrotic area lies in the periphery of the gland, duct irregularities (with occasional calculus formation) may only be found in the duct tributaries that are involved in scarring. In about half of the cases, pseudocysts (BRADLEY 1990) or foci of recent necrosis are present in the vicinity of the scars (KLÖPPEL and MAILLET 1991b).

In advanced chronic pancreatitis, the pancreas is hard and usually shows an irregular contour due to uneven parenchymal scarring with shrinkage. The cut surface has a patchy grayish appearance with loss of normal lobulation. The degree of changes in the main duct, i.e., irregular sacculations and distortions, and the frequency of calculi closely correlate with the extent of parenchymal fibrosis (Fig. 4.11). The calculi vary in diameter from less than 1 mm to more than 1 cm. They are commonly impacted in the ducts and are hence difficult to remove. Spontaneous regression of calcification may occur (AMMANN et al. 1988). Fibrosis in the head of the pancreas may cause a long, tapered stricture of the common bile duct. Thick-walled pseudocysts usually attached to the pancreas are present in a quarter to half of the cases (Fig. 4.12). These vary in size (3–10 cm). The pseudocysts may be connected with the duct system and may infiltrate major portal veins, causing thrombosis, bleeding, and, occasionally, disseminated fat necrosis with subcutaneous nodular panniculitis, polyarthritis, and necrotic bone marrow lesions.

4.4.3.7 Microscopy

In the early stage of the disease, the affected portions of the pancreas show a distinct interlobular (perilobular) fibrosis. Only occasionally does fibrosis involve the entire lobule (intralobular fibrosis) at this stage. The intralobular ducts that are surrounded by fibrotic tissue are distorted and may contain eosinophilic protein concretions. Their epithelium is cuboidal and sometimes hyperplastic. Moderate numbers of lymphocytes, plasma cells, and macrophages are present, either as local collections or diffusely scattered throughout the fibrous tissue. The perilobular fibrosis may also contain patches of resolving fat necrosis surrounded by macrophages and granulocytes. In addition, pseudocysts may be formed. The acinar lobules display well-preserved acinar cells and islets.

In advanced chronic pancreatitis, fibrosis between the lobules, as well as within the lobules, is more widespread and pronounced than in the early stage of the disease. However, there may still be areas that are only slightly affected. The ducts are irregularly distorted and distended, the lumen often being filled with plugs of protein or impacted calculi (Fig. 4.13). Their epithelium is either atrophic or completely replaced by fibrous tissue. Occasionally, a severely dilated duct may form a small retention cyst. Intralobular fibrosis results in a disorderly arrangement of islets, blood vessels, nerves, and remnants of atrophic acinar cells. The islets aggregate and vary in

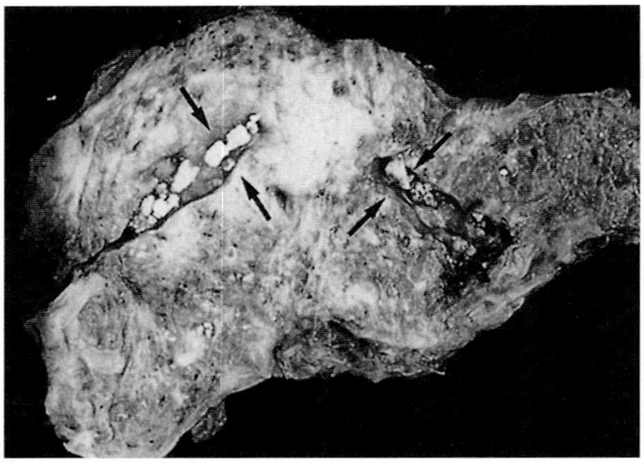

Fig. 4.11. Advanced stage of chronic pancreatitis with irregular scarring in the head of the pancreas and severe distortion of the main pancreatic duct. Note the numerous calculi in the pancreatic duct (*arrows*)

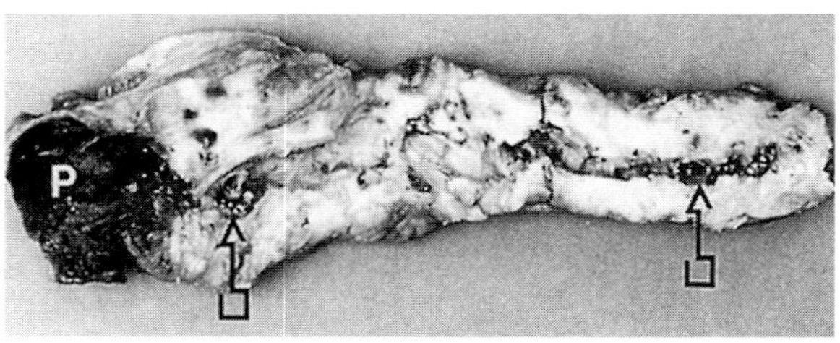

Fig. 4.12. Advanced chronic pancreatitis with calculi in the irregularly dilated main duct (*arrows*), sclerosis of the parenchyma, and pseudocyst (*P*) filled with hemorrhagic debris in the head region

size, and often intra-islet fibrosis causes their cells to separate into a ribbon-like arrangement. The intima of the small arteries is thickened and the nerve trunks are prominent and irregularly distributed within the fibrous tissue. Characteristically, there is only scant lymphocytic infiltration, which is predominantly periductal, but occasionally perineural.

4.4.3.8 Complications

Local complications are pseudocysts (50%), obstruction of the common bile duct (29%), and, in rare cases, obstructions of the small and large intestine due to inflammation of their walls. Systemic complications may be exocrine failure of the gland resulting in maldigestion. Approximately 20%–60% of patients develop diabetes mellitus.

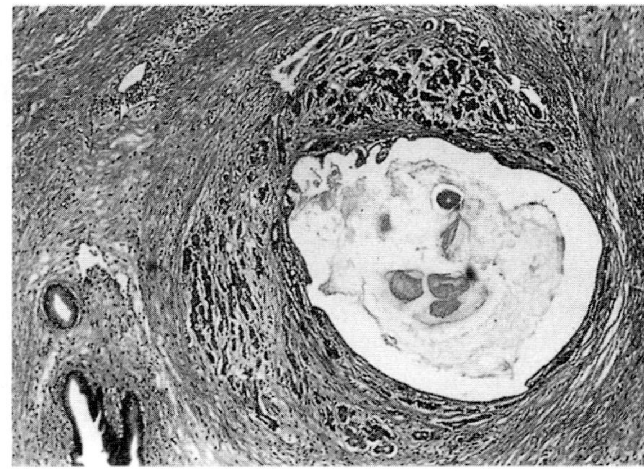

Fig. 4.13. Advanced chronic pancreatitis: dilated duct containing calcified secretions and surrounded by fibrotic tissue and some acinar remnants. H&E, ×65

4.4.3.9 Prognosis

About 20%–30% of patients die during a period of 6–8 years following diagnosis due to marasmus, alcoholic cirrhosis of the liver, local complications, or due to extrapancreatic carcinomas.

4.4.4 Special Types of Chronic Pancreatitis

4.4.4.1 Hereditary Pancreatitis

Hereditary pancreatitis is discussed in more detail elsewhere (see Sect. 4.3.4).

4.4.4.2 Autoimmune Chronic Pancreatitis

Chronic pancreatitis associated with autoimmune diseases such as autoimmune sialadenitis, primary sclerosing cholangitis, or idiopathic inflammatory bowel disease, has been described in a few patients (Ball et al. 1950; Kawagushi et al. 1991; Lászik et al. 1988; Lysy and Goldin 1992; Marrano et al. 1996; Seyrig et al. 1985; Sjögren et al. 1979; Sood et al. 1995; Waldram et al. 1975). The pancreatic changes are characterized by an intense mononuclear inflammation around interlobular ducts, leading to periductal fibrosis and, occasionally, ductal destruction. Calcifications do not occur. In some cases, the inflammation also involves the intrapancreatic segment of the bile duct. The ductal lesions may resemble those seen in the liver in primary sclerosing cholangitis or the salivary glands in autoimmune sialadenitis (Sjögren's syndrome). We termed this type of pancreatic inflammation chronic duct-destructive pancreatitis (Ectors et al. 1997). Because we also observed chronic duct destructive pancreatitis in patients without any associated autoimmune disease, we assume that this type of chronic pancreatitis is the morphologic substrate of many cases of idiopathic chronic pancreatitis. Clinically and macroscopically, chronic duct destructive pancreatitis is commonly mistaken for carcinoma. To date, not much is known about its course and outcome.

4.4.4.3 *Tropical Pancreatitis*

So-called tropical pancreatitis has been described particularly in India, Indonesia, and Nigeria and seems to be related to low-protein diets combined with an as yet unknown toxin (Viswanathan 1980; Zuidema 1959). Grossly and microscopically, tropical pancreatitis is indistinguishable from the classic chronic pancreatitis of Western countries. In tropical countries, chronic pancreatitis is predominantly a disease of youth, often already starting in the first decade of life. It is also more common in men than in women.

4.4.4.4 *Obstructive Chronic Pancreatitis*

The most common cause of duct obstruction is a tumor in the head of the pancreas. Rare causes include intraductal tumors, some cystic and endocrine tumors, and congenital or acquired strictures of the pancreatic duct. Focal obstruction of the main pancreatic duct leads to duct dilatation proximal to the stenosis, as well as atrophy and, finally, disappearance of the acinar cells with replacement by fibrous tissue. Formation of calculi in the dilated duct system is very rare and only occurs in cases with incomplete obstruction.

4.4.4.5 *Chronic Pancreatitis Due to Duodenal Wall Cysts*

Duodenal wall cysts are rare, single, or multiple lesions occurring in the submucosal or intramuscular layers of the duodenum in close proximity to the ampulla of Vater and the intrapancreatic portion of the common bile duct (Fig. 4.14). Histologically, they are lined by columnar mucin-producing cells and may represent heterotopic gastrointestinal structures or pancreatic tissue (Stolte et al. 1982, 1983). Chronic inflammation within the heterotopic tissue may lead to submucosal cyst formation, compression of the common bile duct and chronic inflammatory changes in the surrounding pancreatic tissues (Holstege et al. 1985; Stolte et al. 1983). Clinically, this results in pain, vomiting, and eventually jaundice.

4.4.5 Pancreatic Lobular Fibrosis in Elderly Persons

With increasing age the pancreas may show areas with lobular fibrosis, often combined with some degree of lipomatosis. These alterations are closely associated with ductal changes consisting in mucinous hypertrophy and ductal papillary hyperplasia obstructing the duct lumen. It is therefore most likely that the lobular pancreatic fibrosis in elderly persons is the result of obstructions of small ductal tributaries by nonneoplastic changes in the duct epithelium. The occurrence of small calculi in single secondary ducts of the pancreas in elderly persons also seems to be related to the above-mentioned duct changes (Nagai and Ohtsubo 1984). The latter observations are of particular interest for the pathogenesis of calculus formation in the pancreas (pancreatic lithiasis).

4.5 Pancreatic Pathology in Diabetes Mellitus

Diabetes mellitus is a syndrome of heterogeneous pathogenesis. The syndrome is characterized by impaired utilization of carbohydrates and altered metabolism of fat and proteins due to absolute or relative insulin deficiency.

Between 98% and 99% of cases of diabetes are cases of so-called primary diabetes, including insulin-dependent (IDDM, or type 1) and non-insulin-dependent (NIDDM, or type 2) diabetes mellitus. Type 2 diabetes is ten times more common than type 1. As a secondary event, diabetes occurs due to chronic pancreatitis, hemochromatosis, cystic fibrosis, acromegaly, Cushing's syndrome, and glucagon-secreting endocrine tumors.

From a morphologic point of view, the islet changes associated with the various types of diabetes

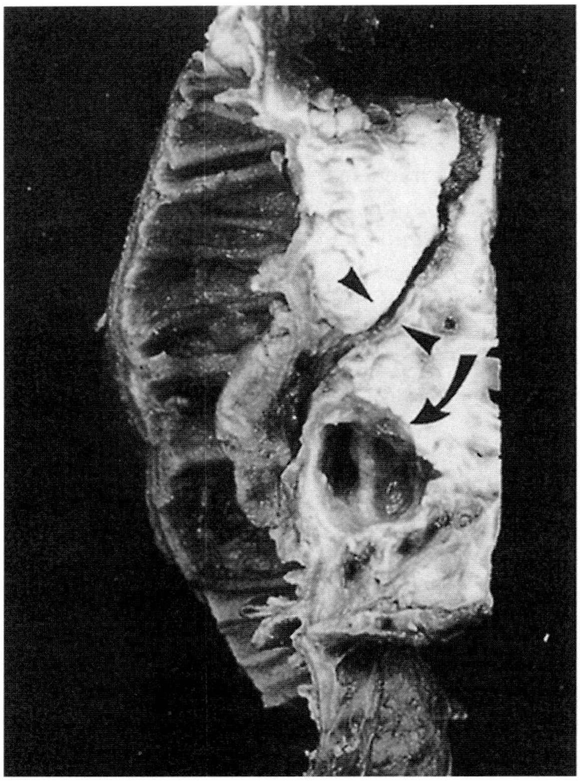

Fig. 4.14. Duodenal wall cyst in the region of the ampulla of Vater (*arrow*). The adjacent pancreatic tissue shows intensive scarring with stenosis of the bile duct (*arrowheads*)

can be divided into those with and those without severe (to absolute) b cell loss. Severe b cell loss is found in type 1 diabetes, while islets without a severe loss of b cells are encountered in type 2 diabetes and in secondary forms of diabetes. A hallmark of the islet changes in type 2 diabetes is the deposition of amylin (islet amyloidosis). A special feature of the pancreas in type 1 diabetes with long-standing disease is the atropy of the entire gland. This does not occur in type 2 diabetes. For a more detailed description of the pancreatic changes in diabetes mellitus and the pathogenesis of the different types, the reader is referred to a recent review (Klöppel et al. 1998).

4.6 Exocrine Pancreatic Tumors

4.6.1 General Considerations and Classification

Epithelial neoplasms of the pancreas include tumors that arise from ductal, acinar, or endocrine cells. Histologic typing of pancreatic exocrine tumors reveals that 80%–90% of all tumors of the pancreas are ductal adenocarcinomas. This tumor, therefore, is the prototype of pancreatic cancer and is intended whenever pancreatic cancer is discussed. All other epithelial tumors are uncommon, but they include a number of neoplasms with special morphologic and biologic features. Nonepithelial tumors of the pancreas are exceedingly rare (Lüttges et al. 1997; Solcia et al. 1997).

The recently published World Health Organization (WHO) classification of exocrine pancreatic tumors (Klöppel et al. 1996) is used in this chapter (Table 4.1). It divides the tumors on the basis of their histologic composition and biologic behavior into benign tumors, borderline tumors (uncertain malignant potential), and malignant tumors.

4.6.2 Serous Cystic Tumor

Serous cystic tumor is a cystic neoplasm composed of multiple, usually small cysts (1–2 mm) which are lined by cuboidal epithelium with clear, glycogen-rich cytoplasm. The majority of serous cystic tumors are benign. Malignant tumors (serous cystadenocarcinoma) are very rare (George et al. 1989; Yoshima et al. 1992). Serous cystadenoma can be divided into a microcystic and an oligocystic-macrocystic type (Solcia et al. 1997). The serous microcystic type occurs almost exclusively in elderly women in their sixth and seventh decade of life (Becker et al. 1965; Bogomoletz et al. 1980). Usually, the tumor is found incidentally, either at laparotomy or at autopsy. It accounts for 1% or less of pancreatic exocrine tumors and comprises 4%–10% of all cystic lesions of the pancreas (Didolkar et al. 1975). The oligocystic-macrocystic type affects both sexes equally, and is usually also an incidental finding, but may occasionally compress the common bile duct (Egawa et al. 1994; Lewandrowski et al. 1992). Serous cystic tumors account for 1% of all exocrine tumors and 4%–10% of all cystic lesions of the pancreas (Didolkar et al. 1975).

Macroscopically, serous microcystic adenoma is a large multiloculated cystic tumor (size range 6–11 cm), containing watery fluid and displaying a central stellate scar (Compagno and Oertel 1978a) (Fig. 4.15). The fibrous stroma occasionally shows a sunburst-like calcification. The tumors are well demarcated and two thirds occur in the body/tail portion of the gland. Serous oligocystic adenoma is

Table 4.1. Histologic classification of epithelial tumors of the exocrine pancreas (KLÖPPEL et al. 1996)

A	Benign
	1. Serous cystadenoma 2. Mucinous cystadenoma 3. Intraductal papillary-mucinous adenoma 4. Mature teratoma
B	Borderline (uncertain malignant potential)
	1. Mucinous cystic tumor with moderate dysplasia 2. Intraductal papillary-mucinous tumor with moderate dysplasia 3. Solid-pseudopapillary tumor
C	Malignant
	1. Severe ductal dysplasia/carcinoma in situ 2. Ductal adenocarcinoma 3. Mucinous noncystic carcinoma 4. Signet-ring cell carcinoma 5. Adenosquamous carcinoma 6. Undifferentiated (anaplastic) carcinoma 7. Mixed ductal-endocrine carcinoma 8. Osteoclast-like giant cell tumor 9. Serous cystadenocarcinoma 10. Mucinous cystadenocarcinoma 11. Intraductal papillary-mucinous carcinoma 12. Acinar cell carcinoma 13. Acinar cell cystadenocarcinoma 14. Mixed acinar-endocrine carcinoma 15. Pancreatoblastoma 16. Solid-papillary carcinoma 17. Miscellaneous carcinoma

poorly demarcated and shows no central stellate scar.

Histologically, the cysts are lined by flattened epithelium with clear, glycogen-rich cytoplasm that fails to stain for mucins and carcinoembryonic antigen (CEA) (BÄTGE et al. 1986).

4.6.3 Mucinous Cystic Tumor

The term „mucinous cystic tumor" or „neoplasm" includes mucinous cystadenomas, borderline lesions, and cystadenocarcinomas. By definition, mucinous cystadenomas show only columnar epithelium with little or no dysplasia. Borderline lesions may show moderate epithelial dysplasia, and mucinous cystadenocarcinoma severe dysplasia to carcinomatous changes, with or without invasion (KLÖPPEL et al. 1996). Because there are several lines of evidence that mucinous cystadenomas are potentially malignant and may transform into cystadenocarcinomas, particularly if treated by drainage (COMPAGNO and OERTEL 1978b), the unifying term „mucinous cystic neoplasm with latent or overt malignancy" has been suggested. Mucinous cystic tumors account for approximately 1%–2% of pancreatic exocrine tumors (KLÖPPEL 1984). The patients are predominantly women, usually between the ages of 40 and 60.

The tumors have diameters between 2–30 cm and consist of a unilocular cyst or multiple separate cysts filled with viscous mucin (Fig. 4.16). The thick fibrous capsule often contains smaller cysts and calcifications. The inner surface of the cysts may display papillary excrescences and solid tissue. The cysts usually do not communicate with the pancreatic duct (WARSHAW et al. 1990; YAMADA et al. 1991). The tumors occur frequently in the body and the tail. Histologically, the cysts are lined by mucinous columnar epithelium that may show an intestinal phenotype and contain single neuroendocrine cells (ALBORES-SAAVEDRA et al. 1988). The columnar epithelium may only show mild to moderate dysplasia or, in addition, foci of severe dysplasia or even unequivocal invasive adenocarcinoma. Immunocytochemically, the tumors are positive for CEA and CA 19–9, which may also be found in the cyst fluid, sometimes at high levels (WARSHAW et al. 1990).

Patients with mucinous cystic tumors can be cured if complete excision of the tumor can be achieved (ZAMBONI et al. 1998). If the patient already presents with invasive disease or metastasis, the prognosis is similar to that of ductal adenocarcinoma (WARSHAW et al. 1990).

4.6.4 Intraductal Papillary-Mucinous Tumor

In recent years, much attention has focused on those pancreatic tumors that grow exclusively or predom-

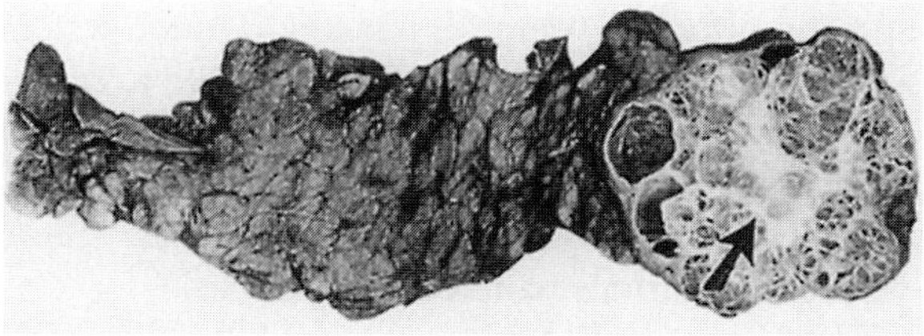

Fig. 4.15. Microcystic serous adenoma in the pancreatic tail, showing a central stellate scar (*arrow*)

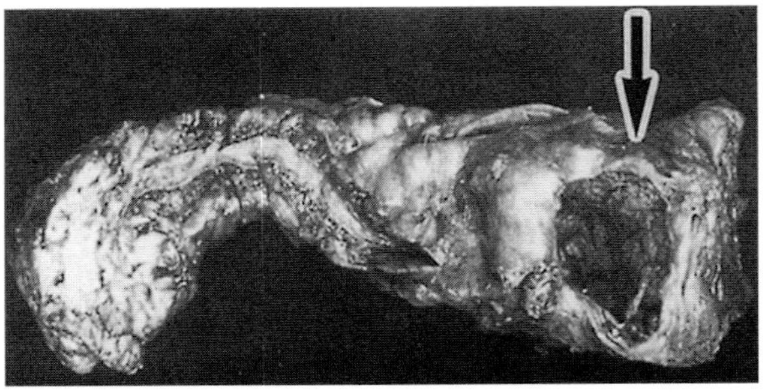

Fig. 4.16. Mucinous cystic tumor in the tail of the pancreas (*arrow*)

inantly within the pancreatic duct system (KLÖPPEL 1984; MOROHOSHI et al. 1983). As gross papillary protrusions are prominent in some of the tumors, while in others mucin hypersecretion is most obvious, two variants of intraductal tumors, the intraductal papillary neoplasm and the intraductal mucin-hypersecreting neoplasm, have been distinguished (MOROHOSHI et al. 1989; RICKAERT et al. 1991). These tumors have also become known under a number of other names [synonyms: intraductal papilloma, villous adenoma of the pancreatic duct, intraductal papillary adenocarcinoma, intraductal carcinoma, early pancreatic carcinoma, intraductal mucin-hypersecreting tumor, mucin producing tumor, and mucinous ductal ectasia (BASTID et al. 1991; CONLEY et al. 1987; Itai et al. 1987; KLÖPPEL 1984; MILCHGRUB et al. 1992; MIZUMOTO et al. 1988; WARSHAW et al. 1987)].

Intraductal papillary-mucinous tumors of the pancreas account for approximately 1%–2% of pancreatic exocrine tumors. They have been observed particularly in Japan (ITAI et al. 1987; OBARA et al. 1991; YAMADA et al. 1991; YAMAGUCHI and TANAKA 1991), but recently some large series have also been reported in Europe and the United States (AZAR et al. 1996; LOFTUS et al. 1996). They affect elderly patients of either sex.

Macroscopically, the lesion is focal (usually involving the main pancreatic duct in the head of the pancreas and only rarely a secondary duct), or spreads diffusely over the pancreatic duct system and may even extend to the ampulla. Due to intensive papillary growths and/or massive discharge of mucin, the main duct is ectatic or even cystic (Fig. 4.17), and the remaining pancreas shows obstructive chronic pancreatitis.

Histologically, all tumors show papillary proliferations of mucin-secreting cells along the duct system (Fig. 4.18). In carcinomas, which account for up to one third of the tumors (AZAR et al. 1996), severe atypia-carcinoma in situ changes are present (CONLEY et al. 1987; CUBILLA and FITZGERALD 1984; MILCHGRUB et al. 1992; MIZUMOTO et al. 1988; MOROHOSHI et al. 1989; YAMADA et al. 1991), which may be accompanied by invasive growth with or without metastatic spread (MIZUMOTO et al. 1988; YAMADA et al. 1991). Immunocytochemically, the tumors stain for CEA and CA 19–9. Mutated K-*ras* gene may be found in a large percentage of cases (SESSA et al. 1994; TADA et al. 1991).

Because the intraductal papillary proliferations and/or the sticky mucin causes obstruction of the main duct, the patients have pancreatitis-like symptoms that may be present several years before the diagnosis (RICKAERT et al. 1991). The overall prognosis seems to be good after extirpation of the tumor, and disease-free survival for more than 10 years has been reported (AZAR et al. 1996; RICKAERT et al. 1991).

4.6.5 Ductal Adenocarcinoma

Ductal adenocarcinoma with its variants accounts for around 90% of all pancreatic tumors. All epidemiological data on „pancreatic carcinoma“, therefore, refer to ductal adenocarcinoma. Between 1930 and 1970, the incidence tripled in the US, in England and Wales it doubled, and in Japan it quadrupled. Currently, between 3% and 7% of all cancer deaths can be attributed to pancreatic carcinoma (KLÖPPEL 1984). In autopsy studies, it accounts for about 2% of cases (MOROHOSHI et al. 1983). The peak number of patients occurs between 60 and 70 years of age. Only

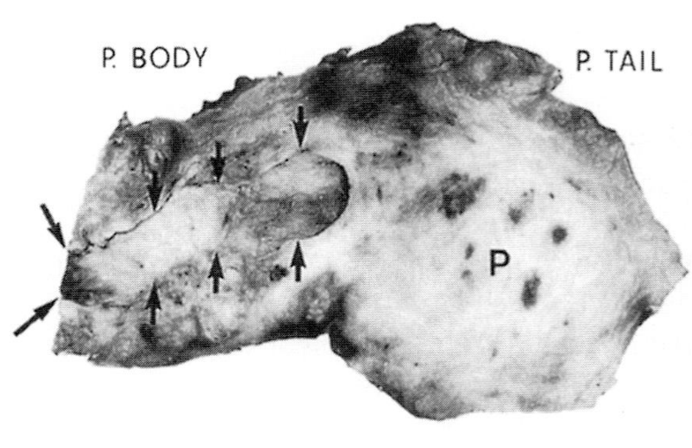

Fig. 4.17. Intraductal papillary tumor of the pancreas. Left-sided resection specimen with a dilated main duct filled with tumor tissue (*arrows*). The remainder of the parenchyma (*P*) is sclerosed

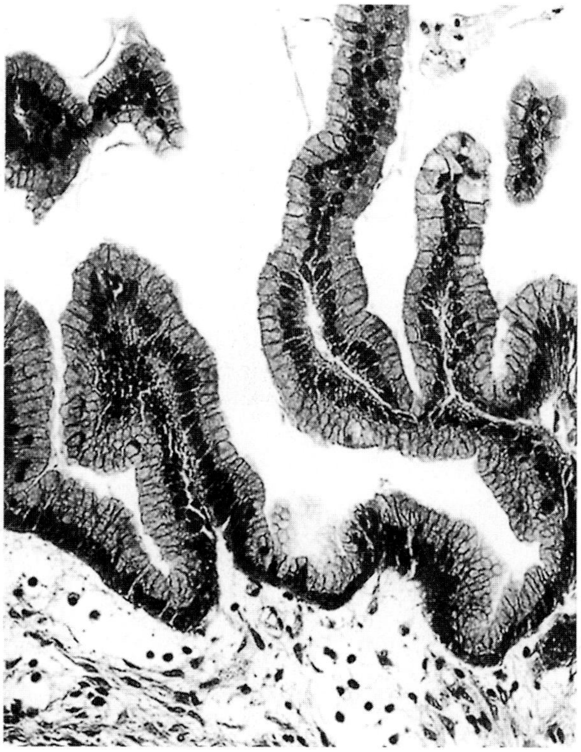

Fig. 4.18. Intraductal papillary tumor. The surface of the main duct shows papillary projections lined by well-differentiated mucin-producing duct cells. H&E, ×125

1%–4% of patients are under 45 years of age. Men predominate over women by a ratio varying between 2.0:1.0 and 1.1:1.0. The mortality rate in the first year after diagnosis is more than 90%.

Ductal adenocarcinomas of the head of the pancreas usually present with jaundice, weight loss, and abdominal pain. Tumors of the body and tail of the pancreas grow more insidiously and often have metastasized by the time the diagnosis is established. Ductal adenocarcinomas can be associated with acute pancreatitis, venous thromboses, or diabetes mellitus, and may lead to gastrointestinal hemorrhages and peritoneal carcinomatosis with ascites.

4.6.5.1 Macroscopy

Between 60% and 70% of cases are localized in the head of the pancreas (Fig. 4.19). Whereas tumors in the upper dorsal region of the head of the pancreas mainly obstruct the bile duct, tumors at other sites of the head also occlude the main pancreatic duct and lead to severe obstructive pancreatitis (Fig. 4.19). The size of carcinomas in resected Whipple specimens usually ranges from 1.5 to 5 cm, with a median diameter varying from around 2.5–3.5 cm. In autopsy series, the tumor size averages 4–6 cm (Cubilla and Fitzgerald 1984; Klöppel et al. 1985; Morohoshi et al. 1983). At diagnosis, carcinomas of the body and/or tail are generally larger than carcinomas of the head (Cubilla and Fitzgerald 1984) (Fig. 4.20). The tumors show a poorly demarcated yellowish-white to gray cut surface and a hard consistency. Hemorrhage and necrosis are usually absent. Microcystic structures may be present and are indicative of a well-differentiated ductal adenocarcinoma.

4.6.5.2 Microscopy and Grading

In their histologic and cytologic appearance, many carcinomas strongly resemble normal pancreatic duct and bile duct structures. Well-differentiated ductal adenocarcinomas grow in tubular and glandular patterns and produce abundant dense stroma (Fig. 4.21a). The irregular glands are lined by cylindrical to cuboidal cells that produce mucin in variable amounts and show irregularly sized nuclei (Fig. 4.21b). In the poorly differentiated tumors, the glandular pattern is more bizarre, the epithelial anaplasia prominent, the mucus production reduced, and the desmoplastic response less pronounced (Fig. 4.21c). According to the histologic differentiation of the carcinomas, three grades of malignancy are distinguished (Klöppel et al. 1985) (Table 4.2).

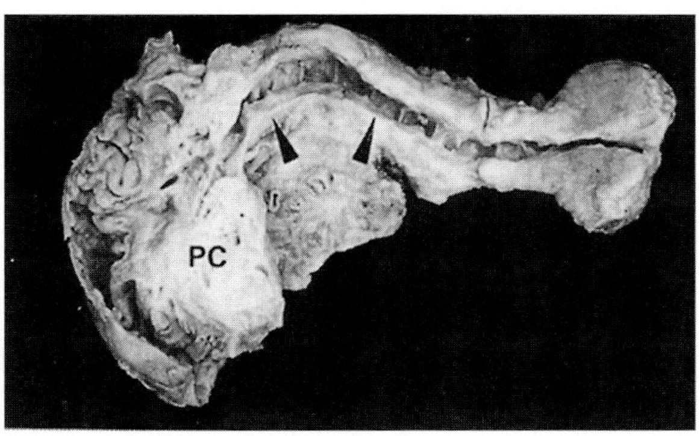

Fig. 4.19. Ductal adenocarcinoma of the pancreas. A tumor in the head of the pancreas (*PC*) obstructs the main pancreatic duct, leading to upstream duct dilatation (*arrowheads*) and exocrine atrophy

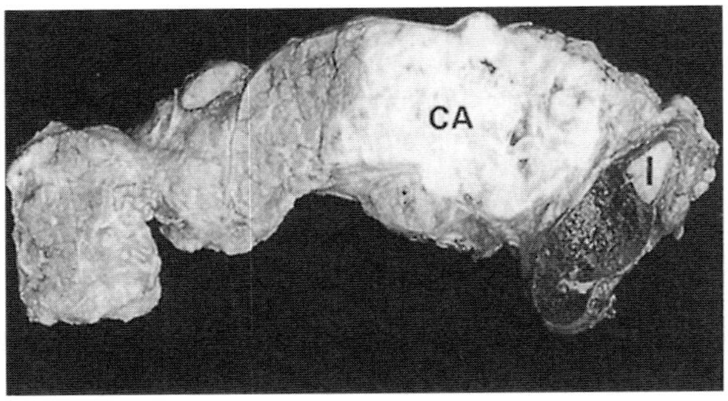

Fig. 4.20. Ductal adenocarcinoma (*CA*) located in the tail of the pancreas. The spleen was infarcted (*I*)

4.6.5.3 Markers

Among the immunocytochemical markers for ductal adenocarcinoma, CA 19–9 (recognizing a carbohydrate structure shared by a monosialoganglioside and a mucin), CEA, DU-PAN-2 [a highly glycosylated mucin-related carbohydrate antigen (Metzgar et al. 1982; Tempero et al. 1989)], and SPan-1 (Kim et al. 1990; Takeda et al. 1991) are those most often used. For unknown reasons, CA 19–9 proved to be superior to CEA for the serologic recognition of pancreatic carcinoma (Fig. 4.22). CA 19–9 has been found to be markedly increased in the serum of 70%–80% of patients with pancreatic carcinoma, though at the tissue level this antibody does not discriminate between normal pancreatic ducts and neoplastic glands (Atkinson et al. 1982; Iwase et al. 1986; Nagakawa et al. 1994). In contrast, monoclonal antibodies directed against epitopes present on both CEA and the CEA-related antigen, nonspecific cross-reacting antigen 95 (NCA 95), are capable of discriminating between reactive duct changes and carcinoma structures, as well as duct-type adenocarcinomas and nonduct-type neoplasms such as acinar cell carcinoma and endocrine tumors (Bätge et al. 1986; Klöppel et al. 1987).

Recently, several genetic alterations have been described in pancreatic carcinomas. Point mutations at codon 12 of the K-*ras* gene have been found in 75%–95% of the tumors (Almoguera et al. 1988; Lemoine et al. 1992; Mariyama et al. 1989), while a mutated p53 tumor suppressor gene was present in approximately 60% of the cases (Barton et al. 1919). There appears to be no correlation between the K-*ras* mutations and tumor grade or tumor stage (Grünewald et al. 1989). Other genetic changes include mutations and deletions of the p16 gene and the DPC4 gene (Klöppel 1994).

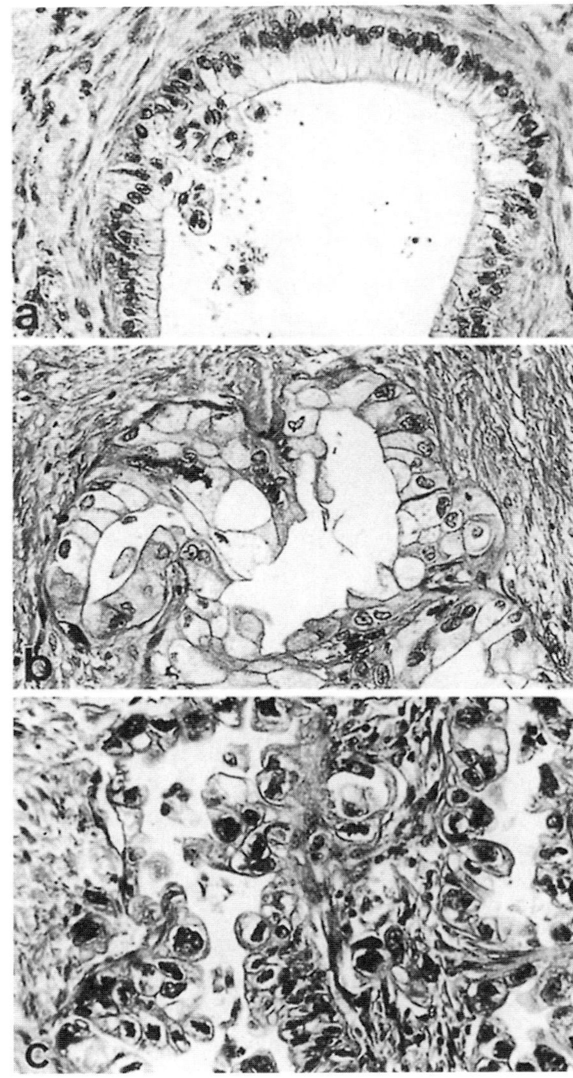

Fig. 4.21a–c. Histologic differentiation in ductal adenocarcinoma of the pancreas. **a** Well-differentiated (grade 1) tumor; **b** moderately differentiated (grade 2) tumor; **c** poorly differentiated (grade 3) tumor. H&E, ×250

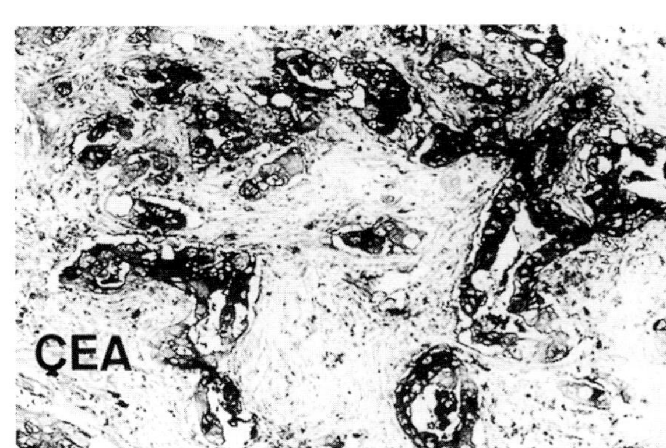

Fig. 4.22. Immunostaining for carcinoembryonic antigen (CEA) in a ductal adenocarcinoma of the pancreas. H&E,

Table 4.2. Histologic grading of pancreatic duct cell adenocarcinoma

Tumor grade	Glandular differentiation	Mucin production	Mitosis (per 10 HPF)	Nuclear anaplasia
1	Well-differentiated duct-like gland; polar arrangement	Intensive	1–5	Little polymorphism
2	Moderately differentiated duct-like and tubular glands	Irregular	6–10	Some polymorphism
3	Poorly differentiated glands; mucoepidermoid and pleomorphic structures	Abortive	>10	Marked pleomorphism and increased nuclear size

4.6.5.4
Intrapancreatic and Extrapancreatic Tumor Extension

Foci of intraductal carcinoma or carcinoma in situ were found in up to 24% of resected pancreases with ductal adenocarcinoma. Such foci were usually located within a few centimeters of the primary tumor (Cubilla and Fitzgerald 1976; Klöppel et al. 1980). These lesions most likely represent intraductal branches of otherwise invasive tumors. Multicentric development of duct carcinoma in the pancreas has been reported in 15%–40% of the cases (Ihse et al. 1977; Pliam and ReMine 1975; Tryka and Brooks 1979; van Heerden 1984). In a study of 37 total pancreatectomy specimens with carcinoma of the pancreatic head (Klöppel et al. 1987), we found no skip development and only three cases (8%) with continuous spread throughout the main pancreatic duct of the head, body, and tail. All of the carcinomas with pronounced intraductal involvement proved to be well-differentiated adenocarcinomas. On the basis of these examinations, we believe that multicentricity may not be as frequent as has been thought (Tryka and Brooks 1979; van Heerden 1984). The pancreatic remnant after a Whipple resection for pancreatic carcinoma is therefore probably rarely the origin of tumor recurrence.

Direct extension beyond the gland is common, even when the primary carcinoma is small (Nagai et al. 1986). It is therefore an exception to find a resected carcinoma that is still limited to the pancreas. In head carcinomas, peripancreatic tumor invasion primarily involves the retroperitoneal fatty tissue behind the pancreas head surrounding the large mesenteric vessels and the nerve plexus. In advanced cases, the walls of veins, neighboring organs, and/or the retroperitoneum are invaded. The duodenum is the organ most often involved by cancer of the head of the pancreas. The stomach, the peritoneum, and the gallbladder are also infiltrated in advanced cases. In carcinomas of the body and tail, local extension is usually greater, because of delayed tumor detection, and includes involvement of the liver, peritoneum, spleen, stomach, colon, and left adrenal gland (Cubilla and Fitzgerald 1984; Klöppel 1984).

Lymphatic spread usually precedes hematogenous spread. The lymph nodes most commonly involved in pancreatic head carcinoma are, in descending order, the retroduodenal (posterior pancreaticoduodenal) and the superior and inferior pancreatic head groups (Cubilla et al. 1978). These lymph nodes are usually resected together with the head of the pancreas by a standard Whipple resection. More distal nodal metastases may be found along the hepatoduodenal ligament, the celiac trunk, the superior mesenteric artery, and on both sides of the aorta at the level of the renal arteries (Lüttges et al. 1998).

Carcinomas of the body and tail metastasize especially to the superior body and tail lymph node groups and the splenic hilus lymph nodes. They may also spread via lymphatic channels to pleura and lung. Hematogenous metastases occur in descending order of frequency in the liver, lungs, adrenals, kidneys, bones, brain, and skin. In 5%–15% of autopsy specimens, there are no hematogenous metastases (Cubilla and Fitzgerald 1984; Klöppel 1984; Mikal and Campbell 1950).

4.6.5.5
Recurrence

Local tumor recurrence seems to be the major factor determining survival after resection of pancreatic ductal carcinoma. The most important sites for tumor residues and recurrences are the tissues surrounding the large mesenteric vessels (Guthoff et al. 1987; KAYAHARA et al. 1993; KLÖPPEL 1993; NAGAI et al. 1986; TEPPER et al. 1976). The retroperitoneal resection margins are therefore of utmost importance if a „curative" (R0) resection is to be achieved (LÜTTGES et al. 1998). Second in frequency are recurrences arising from lymph node or liver metastases that were too small to be detected during surgery.

4.6.6 Potential Precursor Lesions in the Duct System

The discussion of precursor lesions of the ductal adenocarcinoma focuses on changes in the duct epithelium and the ducts. Four such changes can be distinguished: squamous metaplasia, mucinous cell hypertrophy, ductal papillary hyperplasia, and adenomatoid duct hyperplasia (KLÖPPEL 1993; OERTEL et al. 1989; SOLCIA et al. 1997). All lesions occur in the normal or inflamed pancreas, as well as in association with pancreatic tumors. Among these lesions, mucinous cell hypertrophy and ductal papillary hyperplasia have been discussed as precursors of ductal adenocarcinoma because of: (1) their resemblance to carcinoma in situ changes, (2) their increased incidence in association with ductal carcinoma (CHEN and BAITHUN 1985; CUBILLA and FITZGERALD 1976; KLÖPPEL et al. 1980), and (3) their rather frequent expression of a mutated K-*ras* gene, which appears to be a molecular marker of ductal carcinomas (KLÖPPEL 1994). However, it must be emphasized that a definite transition from ductal papillary hyperplasia to carcinoma in situ and invasive carcinoma has not yet been unequivocally demonstrated. A de novo origin, therefore, remains an alternative for the development of ductal adenocarcinoma.

4.6.7 Variants of Ductal Adenocarcinoma

Mucinous noncystic carcinoma, adenosquamous carcinoma, including mucoepidermoid carcinoma and squamous carcinoma, and undifferentiated carcinoma with and without osteoclast-like cells are considered variants of ductal adenocarcinoma (CUBILLA and FITZGERALD 1984; KLÖPPEL 1984; SOLCIA et al. 1997).

In mucinous noncystic carcinoma, excessive mucin production within the tumor tissue results in a gelatinous cut surface („colloid" or gelatinous carcinoma). Most of the mucinous carcinomas show rather well-differentiated cuboidal cells lining cystic spaces or floating free in the mucus, some of them of the signet-ring cell type (Fig. 4.23). Pure signet-ring cell carcinoma is very rare. Mucinous noncystic carcinomas and ductal adenocarcinomas occur in similar locations and in patients of similar age. Patients with mucinous noncystic carcinoma might have a better prognosis, possibly roughly proportional to the amount of mucin produced, than patients with ductal adenocarcinoma (CUBILLA and FITZGERALD 1984).

In adenosquamous carcinoma, the components of glandular and squamous cell carcinoma are mixed and variably distributed in the tumor. Pure squamous cell carcinomas, if they ever exist, are rare, since an intensive workup of these tumors usually reveals some foci of glandular structures (Fig. 4.24). In addition, there may be anaplastic and spindle cell foci. In gross appearance, male/female ratio, and localization, adenosquamous carcinoma resembles ductal adenocarcinoma. As almost all of these carcinomas are of grade 3, they usually have a very poor prognosis.

In undifferentiated carcinoma (synonyms: giant cell, pleomorphic large cell, or anaplastic carcinoma), a pattern of extreme anaplasia with bizarre cellular pleomorphism and numerous mitoses is found (Fig. 4.25). However, focal glandular elements are also a common component of this tumor type, providing evidence of its duct cell origin (CUBILLA and FITZGERALD 1984; TREPETA et al. 1981). The epithelial nature of the pleomorphic and occasionally spindle-shaped cells is revealed by the immunocytochemical demonstration of keratin (HOORENS et al. 1998). At the time of diagnosis, these tumors are usually large and of soft consistency, prominent features being necrosis and hemorrhage (Fig. 4.25). There is

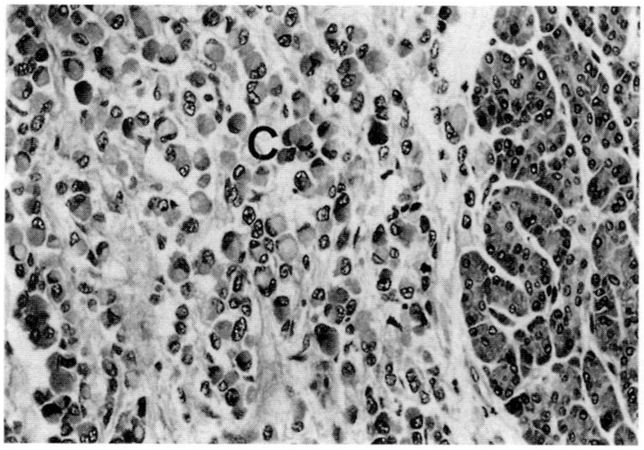

Fig. 4.23. Mucinous noncystic carcinoma (*C*) of the pancreas composed of signet-ring cells. H&E, ×250

no age or sex predilection. Their prognosis is very poor. This is most likely also true of the giant cell tumor with osteoclast-like cells (YAMAGUCHI and ENJOJI 1987), although initial reports suggested that this tumor type behaves less aggressively than ordinary duct cell carcinoma (ROSAI 1968). The role and origin of the osteoclast-like cells in these tumors are obscure (FISHER et al. 1988; GOLDBERG et al. 1991).

4.6.8 Acinar Cell Carcinoma

Acinar cell carcinomas range in size from 2 to 16 cm and are equally distributed in the pancreas. The lobulated tumor masses are fairly well demarcated and brown to yellow, with soft consistency and areas of necrosis. A cystic variant also exists (CANTRELL et al. 1981; STAMM et al. 1987). Metastases are found mainly in the regional lymph nodes, the liver, and the lungs. Histologically, the tumors show an acinar pattern, supported by scanty stroma (Fig. 4.26). However, tumors with solid patterns also occur and these are reminiscent of endocrine tumors. On immunocytochemistry and electron microscopy, pancreatic enzymes and zymogen granules can be demonstrated (KLIMSTRA et al. 1992; MOROHOSHI et al. 1987). In addition, a small number of tumors also contain scattered neuroendocrine cells (positive for chromogranin A and/or synaptophysin) (HOORENS et al. 1992; KLIMSTRA et al. 1994). Acinar cell carcinomas

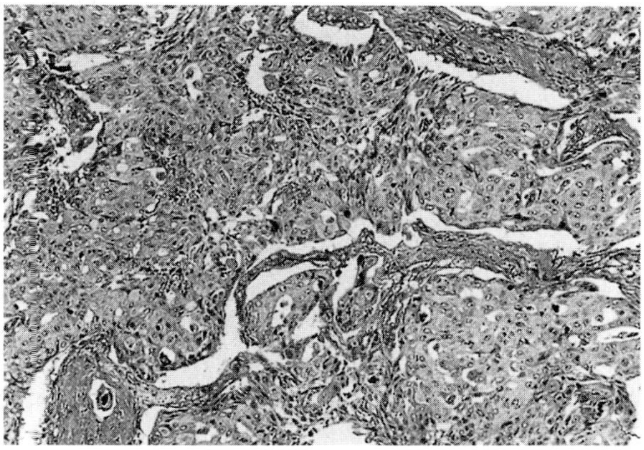

Fig. 4.24. Adenosquamous carcinoma of the pancreas. H&E, ×125

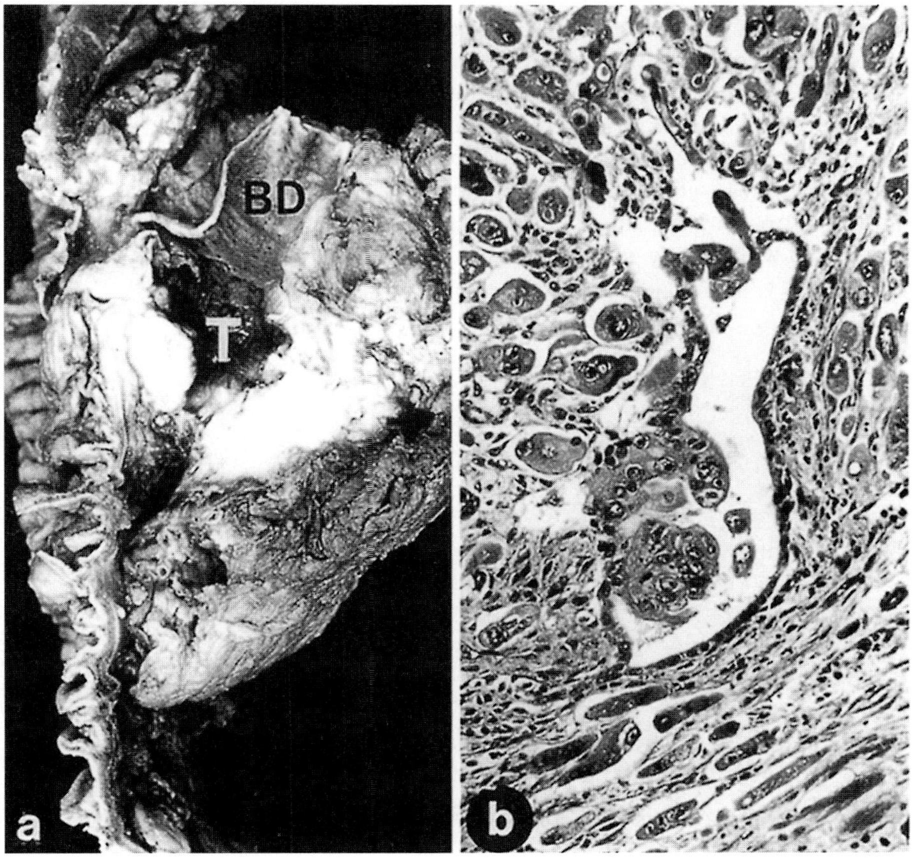

Fig. 4.25a,b. Giant cell carcinoma of the pancreas. **a** Tumor in the head of the pancreas with central necrosis (*T*) and obstruction of the biliary duct (*BD*). **b** Large anaplastic tumor cells forming an irregular gland. H&E, ×250

occur mostly in elderly patients of either sex (Morohoshi et al. 1987), but some rare examples have also been reported in children. Many patients present clinically with distant metastases from an occult carcinoma (Cubilla and Fitzgerald 1984). Individual patients may show disseminated subcutaneous fat necrosis, polyarthralgia, and blood eosinophilia. These lesions presumably result from the release of lipase by the tumor.

4.6.9 Pancreatoblastoma

Pancreatoblastomas are large, soft, rounded tumors (size range 7–12 cm), the cut surfaces of which disclose lobulated yellowish-brown areas and central pseudocystic foci of necrosis. The tumors occur in the pancreas or are attached to it. Histologically, there is either an acinar cell pattern (Horie et al. 1987; Klimstra et al. 1995; Morohoshi et al. 1987) with squamoid nests or a more primitive mixture of epithelial and mesenchymal components (Cubilla and Fitzgerald 1984). Ultrastructurally, zymogen granules can be identified (Klimstra et al. 1995). Some tumors produce a-fetoprotein (Horie et al. 1987) and contain single endocrine cells. Pancreatoblastomas are rare and occur predominantly in young children of between 1 and 8 years of age (Horie et al. 1987). Boys appear to be more frequently affected than girls. Recently, such tumors have also been observed in adults (Hoorens et al. 1992; Palosaari et al. 1986). If the tumor is well encapsulated, complete surgical removal seems to be associated with a fairly good prognosis.

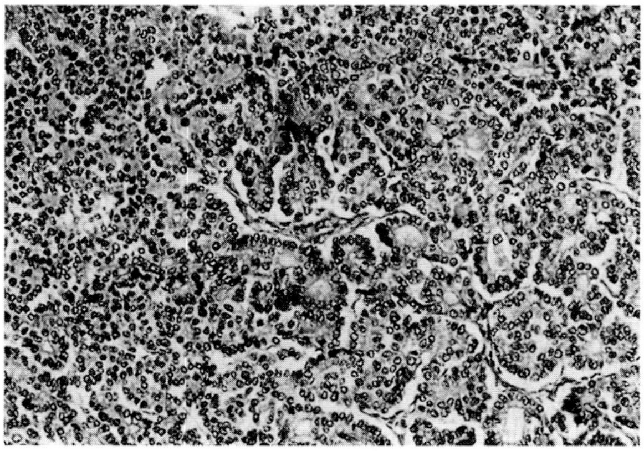

Fig. 4.26. Acinar cell carcinoma showing an admixture of acinar and solid structures. H&E, ×125

4.6.10 Solid-Pseudopapillary Tumor

Solid-pseudopapillary tumors present as large round masses (size range: 3–20 cm in diameter, average size 8 cm) which are well demarcated from the remaining pancreas. The cut surface reveals lobulated, light brown solid areas admixed with pseudocystic areas filled with hemorrhagic and necrotic debris (Fig. 4.27). Histologically, the solid parts consist of monomorphous cells that may form pseudopapillary patterns with variable sclerosis (Fig. 4.28). Some tumor cells stain distinctly with al-antitrypsin. In recent immunocytochemical and ultrastructural studies, acinar, endocrine, and ductal features were noted (Chott et al. 1987; Klöppel et al. 1981; Lieber et al. 1987; Morohoshi et al. 1987). In the vast majority of cases, the tumor occurs in adolescent girls and young women. Clinically, the patients are asymptomatic or complain of upper abdominal discomfort. The prognosis of this tumor is favorable, as most of the patients are cured by tumor resection. Local recurrence is rare and usually only occurs in patients with incomplete resection (Lieber et al. 1987; Mollenhauer et al. 1987; Ulich et al. 1982). Metastases to the liver have been described in a few patients (Masi et al. 1965).

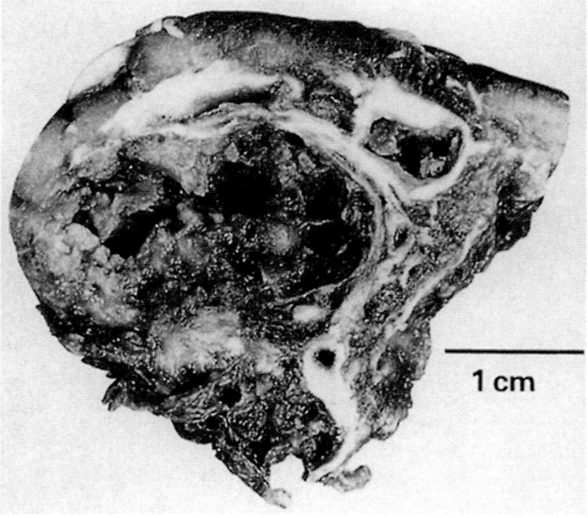

Fig. 4.27. Solid-cystic (papillary-cystic) tumor of the pancreas: fragment of a tumor with central pseudocystic degeneration

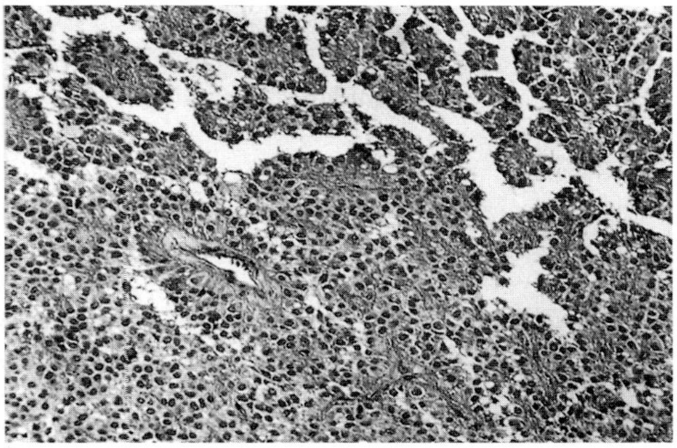

Fig. 4.28. Solid-cystic (papillary-cystic) tumor showing a solid and pseudopapillary pattern. H&E, ×125

4.6.11 Miscellaneous Carcinomas

Carcinomas of the pancreas that do not fit totally into one of the above categories include tumors such as small cell carcinoma (REYES and WANG 1981), ciliated cell carcinoma, oncocytic carcinoma, clear cell carcinoma (CUBILLA and FITZGERALD 1984; LÜTTGES et al. 1998), and mixed endocrine-exocrine tumors (mucinous carcinoid tumors) (EUSEBI et al. 1981). The so-called microadenocarcinomas (CUBILLA and FITZGERALD 1984) probably do not form an entity, but belong to either the endocrine or the acinar tumors (LONARDO et al. 1996).

4.6.12 Nonepithelial Tumors

Primary nonepithelial malignant tumors of the pancreas are extremely uncommon. Those that have been reported include examples of almost all known histologic types of malignant soft tissue tumors (LÜTTGES et al. 1997). Malignant lymphomas and plasmacytomas only rarely arise in the pancreas, whereas secondary involvement of the pancreas by advanced lymphomas is not infrequent. Benign lymphoepithelial cysts of the pancreas are recently described rare lesions that microscopically resemble their counterpart in salivary glands (SOLCIA et al. 1997).

4.7 Endocrine Tumors

4.7.1 General Considerations

Pancreatic endocrine tumors are composed of neuroendocrine cells characterized by the expression of neuroendocrine markers (neuron-specific enolase, synaptophysin, chromogranins, and others) (KLÖPPEL and HEITZ 1988; KLÖPPEL et al. 1993).

The tumors are also referred to as islet cell tumors. This term, however, is unsatisfactory because of the capacity of many of these tumors to produce hormones not normally present in islet cells.

Pancreatic endocrine tumors can be subdivided into those producing symptoms by inappropriate hormone secretion (functioning or hormonally active tumors) and nonfunctioning tumors without known hormonal symptoms. The most common functioning tumor is insulinoma (i.e., a tumor causing hyperinsulinemic hypoglycemia), followed by gastrinoma [i.e., a tumor inducing the Zollinger-Ellison syndrome (ZES)], glucagonoma (i.e., a tumor associated with the glucagonoma syndrome), and VIPoma (VIP, vasoactive intestinal polypeptide) [i.e., a tumor associated with a WDHA (watery diarrhea, hypokalemia, and achlorhydria) syndrome].

Very rare functioning tumors are those inducing Cushing's syndrome, acromegaly, hypercalcemia, or carcinoid syndrome by secretion of adrenocorticotropic hormone (ACTH), growth hormone-releasing hormone (GH-RH), parathyroid hormone-releasing hormone (PTHrH), and serotonin, respectively.

4.7.2 Epidemiology

The prevalence of pancreatic endocrine tumors is estimated at less than one in a population of 100 000 (MOLDOW and CONNELLY 1968; SCHEIN et al. 1973), whereas the incidence of these tumors with relatively good prognosis is substantially lower. At autopsy, pancreatic endocrine tumors are found in 0.4–1.5% of unselected specimens, if systematically sought. Most of these tumors are less than 0.2 cm in diameter and are clinically silent.

Virtually all pancreatic endocrine tumors occur in adults, most frequently between the ages of 30 and 70. They are exceptional in children. Females are affected slightly more often than males.

4.7.3 Macroscopy

Grossly, most hormonally active pancreatic endocrine tumors are solitary, more or less well circumscribed nodules with a diameter of between 1 and 4 cm (Fig. 4.29). They are often difficult to localize prior to surgery. The amount of fibrous stroma is variable; some of the tumors are soft and red, while others are firm and white. Some functioning tumors, and the majority of nonfunctioning tumors, grow to a larger size.

Rarely, more than one endocrine tumor is found. This is strongly indicative of a multiple endocrine neoplasia, type 1 (MEN-1) syndrome, especially if multiple small tumors are present.

4.7.4 Microscopy

In principle, a trabecular architecture including glandular and gyriform structures (Fig. 4.30) can be distinguished from a solid pattern. In most tumors, the cells forming the trabeculae and solid nests are remarkably uniform, with easily recognizable cell borders and small, round or elongated nuclei. Mitoses are usually rare. In cytologic smears, a tentative diagnosis of endocrine tumor can be made in the presence of uniform, dispersed, small tumor cells with little variation in nuclear size and formation of rosette-like clusters.

In a small number of endocrine tumors, cell polymorphism is pronounced and mitoses are common. These tumors are sometimes difficult to distinguish from undifferentiated carcinomas, and immunocytochemistry may be necessary to reveal their endocrine nature. Diagnostic problems arise if the whole tumor is composed of small cells, consequently bearing a resemblance to small cell carcinoma of the lung.

The amount of connective tissue is variable. It may consist only of a rich network of thin-walled vessels, or may be abundant with large areas of hyalinized collagenous stroma, widely separating the remaining small strands of tumor parenchyma. Tiny calcifications may be present and sometimes take the form of laminated psammoma bodies.

4.7.5 Criteria of Malignancy

Endocrine tumors of the pancreas are, in general, slowly growing neoplasms. It is not known whether all tumors are basically malignant and will metastasize if given enough time, or whether some tumors remain benign.

There are only a few reliable signs of malignancy. Among these are the presence of lymph node metastases, invasion of adjacent organs, vascular invasion,

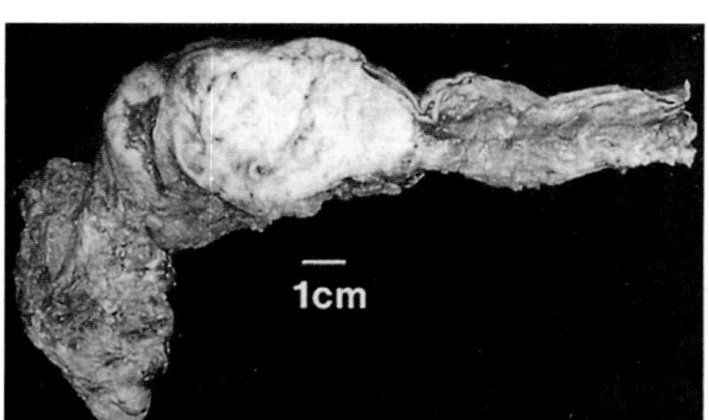

Fig. 4.29. Well-demarcated endocrine tumor in the body of the pancreas

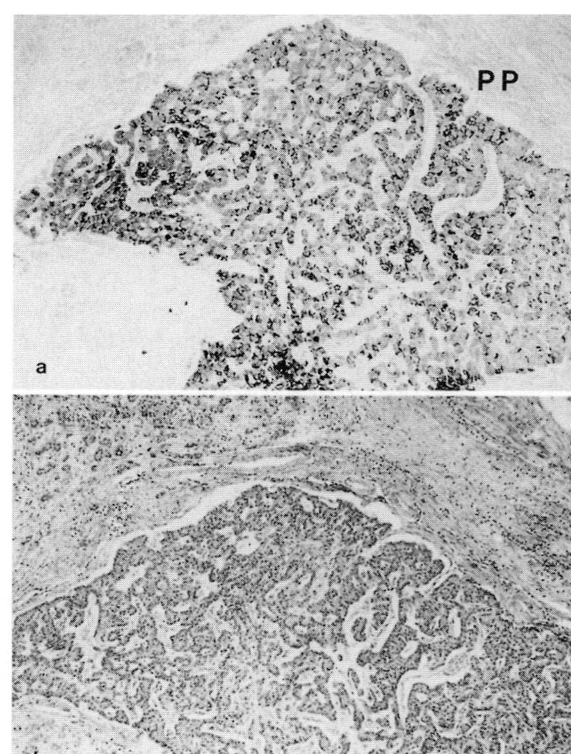

Fig. **4.30a,b.** Pancreatic endocrine tumor. **a** Immunostaining for pancreatic polypeptide (*PP*). **b** Well-demarcated tumor with trabecular pattern

and poor histologic differentiation. In addition, there are criteria which are strongly suggestive of malignancy, i.e., proliferation index, number of mitoses, tumor size, and associated hormonal syndrome (Capella et al. 1997). Using most of these criteria, a new prognostic classification has recently been proposed (Capella et al. 1995) (Table 4.3).

Long survival, even of patients with liver metastases, is not exceptional. Metastases are first found in the locoregional lymph nodes of the pancreas and in the liver. Metastases located elsewhere are uncommon and only to be expected in more advanced stages of the disease. The mean survival rate of patients with metastases is approximately 4 years, though a patient who survived for 19 years has been reported (Cubilla and Hajdu 1975).

Table 4.3. Clinicopathologic classification of endocrine tumors of the pancreas

1.1 Well-differentiated endocrine tumor
– Benign behavior: confined to pancreas, nonangioinvasive, <2 cm in size • Functioning Insulinoma • Nonfunctioning – Uncertain behavior: confined to pancreas, ≥2 cm in size or angioinvasive • Functioning Gastrinoma, insulinoma, VIPoma, glucagonoma, somatostatinoma or other tumors[a] • Nonfunctioning
1.2 Well-differentiated endocrine carcinoma
– Low grade malignant with gross local invasion and/or metastases • Functioning Gastrinoma, insulinoma, glucagonoma, VIPoma, somatostatinoma or other tumors[a] • Nonfunctioning
2. Poorly differentiated endocrine carcinoma
– High grade malignant (small to intermediate cell) carcinoma

[a] Cushing (ACTH, adrenocorticotropic hormone), acromegaly or gigantism (GH), etc.

4.7.6 Individual Types of Endocrine Tumors

4.7.6.1 *Insulinoma*

Insulinomas are frequently discovered while still small (diameter 1–2 cm). Virtually all of them occur in the pancreas (with no preferential localization) or are attached to it. About two thirds of patients can be cured by resection of the tumor. Insulinomas are rarely malignant (5%–10%). Viewed with a light microscope, the tumor cells resemble more or less normal b cells. Most insulinomas store insulin in sufficient amounts to be easily visualized by immunocytochemistry.

Newborns with persistent hyperinsulinemic hypoglycemia suffer from nesidioblastosis, i.e., diffuse or focal islet hyperplasia with B-cell hyperfunction (Goossens et al. 1989).

4.7.6.2 *Gastrinoma*

Gastrinomas are associated with ZES, in which persistent hypersecretion of acid gastric juice leads to duodenal and even jejunal peptic ulcerations. A total of 70% of gastrinomas occur sporadically, while 30% are associated with multiple endocrine neoplasia type 1 (see Sect. 4.7.7). Approximately 50%–70% of gastrinomas associated with the sporadic form of ZES occur in the pancreas, particularly in the head, while the remainder are found in the duodenum (Donow et al. 1991). In the pancreas, they usually have a diameter of 2 cm or more, whereas in the duodenum most gastrinomas are smaller than 1 cm. The gastrinomas associated with MEN-1 are located predominantly in the duodenum; these tumors are also usually smaller than 1 cm and often multicentric (Donow et al. 1991; Pipeleers-Marichal et al. 1990). Pancreatic gastrinomas associated with MEN-1 appear to be exceptions; while the pancreas of these patients usually contains multiple endocrine tumors, the latter virtually never produce gastrin (see Sect. 4.9.8).

Metastasis to regional lymph nodes is found in approximately 60% of patients with pancreatic gastrinomas, but only a relatively small percentage of these patients develop liver metastasis. Duodenal gastrinomas appear to have a somewhat lower malignancy rate than pancreatic gastrinomas. Nevertheless, they can metastasize while still very small and give rise to periduodenal node metastases which may be larger than the primary tumor (Donow et al. 1991).

4.7.6.3 VIPoma

VIPomas are large tumors with a diameter varying from 4 to 10 cm. The majority of VIPomas are malignant. VIP is the principal hormone produced by these tumors and causes the WDHA syndrome (Verner and Morrison 1974).

4.7.6.4 Glucagonoma

Glucagonomas are large and commonly malignant tumors. The clinical manifestations of the syndrome include migratory necrolytic erythema, glossitis, diabetes, and weight loss.

4.7.6.5 Rare Tumors

Tumors producing ectopic hormones such as ACTH, calcitonin, serotonin, parathyroid hormone, or growth hormone-releasing factor are uncommon and almost always large and malignant.

4.7.6.6 Nonfunctioning Tumors

Surgically removed nonfunctioning tumors are frequently more than 5 cm in diameter and malignant. They represent 20%–30% of the endocrine tumors of the pancreas and reveal themselves by nonspecific symptoms such as pain, bleeding, obstruction of the small intestine, or the appearance of metastases. In some of these tumors, small amounts of hormones can be demonstrated by immunocytochemistry.

4.7.7 Multiple Endocrine Neoplasia

Pancreatic endocrine neoplasms are part of the inherited (autosomal dominant) MEN-1 syndrome. Morphologic examination of the pancreas typically reveals one or several grossly recognizable tumors and multiple small adenomas (microadenomatosis) (Komminoth et al. 1998). Some of the small tumors are hardly larger than a normal islet. The hormones most frequently found in these tumors are pancreatic polypeptide, glucagon, and insulin. ZES, which frequently occurs in patients suffering from MEN-1 syndrome, is usually caused by small duodenal gastrinomas and not by pancreatic tumors (Pipeleers-Marichal et al. 1990).

References

Acosta JM, Ledesma CL (1974) Gall stone migration as a cause of acute pancreatitis. N Engl J Med 290:484–487

Aho HJ, Nevalainen TJ, Havia VT, Heinomen RJ, Aho AJ (1982) Human acute pancreatitis. A light and elctron microscopic study. Acta Pathol Microbiol Scand [A] 90:367–373

Aho HJ, Putzke HP, Nevalainen TJ, Löbel D, Pelliniemi LJ, Dummler W, Suonpää AK, Tessenow W (1983) Immunohistochemical localization of trypsinogen and trypsin in acute and chronic pancreatitis. Digestion 27:21–28

Albores-Saavedra J, Nadji M, Henson DE, Angeles-Angeles A (1988) Enteroendocrine cell differentiation in carcinomas of the gallbladder and mucinous cystadenocarcinoma of the pancreas. Pathol Res Pract 183:169–175

Almoguera C, Shibata D, Forrester K, Martin J, Arnheim N, Perucho M (1988) Most human carcinomas of the exocrine pancreas contain mutant c-K-ras genes. Cell 53:549–554

Ammann R (1976) Acute pancreatitis. In: Bockus HL (ed) Gastroenterology, vol 3, 3rd edn. Philadelphia, Saunders, pp 1020–1039

Ammann RW, Akovbiantz A, Largiader F, Schueler G (1984) Course and outcome of chronic pancreatitis. Longitudinal study of a mixed medical-surgical series of 245 patients. Gastroenterology 86:820–828

Ammann RW, Heitz PU, Klöppel G (1996) Course of alcoholic chronic pancreatitis: a prospective clinicomorphological long-term study. Gastroenterology 111:224–231

Ammann RW, Muench R, Otto R, Buehler H, Freiburghaus AU, Siegenthaler W (1988) Evolution and regression of pancreatic calcification in chronic pancreatitis. A prospective long-term study of 107 patients. Gastroenterology 95:1018–1028

Atkinson BF, Ernst C, Herlyn M, Steplewski Z, Sears HF, Koprowski H (1982) Gastrointestinal cancer-associated antigen in immunoperoxidase assay. Cancer Res 42:4820–4823

Azar C, Van de Stadt J, Rickaert F, Devière J, Delhaye M, Baize M, Klöppel G, Gelin M, Cremer M (1996) Intraductal papillary mucinous tumours of the pancreas. Clinical and therapeutic issues in 32 patients. Gut 39:457–464

Ball WP, Baggenstoss AH, Bargen JA (1950) Pancreatic lesions associated with chronic ulcerative colitis. Arch Pathol 50:347–358

Bank S (1986) Chronic pancreatitis: clinical features and medical management. Am J Gastroenterol 81:153–167

Barton CM, Staddon SL, Hughes CM, Hall PA, O'Sullivan C, Klöppel G, Theis B, Russell RCG, Neoptolemos JP, Williamson RCN, Lane DP, Lemoine NR (19919) Abnormalities of the p53 tumour suppressor gene in human pancreatic cancer. Br J Cancer 64:1076–1082

Bastid C, Bernard JP, Sarles H, Payan MJ, Sahel J (1991) Mucinous ductal ectasia of the pancreas: a premalignant disease and a cause of obstructive pancreatitis. Pancreas 6:15–22

Bätge B, Bosslet K, Sedlacek HH, Kern HF, Klöppel G (1986) Monoclonal antibodies against CEA-related components discriminate between pancreatic duct type carcinomas and nonneoplastic duct lesions as well as nonduct type neoplasias. Virchows Arch [A] Pathol Anat 408:361–374

Becker V (1981) Morphology of chronic pancreatitis. In: Scuro LA, Dagradi A (eds) Topics in acute and chronic pancreatitis. Springer, Berlin Heidelberg New York, pp 161–171

Becker WF, Welsh RA, Pratt HS (1965) Cystadenoma and cystadenocarcinoma of the pancreas. Ann Surg 161:845–860

Bockman DE, Büchler M, Beger HG (1987) Ultrastructure of human acute pancreatitis. Int J Pancreatol 1:141–153

Bogomoletz WV, Adnet JJ, Widgren S, Stavrrou M, McLaughlin JE (1980) Cystadenoma of the pancreas: a histological, histochemical and ultrastructural study of seven cases. Histopathology 4:309–320

Bordalo O, Bapista A, Dreiling D, Noronha M (1984) Early pathomorphological pancreatic changes in chronic alcoholism. In: Gyr KE, Singer MV, Sarles H (eds) Pancreatitis – concepts and classification. Elsevier, Amsterdam (Exerpta Medica, international congress series no 642)

Bradley EL III (1990) Pseudocysts in chronic pancreatitis: development and clinical implications. In: Beger HG, Büchler M, Ditschuneit H, Malfertheiner P (eds) Chronic pancreatitis. Springer, Berlin Heidelberg New York, pp 260–268

Bradley EL III (1993) A clinically based classification system for acute pancreatitis: summary of the international symposium on acute pancreatitis, Atlanta 1992. Arch Surg 128:586–590

Braganza JM (1983) Pancreatic disease: a casualty of hepatic „detoxification"? Lancet ii:1000–1003

Cantrell BB, Cubilla AL, Erlandson RA, Fortner J, Fitzgerald PJ (1981) Acinar cell cystadenocarcinoma of human pancreas. Cancer 47:410–416

Capella C, Heitz PU, Höfler H, Solcia E, Klöppel G (1995) Revised classification of neuroendocrine tumours of the lung, pancreas and gut. Virchows Arch 425:547–560

Capella C, La Rosa S, Solcia E (1997) Criteria for malignancy in pancreatic endocrine tumors. Endocr Pathol 8:87–90

Capner P, Lendrum R, Jeffries DJ, Walker G (1975) Viral antibody studies in pancreatic disease. Gut 16:866–870

Caselitz J, Klöppel G, Delling G, Grüttner R, Holdhoff U, Stern M (1979) Shwachman's syndrome and leukemia. Virchows Arch [A] Pathol Anat 385:109–116

Chen J, Baithun SI (1985) Morphological study of 391 cases of exocrine pancreatic tumours with special reference to the classification of exocrine pancreatic carcinoma. J Pathol 146:17–29

Cheng TY, Su CH, Shyr YM, Lui WY (1997) Management of pancreatic lesions in von Hippel-Lindau disease. World J Surg 21:307–312

Chott A, Klöppel G, Buxbaum P, Heitz PU (1987) Neuron specific enolase demonstration in the diagnosis of a solid-cystic (papillary cystic) tumour of the pancreas. Virchows Arch [A] Pathol Anat 410:397–402

Comfort MW, Gambill EE, Baggenstoss AH (1946) Chronic relapsing pancreatitis. A study of 29 cases without associated disease of the biliary or gastrointestinal tract. Gastroenterology 6:239–285 and 376–408

Compagno J, Oertel JE (1978a) Microcystic adenomas of the pancreas (glycogen-rich cystadenomas): a clinicopathologic study of 34 cases. Am J Clin Pathol 69:289–298

Compagno J, Oertel JE (1978b) Mucinous cystic neoplasms of the pancreas with overt and latent malignancy (cystadenocarcinoma and cystadenoma). A clinicopathologic study of 41 cases. Am J Clin Pathol 69:573–580

Conley CR, Scheithauer BW, Weiland LH, van Heerden JA (1987) Diffuse intraductal papillary adenocarcinoma of the pancreas. Ann Surg 205:246–249

Creutzfeldt W, Schmidt H (1976) Etiology and pathogenesis of pancreatitis. In: Bockus HL (ed) Gastroenterology, 3rd edn. Saunders, Philadelphia, pp 1005–1019

Cubilla A, Hajdu SI (1975) Islet cell carcinoma of the pancreas. Arch Pathol 99:204–207

Cubilla AL, Fitzgerald PJ (1976) Morphological lesions associated with human primary invasive nonendocrine pancreas cancer. Cancer Res 36:2690–2698

Cubilla AL, Fitzgerald PJ (1984) Tumors of the exocrine pancreas. Armed Forces Institute of Pathology, Washington DC

Cubilla AL, Fortner JG, Fitzgerald PJ (1978) Lymph node involvement in carcinoma of the head of the pancreas area. Cancer 41:880–887

Delhaye M, Engelholm L, Craemer M (1985) Pancreas divisum: congenital anatomic variant or anormality? Contribution of endoscopic retrograde dorsal pancreatography. Gastroenterology 89:951–958

Didolkar MSD, Malhotra Y, Holyoke ED, Elias G (1975) Cystadenoma of the pancreas. Surg Gynecol Obstet 140:925–928

DiMagno EP, Layer P, Clain JE (1993) Chronic pancreatitis. In: Go VLW, DiMagno EP, Gardner JD, Lebenthal E, Reber HA, Scheele GA (eds) The pancreas: biology, pathobiology, and disease, 2nd edn. Raven, New York, pp 665–706

Dolan RV, ReMine WH, Dockerty MB (1974) The fate of heterotopic pancreatic tissue. Arch Surg 109:762–765

Donow C, Pipeleers-Marichal MA, Schroder S, Stamm B, Heitz PU, Klöppel G (1991) Surgical pathology of gastrinoma. Site, size, multicentricity, association with multiple endocrine neoplasia type 1, and malignancy. Cancer 68:1329–1334

Durbec JP, Sarles H (1978) Multicenter survey on the etiology of pancreatic diseases. Relationship between the relative risk of developing chronic pancreatitis and alcohol, protein, and lipid consumption. Digestion 18:337–350

Dürr GHK (1979) Acute pancreatitis. In: Howat HAT, Sarles H (eds) The exocrine pancreas. Saunders, London, pp 352–401

Ectors N, Maillet B, Aerts R, Geboes K, Donner A, Borchard F, Lankisch P, Stolte M, Lüttges J, Kremer B, Klöppel G (1997) Non-alcoholic duct destructive chronic pancreatitis. Gut 41:263–268

Egawa N, Maillet B, Schröder S, Foulis A, Mukai K, Klöppel G (1994) Serous oligocystic and ill-demarcated adenoma of the pancreas: a variant of serous cystic adenoma. Virchows Arch 424:13–17

Elfring G, Hästbacka J (1965) Pancreatic heterotopia and its clinical importance. Acta Chir Scand 130:593–602

Eusebi V, Capella C, Bondi A, Sessa F, Vezzadini P, Mancini AM (1981) Endocrine-paracrine cells in pancreatic exocrine carcinomas. Histopathology 5:599–613

Feldman M, Weinberg T (1952) Aberrant pancreas: a cause of heterotopic pancreatic tissue. JAMA 148:893–898

Fischer HP, Altmannsberger M, Kracht J (1988) Osteoclast-type giant cell tumour of the pancreas. Virchows Arch [A] Pathol Anat 412:247–253

Fishman RS, Bartholomew LG (1979) Severe pancreatic involvement in three generations in von Hippel-Lindau disease. Mayo Clin Proc 54:329–331

Foulis AK (1980) Histological evidence of initiating factors in acute necrotising pancreatitis in man. J Clin Pathol 33:1125–1131

Froboese C (1949) Beiträge zur Stütze der rheumatischen Ätiologie der Periarteriitis nodosa und zum subtotalen Pankreasinfarkt. Virchows Arch [A] Pathol Anat 317:430–448

Gadrat J, Ribet A, Suduca P, Bertrand J (1965) Pancréas aberrants intrahépatiques. Deux cas diagnostiqués par ponction-biopsie sous controle laparoscopique chez deux cirrhotiques. Arch Mal Appar Dig Nutr 54:1143–1148

George DH, Murphy F, Michalski R, Ulmer BG (1989) Serous cystadenocarcinoma of the pancreas: A new entity? Am J Surg Pathol 13:61–66

Goldberg RD, Michelassi F, Montag AG (1991) Osteoclast-like giant cell tumor of the pancreas: immunophenotypic similarity to giant cell tumor of bone. Hum Pathol 22:618–622

Goossens A, Gepts W, Saudubray JM, Bonnefont JP, Nihoul-Fekete C, Heitz PU, Klöppel G (1989) Diffuse and focal nesidioblastosis: a clinicopathological study of 24 patients with persistent neonatal hyperinsulinemic hypoglycemia. Am J Surg Pathol 13:766–775

Gorry MC, Gabbaizedeh D, Furey W, Gates LK, Jr., Preston RA, Aston CE, Zhang Y, Ulrich C, Ehrlich GD, Whitcomb DC (1997) Mutations in the cationic trypsinogen gene are associated with recurrent acute and chronic pancreatitis. Gastroenterology 113:1063–1068

Gregg JA (1977) Pancreas divisum: its association with pancreatitis. Am J Surg 134:539–543

Grünewald K, Lyons J, Fröhlich A, Feichtinger H, Weger RA, Schwab G, Janssen JW, Bartram CR (1989) High frequency of Ki-ras codon 12 mutations in pancreatic adenocarcinomas. Int J Cancer 43:1037–1041

Guthoff A, Rothe B, Klapdor R, Klöppel G, Greten H (1987) Site of recurrence after resection for pancreatic carcinoma. Dig Dis Sci 32:1168

Gyr K, Singer MV, Sarles H (1984) Pancreatitis. Concepts and classification. Proceedings of the second international symposium on the classification of pancreatitis. Excerpta Medica, Amsterdam

Hashida Y, Jaffe R, Yunis EJ (1983) Pancreatic pathology in trisomy 13: specificity of the morphologic lesion. Pediatr Pathol 1:168–178

Hayakawa T, Naruse S, Kitagawa M, Nakae Y, Harada H, Ochi K, Kuno N, Kurimoto K, Hayakawa S (1995) Pancreatic stone protein and lactoferrin in human pancreatic juice in chronic pancreatitis. Pancreas 10:137–142

Hess W (1976) Verletzungen des Pankreas. In: Forell M (ed) Pankreas. Springer, Berlin Heidelberg New York (Handbuch der Inneren Medizin, vol 3/6)

Holstege A, Barner S, Brambs HJ, Wenz W, Gerok W, Farthmann EH (1985) Relapsing pancreatitis associated with duodenal wall cysts, diagnostic approach and treatment. Gastroenterology 88:814–819

Honicky RE, de Papp EW (1973) Mediastinal teratoma with endocrine function. Am J Dis Child 126:350–357

Hoorens A, Rickaert F, Morohoshi T, Kamisawa T, Heitz PU, Stamm B, McLellan E, Lemoine NR, Rüschoff J, Klöppel G (1992) Pancreatic acinar cell tumours: their histologic, immunocytochemical and ultrastructural features. J Pathol 167 [Suppl]:149A

Hoorens A, Prenzel K, Lemoine NR, Klöppel G (1998) Undifferentiated carcinoma of the pancreas: analysis of intermediate filament profile and Ki-ras mutations provides evidence of a ductal origin. J Pathol 185:53–60

Horanyi J, Füsy F (1963) Nebenpankreas in der Gallenblasenwand. Zentralbl Chir 88:1414–1418

Horie A, Haratake J, Jimi A, Matsumoto M, Ishii N, Tsutsumi Y (1987) Pancreatoblastoma in Japan, with differential diagnosis from papillary cystic tumour (ductuloacinar adenoma) of the pancreas. Acta Pathol Jpn 37:47–63

Höfler H (1978) Über die Häufigkeit, Ätiologie und Komplikationen der akuten Pankreatitis – eine retrospektive Studie. Inn Med 5:273–279

Ihse I, Lilja P, Arnesjö B, Bengmark S (1977) Total pancreatectomy for cancer: an appraisal of 65 cases. Ann Surg 186:675–680

Imrie CW, Ferguson JC, Sommerville RG (1985) Coxsackie and mumps virus infection in a prospective study of acute pancreatitis. Gut 18:53–56

Imrie JR, Fagan DG, Sturgess JM (1979) Quantitative evaluation of the development of the exocrine pancreas in cystic fibrosis and control infants. Am J Pathol 95:697–707

Itai Y, Kokubo T, Terano A (1987) Mucin-hypersecreting carcinoma of the pancreas. Radiology 165:51–55

Iwase K, Kato K, Nagasaka A, Miura K, Kawase K, Miyakawa S, Tei T, Ohtani S, Inagaki M, Shinoda S et al (1986) Immunohistochemical study of neuron-specific enolase and CA 19–9 in pancreatic disorders. The value of neuron-specific enolase as a marker for islet cell and nerve tissue. Gastroenterology 91:576–580

Jansen HH, Rothemund E (1965) Stenosierendes Nebenpankreas des Dünndarms mit tödlichem Invaginationsileus bei einem Säugling. Chirurg 36:519–520

Jenson AB, Rosenberg HS, Notkins AL (1980) Pancreas islet-cell damage in children with fatal viral infections. Lancet ii:354–358

Jeune MC, Beraud C, Carron R (1955) Dystrophie thoracique asphyxiante de caractère familial. Arch Franc Pediatr 12:886–891

Kawagushi K, Koike M, Tsuruta K, Okamoto A, Tabata I, Fukita N (1991) Lymphoplasmacytic sclerosing pancreatitis with cholangitis: a variant of primary sclerosing cholangitis extensively involving pancreas. Hum Pathol 22:387–395

Kayahara M, Nagakawa T, Ueno K, Ohta T, Takeda T, Miyazaki I (1993) An evaluation of radical resection for pancreatic cancer based on the mode of recurrence as determined by autopsy and diagnostic imaging. Cancer 72:2118–2123

Käufer C (1967) Zur stumpfen Pankreasverletzung im Kindesalter. Zentralbl Chir 92:3074–3080

Kim JH, Ho SB, Montgomery CK, Kim YS (1990) Cell lineage markers in human pancreatic cancer. Cancer 66:2134–2143

Kimura W, Ohtsubo K (1989) Clinical and pathological features of acute interstitial pancreatitis in the aged. Int J Pancreatol 5:1–9

Klimstra DS, Heffess CS, Oertel JE, Rosai J (1992) Acinar cell carcinoma of the pancreas: a clinicopathologic study of 28 cases. Am J Surg Pathol 16:815–837

Klimstra DS, Rosai J, Heffess CS (1994) Mixed acinar-endocrine carcinomas of the pancreas. Am J Surg Pathol 18:765–778

Klimstra DS, Wenig BM, Adair CF, Heffess CS (1995) Pancreatoblastoma. A clinicopathologic study and review of the literature. Am J Surg Pathol 19:1371–1389

Klöppel G (1983) Development of pancreatic morphological lesions in cystic fibrosis. In: Kaiser D (ed) Approaches to cystic fibrosis research. Maizena, Heilbronn

Klöppel G (1984) Pancreatic, non-endocrine tumours. In: Klöppel G, Heitz PU (eds) Pancreatic pathology. Churchill Livingstone, Edinburgh, pp 79–113

Klöppel G (1986) Pathomorphology of chronic pancreatitis. In: Malfertheiner P, Ditschuneit H (eds) Diagnostic procedures in pancreatic disease. Springer, Berlin Heidelberg New York, pp 135–139

Klöppel G (1993) Pathology of nonendocrine pancreatic tumors. In: Go VLW, DiMagno EP, Gardner JD, Lebenthal E, Reber HA, Scheele GA (eds) The pancreas: biology, pathobiology, and disease, 2nd edn. Raven, New York, pp 871–897

Klöppel G (1994) Gene changes and pancreatic carcinoma: the significance of K-ras. Dig Surg 11:164–169

Klöppel G, Heitz PU (1988) Pancreatic endocrine tumors. Pathol Res Pract 183:155–168

Klöppel G, Maillet B (1991a) Chronic pancreatitis: evolution of the disease. Hepatogastroenterology 38:408–412

Klöppel G, Maillet B (1991b) Pseudocysts in chronic pancreatitis: a morphological analysis of 57 resection specimens and 9 autopsy pancreata. Pancreas 6:266–274

Klöppel G, Maillet B (1992) The morphological basis for the evolution of acute pancreatitis into chronic pancreatitis. Virchows Arch [A] Pathol Anat 420:1–4

Klöppel G, Maillet B (1993) Pathology of acute and chronic pancreatitis. Pancreas 8:659–670

Klöppel G, Bommer G, Rückert K, Seifert G (1980) Intraductal proliferation in the pancreas and its relationship to human and experimental carcinogenesis. Virchows Arch [A] Pathol Anat 387:221–233

Klöppel G, Morohoshi T, John HD, Oehmichen W, Opitz K, Angelkort A, Lietz H, Rückert K (1981) Solid and cystic acinar cell tumour of the pancreas. A tumour in young women with favourable prognosis. Virchows Arch [A] Pathol Anat 392:171–183

Klöppel G, von Gerkan R, Dreyer T (1984) Pathomorphology of acute pancreatitis. Analysis of 367 autopsy cases and 3 surgical specimens. In: Gyr KE, Singer MV, Sarles H (eds) Pancreatitis – concepts and classification. Elsevier, Amsterdam, pp 29–35

Klöppel G, Lingenthal G, von Bülow M, Kern HF (1985) Histological and fine structural features of pancreatic ductal adenocarcinomas in relation to growth and prognosis: studies in xenografted tumours and clinicohistopathologic correlation in a series of 75 cases. Histopathology 9:841–856

Klöppel G, Dreyer T, Willemer S, Kern HF, Adler G (1986) Human acute pancreatitis: its pathogenesis in the light of immunocytochemical and ultrastructural findings in acinar cells. Virchows Arch [A] Pathol Anat 409:791–803

Klöppel G, Lohse T, Bosslet K, Rückert K (1987) Ductal adenocarcinoma of the head of the pancreas: incidence of tumour involvement beyond the Whipple resection line. Histological and immunocytochemical analysis of 37 total pancreatectomy specimens. Pancreas 2:170–175

Klöppel G, Höfler H, Heitz PU (1993) Pancreatic endocrine tumours in man. In: Polak JM (ed) Diagnostic histopathology of neuroendocrine tumours, chap 5. Churchill Livingstone, Edinburgh, pp 91–121

Klöppel G, Solcia E, Longnecker DS, Capella C, Sobin LH (1996) Histological typing of tumours of the exocrine pancreas, 2nd edn. WHO International histological classification of tumours. Springer, Berlin Heidelberg New York

Klöppel G, In't Veld PA, Komminoth P, Heitz PU (1998) The endocrine pancreas. In: Kovacs K, Asa SL (eds) Functional endocrine pathology, 2nd edn. Blackwell, Boston, pp 415–487

Komminoth P, Heitz PU, Klöppel G (1998) Pathology of MEN-1: morphology, clinicopathologic correlations and tumour development. J Intern Med 243:455–464

Korc M, Friess H, Yamanaka Y, Kobrin MS, Buchler M, Beger HG (1994) Chronic pancreatitis is associated with increased concentrations of epidermal growth factor receptor, transforming growth factor a, and phospholipase Cgamma. Gut 35:1468–1473

Kubota K (1955) A case of rare type of an accessory pancreas. Okajimas Folia Anat Jpn 27:193–196

Laszik GZ, Pap A, Farkas G (1988) A case of primary sclerosing cholangitis mimicking chronic pancreatitis. Int J Pancreatol 3:503–508

Layer P, Singer MV (1990) Non-alcohol-related etiologies in chronic pancreatitis. In: Beger HG, Büchler M, Ditschuneit H, Malfertheiner P (eds) Chronic pancreatitis. Springer, Berlin Heidelberg New York, pp 35–40

Lebenthal E, Shwachman H (1977) The pancreas development, adaption and malfunction in infancy and childhood. Clin Gastroenterol 6:397–413

Lemoine NR, Jain S, Hughes CM, Staddon SL, Maillet B, Hall PA, Klöppel G (1992) Ki-ras oncogene activation in preinvasive pancreatic cancer. Gastroenterology 102:230–236

Lewandrowski K, Warshaw A, Compton C (1992) Macrocystic serous cystadenoma of the pancreas: a morphologic variant differing from microcystic adenoma. Hum Pathol 23:871–875

Lieber MR, Lack EE, Roberts JR, Merino MJ, Paterson K, Restrepo C, Solomon D, Chandra R, Triche TJ (1987) Solid and papillary epithelial neoplasm of the pancreas. An ultrastructural and immunohistochemical study of six cases. Am J Surg Pathol 11:85–93

Loftus EV Jr, Olivares-Pakzad BA, Batts KP, Adkins MC, Stephens DH, Sarr MG, DiMagno EP, Members of the Pancreas Clinic, Pancreatic surgeons of Mayo Clinic (1996) Intraductal papillary-mucinous tumors of the pancreas: clinicopathologic features, outcome, and nomenclature. Gastroenterology 110:1909–1918

Lonardo F, Cubilla AL, Klimstra DS (1996) Microadenocarcinoma of the pancreas – morphologic pattern or pathologic entity? Am J Surg Pathol 20:1385–1393

Lüttges J, Pierré E, Zamboni G, Weh G, Lietz H, Kussmann J, Klöppel G (1997) Maligne nicht-epitheliale Tumoren des Pankreas. Pathologe 18:233–237

Lüttges J, Vogel I, Menke M, Henne-Bruns D, Kremer B, Klöppel G (1998) The retroperitoneal resection margin and vessel involvement are important factors determining survival after pancreaticoduodenectomy for ductal adenocarcinoma of the head of the pancreas. Virchows Arch (in press)

Lysy J, Goldin E (1992) Pancreatitis in ulcerative colitis. J Clin Gastroenterol 15:336–339

Mack DR, Forstner GG, Wilschanski M, Freedman MH, Durie PR (1996) Shwachman syndrome: exocrine pancreatic dysfunction and variable phenotypic expression. Gastroenterology 111:1593–1602

MacKinnon D, Nash FW (1957) Pyloric obstruction due to pancreatic heterotopia in a child. Br Med J 5010:87–88

MacLean JM (1979) Embryology of the pancreas. In: Howat HAT, Sarles H (eds) The exocrine pancreas. Saunders, London

Malagelada JF (1986) The pathophysiology of alcoholic pancreatitis. Pancreas 1:270–278

Mariyama M, Kishi K, Nakamura K, Obata H, Nishimura S (1989) Frequency and types of point mutation at the 12th codon of the c-K-ras gene found in pancreatic cancers from Japanese patients. Jpn J Cancer Res 80:622–626

Marks IN (1990) Alcohol, the alimentary tract and pancreas: facts and controversies. In: Beger HG, Büchler M, Ditschuneit H, Malfertheiner P (eds) Chronic pancreatitis. Springer, Berlin Heidelberg New York, pp 26–34

Marks IN, Bornman PC (1994) Acute alcoholic pancreatitis: a South African view point. In: Bradley EL III (ed) Acute pancreatitis: diagnosis and therapy. Raven, New York, pp 271–277

Marrano D, Gullo L, Casadei T, Santini D, Leone O, Campione O (1996) An unusual case of chronic pancreatitis of possible immune origin. Letter to the editor. Pancreas 12:202–213

Masi AT, Hartmann WH, Hahn BN, Abbey H, Shulman LE (1965) Hashimoto's disease – a clinicopathological study with matched controls. Lancet i:123–126

Metzgar RS, Gaillard MT, Levine SJ, Tuck FL, Bossen EH, Borowitz MJ (1982) Antigens of human pancreatic adenocarcinoma cells defined by murine monoclonal antibodies. Cancer Res 42:601–608

Mikal S, Campbell AJA (1950) Carcinoma of the pancreas. Diagnostic and operative criteria based on one hundred consecutive autopsies. Surgery 28:963–969

Milchgrub S, Campuzano M, Casillas J, Albores-Saavedra J (1992) Intraductal carcinoma of the pancreas. Cancer 69:651–656

Mizumoto K, Inagaki T, Koizumi M, Uemura M, Ogawa M, Kitazawa S, Tsutsumi M, Toyokawa M, Konishi Y (1988) Early pancreatic duct adenocarcinoma. Hum Pathol 19:242–244

Moldow RE, Connelly RR (1968) Epidemiology of pancreatic cancer in Connecticut. Gastroenterology 55:677–686

Mollenhauer J, Roether I, Kern HF (1987) Distribution of extracellular matrix proteins in pancreatic ductal adenocarcinoma and its influence on tumor cell proliferation in vitro. Pancreas 2:14–24

Morohoshi T, Held G, Klöppel G (1983) Exocrine pancreatic tumours and their histological classification. A study based on 167 autopsy and 97 surgical cases. Histopathology 7:645–661

Morohoshi T, Kanda M, Horie A, Chott A, Dreyer T, Klöppel G, Heitz PU (1987) Immunocytochemical markers of uncommon pancreatic tumors. Acinar cell carcinoma, pancreatoblastoma, and solid cystic (papillary-cystic) tumor. Cancer 59:739–747

Morohoshi T, Kanda M, Asanuma K, Klöppel G (1989) Intraductal papillary neoplasms of the pancreas. A clinicopathologic study of six patients. Cancer 64:1329–1335

Mössner J (1993) Epidemiology of chronic pancreatitis. In: Beger HG, Büchler M, Malfertheiner P (eds) Standards in pancreatic surgery. Springer, Berlin Heidelberg New York, pp 263–271

Multigner I, Sarles H, Lombardo D, de Caro A (1985) Pancreatic stone protein II: Implication in stone formation during the course of chronic calcifying pancreatitis. Gastroenterology 89:387–391

Naficy K, Nategh R, Ghadimi (1973) Mumps pancreatitis without parotitis. Br Med J I:529

Nagai H, Ohtsubo K (1984) Pancreatic lithiasis in the aged. Its clinicopathology and pathogenesis. Gastroenterology 86:331–338

Nagai H, Kuroda A, Morioka Y (1986) Lymphatic and local spread of T1 and T2 pancreatic cancer. A study of autopsy material. Ann Surg 204:65–71

Nagakawa T, Kobayashi H, Ueno K, Ohta T, Kayahara M, Miyazaki I (1994) Clinical study of lymphatic flow to the paraaortic lymph nodes in carcinoma of the head of the pancreas. Cancer 73:1155–1162

Nevalainen TJ, Aho HJ, Eskola JU, Suonpää AK (1983) Immunohistochemical localization of phospholipase A2 in human pancreas in acute and chronic pancreatitis. Acta Pathol Microbiol Scand [A] 91:97–102

Nicolesco ST, Velciu V (1968) Contribution à l'étude morphopathologique des hétérotopies pancréatiques du tractus digestif. Arch Anat Cytol Pathol 16:271–280

Noronha M, Bordalo O, Dreiling DA (1981) Alcohol and the pancreas. II. Pancreatic morphology of advanced alcoholic pancreatitis. Am J Gastroenterol 76:120–124

Obara T, Maguchi H, Saitoh Y, Ura H, Koike Y, Kitazawa S, Namiki M (1991) Mucin-producing tumour of the pancreas: a unique clinical entity. Am J Gastroenterol 86:1619–1625

Oertel JE, Heffess CS, Oertel YC (1989) Pancreas. Diagn Surg Pathol 2:1057–1093

Opie EL (1901) The relation of cholelithiasis to disease of the pancreas and to fat necrosis. Am J Med Sci 121:27–43

Palosaari D, Clayton F, Seaman J (1986) Pancreatoblastoma in an adult. Arch Pathol Lab Med 110:650–652

Pipeleers-Marichal MA, Somers G, Willems G, Foulis A, Imrie C, Bishop AE, Polak JM, Häcki WH, Stamm B, Heitz PU (1990) Gastrinomas in the duodenums of patients with multiple endocrine neoplasia type 1 and the Zollinger-Ellison syndrome. N Engl J Med 322:723–727

Pliam MB, ReMine WH (1975) Further evaluation of total pancreatectomy. Arch Surg 110:506–512

Pollak OJ (1968) Human pancreatic arteriosclerosis. Ann NY Acad Sci 149:928–931

Renner IG, Savage WT, Pantoja JL, Renner VJ (1985) Death due to acute pancreatitis. A retrospective analysis of 405 autopsy cases. Dig Dis Sci 30:1005–1018

Reyes CV, Wang T (1981) Undifferentiated small cell carcinoma of the pancreas: A report of five cases. Cancer 47:2500–2502

Rickaert F, Cremer M, Devière J, Tavares L, Lambilliotte JP, Schröder S, Wurbs D, Klöppel G (1991) Intraductal mucin-hypersecreting neoplasms of the pancreas. A clinicopathologic study of eight patients. Gastroenterology 101:512–519

Rosai J (1968) Carcinoma of pancreas simulating giant cell tumor of bone. Electron-microscopic evidence of its acinar cell origin. Cancer 22:333–344

Sarles H, Muratore R, Sarles JC, Gaini M, Camatte R, Pastor J, Guien C (1965) Aetiology and pathology of chronic pancreatitis. In: Sarles H (ed) Pancreatitis. Karger, Basel, pp 75–120 (Bibliotheca Gastroenterologica no 7)

Sarles H, Bernard JP, Gullo L (1990) Pathogenesis of chronic pancreatitis. Gut 31:629–632

Sarles H, Payan H, Tasso F, Sahel J (1976) Chronic pancreatitis, relapsing pancreatitis, calcification of the pancreas. In: Bockus HL (ed) Gastroenterology, 2nd edn. Saunders, Philadelphia, pp 1040–1051

Scheele GA, Adler G, Kern HF (1984) Role of lysosomes in the development of acute pancreatitis. In: Gyr KE, Singer MV, Sarles H (eds) Pancreatitis – concepts and classification. Excerpta Medica, Amsterdam, pp 17–23

Schega W, Dennhardt D (1971) Pankreasverletzungen im Kindesalter. Dtsch Med Wochenschr 96:1662–1667

Schein PS, DeLellis RA, Kahn CR, Gorden P, Kraft AR (1973) Islet cell tumors. Current concepts and management. Ann Intern Med 79:239–257

Schlumberger HF (1946) Teratoma of anterior mediastinum in the group of military age: a study of 16 cases, and a review of theories of genesis. Arch Pathol Lab Med 41:398–444

Schmiegel W (1993) PSP, PTP, or REG protein? The role of pancreatic stone protein. In: Beger HG, Büchler M, Malfertheiner P (eds) Standards in pancreatic surgery. Springer, Berlin Heidelberg New York, pp 281–289

Schmiegel W, Burchert M, Kalthoff H, Roeder C, Bützow G, Grimm H, Kremer B, Soehendra N, Schreiber HW, Thiele HG, Greten H (1990) Immunochemical characterization and quantitative distribution of pancreatic stone protein in sera and pancreatic secretions in pancreatic disorders. Gastroenterology 99:1421–1430

Schmitz-Moormann P (1981) Comparative radiological and morphological study of the human pancreas. IV. Acute necrotizing pancreatitis in man. Pathol Res Pract 171:325–335

Seifert G (1959) Lipomatöse cystische Pankreasfibrose und lipomatöse Pankreasatrophie des Kindesalters. Beitr Pathol Anat 121:64–80

Seifert G (1984) Congenital anomalies. In: Klöppel G, Heitz PU (eds) Pancreatic pathology. Churchill Livingstone, London

Seifert G, Klöppel G (1984) Diagnostic value of pancreatic biopsy. Pathol Res Pract 164:357–384

Seligson U, Cho JW, Ihse I, Lundh G (1982) Clinical course and autopsy findings in acute and chronic pancreatitis. Acta Chir Scand 148:269–274

Sessa F, Solcia E, Capella C, Bonato M, Scarpa A, Zamboni G, Pellegata NS, Ranzani GN, Rickaert F, Klöppel G (1994) Intraductal papillary-mucinous tumours represent a distinct group of pancreatic neoplasms: an investigation of tumour cell differentiation and K-ras, p53, and c-erbB-2 abnormalities in 26 patients. Virchows Arch 425:357–367

Seyrig JA, Jian R, Modigliani R, Golfain D, Florent C, Messing B, Bitoun A (1985) Idiopathic pancreatitis as associated with inflammatory bowel disease. Dig Dis Sci 30:1121–1126

Shwachman H, Diamond LK, Oski FA, Khaw KT (1964) The syndrome of pancreatic insufficiency and bone marrow dysfunction. J Pediatr 65:645–663

Sibert JR (1975) Pancreatitis in children. A study in the north of England. Arch Dis Child 50:443–448

Sjögren I, Wengle B, Korsgren M (1979) Primary sclerosing cholangitis associated with fibrosis of the submandibular glands and the pancreas. Acta Med Scand 205:139–141

Solcia E, Capella C, Klöppel G (1997) Tumors of the pancreas. AFIP atlas of tumor pathology, 3rd ser, fascicle 20. Armed Forces Institute of Pathology, Washington DC

Sood S, Fossard DP, Shorrock K (1995) Chronic sclerosing pancreatitis in Sjögren's syndrome: a case report. Pancreas 10:419–421

Stamm B, Burger H, Hollinger A (1987) Acinar cell cystadenocarcinoma of the pancreas. Cancer 60:2542–2547

Starck D (1965) Ein Lehrbuch auf allgemein biologischer Grundlage. Thieme, Stuttgart

Steer ML (1989) Classification and pathogenesis of pancreatitis. Surg Clin North Am 69:467–480

Stern RC (1997) The diagnosis of cystic fibrosis. N Engl J Med 336:487–491

Stoffers DA, Zinkin NT, Stanojevic V, Clarke WL, Habener JF (1997) Pancreatic agenesis attributable to a single nucleotide deletion in the human IPF1 gene coding sequence. Nat Genet 15:106–110

Stolte M, Weiss W, Volkholz H, Rösch W (1982) A special form of segmental pancreatitis: „groove pancreatitis“. Hepatogastroenterology 29:198–208

Stolte M, Zink W, Schaffner O (1983) Duodenalwandzysten und Erkrankungen der Bauchspeicheldrüsen. Leber Magen Darm 13:140–149

Storck G, Pettersson G, Edlund Y (1976) A study of autopsies upon 116 patients with acute pancreatitis. Surg Gynecol Obstet 143:241–245

Stömmer P (1980) Lipomatöse Pankreasfibrose – eine Sonderform der Mukoviszidose. Inn Med 7:95–100

Suda K, Mizuguchi K, Hebisawa A, Wakabayashi T, Saito S (1984) Pancreatic tissue in teratoma. Arch Pathol Lab Med 108:835–837

Sugawa G, Walt AJ (1979) Endoscopic retrograde pancreatography in the surgery of pancreatic pseudocysts. Surgery 86:639–647

Tabata T, Fujimoro T, Maeda S, Yamamoto M, Saitoh Y (1993) The role of ras mutation in pancreatic cancer, precancerous lesions, and chronic pancreatitis. Int J Pancreatol 14:237–244

Tada M, Omata M, Ohto M (1991) Ras gene mutations in intraductal papillary neoplasms of the pancreas. Analysis in five cases. Cancer 67:634–637

Takeda S, Nakao A, Ichihara T, Suzuki Y, Nonami T, Harada A, Kohhikawa T, Takagi H (1991) Serum concentration and immunohistochemical localization of SPan-1 antigen in pancreatic cancer: a comparison with CA 19–9 antigen. Hepatogastroenterology 38:143–148

Tempero M, Takasaki H, Uchida E, Takiyama Y, Colcher D, Metzgar RS, Pour PM (1989) Co-expression of CA 19–9, DU-PAN-2, CA 125, and TAG-72 in pancreatic adenocarcinoma. Am J Surg Pathol 13:89–95

Tepper J, Nardi G, Suit H (1976) Carcinoma of the pancreas: review of MGH experience from 1963 to 1973. Analysis of surgical failure and implications for radiation therapy. Cancer 37:1519–1524

Thompson RJ, Hinshaw DB (1966) Pancreatic trauma: review of 87 cases. Ann Surg 163:153–160

Torrance B (1979) Traumatic lesions of the pancreas. In: Howat HAT, Sarles H (eds) The exocrine pancreas. Saunders, London

Trapnell JE (1971) Complications of acute pancreatitis. Ann Roy Coll Surg Engl 49:361–372

Trepeta RW, Mathur B, Lagin S, LiVolsi VA (1981) Giant cell tumor („osteoclastoma“) of the pancreas: a tumor of epithelial origin. Cancer 48:2022–2028

Tryka AF, Brooks JR (1979) Histopathology in the evaluation of total pancreatectomy for ductal carcinoma. Ann Surg 190:373–379

Ulich T, Cheng L, Lewin KJ (1982) Acinar-endocrine cell tumor of the pancreas. Report of a pancreatic tumor containing both zymogen and neuroendocrine granules. Cancer 50:2099–2105

Uys CJ, Bank S, Marks IN (1973) The pathology of chronic pancreatitis in Cape Town. Digestion 9:454–468

van Heerden JA (1984) Pancreatic resection for carcinoma of the pancreas: whipple versus total pancreatectomy – an institutional perspective. World J Surg 8:88–88 van Laethem JL, Devière J, Resibois A, Rickaert F, Vertongen P, Ohtani H, Cremer M, Miyazono K, Robberecht P (1995) Localizing of transforming growth factor b1 and its latent binding protein in human chronic pancreatitis. Gastroenterology 108:1873–1881

Verner JV, Morrison AB (1974) Endocrine pancreatic islet disease with diarrhoea. Report of a case due to diffuse hyperplasia of non beta islet tissue with a review of 54 additional cases. Arch Intern Med 133:492–500

Viswanathan M (1980) Pancreatic diabetes in India: an overview. In: Podolsky S, Viswanathan M (eds) Secondary diabetes: the spectrum of the diabetic syndromes. Raven, New York, pp 105–116

Waldram R, Kopelman H, Tsantoulas D, Williams R (1975) Chronic pancreatitis, sclerosing cholangitis, and sicca complex in two siblings. Lancet 550–552

Warkany JE, Passarge E, Smith LB (1966) Congenital malformations in autosomal trisomy syndromes. Am J Dis Child 112:502–517

Warshaw AL, Berry J, Gang DL (1987) Villous adenoma of the duct of Wirsung. Dig Dis Sci 32:1311–1313

Warshaw AL, Simeone JF, Schapiro RH, Flavin-Warshaw B (1990) Evaluation and treatment of the dominant dorsal duct syndrome (pancreas divisum redefined). Am J Surg 159:59–66

Whitcomb DC, Preston RA, Aston CE, Sossenheimer MJ, Barua PS, Zhang Y, Wong-Chong A, White GJ, Wood PG, Gates LK Jr, Ulrich C, Martin SP, Post JC, Ehrlich GD (1996) A gene for hereditary pancreatitis maps to chromosome 7q35. Gastroenterology 110:1975–1980

Willemer S, Adler G (1989) Histochemical and ultrastructural characteristics of tubular complexes in human acute pancreatitis. Dig Dis Sci 34:46–55

Willemer S, Klöppel G, Kern HF, Adler G (1989) Immunocytochemical and morphometric analysis of acinar zymogen granules in human acute pancreatitis. Virchows Arch [A] Pathol Anat 415:115–123

Witte CL, Schanzer CB (1968) Pancreatitis due to mumps. JAMA 203:1068–1069

Worning H (1984) Chronic pancreatitis: pathogenesis, natural history and conservative treatment. Clin Gastroenterol 13:871–894

Worning H (1990) Incidence and prevalence of chronic pancreatitis. In: Beger HG, Büchler M, Ditschuneit H, Malfertheiner P (eds) Chronic pancreatitis. Springer, Berlin Heidelberg New York, pp 8–14

Wöckel W, Scheibner K (1977) Aplasie des Pankreas mit Diabetes mellitus, intrahepatischer Gallengangsaplasie und weiteren Missbildungen bei einem hypotrophen Neugeborenen. Zentralbl Allg Pathol Pathol Anat 121:186–194

Yamada M, Kozuka S, Yamao K, Nakazawa S, Naitoh Y, Tsukamoto Y (1991) Mucin-producing tumour of the pancreas. Cancer 68:159–168

Yamaguchi K, Enjoji M (1987) Cystic neoplasm of the pancreas. Gastroenterology 92:1934–1943

Yamaguchi K, Tanaka M (1991) Mucin-hypersecreting tumor of the pancreas with mucin extrusion through an enlarged papilla. Am J Gastroenterol 86:835–839

Yoshimi N, Sugie S, Tanaka T, Aijin W, Bunai Y, Tatematsu, Okada T, Mori H (1992) A rare case of serous cystadenocarcinoma of the pancreas. Cancer 69:2449–2453

Zamboni G, Scarpa A, Bogina G, Iacono C, Bassi C, Talamini G, Sessa F, Capella C, Solcia E, Rickaert F, Mariuzzi GM, Klöppel G (1998) Mucinous cystic tumors of the pancreas: clinicopathological features, prognosis and relationship to other mucinous cystic tumors. Am J Surg Pathol (in press)

Zuidema PJ (1959) Cirrhosis and disseminated calcification of the pancreas in patients with malnutrition. Trop Geog Med 11:70–74

5 Pancreatic Diseases in Childhood

J.F. Chateil, M. Brun, and F. Diard

CONTENTS

J.F. Chateil, MD
Service de Radiologie A, Hôpital Pellegrin, Place A Raba Léon, F-33076 Bordeaux, France
M. Brun, MD
Service de Radiologie A, Hôpital Pellegrin, Place A Raba Léon, F-33076 Bordeaux, France
F. Diard, MD
Professeur de Radiologie, Service de Radiologie A, Hôpital Pellegrin, Place A Raba Léon, F-33076 Bordeaux, France

5.1 Introduction

Diseases of the pancreas in children can be of congenital, inflammatory, or, more rarely, tumoral origin. The most frequent condition is pancreatitis regardless of its origin.

5.2 Investigative Methods and Normal Radiological Findings in Children

5.2.1 Plain Films of the Abdomen

The pancreas is not directly visualized on plain films of the abdomen. Calcifications in the pancreatic region or biliary lithiasis can sometimes be demonstrated. The existence of adynamic ileus of duodenum and the proximal small bowel loops (sentinel loop), or a generalized ileus, can be associated signs in acute disorders.

5.2.2 Ultrasonography

Ultrasonography is currently the easiest way of examining the pancreas in children, and the pancreas can be well evaluated in most cases (Berrocal et al. 1995a). The left liver lobe is more prominent than in the adult and is therefore an excellent acoustic window for the study of the head and body of the pancreas. In the same way, the spleen can allow excellent visualization of the pancreatic tail. The examination is best performed in children who have fasted for 3–4 h in order to avoid superimposition of the stomach. Children are examined supine or, sometimes, sitting or standing. Ingestion of water can be useful. If there is a significant adynamic ileus, placement of a gastric tube and aspiration of the digestive secretions may be necessary for better exploration of the pancreas.

In children, the pancreas has an almost horizontal orientation so that the entire gland can be visualized on one transverse scan (Fig. 5.1). The head and the tail are somewhat more voluminous than the body. In Table 5.1, the transverse dimensions of the pancreas as a function of pediatric age are given, according to SIEGEL et al. (1987).

The pancreatic parenchyma is homogeneous, with mild echogenicity. It is usually somewhat more echogenic than adjacent liver at the same level, but can also be isoechoic or relatively hypoechoic (FLEISCHER et al. 1983; SIEGEL et al. 1987). In the newborn, and especially in the premature infant, the greater echogenicity of the pancreas compared with the liver is more pronounced due to the abundance of connective tissue (WALSH et al. 1990). This feature progressively disappears with age, but returns in adults with the growth of fatty tissue. It is hazardous to rely on alterations in the echogenicity of the pancreas alone to make the diagnosis of pancreatic disease. The pancreatic duct can be visible as either one or two hyperechoic lines at the level of the head and body. The lumen is very small and often not clearly visible; normal ductal diameter should be no larger than 1–2 mm (SIEGEL and SIVIT 1997).

Ultrasonographic study of the pancreas always includes examination of the biliary ducts, liver, and spleen. The vessels must also be analyzed, in particular the portal vein and its tributaries. Examination of the vascular flow with pulsed Doppler or color Doppler can also be useful.

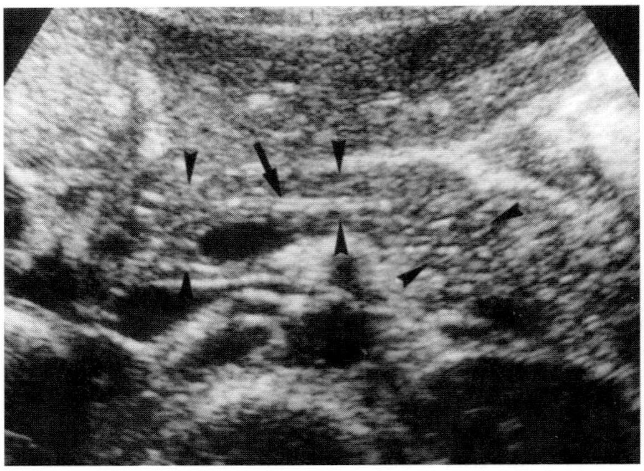

Fig. 5.1. Normal pancreas in a 9-year-old child: transverse sonogram. The *arrowheads* indicate the limits of the pancreas at the level of the head, the body, and the tail, corresponding to the normal measurements as shown in Table 5.1. The parenchyma is isoechoic with the liver; the pancreatic duct is clearly visible as two parallel hyperechoic lines (*arrow*)

5.2.3 Barium Studies of the Upper Digestive Tract

Barium studies are rarely used nowadays when there is a suspicion of pancreatic disease and have been largely replaced with ultrasonography and computed tomography (CT). They remain of some interest in occlusive neonatal syndromes where an anomaly of the pancreas can be associated with duodenal anomalies (SMITH 1982).

Table 5.1. Normal dimensions of the pancreas as a function of age (SIEGEL et al. 1987)

Age	Maximal anteroposterior dimensions of pancreas (cm±1 SD)		
	Head	Body	Tail
<1 month	1.0±0.4	0.6±0.2	1.0±0.4
1 month–1 year	1.5±0.5	0.8±0.3	1.2±0.4
1–5 years	1.7±0.3	1.0±0.2	1.8±0.4
5–10 years	1.6±0.4	1.0±0.3	1.8±0.4
10–19 years	2.0±0.5	1.1±0.3	2.0±0.4

5.2.4 Computed Tomography

In the study of pediatric pancreas, CT is a method of second choice and is reserved for those cases in which ultrasonography does not allow a precise diagnosis. The interpretation is not always easy in children due to the low amount of fat in the retroperitoneal and pancreatic area.

The introduction of spiral CT has improved the usefulness of the exam. In the young child, the examination needs to be performed, in most cases, with the patient under sedation, even though total time scanning is shortened in a helical CT study, and can reduce the need for sedation (FRUSH et al. 1997). It is also important to obtain a good opacification of the digestive tract. Specific preparation of diluted barium sulfate (1%–2% solution), or a dilute solution of water-soluble iodine-based contrast mixed with soft drinks to avoid an unpleasant taste can be used. The amounts of contrast material by age are given in Table 5.2, according to FRUSH et al. (1997). New negative oral contrast material is currently being evaluated for the study of the intestinal tract. If sedation is necessary, no oral contrast material can be administered.

Most CT examinations of the abdomen are performed with intravenous contrast material. Optimal

Table 5.2. Doses of oral contrast material for spiral computed tomography by patient age (FRUSH et al. 1997)

Age	Amount given 45 min before scanning (ml)	Amount given 15 min before scanning (ml)
<1 month	60–90	30–45
1 month–1 year	120–240	60–120
1–5 years	240–360	120–180
6–12 years	360–480	180–240
13–15 years	480–600	240–300
16–18 years	720	360

parenchymal enhancement depends on the amount of contrast material and the injection rate used. The dose of contrast material is 2 ml/kg. Manual injection is frequently used for pediatric CT examinations, but a power injector can also be used. The injection rate is difficult to determine with manual injection. Optimal enhancement also depends on time of scanning. In most cases, this occurs after 100% of the dose of contrast material has been administered. A delay of 10 s following completion of the injection, with contrast injected as rapidly as possible, can be recommended (WHITE 1996). The contrast enhancement can also be monitored to determine the beginning of the scanning. For a study of the pancreas, the slices have to be adjacent (pitch 1:1) with a slice thickness of 3–5 mm and a scan time as short as possible. If image reconstruction is needed, overlapping slices may be necessary. Spiral CT cholangiography with three-dimensional (3D) reconstruction using surface rendering or maximum intensity projection (MIP) can be performed; CT has to be obtained 1 h after intravenous injection of iodipamide (BOROCCO et al. 1996b).

The pancreas is of homogeneous density, slightly inferior to that of the liver, and enhances after intravenous injection of contrast material. The pancreas has regular contours, but discrete lobulations of the head and neck of the pancreas are normal variants, representing a spectrum of fusion patterns of the dorsal and ventral buds of the pancreas (ROSS et al. 1996). The pancreatic duct is rarely visible. The normal bile duct can be recognized at the level of the head of the pancreas (VEYRAC et al. 1987).

5.2.5 Magnetic Resonance Imaging

Magnetic resonance imaging (MRI) of the pancreas in children remains difficult to perform and to interpret since numerous artifacts result from the long duration of the examination and the presence of intestinal peristalsis. The development of short acquisition sequences progressively allows utilization of this technique as a complement or a substitute for CT.

Magnetic resonance cholangiopancreatography (MRCP) can be of interest in the evaluation of the normal and abnormal pancreatic duct. The MRCP technique is based on heavily T2-weighted pulse sequences (gradient-echo or fast spin-echo sequences), with two-dimensional (2D) or 3D sequences (Fig. 5.2). Breath-hold imaging techniques with rapid acquisition by repeated echoes (RARE sequence) are also evaluated (ICHIKAWA et al. 1996). Image interpretation can use native images, multiplanar reconstruction or 3D MIP. With such a technique, the main pancreatic duct can be identified in children in most MR pancreatograms. The presence of anatomic variants and bile duct obstruction can be evaluated in neonates and infants (GUIBAUD et al. 1995, 1998; REINHOLD and BRET 1996; MIYAZAKI et al. 1998).

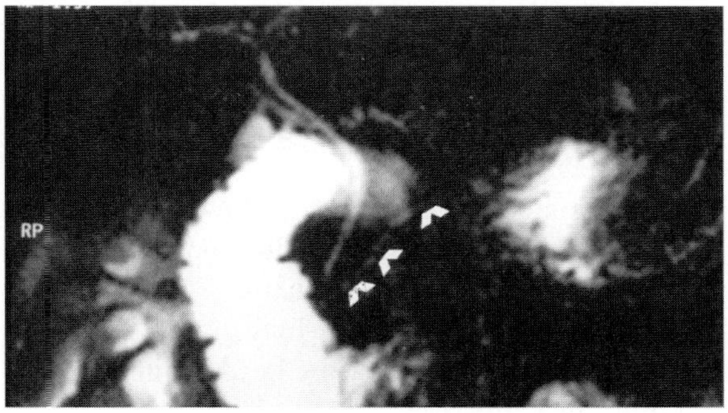

Fig. 5.2. Magnetic resonance cholangiopancreatography (T2-weighted turbo spin echo sequence) in a 13-year-old child. The normal bile duct is clearly delineated; the pancreatic duct is also visible (*arrowheads*). (Courtesy of Dr. Lescene)

5.2.6 Endoscopic Retrograde Cholangiopancreatography (ERCP)

Retrograde catheterization of the papilla is less easy than in the adult, but with new, small endoscopic instruments, ERCP can be performed in infants. It is indicated in cases of pancreatitis of unknown origin, to detect post-traumatic or post-pancreatitis complications, or to diagnose an anatomic abnormality of the pancreatic ducts (ALLENDORPH et al. 1987;

Teele and Share 1991; Lerner et al. 1996). Therapeutic endoscopic intervention can also been performed (Tagge et al. 1997).

5.2.7 Other Investigations

Angiography is rarely indicated in children. Selective pancreatic venous sampling has been described in the study of children with hyperinsulinism (Brunelle et al. 1989). The use of an artificial pancreas may be of value to appreciate immediate variations in glycemia pre- and peroperatively (Gin et al. 1987). Ultrasonography and opacification of the pancreatic ducts can also be performed perioperatively.

The biologic examinations must always guide the indications for and interpretations of the imaging studies. The serum and urine levels of amylase and lipase serve as indicators of pancreatic cytolysis. The detection of steatorrhea is essential in the evaluation of exocrine function.

5.3 Congenital Anomalies of the Pancreas

From an embryological point of view, it is essential to remember that the pancreas develops in the four-week embryo from two diverticula of the primitive digestive foregut. The dorsal bud gives rise to the body, the tail, and a part of the head, while the ventral bud forms the rest of the head and the uncinate process. At the end of the sixth week of gestation, these two buds fuse after the rotation of the duodenum to the right. The ventral bud circles around the duodenum from the right side. Each bud is drained by an independent duct, the two ducts fusing to form the pancreatic duct. This duct joins the common bile duct at the level of the ampulla of Vater. Different embryological anomalies can occur during organogenesis.

5.3.1 Aplasia, Hypoplasia, and Dysplasia of the Pancreas

Complete agenesis of the pancreas is extremely rare, and it is usually incompatible with life. In partial agenesis, there is a incomplete development of the dorsal bud (congenital short pancreas). It can be associated with polysplenia (Herman and Siegel 1991). In hypoplasia, the normal epithelial cells are replaced by fatty tissue. In dysplasia, embryological development is normal, but there is ineffective cellular differentiation: the parenchyma is disorganized with duct dilatation and fibromuscular abundance (Durie 1996). The clinical presentation is variable, and includes intra-uterine retardation, failure to thrive, and pancreatic origin malabsorption. Sometimes, the residual pancreatic capacity is sufficient, and the disease may not be symptomatic. Ultrasonography and CT are helpful for diagnosis (Lerner et al. 1996).

5.3.2 Annular Pancreas

Annular pancreas consists in the presence of a band of pancreatic parenchyma around a section of the second part of the duodenum. This band can be complete or incomplete. When it is complete, it is most frequently associated with stenosis or atresia of the duodenum: annular pancreas is found in one third of these cases. The primary embryological anomaly is most probably situated at the level of the duodenum, causing persistence or malrotation of the ventral pancreatic bud, which remains circumferential at the level of the duodenum. This malformation can be isolated or can be accompanied by a digestive tract malrotation, atresia of the esophagus, anorectal malformation, Meckel's diverticulum, spinal defects, and cardiac anomalies (Ökten et al. 1994; Summer et al. 1997). Its frequency is also increased in trisomy 21.

The diagnosis can be suggested on prenatal ultrasonography by the demonstration of two constant liquid-containing abdominal structures, possibly accompanied by hydramnios. If such an anomaly is discovered, a fetal karyotype has to be performed in order to exclude Down's syndrome. After birth, the clinical presentation depends on the degree of duodenal obstruction. If duodenal obstruction is complete, the diagnosis is rapidly evident due to the presence of occlusion in the neonate with little or no upper abdominal distention (Fig. 5.3). The plain film of the abdomen shows the classic „double bubble", with two asymmetrical air-fluid levels, one gastric, on the left side, the other duodenal (Smith 1982). If there is only a stenosis or diaphragm of the duodenum, contrast study of the bowel will allow the diagnosis by showing a reduction in the caliber and by

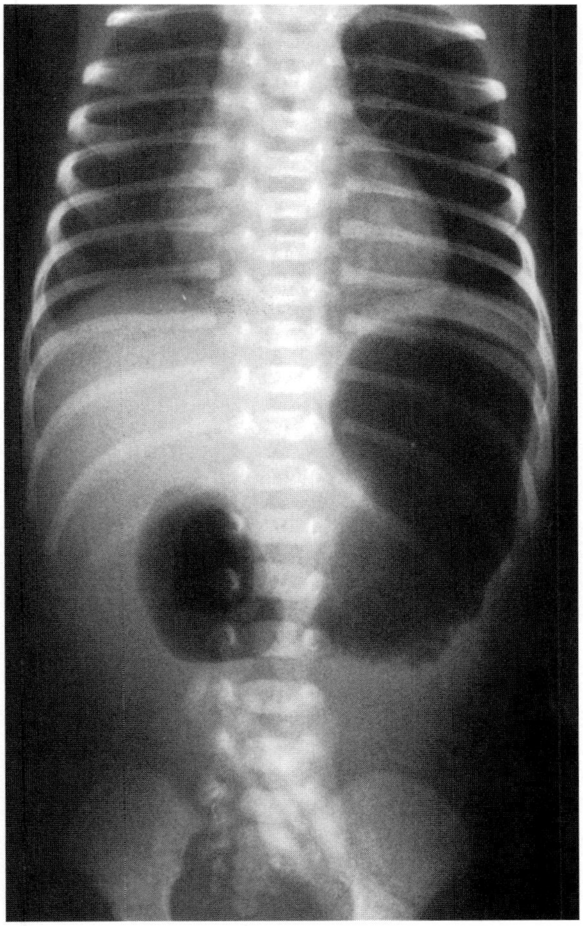

Fig. 5.3. Annular pancreas associated with duodenal atresia in a 1-day-old neonate with clear vomit. The anteroposterior thoracoabdominal plain film with the baby in the upright position shows the presence of two air-fluid levels, one corresponding to the stomach, the other to the duodenum. There is no air in the more distal bowel loops, indicating a complete obstruction. Surgical intervention confirmed atresia of the second duodenum, with a circumferential band of pancreatic parenchymal tissue

demonstrating the level of the obstruction. This anomaly can also be suspected by ultrasonography (TEELE and SHARE 1991) The MR appearance of annular pancreas has been described in an adolescent boy, with pancreatic tissue surrounding the second portion of the duodenum demonstrated with T2-weighted images; despite this case, MRI should not be used routinely in such patients (REINHART et al. 1994). Treatment is always surgical.

On the other hand, this anomaly can be diagnosed later, particularly in the adult, in the presence of signs of incomplete obstruction of the duodenum, or of pancreatitis (GLAZER and MARGULIS 1979; BERNARD et al. 1984).

5.3.3 Pancreas Divisum and Anomalies of the Pancreatic Duct

Pancreas divisum represents an anomaly of the fusion of the two pancreatic buds. It is the most common congenital anomaly of the pancreas. The two pancreatic ducts end separately in the duodenum. The ventral duct of Wirsung fuses with the common bile duct at the level of the ampulla of Vater. The dorsal duct of Santorini, which drains the body and the tail of the pancreas, terminates more cephalad, at the level of the accessory papilla.

A communication can exist between the two ducts. In the presence of associated atresia of the duodenum, this intrapancreatic anastomosis can be responsible for progression of air into the bowel distal to the obstruction, modifying the findings on plain films of the abdomen (SMITH 1982).

Pancreas divisum is usually asymptomatic, but abdominal pain is sometimes noted. The occurrence of pancreatitis seems to be more specific, resulting from inefficient drainage of the pancreatic secretions by the duct of Santorini, which is too narrow (GOLD et al. 1984; ZEMAN et al. 1988; TEELE and SHARE 1991).

The diagnosis is made by retrograde catheterization and opacification of the pancreatic ducts. A short duct of Wirsung confined to the head of the pancreas and a full-length duct of Santorini are visualized. Thin-section CT has also been proposed to demonstrate the two canals, but this is difficult in children (ZEMAN et al. 1988). MRCP is adequate for diagnosing pancreas divisum, and can be a good examination in children with subacute pancreatitis in whom a pancreas divisum is suspected (SOTO et al. 1995; BRET et al. 1996).

5.3.4 Common Bilio-pancreatic Channel

Other anatomic variants of the pancreatic duct include an excessively proximal junction of the pancreatic duct with the common bile duct, responsible for a common bilio-pancreatic channel, longer than 5 mm. This can lead to the formation of a cyst of the common bile duct (choledochal cyst), due to reflux of pancreatic secretions into the biliary tree (BABBITT et al. 1973; ARIMA and AKITA 1979) Pancreatitis may occur (STRINGER et al. 1995). On the other hand, in this situation, the existence of a functional duct of Santorini may have a protective effect against the occurrence of pancreatitis (Perisic et al. 1991). Association with an annular pancreas has been described (Komura et al. 1993). In the absence of the development of a cyst, intermittent dilatation of the bile tract caused by a protein plug in the common channel may occur (Lachaux et al. 1994). Clinically, occurrence of abdominal pain, nausea, vomiting, jaundice, and acholic stools may be explained by this obstruction. ERCP or opacification during surgery demonstrate the abnormal fusion (Ando et al. 1995; Miyano et al. 1996). In a recent study, the diagnostic accuracy of MRCP was 69% in patients with anomalous connections between the bile and pancreatic ducts (Miyazaki et al. 1998). Surgical treatment relieves symptoms and minimizes the risk of malignancy of the bile duct in later life (Ando et al. 1995; Miyano et al. 1996).

5.3.5 Heterotopic Pancreas

In the case of the ectopic or aberrant pancreas, islands of pancreatic glandular tissue are present in a heterotopic position, i.e., the stomach, duodenum, Meckel's diverticulum, gallbladder fossa, or duplication of a part of the digestive tract (Alessandrini and Derlon 1991; Ueda et al. 1991). The most frequent localizations are the greater curvature of the stomach and the antral region. Extra-abdominal sites have been described. The ectopic pancreatic tissue is presented as a firm regular nodule, with ductal and acinar components. This anomaly can be asymptomatic and a fortuitous finding during a gastrointestinal work-up. The presence of an alkaline secretion in the stomach can provoke epigastric pain and dyspepsia. Intermittent acute abdominal pain due to gastroduodenal prolapse of the ectopic pancreas may occur (Allison et al. 1995). Complications include gastrointestinal bleeding, intussusception, and several cases of carcinoma have been reported. The radiological appearance during a barium study (Fig. 5.4) is frequently characteristic (in two thirds of cases): a mass of 1–4 cm in diameter protrudes under the mucosa, with a central umbilication corresponding to the ostium of the pancreatic duct (Eklöf et al. 1973; Tschäppeler 1990; Sty et al. 1992). Ultrasonography can show a mass within the gastrointestinal wall (Blais and Mass 1995), and endoscopy is sometimes diagnostic, showing a polypoid aspect, mainly in a pyloroantral position, but endoscopic biopsies are not helpful to establish the diagnosis since the lesions are almost always submucosal (Durie 1996).

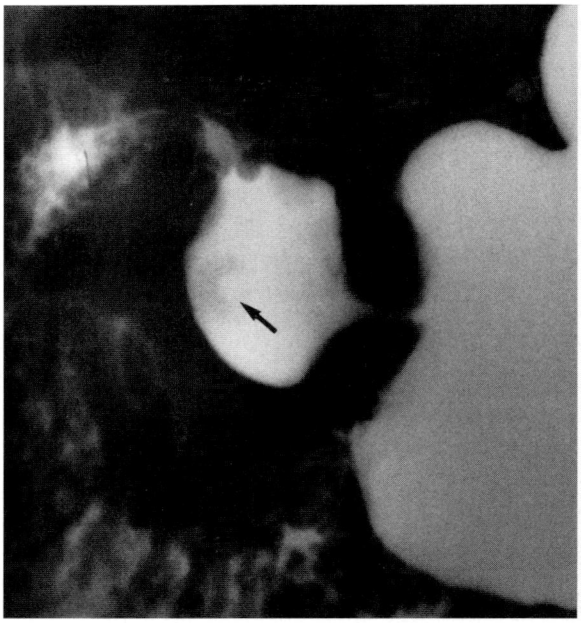

Fig. 5.4. Ectopic pancreas in a 7-year-old girl who presented with vomiting and epigastric pain. The barium study shows a rounded prepyloric lacuna with a more opaque center (*arrow*). Surgical biopsy confirmed pancreatic heterotopia

5.4 Insufficiency of the Exocrine Pancreas

5.4.1 Cystic Fibrosis

Cystic fibrosis is an autosomal recessive hereditary disease. The responsible gene is located on chromosome 7 and codes for a protein cystic fibrosis transmembrane conductance regulator (CFTR) which plays a role in the transmembranous transport of chlorine. The most frequent mutation is the ΔF 508, but more than 500 gene mutations have since been described (Durie 1996). The disease is characterized by condensation of all exocrine secretions, particularly at the level of the digestive tract, the bronchopulmonary system, and the skin (Sarles 1990).

The clinical manifestations are variable and are a function of the patient's age and the severity of the disease. Genetic factors influence the degree of pancreatic disease and its rate of progression, and some patients remain pancreatic-sufficient. In the neonatal period, the disease can be revealed by digestive symptoms, with the occurrence of meconium ileus due to exocrine pancreatic insufficiency and condensed digestive secretions. Later, respiratory signs dominate, with chronic bronchitis and dilatation of the bronchi, which are a determining factor in the prognosis. The diagnosis relies on the sweat test and characterization with molecular biology of the pathologic gene.

Involvement of the exocrine pancreas is a quasi-constant element of the disease. Pancreatic ducts are obstructed by the condensed secretions. The gland is initially hypertrophied, but then evolves progressively towards atrophy and fatty involution. Inflammatory phenomena can be associated with secondary progressive interstitial fibrosis, sometimes accompanied by small cysts. Rarely, these cysts can be more voluminous.

Ultrasonography allows the demonstration of these anomalies in the majority of cases (Spehl-Robberecht et al. 1981, 1986; Mac Hugo et al. 1987). However, in some patients, the pancreas cannot be correctly depicted. Before the age of 2 years, the pancreas has a perfectly normal aspect on ultrasonography. Progressively, the echogenicity of the parenchyma increases. In some cases, a heterogeneous appearance will be present. The dimensions of the gland decrease. The size of the pancreas can be difficult to appreciate since the ultrasonographic distinction between the parenchyma and the adjacent fat is not always easy. Calcifications may appear, which are equally visible on plain film of the abdomen. Rarely, macrocystic formations are observed by ultrasonography (Fig. 5.5), the gland then presenting a multicystic aspect (Hernanz-Schulman et al. 1986). The gallbladder is small with a thick wall, biliary lithiasis may be present. The liver is sometimes involved, with hyperechoic parenchyma due to cirrhosis (Agrons et al. 1996). Liver and biliary tract disease can occur independently of the underlying disease severity and the presence of pancreatic involvement (Waters et al. 1995).

CT shows the same anomalies. In the presence of fatty involution, the pancreas appears hypodense on CT, which can also demonstrate calcifications and macrocysts (Hernanz-Schulman et al. 1986; Veyrac et al. 1987; Sty et al. 1992). MRI shows an enlarged pancreas or atrophic gland with or without fatty replacement (Tjon et al. 1991). On T1-weighted images, four patterns have been described by Ferrozzi: (1) diffuse hyperintensity with residual lobular pattern, (2) homogeneous hyperintensity without residual lobular pattern, (3) hyperintense parenchyma with focal areas of hypointensity, or (4) absence of structural or signal intensity changes. T1 value of the pancreas is lower in patients with marked pancreatic insufficiency. This decrease could be correlated with the degree of clinical compromise (Ferrozzi et al. 1996).

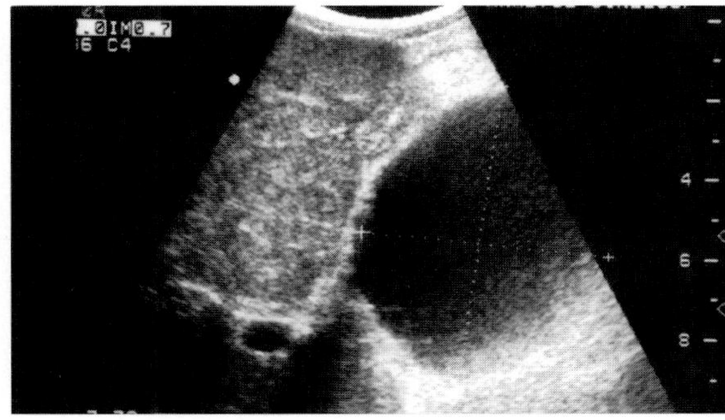
a

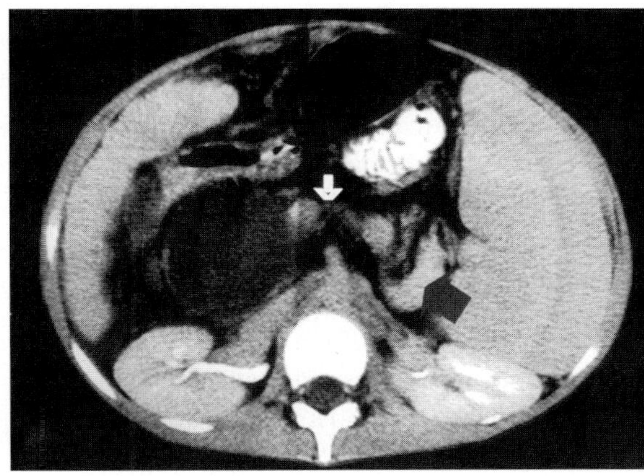
b

Fig. 5.5a,b. A 14-year-old boy with cystic fibrosis. **a** Ultrasonography demonstrates a large cyst within the head of the pancreas. **b** Computed tomography confirms the presence of the cyst; the body of the pancreas is small and hypodense, with fatty involution (*white arrow*). There is a splenomegaly in relation to portal hypertension, with an enlarged splenic vein (*black arrow*) due to liver cirrhosis

In other cases, however, where the pulmonary involvement is predominant, the pancreatic secretions can be normal, with imaging procedures revealing a normal aspect of the gland (Spehl-Robberecht et al. 1986).

5.4.2 Shwachman-Diamond Syndrome

Shwachman-Diamond syndrome is characterized by exocrine pancreatic insufficiency, most frequently associated with neutropenia, which is responsible for relapsing infections; thrombocytopenia and red cell hypoplasia are slightly less common. Growth retardation and metaphyseal dysplasia can be seen. Associated manifestations include dental abnormalities, renal dysfunction, hepatomegaly, abnormal lung function, delayed puberty, and ichthyosis. The suggested mode of inherence is autosomal recessive

(LERNER et al. 1996), but an autosomal dominant pattern with variable expression is present in some families (DURIE 1996). The exocrine glandular tissue undergoes fatty involution, with preservation of the ducts and the islets of Langerhans (ROBBERECHT et al. 1985). Usually, malabsorption is present during infancy.

Ultrasonography demonstrates a pancreas of normal size, with a marked increase in echogenicity due to lipomatous infiltration and fibrosis (Fig. 5.6) (BERROCAL et al. 1995b). CT can also diagnose this anomaly (HIBON and FILIATRAULT 1985; KRIEF et al. 1988; BOM et al. 1993). MRI visualizes a normal-sized or enlarged pancreas, a hyperintense signal on T1- and T2-weighted images, and a null signal on short tan inversion recovery (STIR)-weighted image, characteristic of fat (BOM et al. 1993; LACAILLE et al. 1996).

Skeletal abnormalities include a delay in the osseous age, chondrodysplasia with shortness of the long bones, hypoplasia of the iliac bones, short and wide femoral metaphysis, and cup deformation of the anterior ends of the ribs (TSCHÄPPELER 1990; BERROCAL et al. 1995b).

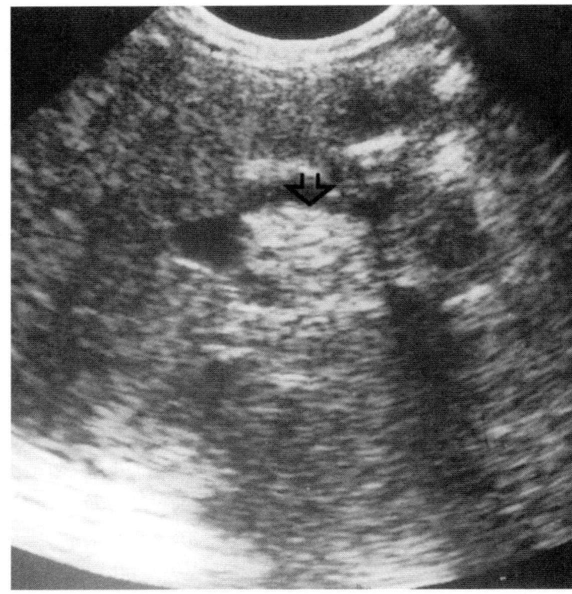

Fig. 5.6. A 5-year-old child with relapsing pulmonary infections due to Shwachman-Diamond syndrome. At ultrasonography, the head of the pancreas appears hyperechoic. (Courtesy of Dr. Avni)

5.4.3 Other Disorders with Pancreatic Insufficiency

Johanson-Blizzard syndrome is a rare autosomal recessive disease, with pancreatic insufficiency, in relation with a primary acinar cell defect, nasal alar hypoplasia, absence of permanent teeth, short stature, congenital deafness, and psychomotor retardation (JONES et al. 1994; DURIE 1996). Other isolated congenital enzyme deficiencies have been described for lipase, colipase, amylase, and trypsinogen (DURIE 1996; LERNER et al. 1996).

5.5 Pancreatitis

Pancreatitis is proportionally less frequent in children than in adults. Most of the cases are acute pancreatitis of inflammatory origin. The etiology is very variable: trauma, infection, intoxication, obstruction of the common bile or pancreatic ducts, but cannot always be identified (HADDOCK et al. 1994; BERNEY et al. 1996). Mild acute pancreatitis is characterized pathologically by interstitial edema. Severe acute pancreatitis is manifested by pancreatic and peripancreatic fat necrosis. Clinical findings consist in acute abdominal pain, vomiting, and abdominal tenderness. Patients with severe disease demonstrate shock, renal failure, gastrointestinal bleeding, and pulmonary insufficiency. The diagnosis is based essentially on the serum and urinary levels of amylase and lipase, and low serum calcium level.

5.5.1 Traumatic Pancreatitis

Lesions of the pancreas can occur in children after moderate (e.g., a fall from a bicycle) or more severe trauma (e.g., a car accident). If the mechanism of trauma is unknown, battered-child syndrome has to be suspected (HILFER and HOLGERSEN 1995). In children, the pancreas is not very deep and there is little fat around it. Thus, it can be easily compressed against the spine, leading to a contusion, a laceration, or a complete fracture of the gland, with injury of the pancreatic duct. The condition can evolve into pseudocyst formation. A lesion of the duodenum or the angle of Treitz can be associated with parietal hematoma or rupture.

In the initial phase, the radiological diagnosis is sometimes difficult. Plain films of the abdomen show adynamic ileus with a sentinel loop in the superior part of the abdomen (Schmittenbecher et al. 1996). Direct visualization on an intraperitoneal fluid collection is rare. Pleural effusion can be demonstrated by chest X-rays.

The presence of ileus can interfere with the quality of ultrasonographic study. This technique can demonstrate an increased pancreatic volume, with heterogeneous parenchyma and zones of variable echogenicity, hypoechogenicity in most cases, corresponding to edema or hemorrhage (Fig. 5.7) (Coleman et al. 1983; Fleischer et al. 1983; Haddock et al. 1994; Schmittenbecher et al. 1996). The wall of the duodenum can be thickened due to hematoma formation. The gallbladder is frequently enlarged and the biliary ducts dilated. The presence of an intraperitoneal effusion can be the consequence of another associated parenchymous lesion, or of a rupture of the pancreatic duct. Chylous ascites have also been reported, presumably due to the disruption of the intestinal trunk of lymphatics at the root of the mesentery (Hilfer and Holgersen 1995). A hyperechoic aspect of the pararenal space is also suggestive of pancreatitis (Swischuk and Hayden 1985).

CT is indicated for a more precise evaluation of the extent of the lesions (Sivit et al. 1992), but this can give false-negative results. Conversely, a false-positive diagnosis of pancreatic rupture can be achieved with thick slices and volume averaging of adjacent bowel. The size of the gland may be normal or enlarged. Heterogeneous enhancement is more characteristic of pancreatic necrosis. Intrapancreatic fluid collections are rare (King et al. 1995). Peripancreatic inflammation with effusion can be seen (Fig. 5.8), particularly in the anterior pararenal space, with thickening of Gerota's fascia, at the level of the lesser sac, lesser omentum, and transverse mesocolon (King et al. 1995; Siegel and Sivit 1997). The presence of fluid between the splenic vein and the pancreas is often seen in conjunction with fluid in the anterior pararenal space, but it is a nonspecific sign of pancreatic injury in children (Sivit and Eichelberger 1995). The association of the signs is suggestive of a pancreatic lesion and can help in the clinical evaluation of whether surgery is indicated or not.

Some authors have reported the use of early ERCP, when CT is suggestive of pancreatic transection, to assess a ductal injury leading to surgical intervention (Rescorla et al. 1995; Tagge et al. 1997).

Follow-up imaging can be performed with sonography, to monitor changes in pancreas size and peripancreatic fluid collection. Pseudocysts develop within 1–3 weeks following trauma in about 30%–60% of cases (Bass et al. 1988; Schmittenbecher et al. 1996; Yeung et al. 1996). They correspond to an accumulation of pancreatic fluids, necrotic tissue, and blood in a newly formed cavity limited by an inflammatory capsule. They are most frequently localized in the lesser sac, to the left of the midline, but they may occur in the pararenal space, left lobe of the liver, juxtasplenic area, retroperi-

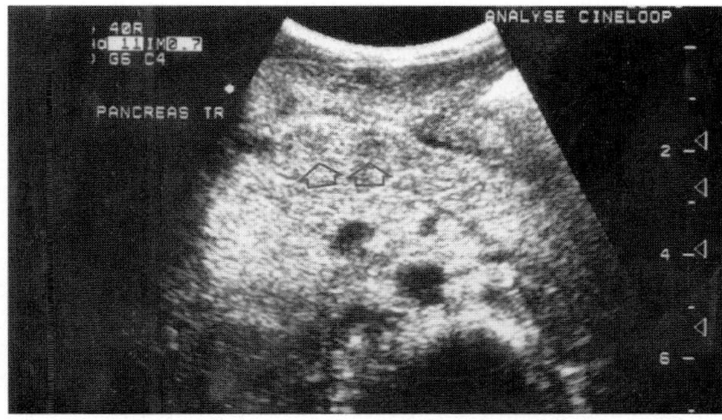

Fig. 5.7. A 7-year-old boy with acute post-traumatic pancreatitis. Transverse ultrasonography shows an enlarged heterogeneous pancreatic head, hyperechoic with hypoechoic foci (*open arrows*)

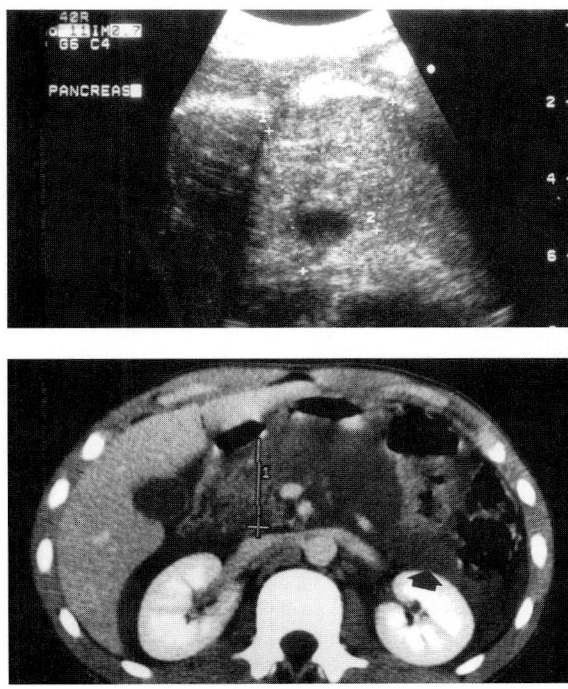

a

b

Fig. 5.8a,b. Post-traumatic pancreatitis in a 15-year-old child. **a** Ultrasonography demonstrates a hyperechoic, enlarged gland (*calipers*). **b** Computed tomography after intravenous infusion confirms the lesion of the pancreas, with a peripancreatic effusion and presence of fluid in the left anterior pararenal space (*arrow*)

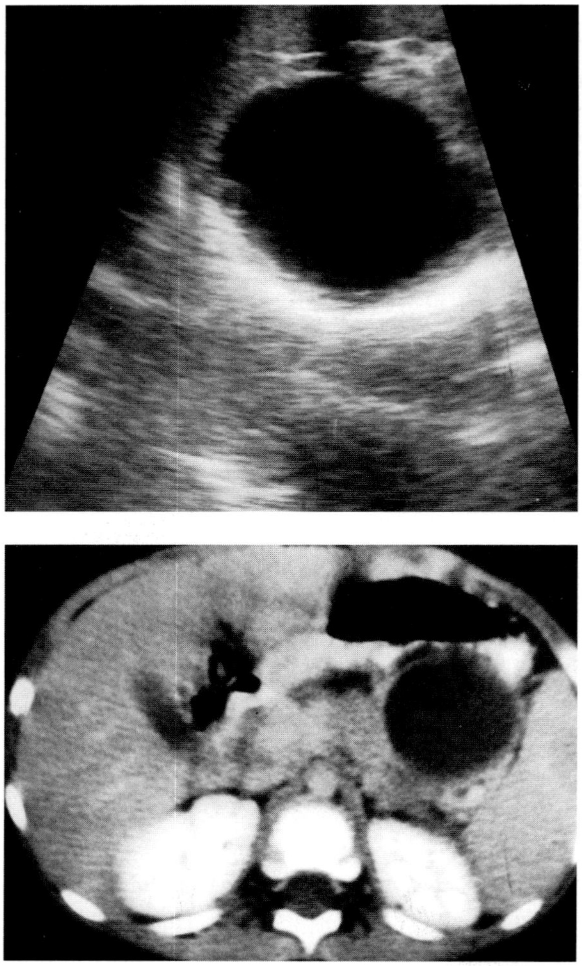

a

b

Fig. 5.9a,b. Post-traumatic pseudocyst of the pancreas in a 4-year-old boy who had suffered abdominal trauma 10 days previously. There was persistent epigastric pain with hyperamylasemia. **a** Ultrasonography shows a fluid-filled mass, 4 cm in diameter, at the level of the splenic hilum. The mass has a slightly irregular wall. **b** Contrast-enhanced computed tomography after bowel opacification confirms the presence of a rounded cyst of the lesser sac. Surgical drainage was performed, with diagnosis of section of the pancreatic duct

toneum, and mediastinum (Siegel and Sivit 1997). Clinically, fever and, more rarely, a palpable mass may be present, in association with persistent hyperamylasemia. The diagnosis is easy when the traumatic context is known and if the signs appear during follow-up. In other cases, the discovery of a mass can be the first delayed sign of traumatic pancreatitis.

In the presence of a pseudocyst, a plain film of the abdomen may show displacement of the stomach in a ventral and upward direction, and downward displacement of the transverse colon. If a bowel contrast study is performed, the displacement of the digestive tract is more evident. Ultrasonography, however, is the best diagnostic method, and its repeated use is therefore essential in the follow-up of traumatic lesions (Fig. 5.9). Pseudocysts are visualized as well-defined, fluid-filled, or sometimes more heterogeneous lesions of variable volume (Teele and Share 1991).

CT can clarify the aspect and topography of the pseudocyst. The thickness of the wall of the pseudocyst can be appreciated and signs of superinfection may be revealed, e.g., a spontaneously dense collection, septation, and significant contrast enhancement of the thickened wall (Veyrac et al. 1987). Bubbles of gas may be noted within the abscess (Siegel and Sivit 1997). Other complications include rupture, obstruction of adjacent bowel or bile ducts, and invasion of the spleen and liver.

The choice of therapy depends on the clinical consequences and the evolution, and comprise simple surveillance, percutaneous drainage, or surgical intervention if section of the pancreatic duct is suspected. If superinfection is present, drainage is necessary (Garel et al. 1983; Bass et al. 1988; Teele and Share 1991).

5.5.2 Nontraumatic Acute Pancreatitis

The etiologies of nontraumatic acute pancreatitis are very varied; in some cases, etiology is evident, according to the clinical signs. In other cases, investigation needs to be carried. Some cases remain idiopathic. The diagnosis of pancreatitis always relies on the association of relevant clinical signs and hyperamylasemia. Nevertheless, serum amylase levels can be elevated without underlying pancreatitis cytolysis as, for instance, in the case of mumps parotitis. Ultrasonography of the abdomen is not always abnormal. In other cases, it demonstrates an increase in the pancreatic volume or abnormal echogenicity, but the latter criterion remains difficult to appreciate. Dilatation of the pancreatic duct seems to be the most specific sign (Teele and Share 1991). CT signs include changes in size and density of the gland, peripancreatic edema, and peritoneal exudate. Anomalies of the biliary or pancreatic ducts, although rare in children, must be systematically investigated. MRCP could be of value in such cases (Miyazaki et al. 1998). As with traumatic pancreatitis, follow-up is necessary in order to detect complications, more particularly the development of a pseudocyst or an abscess.

In children, acute pancreatitis can be secondary to a wide variety of diseases:

1. Infection can be complicated with acute pancreatitis. Mumps is the most frequent. Other infections include septicemia, viral infection [cytomegalovirus, hepatitis A (Shrier et al. 1995; Lerner et al. 1996; Yeung et al. 1996)]. In the HIV-positive child, pancreatitis can be due to dideoxyinosine or pentamidine, antiretroviral drugs used in the treatment of human deficiency virus (Cappell and Marks 1995; Levin et al. 1997). In children with AIDS, pancreatic involvement by opportunistic infections seems to be rare; lymphoplasmacytic infiltration of the gland is also rare (Kahn et al. 1995). In patients with severe combined immunodeficiency or DiGeorge's syndrome, viral pancreatitis may occur, and has to be differentiated from acute graft versus host disease in patients who have undergone bone marrow transplantation (Washington et al. 1994).
2. Inflammatory systemic disease such as hemolytic-uremic syndrome, Schönlein-Henoch purpura, Kawasaki disease, and juvenile dermatomyositis complicated with pancreatitis have been described (Spehl-Robberecht et al. 1986; Lerner et al. 1996; See et al. 1997).
3. Acute pancreatitis can be in relationship with toxins and drugs: glucocorticoids, valproic acid (Kayemba Kay's Kabangu et al. 1991; Rose et al. 1991), chemotherapy with L-asparaginase (Fig. 5.10); extensive necrosis can occur, leading to death (Yeung et al. 1996; Sadoff et al. 1997). Even in children, alcohol intoxication has been described (Yeung et al. 1996).
4. Obstructive causes are less frequent than in adults: choledocho-lithiasis, ascariasis, and duodenopancreatic tumor (Wan et al. 1988; Rocha et al. 1995).
5. Anatomic variants have to be suspected when the etiology of the pancreatitis is not clear. Such abnormalities include pancreas divisum (Allendorph et al. 1987; Sanada et al. 1995), choledochal cyst and common bilio-pancreatic channel (Fig. 5.11) (Okada et al. 1995; Yeung et al. 1996), intra- or juxtapancreatic intestinal duplication (Hélardot et al. 1982; Black et al. 1986; Okada et al. 1995; Demetriadis et al. 1997).
6. Metabolic inhered disorders can be also complicated with pancreatitis: type IA glycogenosis (Herman 1995), organic acidemia: isovaleric acidemia, methylmalonic acidemia, maple syrup urine disease (Kahler et al. 1994). Abnormalities of the pancreas have also been described in type 1 hereditary tyrosinemia, with increased pancreatic volume, and hyper- or hypoechogenic gland (Dubois et al. 1996).

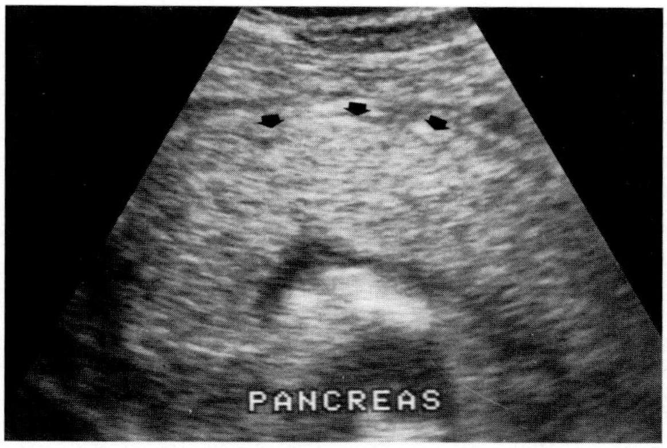

Fig. 5.10. Toxic acute pancreatitis in a 6-year-old girl treated for acute leukemia with asparaginase and prednisone. Abdominal pain, mild jaundice, and hyperamylasemia were present. Ultrasonography demonstrates a globally enlarged pancreas with hyperechoic parenchyma. There was secondary regression

5.5.3 Hereditary Pancreatitis

Hereditary relapsing pancreatitis is a rare disease characterized by an autosomal-dominant mode of inheritance with incomplete penetrance. It is the most frequent cause of recurrent pancreatitis in children (Franken et al. 1984; Spencer et al. 1990). The gene for this disease has recently been mapped to chromosome 7q35, and the defect is believed to be caused by a mutation in the cationic trypsinogen gene (Arg-His substitution at residue 117) (Lowenfels et al. 1997). The etiology appears to be related to a quantitative deficit of pancreatic stone proteins (PSP) that maintain the equilibrium of solutes contained in the pancreatic juice. This deficit promotes the formation of calcium-protein precipitates within the pancreatic ducts (Perrelli et al. 1996). Clinically, relapsing periods of abdominal pain are noted, starting in late childhood or adolescence. The serum amylase level is simultaneously increased. The evolution is generally benign, but the classic complications of pancreatitis are possible, i.e., severe hemorrhagic pancreatitis and formation of pseudocysts. The plain film of the abdomen quite frequently shows calcifications in the pancreatic area as multiple, dense, rounded opacities with a hyperdense center. The calcifications are often situated within the pancreas duct. Ultrasonography and CT can easily detect these calcifications. During the acute episodes, the pancreas swells and the pancreatic duct is usually dilated, as can be confirmed by ERCP (Fig. 5.12). The treatment is symptomatic during

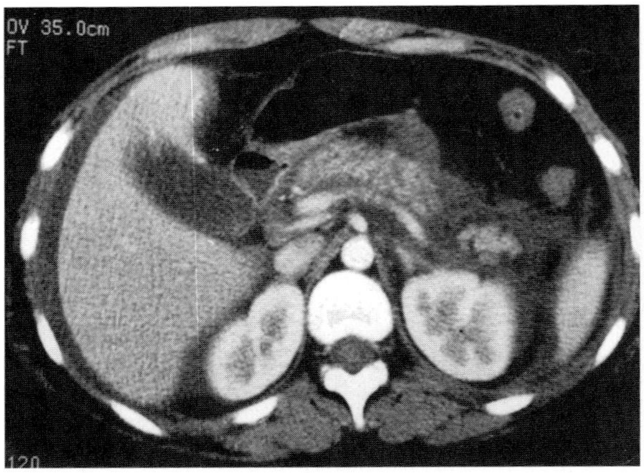

a

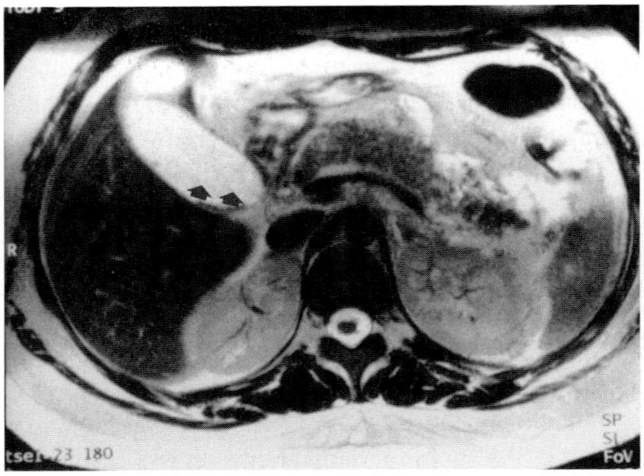

b

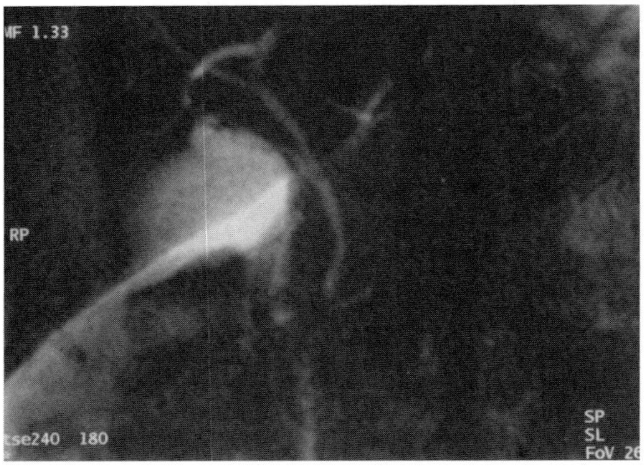

c

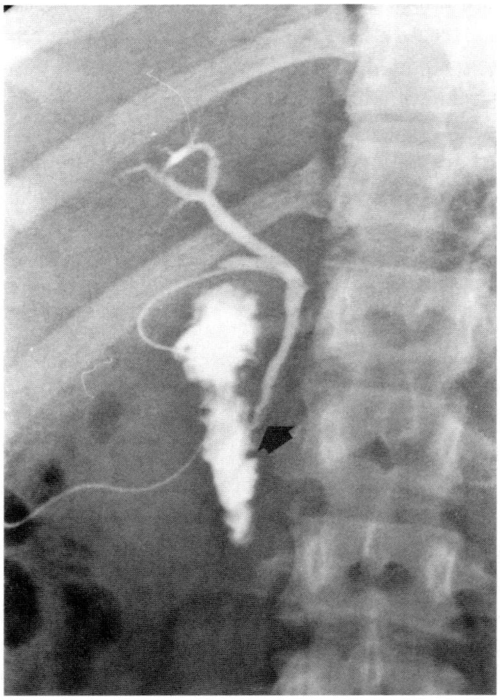

d

Fig. 5.11a–d. Acute pancreatitis in a 14-year-old girl. Ultrasonography has shown gallstones. **a** Computed tomography scan after intravenous infusion demonstrates a peripancreatic and intraperitoneal effusion. **b** Magnetic resonance imaging, transverse T2-weighted image confirms an heterogeneous gland. Declive gallstones are visible in the gallbladder (*arrows*). **c** Magnetic resonance cholangiopancreatography clearly demonstrates the bile duct and the pancreatic duct, but fails to shows the bilio-pancreatic junction (courtesy of Dr. Lescene). **d** Postoperative cholangiography demonstrates a common bilio-pancreatic channel (*arrow*)

acute exacerbations, which tend to decline in frequency once adulthood is reached. ERCP enables the restoration of normal pancreatic flow in cases of obstruction (sphincterotomy, extraction of stones) (Perrelli et al. 1996).

Patients with hereditary pancreatitis have a high risk of pancreatic cancer several decades after the initial onset of pancreatitis (40% at the age of 70). A paternal inheritance pattern increases the probability of developing pancreatic cancer (Lowenfels et al. 1997).

5.5.4 Fibrosing Pancreatitis

Fibrosing pancreatitis is an exceptional disease in children, characterized by interstitial fibrosis around the acini, without ductal involvement (Atkinson et al. 1988).

Clinical features consist in progressive jaundice and abdominal pain (Amerson and Ricketts 1996). Amylase levels are generally normal or mildly elevated. Ultrasonography demonstrates dilatation of the intra- and extrahepatic biliary ducts with an increase in the volume of the pancreatic head or the entire pancreas. Cholangiography or ERCP can specify the site of the obstruction. Differential diag-

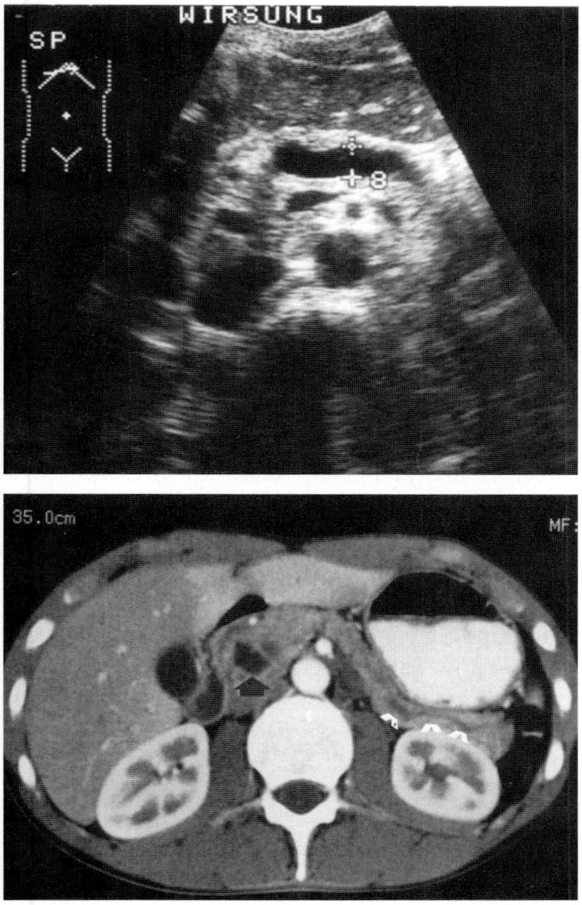

a

b

Fig. 5.12a,b. Recurrent pancreatitis in a 15-year-old child. **a** Transverse ultrasonography demonstrates an enlarged Wirsung canal. **b** Contrast-enhanced computed tomography confirmed the dilatation of the pancreatic duct (*white arrowheads*) and shows a pseudocyst within the head of the gland (*arrow*)

nosis has to be made with a tumor of the pancreatic head and is only possible with anatomopathological examination. The treatment consists in internal drainage of the biliary flow, with bilio-enteric bypass (Amerson and Ricketts 1996).

5.6 Pancreatic Masses

5.6.1 Cystic Lesions

Numerous cystic lesions are postpancreatitis pseudocysts. Primitive cysts are of various origin.

5.6.1.1 Congenital Cysts

Congenital cysts can be found in several diseases:

1. Congenital cysts are sometimes observed in the pancreas in the dominant form of hepatorenal polycystic disease. The diagnosis is easy since multiple lesions are visualized by ultrasonography or CT in the kidneys and the liver. These cysts are rare in children and appear from adolescence onward (Teele and Share 1991).
2. Von Hippel-Lindau disease is an autosomic dominant phakomatosis. Retinal angioma, multiple hemangioblastomas of the cerebellum, medulla oblongata, and spinal cord occur. In the abdomen, renal cell carcinoma, pheochromocytoma, and cysts in pancreas, kidneys, and liver can be discovered (Teele and Share 1991). As in hepatorenal polycystic disease, these lesions are only exceptionally present in children; more often they become apparent at the end of adolescence. Later, there is a higher risk of microcystic adenoma, islet cell tumor, and pancreatic carcinoma (Sty et al. 1992). Screening of the abdomen of patients with a family history of Von Hippel-Lindau disease should begin in the early teens; the presence of multiple pancreatic cysts is diagnostic (Hough et al. 1994).
3. We have also observed a cyst on the pancreatic tail in a child with Beckwith-Wiedemann syndrome, who presented with frequent hypoglycemia (Fig. 5.13), and one other case of pancreatic cyst in a 5-month-old infant, with a storage disease (Niemann-Pick) (Fig. 5.14).

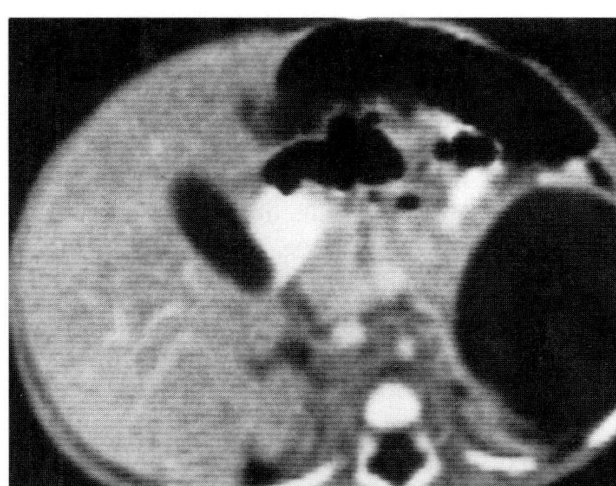

Fig. 5.13. Pancreatic cyst in a 20-day-old girl with hemihypertrophy and relapsing hyperglycemia. Computed tomography shows the presence of a mass within the pancreatic tail. Surgical resection was performed

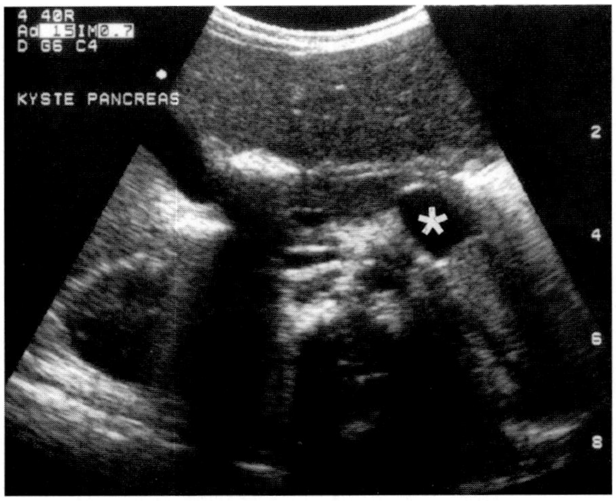

Fig. 5.14. A 5-year-old boy with hepatomegaly in relation with Niemann-Pick disease. Ultrasonography reveals a corporeal pancreatic cyst (*asterisk*)

4. Idiopathic congenital cysts are rare. It is believed that these cysts are caused by anomalous development of the pancreatic ductal system, with sequestered segments giving rise to a cyst. Unilocular or multilocular cysts can occur. Antenatal diagnosis has been described (Baker et al. 1990), and most cases are discovered in newborns. Ultrasonography and CT disclose the cystic mass, showing an uni- or multilocular anechoic tumor, with low attenuation on CT (Auringer et al. 1993).

5.6.1.2 Cystadenoma of the Pancreas

Cystadenoma of the pancreas is an exceptional tumor in childhood (Panuel et al. 1984; Jenkins and Othersen 1992). Besides microcystic forms (serous cystadenoma), macrocystic lesions exist (mucous cystadenoma), these most frequently being multilocular. In an infant, distinction between a serous cystadenoma and a congenital unilocular or multilocular cyst can be difficult.

Exploration of an abdominal mass discloses multiseptated cystic formation. Ultrasonography and CT allow localization of the tumor in the pancreas and detection of a possible solid component. Nevertheless, the diagnosis is rarely made before surgical intervention and anatomopathological examination (Jenkins and Othersen 1992)

5.6.1.3 Hydatid Cysts

Pancreatic localizations of echinococcosis are rare in children; a few such observations have been reported in the literature (Khiari et al. 1994; Barrera et al. 1995; Brown et al. 1995). They can be associated with other visceral localizations, more particularly the liver, or are isolated, making the etiologic diagnosis even more difficult. The mode of infestation is presumed to be hematogenous. Hydatid cysts are usually located in the head of the pancreas. Compression of, or fistulization with, the common bile duct can exist, with jaundice.

Ultrasonography may show the presence of a membranous detachment, the presence of a sediment, or peripheral arciform calcifications that are also visible on plain films (Zakari et al. 1984; Khiari et al. 1994). CT demonstrates a cystic lesion, uni- or multilocular, containing an undulating membrane (Brown et al. 1995). Diagnostic indicators are the geographic or ethnic context, the existence of hypereosinophilia, and positivity of specific serologic tests, but a diagnostic laparotomy can be necessary.

5.6.1.4 Cystic Lesions in the Vicinity of the Pancreas

Other cystic lesions may be contiguous to the pancreas and simulate a pancreatic mass. The exact topographic diagnosis and the relations with the gland can be difficult to establish with ultrasonography and CT:

1. Cystic lymphangioma of the lesser sac can suggest a tumor of the body or the tail of the pancreas. Lymphangioma can also be located within the pancreatic gland (Daltrey and Johnson 1996; Itterbeek et al. 1997). Most frequently, one observes a septated multicystic lesion with variable echogenicity of the cysts, due to a complication such as infection or hemorrhage. CT shows a multicystic mass, with a variable attenuation, depending on the nature of the liquid component (chylous, serous, bloody, or purulent). Contrast-enhanced CT demonstrates an enhancement in the walls of the cysts. Complete excision of the tumor, if possible, is mandatory (Daltrey and Johnson 1996).
2. Duplications of the digestive tract can also simulate a pancreatic mass (Dutheil-Doco et al. 1998). The study of the wall with ultrasonography of the cyst can be indicative of the diagnosis, by

showing two fine hyperechoic lines separated by a hypoechoic layer. This finding, however, is in itself insufficient to allow the diagnosis. A duplication of the digestive tract can obstruct or communicate with the pancreatic ducts and can be at the origin of recurrent pancreatitis (Hélardot et al. 1982; Black et al. 1986; Demetriadis et al. 1997). Communication between the cyst and the bilio-pancreatic duct could be demonstrated by spiral CT cholangiography (Borocco et al. 1996a). In other cases, heterotopic pancreas can be found in the wall of a duplication (Blais and Mass 1995), sometimes complicated with pancreatitis (Fig. 5.15) (Steyaert et al. 1997).

3. Cystic tumors of the left adrenal gland can be difficult to distinguish from a cyst of the pancreatic tail, particularly on ultrasonography.

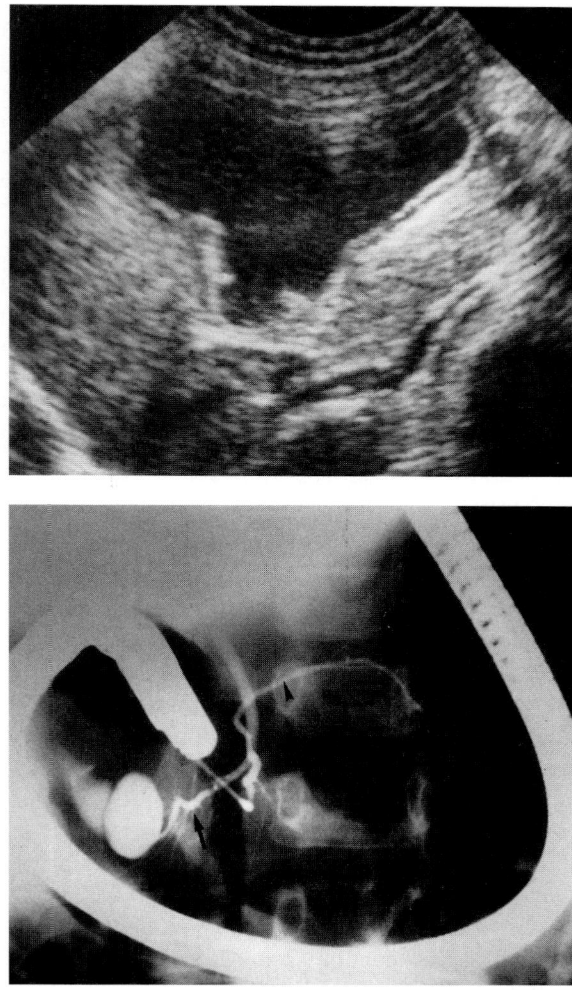

a

b

Fig. 5.15a,b. Duplication of the duodenum with ectopic termination of the duct of Santorini in a 5-year-old child who had suffered several episodes of pancreatitis. **a** A right transverse ultrasonogram shows an irregular hypoechoic mass with a sharply demarcated wall, situated below the liver. **b** Endoscopic retrograde pancreatography, with opacification of the duct of Santorini (*arrow*). There is reflux of contrast in the cystic formation. The pancreatic duct (*arrowhead*) and the common bile duct were opacified earlier. (Courtesy of Dr. Avni)

5.6.2 Solid Tumors

Solid tumors of the pancreas are also rare in childhood. They are secretory tumors originating from the endocrine tissue, or tumors that have developed from the exocrine cells.

5.6.2.1 Lesions of the Endocrine Pancreas

Two diseases can result in severe hypoglycemia in children, namely nesidioblastosis and insulinoma of the pancreas, the most frequent functioning islet cell tumor. Other endocrine tumors are exceptional; some of them are nonfunctioning tumors.

5.6.2.1.1 Nesidioblastosis

Nesidoblastosis is not a real tumor, but rather it involves the persistence, hyperplasia, and dysplasia of primitive cells, i.e., β cells of the islets of Langerhans. It can occur in association with Beckwith-Wiedemann syndrome. Nesidioblastosis is manifested in the neonate or infant by severe hypoglycemia with hyperinsulinism. Since the pancreas is normal macroscopically, imaging techniques and, in particular, ultrasonography fail to demonstrate the lesion (Teele and Share 1991). If hypoglycemia cannot be managed medically, the treatment consists in partial or subtotal pancreatectomy in order to decrease the secretion of insulin (Shilyansky et al. 1997).

5.6.2.1.2 Insulinoma

Insulinoma is, in most cases, benign (90%), but a few cases of islet cell carcinoma have been reported in children (Lobe et al. 1992). It can be solitary or occur in the context of multiple endocrine neoplasia type I (MEN-I). The symptoms are related to the secretion of insulin. The diagnosis of hyperinsulinism can be confirmed by the infusion of increasing doses of insulin in a patient in whom the glycemia is kept constant by an artificial pancreas with infusion of glucose. The presence of high levels of endogenous C peptide indicates the autonomous secretion of insulin (GIN et al. 1987). The insulinoma is usually small in size, and is difficult to demonstrate with ultrasonography. Multiple insulinoma can be found. The nodules are smaller than 2 cm in diameter and are rather hypoechoic. CT may aid in the localization of this lesion, but few cases are described in children. Selective arteriography often fails to demonstrate the tumor in children (ZELLER et al. 1993). Hyperselective venous sampling has also been proposed (BRUNELLE et al. 1989; ZELLER et al. 1993). Perioperative ultrasonography can aid in the detection of the lesion (TELANDER et al. 1986).

5.6.2.1.3
OTHER SECRETORY TUMORS

Other secretory tumors are exceptional in childhood. Most of them are gastrinomas, which are responsible for Zollinger-Ellison syndrome (SMITH 1982; STY et al. 1992). The latter can be a feature of MEN-I syndrome. The hypersecretion of gastrin is responsible for excessive acid production, with the development of peptic ulcer(s). In most of cases, ultrasonography and CT show these tumors. Enhancement after injection can be absent (EIRE et al. 1996).

Among the other tumors, VIPomas, responsible for chronic diarrhea, glucagonomas, and somatostatin-secreting adenomas need to be mentioned (ROSSI et al. 1989).

5.6.2.2 Tumors of the Exocrine Pancreas

Tumors of the exocrine pancreas are also rare. The classification distinguishes ductal cell carcinomas and nonductal carcinomas; among nonductal carcinomas, acinar cell carcinoma, solid cystic epithelial tumor, and pancreatoblastoma can occur.

5.6.2.2.1
DUCTAL CELL AND ACINAR CELL CARCINOMAS

These are usually located in the head of the pancreas. The clinical signs are similar to those encountered in adults, i.e., progressive jaundice, epigastric pain, problems with gastrointestinal transit, and hematemesis.

Barium study can reveal changes in the form and contour of the duodenal loop, but is rarely used. Ultrasonography allows the discovery of a mass that is generally more echogenic than the pancreas, though this is not always the case (Fig. 5.16). Dilatation of the biliary tract, compression of the portal vein and its branches, and hepatic and lymph node metastases need to be sought (ROBEY et al. 1983; TEELE and SHARE 1991). The appearance can be similar to that observed in chronic fibrosing pancreatitis. CT can demonstrate locoregional extension of the tumor and provide more complete information on hepatic and lymph node metastases.

5.6.2.2.2
SOLID CYSTIC EPITHELIAL TUMOR

A solid cystic tumor is also termed papillary-cystic or Frantz's tumor. This lesion occurs in girls and young women. Only a few male patients have been reported in children series (KY et al. 1998). The tumor is usually a well-encapsulated mass with variable degrees of internal hemorrhage and cystic degeneration (BUETOW et al. 1996). Microscopic examination demonstrates papillary architecture

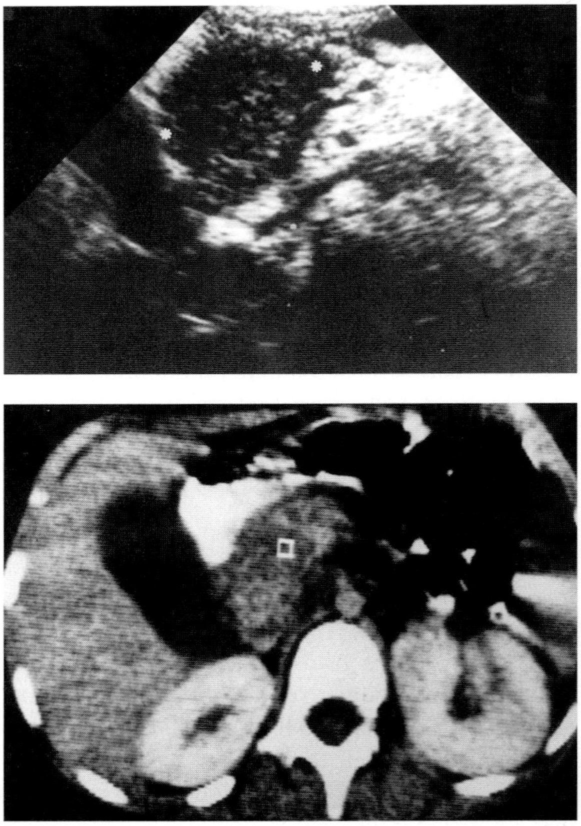

a

b

Fig. 5.16a,b. Adenocarcinoma of the head of the pancreas in a 9-year-old girl with abdominal pain and iron-deficiency anemia due to ulceration of the second duodenum. **a** Transverse ultrasonogram shows a hypoechoic mass of the pancreatic head (*asterisks*). **b** Contrast-enhanced computed tomography confirms the presence of a heterogeneous mass of the pancreatic head (*square*) mixed with solid areas. The mode of presentation includes epigastric pain and a palpable abdominal mass (JAKSIC et al. 1992; KY et al. 1998).

Ultrasonography depicts a well-delineated lesion, with variable echo structure. In most cases, the tumor is hyperechoic. Sometimes, anechoic or hypoechoic areas are seen centrally (Fig. 5.17).

Calcifications are seen with CT in 30% of cases. The lesion can be of soft tissue-, intermediate-, or water-attenuation, with enhancement after injection of contrast media in the soft-tissue attenuating areas. With MRI, T1-weighted images show areas of high signal intensity, corresponding to hemorrhagic necrosis or debris. On T2-weighted images, areas of high intensity are related to solid or cystic hemorrhagic areas (BUETOW et al. 1996).

Solid cystic tumor is a low-grade malignant tumor, and complete resection is usually adequate for treatment (WÜNSCH et al. 1997). Liver and lymph node metastases, although rare, have been described, with successful treatment after surgery in most of cases (JAKSIC et al. 1992; HORISAWA et al. 1995; KY et al. 1998).

5.6.2.2.3
PANCREATOBLASTOMA

Pancreatoblastoma is a well-differentiated tumor of embryological origin. The pathologic diagnosis is made on the basis of an organoid cell pattern with areas of fibrous stroma and the presence of zymogen-like granules on electron microscopy (JAKSIC et al. 1992; LEE et al. 1996). The lesion is most frequently localized in the head of the pancreas (STY et al. 1992). Prognosis after surgery in localized tumor is usually good, but it is rather poor when metastatic disease is present. The most frequent site of metastases is the liver. Initial symptoms include palpable mass, anorexia, and vomiting (LEE et al. 1996).

Ultrasonography demonstrates a well-delineated mass; the echo structure is heterogeneous, with mixed echogenicity. A multiloculated appearance with echogenic septation can be seen. CT findings include a large, well-defined tumor with variable degrees of lobulation. After infusion of contrast media, some lesions demonstrated a multiloculated aspect by enhancing septa (LEE et al. 1996). Localized and nonmetastatic tumors must be completely resected. Metastatic spread, primarily inoperable conditions, or relapse need the use of chemotherapy (WILLNOW et al. 1996).

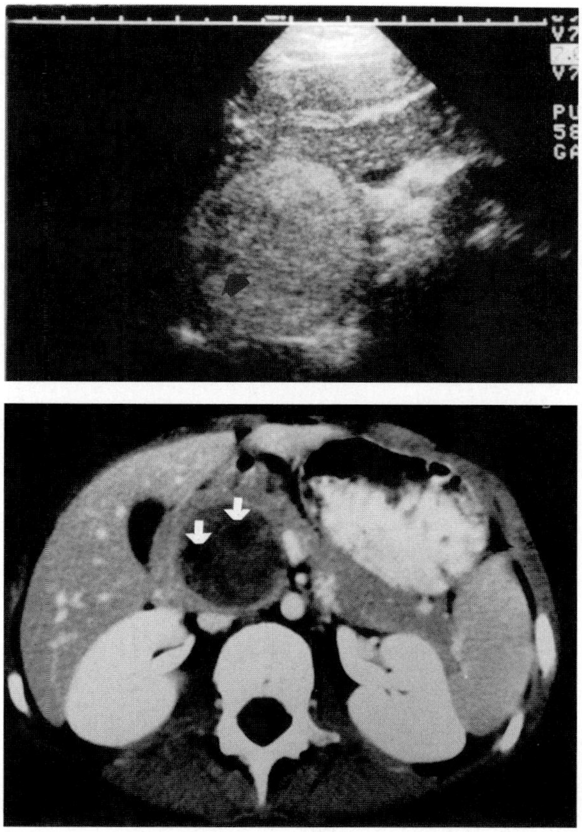
a
b

Fig. 5.17a,b. Frantz's tumor in an adolescent girl. **a** Transverse ultrasonogram shows a rounded hyperechoic mass, with hypoechoic foci (*arrow*). **b** Contrast-enhanced computed tomography demonstrates a well-delineated tumor, with a non-enhanced cystic component (*arrows*). (Courtesy of Dr. Panuel)

5.6.2.3
Solid Tumors in the Vicinity of the Pancreas

The pancreas can be invaded by an adjacent malignant tumor. In these cases, it is difficult to individualize the gland with imaging techniques and to study the tumoral relations, especially if the mass is retroperitoneal.

Neuroblastoma, being of celiomesenteric or adrenal origin, can invade all the structures of the median retroperitoneum (GALIFER et al. 1983). This tumor develops from the cells of the neural crest. It usually occurs during the first 5 years of life. The level of urinary catecholamines is increased in most cases. The retroperitoneal location, the presence of multiple fine calcifications, and the encasement of large vessels (aorta, mesenteric artery, vena cava, etc.) are important features. Use of metaiodobenzyl-

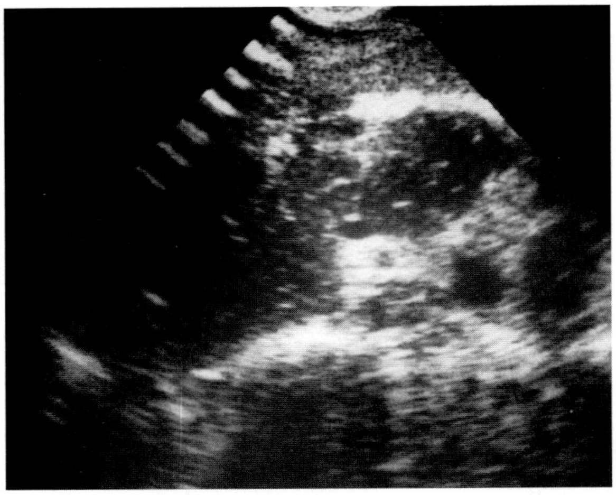

a

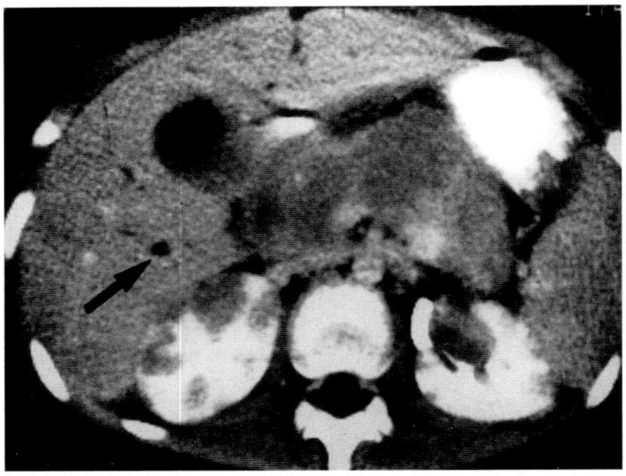

b

Fig. 5.18a,b. Lymphomatous infiltration of the pancreas in an 11-year-old boy with jaundice and impaired general condition. **a** Transverse ultrasonogram shows the pancreas to be increased in volume and very heterogeneous. **b** On contrast-enhanced computed tomography, the pancreas is seen to be infiltrated and heterogeneous. The intrahepatic ducts are dilated (*arrow*). Multiple nodules are present in both kidneys. Cytology of the ascitic liquid led to the diagnosis of Burkitt's lymphoma

guanidine (MIBG) scanning shows an increased uptake of the lesion.

Lymphomas can have a pancreatic localization, either by infiltration of the gland itself or by contiguity (Wan et al. 1988; Ng et al. 1994). In children, abdominal Burkitt lymphomas are the most common (Fig. 5.18). Ultrasonography shows an increase in the volume of the pancreas, which is rarely isolated. The diagnosis is favored by the existence of ascites, a pleural effusion, other intraperitoneal tissular masses involving the gut, lymphadenopathies, renal involvement; retroperitoneal lymph node enlargement is rarely associated with pancreatic involvement (Ng et al. 1994). It is confirmed by cytological analysis of the ascitic fluid or fine-needle biopsy of one of the masses.

References

Agrons GA, Corse WR, Markowitz RI, Suarez ES, Perry DR (1996) Gastrointestinal manifestations of cystic fibrosis: radiologic-pathologic correlation. Radiographics 16:871–893

Alessandrini P, Derlon S (1991) Gastric duplication communicating with an aberrant pancreas. Eur J Pediatr Surg 1:309–311

Allendorph M, Werlin SL, Geenen JE, Hogan WJ, Venu RP, Stewart ET, Blank E (1987) Endoscopic retrograde cholangiopancreatography in children. J Pediatr 110:206–211

Allison JW, Johnson JFr, Barr LL, Warner BW, Stevenson RJ (1995) Induction of gastroduodenal prolapse by antral heterotopic pancreas. Pediatr Radiol 25:50–51

Amerson JL, Ricketts RR (1996) Idiopathic fibrosing pancreatitis: a rare cause of obstructive jaundice in children. Am Surg 62:295–299

Ando H, Ito T, Nagaya M, Watanabe Y, Seo T, Kaneko K (1995) Pancreaticobiliary maljunction without choledochal cysts in infants and children: clinical features and surgical therapy. J Pediatr Surg 30:1658–1662

Arima E, Akita H (1979) Congenital biliary tract dilatation and anomalous junction of the pancreatico-biliary ductal system. J Pediatr Surg 14:9–15

Atkinson GO, Wyly JB, Gay BB, Ball TI, J WK (1988) Idiopathic fibrosing pancreatitis: a cause of obstructive jaundice in childhood. Pediatr Radiol 18:28–31

Auringer ST, Ulmer JL, Sumner TE, Turner CS (1993) Congenital cyst of the pancreas. J Pediatr Surg 28:1570–1571

Babbitt DP, Starshak RJ, R CA (1973) Choledochal cyst: A concept of etiology. AJR 119:57–62

Baker LL, Hartman GE, Northway W (1990) Sonographic detection of congenital pancreatic cysts in the newborn: report of a case and review of the literature. Pediatr Radiol 20:488–490

Barrera MC, Villanua J, Barrena JF, Nogues A (1995) Pancreatic hydatid disease. Pediatr Radiol 25 [Suppl 1]:S169–S170

Bass J, Di Lorenzo M, Desjardins JG, Grignon A, Ouimet A (1988) Blunt pancreatic injuries in children: the role of percutaneous external drainage in the treatment of pancreatic pseudocysts. Pediatr Surg 23:721–724

Bernard C, Regent D, Delgoffe C, Boissel P, Claudon M, Chaulieu C, Treheux A (1984) Apport de la radiologie au diagnostic des formes compliquées de pancréas annulaire chez l'adulte. J Radiol 65:839–843

Berney T, Belli D, Bugmann P, Beghetti M, Morel P, LeCoultre C (1996) Influence of severe underlying pathology and hypovolemic shock on the development of acute pancreatitis in children. J Pediatr Surg 31:1256–1261

Berrocal T, Prieto C, Pastor I, Gutierrez J, al-Assir I (1995a) Sonography of pancreatic disease in infants and children. Radiographics 15:301–313

Berrocal T, Simòn MJ, al-Assir I, Prieto C, Pastor I, de Pablo L, Lama R (1995b) Shwachman-Diamond syndrome: clinical, radiological and sonographic findings. Pediatr Radiol 25:356–359

Black PR, Welch KJ, Eraklis AJ (1986) Juxtapancreatic intestinal duplications with pancreatic ductal communication: a cause of pancreatitis and recurrent abdominal pain in childhood. J Pediatr Surg 21:257–261

Blais C, Mass S (1995) Preoperative ultrasound diagnosis of a gastric duplication cyst with ectopic pancreas in a child. J Pediatr Surg 30:1384–1386

Bom EP, van der Sande FM, Tjon RT, Tham A, Hillen HF (1993) Shwachman syndrome: CT and MR diagnosis. J Comput Assist Tomogr 17:474–476

Borocco A, Bosson N, Ducou le Pointe H, Josset P, Gruner M, Picamoles P, Montagne JP (1996a) A case of intrapancreatic duodenal duplication communicating with the biliopancreatic channel. J Radiol 77:49–51

Borocco A, Bosson N, Leroux C, Ducou le Pointe H, Montagne JP (1996b) Spiral cholangioscanners and tridimensional reconstructions of the biliary tract in children. J Radiol 77:663–666

Bret PM, Reinhold C, Taourel P, Guibaud L, Atri M, Barkun AN (1996) Pancreas divisum: evaluation with MR cholangiopancreatography. Radiology 199:99–103

Brown RA, Millar AJ, Steiner Z, Krige JE, Burkimsher D, Cywes S (1995) Hydatid cyst of the pancreas – a case report in a child. Eur J Pediatr Surg 5:121–123

Brunelle F, Negre V, Barth MO, Fekete CN, Czernichow P, Saudubray JM, Kuntz F, Tach T, Lallemand D (1989) Pancreatic venous samplings in children and children with primary hyperinsulinism. Pediatr Radiol 19:100–103

Buetow PC, Buck JL, Pantongrag-Brown L, Beck KG, Ros PR, Adair CF (1996) Solid and papillary epithelial neoplasm of the pancreas: imaging-pathologic correlation on 56 cases. Radiology 199:707–711

Cappell MS, Marks M (1995) Acute pancreatitis in HIV-seropositive patients: a case control study of 44 patients. Am J Med 98:243–8

Coleman BG, Arger PH, Rosenberg HK, Mulhern CB, Ortega W, Stauffer D (1983) Gray-scale sonographic assessment of pancreatitis in children. Radiology 146:145–150

Daltrey IR, Johnson CD (1996) Cystic lymphangioma of the pancreas. Postgrad Med J 72:564–566

Demetriadis D, Ververidis M, Papathanasiou D, Bania D, Giannoulopoulos G (1997) Pancreatitis due to cystic duodenal duplication in a 12- year-old child. Eur J Pediatr Surg 7:109–111

Dubois J, Garel L, Patriquin H, Paradis K, Forget S, Filiatrault D, Grignon A, Russo P, St-Vil D (1996) Imaging features of type 1 hereditary tyrosinemia: a review of 30 patients. Pediatr Radiol 26:845–851

Durie PR (1996) Inherited and congenital disorders of the exocrine pancreas. Gastroenterologist 4:169–187

Dutheil-Doco A, Ducou-Lepointe H, Larroquet M, Ben Lagha N, Montagne JP (1998) A case of perforated cystic duplication of the transverse colon. Pediatr Radiol 28:20–22

Eire PF, Rodriguez Pereira C, Barca Rodriguez P, Varela Cives R (1996) Uncommon case of gastrinoma in a child. Eur J Pediatr Surg 6:173–174

Eklöf O, Lassrich A, Stanley P, Chrispin AR (1973) Ectopic pancreas. Pediatr Radiol 1:24–27

Ferrozzi F, Bova D, Campodonico F, De Chiara F, Uccelli M, Bacchini E, Grinzcich R, dé Angelis GL, Battistini A (1996) Cystic fibrosis: MR assessment of pancreatic damage. Radiology 198:875–879

Fleischer AC, Parker P, Kirchner SG, James AE (1983) Sonographic findings of pancreatitis in children. Radiology 146:151–155

Franken EA, Chiu LC, Smith WL, Lu CH (1984) La pancréatite héréditaire de l'enfant. Ann Radiol 27:130–137

Frush DP, Siegel MJ, Bisset GS (1997) Challenges of pediatric spiral CT. Radiographics 17:939–959

Galifer RB, Margueritte G, Balmes M, Barneon G, Rieu D (1983) Ganglioneuroblastome de la tête du pancréas Présentation d'un cas chez un garçon de 2 ans. Chir Pediatr 24:396–400

Garel L, Brunelle F, Lallemand D, Sauvegrain J (1983) Pseudocysts of the pancreas in children: wich cases require surgery? Pediatr Radiol 13:120–124

Gin H, Brottier E, Dupuy B, Guillaume D, Ponzo J, Aubertin J (1987) Use of the glucose clamp technique for confirmation of insulinoma autonomous hyperinsulinism. Arch Intern Med 147:985–987

Glazer GM, Margulis AR (1979) Annular pancreas: etiology and diagnosis using endoscopic retrograde cholangiopancreatography. Radiology 133:303–306

Gold RP, Berman H, Fakhry J, Heier S, Rosenthal W, Delguercio L (1984) Pancreas divisum with pancreatitis and pseudocyst. AJR 143:1343–1344

Guibaud L, Bret PM, Reinhold C, Atri M, Barkun AN (1995) Bile duct obstruction and choledocholithiasis: diagnosis with MR cholangiography. Radiology 197:109–115

Guibaud L, Lachaud A, Touraine R, Guibal AL, Pelizzari M, Basset T, Pracros JP (1998) MR cholangiography in neonates and infants: feasibility and preliminary applications. AJR Am J Roentgenol 170:27–31

Haddock G, Coupar G, Youngson GG, MacKinlay GA, Raine PA (1994) Acute pancreatitis in children: a 15-year review. J Pediatr Surg 29:719–722

Hélardot PG, Van Kote G, Barbet P, Godefroy Y, Bienaymé J (1982) Les duplications gastriques séparées de l'estomac et en relation avec le pancréas. Chir Pediatr 23:363–368

Herman TE (1995) Type IA glycogenosis with acute pancreatitis. J Radiol 76:51–53

Herman TE, Siegel MJ (1991) Polysplenia syndrome with congenital short pancreas. AJR 156:799–800

Hernanz-Schulman M, Teele RL, Perez-Atayde A, Zollars L, Levine J, Black P, Kuligowska E (1986) Pancreatic cystosis in cystic fibrosis. Radiology 158:629–631

Hibon D, Filiatrault D (1985) Le syndrome de Shwachman. Aspects échographiques et tomodensitométriques. A propos de 3 cas. Ann Radiol 28:469–473

Hilfer CL, Holgersen LO (1995) Massive chylous ascites and transected pancreas secondary to child abuse: successful non-surgical management. Pediatr Radiol 25:117–119

Horisawa M, Niinomi N, Sato T, Yokoi S, Oda K, Ichikawa M, Hayakawa S (1995) Frantz's tumor (solid and cystic tumor of the pancreas) with liver metastasis: successful treatment and long-term follow-up. J Pediatr Surg 30:724–726

Hough DM, Stephens DH, Johnson CD, Binkovitz LA (1994) Pancreatic lesions in von Hippel-Lindau disease: prevalence, clinical significance, and CT findings. AJR Am J Roentgenol 162:1091–1094

Ichikawa T, Nitatori T, Hachiya J, Mizutani Y (1996) Breath-held MR cholangiopancreatography with half-averaged single shot hybrid rapid acquisition with relaxation enhancement sequence: comparison of fast GRE and SE sequences. J Comput Assist Tomogr 20:798–802

Itterbeek P, Vanclooster P, de Gheldere C (1997) Cystic lymphangioma of the pancreas: an unusual cause of the acute surgical abdomen. Acta Chir Belg 97:297–298

Jaksic T, Yaman M, Thorner P, Wesson DK, Filler RM, Shandling B (1992) A 20-year review of pediatric pancreatic tumors. J Pediatr Surg 27:1315–1317

Jenkins JM, Othersen HB (1992) Cystadenoma of the pancreas in a newborn. J Pediatr Surg 27:1569

Jones NL, Hofley PM, Durie PR (1994) Pathophysiology of the pancreatic defect in Johanson-Blizzard syndrome: a disorder of acinar development. J Pediatr 125:406–408

Kahler SG, Sherwood WG et al (1994) Pancreatitis in patients with organic acidemias. J Pediatr 124:239–243

Kahn E, Anderson VM, Greco MA, Magid M (1995) Pancreatic disorders in pediatric acquired immune deficiency syndrome. Hum Pathol 26:765–770

Kayemba Kay's Kabangu S, Bovier Lapierre M, Jalaguier E (1991) Pancréatite aiguë et acide valproïque. Pediatrie 46:839–843

Khiari A, Mzali R, Ouali M, Kharrat M, Kechaou MS, Beyrouti MI (1994) Hydatid cyst of the pancreas. Apropos of 7 cases. Ann Gastroenterol Hepatol (Paris) 30:87–91

King LR, Siegel MJ, Balfe DM (1995) Acute pancreatitis in children: CT findings of intra- and extrapancreatic fluid collections. Radiology 195:196–200

Komura J, Yano H, Tanaka Y, Tsuru T (1993) Annular pancreas associated with pancreaticobiliary maljunction in an infant. Eur J Pediatr Surg 3:244–247

Krief S, Turck D, Lefebvre R, Lemaitre L (1988) Syndrome de Shwachman (Rubrique iconographie). Arch Fr Pediatr 45:275–276

Ky A, Shilyansky J, Gerstle J, Taylor G, Filler RM, Grace N, Superina R (1998) Experience with papillary and solid epithelial neoplasms of the pancreas in children. J Pediatr Surg 33:42–44

Lacaille F, Mamou-Mani T, Brunelle F, Lallemand D, Schmitz J (1996) Magnetic resonance imaging for diagnosis of Shwachman's syndrome. J Pediatr Gastroenterol Nutr 23:599–603

Lachaux A, Fournier V, Ponchon T, Loras I, Hermier M (1994) Common bilio-pancreatic channel. Apropos of a case with intermittent dilatation of the biliary tracts. Arch Pediatr 1:38–41

Lee JY, Kim IO, Kim WS, Kim CW, Yeon KM (1996) CT and US findings of pancreatoblastoma. J Comput Assist Tomogr 20:370–374

Lerner A, Branski D, Lebenthal E (1996) Pancreatic diseases in children. Pediatr Clin North Am 43:125–156

Levin TL, Berdon WE, Tang HB, Haller JO (1997) Dideoxyinosine-induced pancreatitis in human immunodeficiency virus-infected children. Pediatr Radiol 27:189–191

Lobe TE, Vera SR, Bowman LC, Fontanesi J, Britt LG, Gaber AO (1992) Hepaticopancreaticogastroduodenectomy with transplantation for metastatic islet cell carcinoma in childhood. J Pediatr Surg 27:227–229

Lowenfels AB, Maisonneuve P, DiMagno EP, Elitsur Y, Gates LK, Jr., Perrault J, Whitcomb DC (1997) Hereditary pancreatitis and the risk of pancreatic cancer. International Hereditary Pancreatitis Study Group. J Natl Cancer Inst 89:442–446

Mac Hugo JM, Mac Keown C, Brown MT, Weller P, Shah KJ (1987) Ultrasound findings in children with cystic fibrosis. Br J Radiol 60:137–141

Miyano T, Ando K, Yamataka A, Lane G, Segawa O, Kohno S, Fujiwara T (1996) Pancreaticobiliary maljunction associated with nondilatation or minimal dilatation of the common bile duct in children: diagnosis and treatment. Eur J Pediatr Surg 6:334–337

Miyazaki T, Yamashita Y, Tang Y, Tsuchigame T, Takahashi M, Sera Y (1998) Single-shot MR cholangiopancreatography of neonates, infants, and young children. AJR Am J Roentgenol 170:33–37

Ng YY, Healy JC, Vincent JM, Kingston JE, Armstrong P, Reznek RH (1994) The radiology of non-Hodgkin's lymphoma in childhood: a review of 80 cases. Clin Radiol 49:594–600

Okada A, Higaki J, Nakamura T, Fukui Y, Kamata S (1995) Pancreatitis associated with choledochal cyst and other anomalies in childhood. Br J Surg 82:829–832

Ökten A, Demirci A, Sahuran H, Mocan H, Karagüzel G (1994) Dorsal mesodermal sinus associated with annular pancreas and meconium pancreatitis. Pediatr Radiol 24:302–303

Panuel M, Devred P, Delarue A, Faure F, Grangier ML, Padovani J (1984) Cystadénome multiloculaire du pancréas. Une tumeur exceptionnelle chez l'enfant. J Radiol 65:275–278

Perisic VN, Mihailovic T, Tomomasa T, Milovanovic D, Kuroume T (1991) The role of accessory pancreatic duct of Santorini in pancreatic drainage in children (with emphasis on choledochal cyst patients). Pediatr Radiol 21:258–261

Perrelli L, Nanni L, Costamagna G, Mutignani M (1996) Endoscopic treatment of chronic idiopathic pancreatitis in children. J Pediatr Surg 31:1396–1400

Reinhart RD, Brown JJ, Foglia RP, Aliperti G (1994) MR imaging of annular pancreas. Abdom Imaging 19:301–303

Reinhold C, Bret PM (1996) Current status of MR cholangiopancreatography. Am J Roentgenol 166:1285–1295

Rescorla FJ, Plumley DA, Sherman S, Scherer LR, West KW, Grosfeld JL (1995) The efficacy of early ERCP in pediatric pancreatic trauma. J Pediatr Surg 30:336–340

Robberecht E, Nachtegaele P, Van Rattinghe R, Afschrift M, Kunnen M, Verhaaren R (1985) Pancreatic lipomatosis in the Shwachman-Diamond syndrome. Identification by sonography and CT-scan. Pediatr Radiol 15:348–349

Robey G, Daneman A, Martin DJ (1983) Pancreatic carcinoma in a neonate. Pediatr Radiol 13:284–286

Rocha MdS, Costa NS, Costa JC, Angelo MT, Lessa Angelo JR, Sonoda L, de Andrade MR, Scatigno Neto A (1995) CT identification of ascaris in the biliary tract. Abdom Imaging 20:317–319

Rose E, De Miscault G, Thome M, Boussard N (1991) Pancréatite aigu' au valproate de sodium Revue de la littérature. A propos d'un cas chez l'enfant. Pediatrie 46:831–837

Ross BA, Jeffrey RB Jr, Mindelzun RE (1996) Normal variations in the lateral contour of the head and neck of the pancreas mimicking neoplasm: evaluation with dual-phase helical CT. AJR Am J Roentgenol 166:799–801

Rossi P, Allison DJ, Bezzi M (1989) Endocrine tumors of the pancreas. Radiol Clin North Am 27:129–161

Sadoff J, Hwang S, Rosenfeld D, Ettinger L, Spigland N (1997) Surgical pancreatic complications induced by L-asparaginase. J Pediatr Surg 32:860–863

Sanada Y, Yoshizawa Y, Chiba M, Nemoto H, Midorikawa T, Kumada K (1995) Ventral pancreatitis in a patient with pancreas divisum. J Pediatr Surg 30:665–667

Sarles J (1990) Les affections du pancréas exocrine de l'enfant. Pédiatrie 45:99–104

Schmittenbecher PP, Rapp P, Dietz HG (1996) Traumatic and non-traumatic pancreatitis in pediatric surgery. Eur J Pediatr Surg 6:86–91

See Y, Martin K, Rooney M, Woo P (1997) Severe juvenile dermatomyositis complicated by pancreatitis. Br J Rheumatol 36:912–916

Shilyansky J, Fisher S, Cutz E, Perlman K, Filler RM (1997) Is 95% pancreatectomy the procedure of choice for treatment of persistant hyperinsulinemic hypoglycemia in the neonate ? J Pediatr Surg 32:342–346

Shrier LA, Karpen SJ, McEvoy C (1995) Acute pancreatitis associated with acute hepatitis A in a young child. J Pediatr 126:57–59

Siegel MJ, Sivit CJ (1997) Pancreatic emergencies. Radiol Clin North Am 35:815–830

Siegel MJ, Martin KW, Worthington JL (1987) Normal and abnormal pancreas in children: US studies. Radiology 165:15–18

Sivit CJ, Eichelberger MR (1995) CT diagnosis of pancreatic injury in children: significance of fluid separating the splenic vein and the pancreas. AJR 165:921–924

Sivit CJ, Eichelberger MR, Taylo GA, Bulas DI, Gotschall CS, Kushner DC (1992) Blunt pancreatic trauma in children : CT diagnosis. AJR 158:1097–1100

Smith WL (1982) The pancreas. In: Franken EA, Smith WL (eds) Gastrointestinal imaging in pediatrics. Harper and Row, Philadelphia, pp 459–467

Soto JA, Barish MA, Yucel EK, Clarke P, Siegenberg D, Chuttani R, Ferrucci JT (1995) Pancreatic duct: MR cholangiopancreatography with a three- dimensional fast spin-echo technique. Radiology 196:459–464

Spehl-Robberecht M, Baran D, Dab I, Perlmutter-Cremer N (1981) Ultrasonic study of pancreas in cystic fibrosis. Ann Radiol 24:49–52

Spehl-Robberecht M, Garel L, Lallemand D (1986). Le pancréas. In: Kalifa G (ed) Echographie pédiatrique. Vigot, Paris, pp 175–190

Spencer JA, Lindsell DRM, Isaacs D (1990) Hereditary pancreatitis: early ultrasound appearances. Pediatr Radiol 20:293–295

Steyaert H, Voigt JJ, Brouet P, Vaysse P (1997) Uncommon complication of gastric duplication in a three-year-old child. Eur J Pediatr Surg 7:243–244

Stringer MD, Dhawan A, Davenport M, Mieli-Vergani G, Mowat AP, Howard ER (1995) Choledochal cysts: lessons from a 20 year experience. Arch Dis Child 73:528–531

Sty JR, Wells RG, Starshak RJ, Gregg DC (1992). The pancreas. In: Diagnostic imaging of infants and children. Aspen, Gaithersburg, pp 310–325

Summer TE, Auringer ST, Cox TD (1997) A complex communicating bronchopulmonary foregut malformation: diagnostic imaging and pathogenesis. Pediatr Radiol 27:799–801

Swischuk LE, Hayden CK (1985) Pararenal space hyperechogenicity in childhood pancreatitis. AJR 145:1085–1086

Tagge EP, Tarnasky PR, Chandler J, Tagge DU, Smith C, Hebra A, Hawes RH, Cotton PB, Othersen HB Jr (1997) Multidisciplinary approach to the treatment of pediatric pancreaticobiliary disorders. J Pediatr Surg 32:158–164

Teele RL, Share JC (1991) The pancreas. In: Ultrasonography of infants and children. Saunders, Philadelphia, pp 389–404

Telander RL, Charboneau JW, Haymond MW (1986) Intraoperative ultrasonography of the pancreas in children. Pediatr Surg 21:262–266

Tjon A, Tham RTO, Heyerman HGM, Falke THM, Zwinderman AH, Bloem JL, Bakker W, Lamers CBHW (1991) Cystic fibrosis: MR imaging of the pancreas. Radiology 179:183–186

Tschäppeler H (1990). Les maladies du pancréas chez l'enfant. In: Terrier F, Fuchs WA (eds) Imagerie médicale du pancréas. Vigot, Paris, pp 286–293

Ueda D, Taketazu M, Itoh S, Azuma H, Oshima H (1991) A case of gastric duplication cyst with aberrant pancreas. Pediatr Radiol 21:379–380

Veyrac C, Couture A, Baud C, L FJ (1987). Le pancréas. In: Montagne JP, Couture A (Eds) Tomodensitométrie pédiatrique. Vigot, Paris, pp 345–352

Walsh E, Cramer B, Pushpanathan C (1990) Pancreatic echogenicity in premature and newborn infants. Pediatr Radiol 20:323–325

Wan Y, Chen WJ, Huang SC, Lee TY, Tsai CC (1988) Solitary hepatic burkitt lymphoma presenting as acute pancreatitis. Pediatr Radiol 18:160

Washington K, Gossage DL, Gottfried MR (1994) Pathology of the pancreas in severe combined immunodeficiency and DiGeorge syndrome: acute graft-versus-host disease and unusual viral infections. Hum Pathol 25:908–914

Waters DL, Dorney SF, Gruca MA, Martin HC, Howman-Giles R, Kan AE, De Silva M, Gaskin KJ (1995) Hepatobiliary disease in cystic fibrosis patients with pancreatic sufficiency. Hepatology 21:963–969

White KS (1996) helical/spiral CT scanning: a pediatric radiology perspective. Pediatr Radiol 26:5–14

Willnow U, Willberg B, Schwamborn D, Körholz D, Göbel U (1996) Pancreatoblastoma in children. Case report and review of the literature. Eur J Pediatr Surg 6:369–372

Wünsch LP, Flemming P, Werner U, Gluer S, Bürger D (1997) Diagnosis and treatment of papillary cystic tumor of the pancreas in children. Eur J Pediatr Surg 7:45–47

Yeung CY, Lee HC et al (1996) Pancreatitis in children-experience with 43 cases. Eur J Pediatr 155:458–463

Zakari S, Ajana A, Dhobb OH, Iraqi HS, Imani F (1984) Aspects échographiques du kyste hydatique du pancréas. A propos de deux cas avec revue de la littérature. Ann Radiol 27:607–613

Zeller J, Roche A, Rahier J, Adamsbaum C, Carel JC, Hélardot P, Bougnères PF (1993) Localizing of Langerhans islets adenoma by transhepatic portal catheterization. Arch Fr Pediatr 50:675–680

Zeman RK, McVay LV, Silverman PM, Cattau EL, Benjamin SB, Fleischer D, Garra BS, Jaffe MH (1988) Pancreas divisum: thin-section CT. Radiology 169:395–398

6 Acute Pancreatitis

R. LECESNE, J. DROUILLARD

CONTENTS

R. LECESNE, MD
Service d'Imagerie Médicale, Radiologie Diagnostique et Thérapeutique, Université de Bordeaux II, Hôpital Haut Lévêque, USN, C.H.U. Bordeaux, Avenue de Magellan, F-33604 Pessac, France
J. DROUILLARD, MD
Professor of Radiology, Service d'Imagerie Médicale, Radiologie Diagnostique et Thérapeutique, Université de Bordeaux II, Hôpital Haut Lévêque, USN, C.H.U. Bordeaux, Avenue de Magellan, F-33604 Pessac, France

6.1 Introduction

Acute pancreatitis, an acute inflammatory process of the pancreas, can be triggered by numerous etiologic factors. Most patients have self-limiting pancreatitis requiring nothing beyond ordinary supportive care; however, 1% of patients will have more severe disease with potentially devastating local and systemic consequences. An international symposium was held in Atlanta in 1992 to establish a clinically based classification system for acute pancreatitis, with a precisely defined clinical and morphologic nomenclature (BRADLEY 1993). On the basis of the severity of pathologic changes, clinical manifestations, and laboratory values, acute pancreatitis is classified as mild or severe acute pancreatitis (BALTHAZAR et al. 1994).

In mild cases of pancreatitis, interstitial edema of the pancreatic tissue predominates in association with only a few foci of necrosis; in severe forms, extensive pancreatic necrosis and inflammation of the peripancreatic fat are present that may evolve towards the formation of fluid collections. However, a variable spectrum of disease is observed, comprising numerous transitional stages of clinical and pathologic findings.

6.2 Etiology, Physiopathology, and Clinical Background

Since its first clinical description (FITZ 1889), we still do not know how or why this disease occurs. The most common associated etiologic factors are gallstones and heavy alcohol abuse (together these account for 80% of cases). At least 30 or so other causes of pancreatitis have been described and could be subgrouped as follows:

- Metabolic: hyperlipoproteinemia, hypercalcemia, drugs, genetic factors

- Mechanical duct obstruction: pancreatic tumor, duodenal hematoma (Sadry and Hauser 1990), ascariasis (Leung et al. 1987), duodenal obstruction, minor ampullary stenosis associated with pancreas divisum (Topazian 1994)
- Iatrogenic: abdominal surgery, endoscopic retrograde sphincterotomy (Kuhlman et al. 1989), endoscopic retrograde cholangiopancreatography (Thoeni et al. 1990), post-traumatic percutaneous transpancreatic biopsy of adrenal glands (Kane et al. 1991), pancreatic biopsy (Mueller et al. 1988)
- Vascular: cardiopulmonary bypass, periarteritis nodosa, aortic dissection (Pombo et al. 1991), chemoembolization of hepatocellular carcinoma (Kishimoto et al. 1989)
- Infectious and toxic: mumps, Coxsackie virus, scorpion bite.

The physiopathologic nature of the disease has not yet been clearly resolved, but it seems to be related mainly to temporary or permanent blockage of the pancreatic duct with passage of the pancreatic enzymes into the adjacent interstitial tissue. In the presence of underlying cholelithiasis, such blockage is due to the passage of calculi through the papilla of Vater. In alcoholics, the phenomenon could be due to a toxic effect and chemical alteration of the exocrine secretion, intraductal proteins precipitate, leading to obstruction.

Interlobular fat necrosis is the primary lesion in acute pancreatitis and the extent of necrosis defines the severity of the inflammatory process. In severe forms, interlobular fat necrosis involves the lobules within the pancreas and could lead to acinar cell disruption and the release of toxic and vasoactive substances. Bacterial contamination of necrosis often leads to systemic complications.

The clinical picture is quite evocative in a patient who presents with acute abdomen including upper abdominal pain, tenderness, nausea, and vomiting, and who has a past history of heavy alcohol consumption and an elevated serum amylase level.

However, both the clinical presentation and the laboratory findings are sometimes misleading. A normal serum amylase level may be observed if tests are performed a few days after the initial episode.

In addition, hyperamylasemia may occur in association with other acute abdominal conditions, e.g., acute cholecystitis, small bowel obstruction, bowel ischemia, and peptic ulcers. The early diagnosis of severe pancreatitis is missed in 30%–40% of cases when only the clinical picture is considered. Thus, imaging studies are of great help.

Management of patients with acute pancreatitis is based on the severity of the initial attack. The severity of an acute attack of pancreatitis and the prognosis of the disease has been appraised by an objective quantification system using clinical and laboratory parameters. The most widely used system is the application of Ranson criteria (Ranson 1982) (Table 6.1) and Apache II criteria (Knaus et al. 1985). Three or more Ranson criteria or eight or more on the Apache II score at the onset of attack indicate severe acute pancreatitis. These criteria have proved to be reliable predictors of severe pancreatitis, enabling an improvement in patient care and interaction of conservative medical therapy. The Apache II score indicates the severity of the disease at any time during the course of acute pancreatitis, enabling therapy to be evaluated.

Table 6.1. Early prognostic signs used to estimate the risk of major complications from acute pancreatitis. [From Ranson (1982)]

At admission	During initial 48 h
Age over 55 years	Hematocrit fall of greater than 10%
White blood cell count over 16 000/mm3	Blood urea nitrogen rise of more than 5 mg/100 ml
Blood glucose over 11 mmol/l	Serum calcium level below 8 mg/100 ml
Serum lactic dehydrogenase over 350 IU/l	Arterial $P0_2$ below 60 mmHg
Serum glutamic oxaloacetic transaminase over 250 IU/l	Base deficit greater than 4 mEq/l
	Estimated fluid sequestration more than 6000 ml

6.3 Nomenclature of Terminology and Complications

6.3.1 Pancreatic Necrosis

Pancreatic gland necrosis is defined as focal or diffuse areas of nonviable parenchyma which is typically associated with peripancreatic fat necrosis. Pancreatic necrosis develops early in the course of severe acute pancreatitis and is well established by 96 h after the onset of symptoms (Isenmann et al. 1993).

6.3.2 Acute Fluid Collections

These are collections of enzyme-rich pancreatic juice that occur early in the course of acute pancreatitis. They are located mostly near the pancreas. They are limited by the anatomic space without any capsule (Kourtesis et al. 1990). They can resolve spontaneously or evolve into pseudocysts or pancreatic abscesses. The international symposium in Atlanta elected to abandon the use of the term phlegmon since it has been used erroneously.

6.3.3. Pseudocysts

These are round, encapsulated (fibrous-tissue walled) collections of pancreatic fluid. Their incidence following acute pancreatitis has been reported to be 2%–3% (Balthazar 1989). They evolve from acute fluid collections requiring at least 4–6 weeks. They can resolve spontaneously, stabilize, partially resolve, or cause complications. The risk of complications seems to be proportional to the size of pseudocyst.

6.3.4 Sepsis

Acute pancreatitis promotes translocation of gut-derived organisms to the inflamed pancreas and peripancreatic region (Medich et al. 1993). Pancreatic and peripancreatic infection occurs in only 1%–5% of patients with acute pancreatitis (Lumson and Bradley 1990). In severe acute pancreatitis, the frequency of development of sepsis is overall between 40% and 70%, increasing with time after onset of symptoms (Beger et al. 1986).

6.3.4.1 Pancreatic Abscesses

These correspond to circumscribed intra-abdominal collections of pus located in proximity to the pancreas, usually occurring 4 weeks or more after the onset of attack and arising as a secondary infection of limited necrosis (Bittner et al. 1987). These abscesses are associated with a high mortality rate if not treated. Abscesses can be treated effectively with percutaneous catheter drainage.

6.3.4.2 Infected Necrosis

This is defined as infected pancreatic and/or peripancreatic necrotic tissue. The process can be focal or widespread and severe. The risk of mortality associated with infected necrosis is nearly double that for pancreatic abscesses and requires mostly surgical débridement (Büchler et al. 1992).

6.3.5 Hemorrhage

This occurs as a late consequence of vascular injuries produced by extravasated pancreatic enzymes. Injuries to the pancreaticoduodenal artery and branches of the splenic artery prevail. Bleeding is often preceded by the development of a pseudoaneurysm. Selective embolization is the treatment of choice (Vujic 1989).

6.4 Plain Abdominal X-Ray and Conventional Gastrointestinal Examination

6.4.1 Plain Radiographic Evaluation

A plain radiographic evaluation of patients with suspected acute pancreatitis begins with conventional supine and, when possible, upright views of the abdomen. Even in severe cases, the plain film may be normal. Nevertheless, a variety of findings are suggestive of acute pancreatitis. Two signs have been described as particularly valuable in establishing a diagnosis:

- A mottled or homogeneous gas lucency causing displacement of the stomach or transverse colon is evocative of a pancreatic abscess
- Significant gas within the duodenal loop indicates the presence of an adjacent inflammatory process.

Two other signs, although recognized as suggestive of acute pancreatitis, are equally found in other acute abdominal conditions (Safrit and Rice 1989):

- The "sentinel loop sign" due to a focally distended small bowel loop in the left upper quadrant
- The "colon cut off" sign, seen as an abrupt obliteration of the lucency of the transverse colon.

Other less specific and inconstant findings include:
- A soft tissue mass representing enlargement of the pancreas or an associated pseudocyst
- A totally gasless abdomen
- A pleural effusion (more often on the left side)
- Calcified gallstones, ascites, and obliteration of renal or psoas margins.

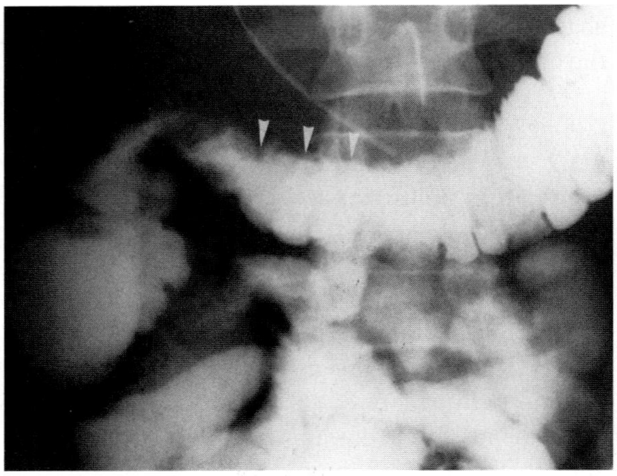

Fig. 6.1. Barium enema. There are asymmetric irregularities (*arrowheads*) of the transverse colon related to acute pancreatitis

6.4.2 Contrast Examination of the Gastrointestinal Tract

This method has been largely replaced by ultrasonography (US) and computed tomography (CT) as a means of evaluating patients with acute pancreatitis. However, barium opacification can detect some abnormalities which are suggestive of the diagnosis:
- Duodenal narrowing or stenosis, which may result from extrinsic compression and/or inflammation of the duodenum (Safrit and Rice 1989)
- Transverse colon: a spectrum of manifestations comprising spasm, edematous fold, stenosis, fistula, and necrosis. The distribution of the lesions is usually asymmetric (Fig. 6.1) owing to their relation to the dissecting pathway of the pancreatic exudates, which tends to involve mainly the inferior borders of the transverse colon at the attachment of the mesocolon (Meyers and Evans 1973).

6.5 Ultrasonography

US is usually the first modality of choice in a patient with acute abdomen, being the most easily and rapidly performed examination. While there are technical limitations during the first 48 h in acute pancreatitis owing to paralytic ileus, the pancreas is more easily visualized during the convalescent phase (Jeffrey 1989).

In the early phase, the goals of US include:
- To suggest an alternative diagnosis (acute cholecystitis, hepatic abscess, or bowel obstruction)
- To evaluate the gallbladder and the biliary tree
- To clarify diagnostic dilemmas in questionable cases of mild pancreatitis
- To diagnose pancreatic and peripancreatic acute fluid collections and to follow-up pseudocysts
- To suggest hemorrhagic fluid collection by demonstrating an echogenic mass.

Although complete assessment of the peripancreatic compartment is seldom possible with US, an optimal scanning technique can facilitate the sonographic evaluation of the upper abdomen, allowing visualization of the pancreas in more than 90% of patients (Freise 1987). Besides conventional, transverse, and longitudinal scanning in the supine position, complementary scanning in the semi-erect position is useful since it allows better visualization of the body of the pancreas and lesser sac. Furthermore, coronal scanning employing a left flank approach is useful for visualization of the anterior pararenal space.

The pancreas can be diffusely enlarged and hypoechoic owing to interstitial edema in approximately one third of cases (Fig. 6.2). However, a normal gland can be observed in the mild form (Jeffrey 1989).

Numerous factors influence the echogenicity of the pancreas in acute pancreatitis; chief among these are the time of scanning and the degree of extrapancreatic spread (Fig. 6.3). Maximal glandular hypoechogenicity occurs 2-5 days following the initial episode (Freise 1987).

The pancreatic duct may be dilated both during the acute episode and later, during the convalescent

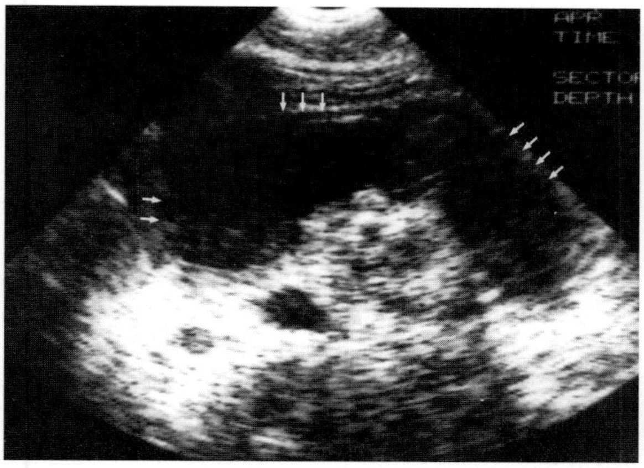

Fig. 6.2. Ultrasonography. Transverse view of a diffusely enlarged pancreatic gland with decreased echogenicity (*small arrows*)

phase (MALFERTHEINER and BÜCHLER 1987). Although the glandular changes in size, echogenicity, and ductal dilatation generally constitute reliable evidence of acute pancreatitis, these signs are not invariably present.

Focal intrapancreatic ill-defined masses can be observed in acute pancreatitis and are due to pancreatic necrosis or hemorrhagic areas (Fig. 6.3). Fluid collections may be identified on the basis of their sonolucency. However, more echoic fluid collections may be difficult to differentiate from carcinoma (NEFF et al. 1984). Focal echogenic masses are more suggestive of hemorrhage (ISIKOFF et al. 1981; HASHIMOTO et al. 1984). Free intraperitoneal fluid should be searched for in the pouches of Morison and Douglas.

Extrapancreatic spread may be present anywhere from the pericardium to the inguinal area and thigh. The most common locations are the lesser sac, the left anterior pararenal space, and the transverse mesocolon (WEILL et al. 1983). Fluid collections of the lesser sac are almost always visible on sagittal slices, while those of the pararenal space can be demonstrated by a coronal flank approach in 75% of cases (Fig. 6.4). The transverse mesocolon is the most difficult peripancreatic compartment to visualize by US owing to frequent gaseous distention. Only one third of cases diagnosed by CT are equally visible on US (JEFFREY et al. 1986). Moreover, thickening of Gerota's fascia, visible on CT, cannot be appreciated by US.

Demonstration of intra- or extrapancreatic fluid collections can be followed up by serial US. Though the majority of masses resolve with time, pseudo-

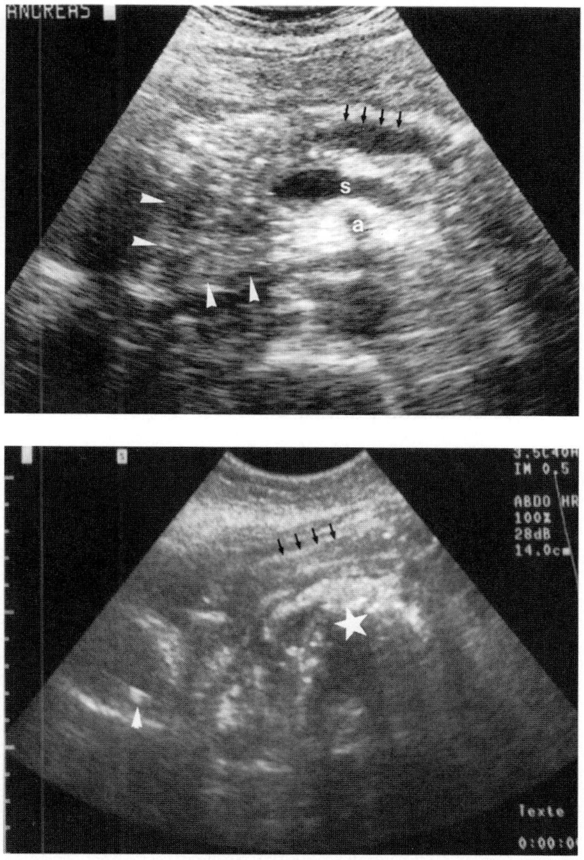

Fig. 6.3a,b. Ultrasonography of acute pancreatitis. **a** Axial epigastric view. Enlargement of the pancreatic head (*arrowheads*) associated with peripancreatic acute fluid collection behind the body of the pancreas (*arrows*). *s*, Splenic vein; *a*, superior mesenteric artery. **b** Axial epigastric view. Heterogeneous hyperechoic mass is depicted (*star*) within the lesser sac displacing the stomach anteriorly (*arrows*). Complex acute fluid collection is strongly suspected. Stone is shown within thick-walled gallbladder (*arrowhead*)

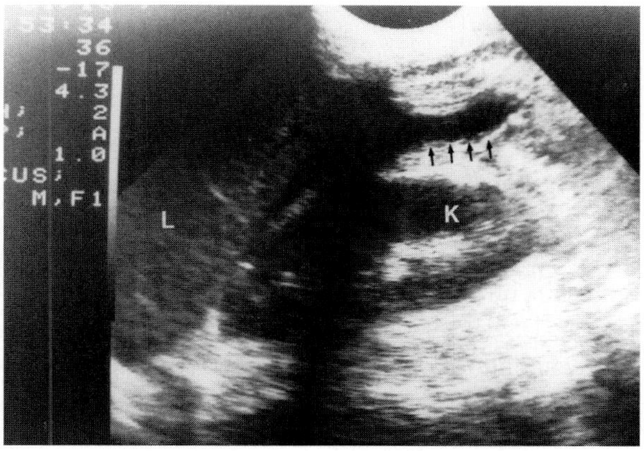

Fig. 6.4. Ultrasonography in a patient with acute pancreatitis. Right intercostal sagittal view. Right anterior pararenal collection (*arrows*) is visible between liver (*L*) and right kidney (*K*)

cysts with fluid content present for more than 6 weeks often do not regress.

Color Doppler US can be performed easily and quickly, but often visualizes the pancreaticobiliary area inadequately because of abundant bowel gas due to paralytic ileus. Color Doppler US evaluation of pancreatitis can aid in diagnosing vascular complications such as gastroduodenal artery pseudoaneurysm or splenic artery pseudoaneurysm (Vujic 1989). Thrombosis of the portal system can occur secondary to acute pancreatitis (Fig. 6.5). Color Doppler US can demonstrate thrombi and/or depict venous collateral pathways.

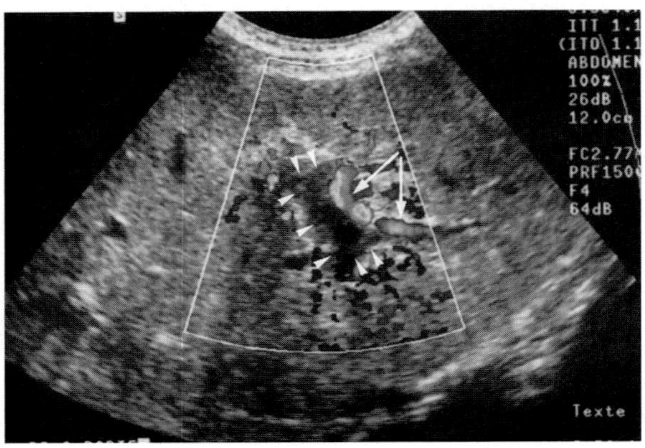

Fig. 6.5. Power Doppler ultrasonography. Transverse epigastric view. Acute thrombosis of the left portal vein (*arrowheads*) which appears enlarged and hypoechoic without any flow color. Flow color is depicted only in the left branch of the hepatic artery (*arrows*)

6.6 Endoscopic US

This is a new imaging technique (Amouyal et al. 1989) which allows adequate visualization and high resolution imaging of the pancreaticobiliary region and can be performed even at the bedside. Endoscopic US is performed under neuroleptanalgesia. An echoendoscope using a 7.5-MHz probe is introduced into the descending duodenum and the pancreaticobiliary areas are scanned while the endoscope is slowly withdrawn. The pancreatic head, extrahepatic bile duct, and gallbladder can be visualized from the duodenum, and the pancreatic body and tail from the stomach.

Endoscopic US has proved potent for differentiating mild and severe pancreatitis; furthermore, it enables clarification of the cause of pancreatitis, such as gallstones and acute exacerbation of chronic pancreatitis. In mild pancreatitis, endoscopic US (Sugiyama et al. 1995) has depicted the pancreas as an enlarged and diffusely hypoechoic structure. In cases of severe pancreatitis, endoscopic US can depict intrapancreatic focal hypoechoic masses interpreted as areas of focal pancreatic necrosis.

Acute fluid collections can be identified as hypoechoic areas. Endoscopic US allows a precise assessment of acute fluid collections adjacent to the pancreas and within the lesser sac. The assessment of extensive retroperitoneal spread with endoscopic US is limited because the maximal display depth does not exceed 5–7 cm from the transducer. An important contribution of US endoscopy has been the ability to determine the etiology of the disease. Endoscopic US can depict choledocholithiasis (Fig. 6.6) in patients in whom conventional US has failed or abnormal liver function does not exist. High sensitivity (97%) and specificity (100%) of endoscopic US for diagnosing common bile duct stones has been reported (Amouyal et al. 1989).

Endoscopic US can visualize subtle abnormalities of the pancreatic ducts or pancreatic parenchyma architecture, enabling the diagnosis of early or advanced chronic pancreatitis. Furthermore, less common etiologies, such as an underlying pancreatic tumor or a pancreas divisum, could be evidenced. Some complications can be detected by endoscopic US. When intrapancreatic focal hyperechoic areas with interspersed hyperechoic spots occur, a pancre-

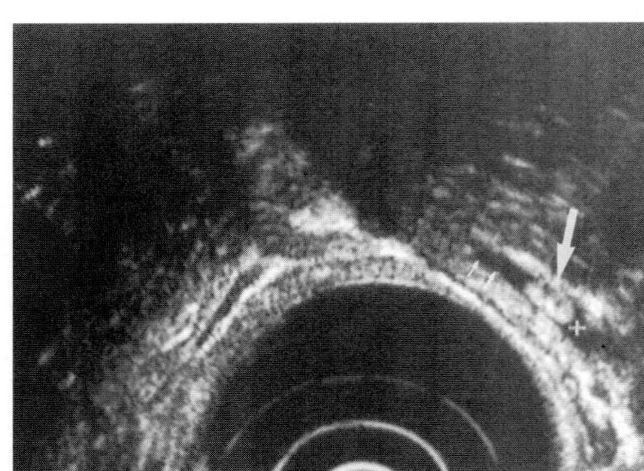

Fig. 6.6. Endoscopic ultrasonography. A small choledocholithiasis (*large arrow*) is depicted within the distal part of the common bile duct (*small arrows*)

atic abscess or an infected necrosis should be diagnosed. Pancreatic pseudocysts are well imaged by endoscopic US.

6.7 Computed Tomography

Contrast-enhanced CT currently plays a critical role in acute pancreatitis: firstly in the diagnosis of the initial process, secondly as an early predictive indicator of severity, thirdly in detecting associated complications, and fourthly to ensure efficacy in percutaneous therapy.

6.7.1 Technique

Fast CT scanners improve the diagnostic capabilities of CT of the pancreas. Helical CT provides excellent depiction of small vessels and high levels of parenchymal enhancement, and avoids respiratory misregistration (DUPUY et al. 1992). Our recent protocol includes no bowel opacification because the patients are fasting. The field of view is chosen to include the entire abdomen. Unenhanced slices are necessary to rule out recent hemorrhage. Contrast-enhanced acquisition is performed after intravenous injection of 2 ml/kg of body weight of iodinated contrast agent (300 mg iodine/ml) using a power injector. Dual-phase helical acquisition was obtained 30 s (collimation, 3 mm; table speed, 4.5 mm/s; pitch, 1.5) and 60 s (collimation, 5 mm; table speed, 7.5 mm/s; pitch, 1.5) after injection of contrast medium with a rate of 3–4 ml/s. Vascularization of the pancreas and peripancreatic inflammatory changes are best evaluated at the peak of pancreatic perfusion (initial phase). The whole abdominal cavity from the diaphragm down to the pelvis is surveyed during the other phase.

6.7.2 CT Findings

CT findings in acute pancreatitis reflect both intra- and extrapancreatic changes, independent of the etiology.

6.7.2.1 Parenchymal Changes

Parenchymal changes vary with the severity of the process. With milder clinical forms, CT shows a normal pancreas or slight to moderate diffuse hypertrophy of the gland. Only a part of the gland may be enlarged in 18% of patients (BALTHAZAR et al. 1985) (Fig. 6.7). The overall incidence of a normal pancreas is reported to vary between 14% and 28 % based on clinical correlations (HILL et al. 1982; BALTHAZAR et al. 1985).

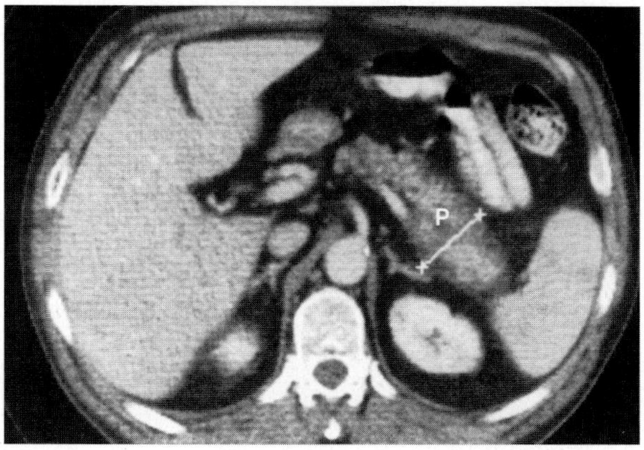

Fig. 6.7. Acute pancreatitis. Enhanced computed tomography. Focal enlargement of the pancreatic tail (*P*) with disappearance of the lobulated contours of the gland. Grade B staging

A focal or diffuse, well marginated area of unenhanced pancreatic parenchyma is considered a reliable CT finding for a diagnosis of pancreatic necrosis (BALTHAZAR et al. 1994). A semiquantitative assessment of pancreatic enhancement can be obtained by comparing splenic attenuation (Fig. 6.8). The two normal organs have similar attenuation. A good correlation has been found between operative and CT findings in respect of glandular necrosis (Fig. 6.9) (KIVISAARI et al. 1984; MAIER 1986; JOHNSON et al. 1991). Necrosis is usually well established by 96 h after the onset of clinical symptoms (ISENMANN et al. 1993). However, it has been shown that most small, unenhanced lesions within the pancreas have disappeared on follow-up CT, indicating that they were due to edema (BENZIANE et al. 1992; WHITE et al. 1986). When the percentage of gland necrosis is more than 30%, CT specificity is 100%; it is 50% if only small areas of necrosis are present (BEGER et al. 1986). Because the CT findings of pancreatic necrosis may be equivocal at the onset of pancreatitis, it has been recommended that the initial CT

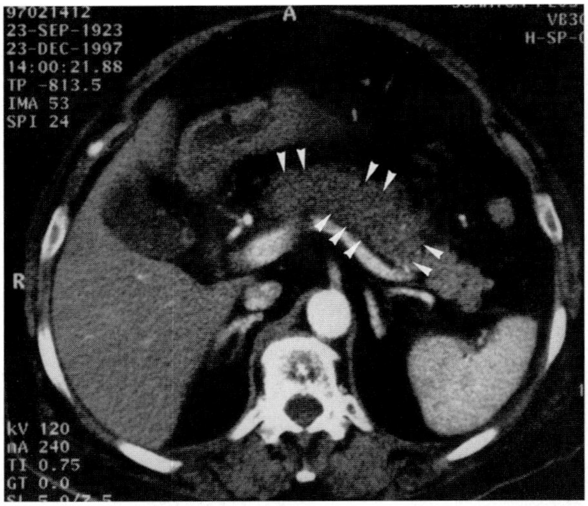

Fig. 6.8. Enhanced computed tomography of acute pancreatitis 24 h after the onset of symptoms. Unenhanced pancreatic parenchyma is depicted comparing splenic attenuation (*arrowheads*). This area is considered as pancreatic necrosis staging between 30% and 50%, but could be due in fact to pancreatic edema

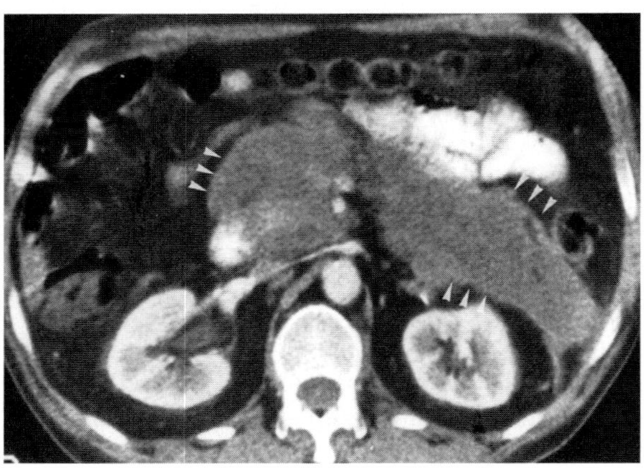

Fig. 6.9. Enhanced computed tomography (CT) of acute pancreatitis 4 days after onset of the attack. Necrosis of the entire pancreatic gland (*arrowheads*) is well established because no enhancement of the gland is observed on the postponed CT

scan be postponed (White et al. 1986; Beger et al. 1986).

Late pancreatic necrosis can develop in an initially normal pancreas (Balthazar et al. 1990). Due to the lack of a well-developed fibrous capsule, peripancreatic changes, caused by extravasation of the pancreatic enzymes, are seen at an early stage. In the mild form, peripancreatic fatty changes and mild thickening of the adjacent facial planes give the pancreatic contour a hazy and dirty appearance, with a slight increase in the density of peripancreatic fat (Fig. 6.9).

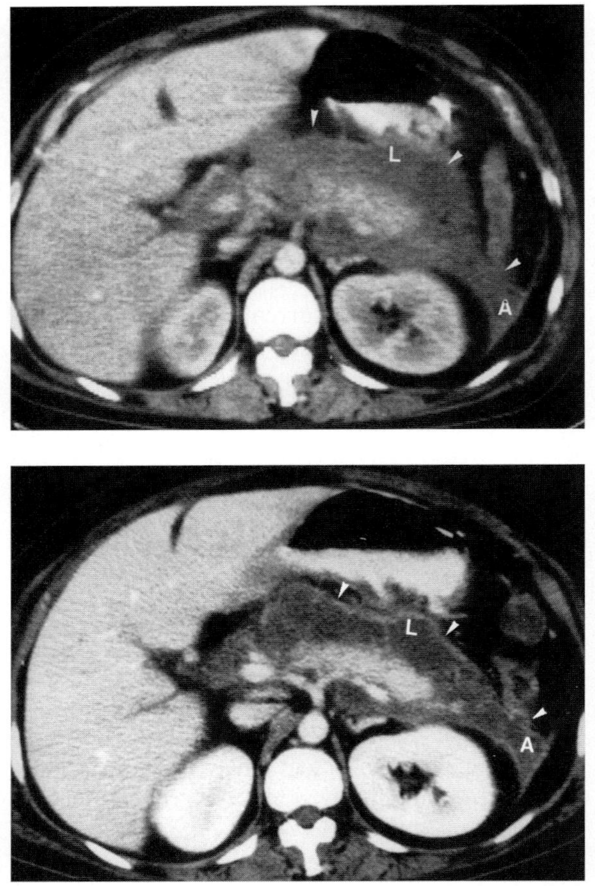

Fig. 6.10a,b. Acute pancreatitis, grade E staging with acute fluid collections within the lesser sac (*L*) and left anterior pararenal space (*A*) (*arrowheads*). **a** Initial enhanced computed tomography (CT) performed 72 h after onset of the attacks. The collections appear as ill-defined masses of low attenuation. **b** Follow-up CT 3 weeks later. The collections appear more hypoattenuated, decreasing in size and developing an enhanced rim (*arrowheads*)

In more severe forms, acute fluid collections (20–40 HU), seen as ill-defined masses of low attenuation, are present within peripancreatic areas. No recognizable capsule or wall distinguishes them from pseudocysts The most common recesses involved are the anterior pararenal space, particularly the left, and the lesser sac (Fig. 6.10) (Fujiwara et al. 1995). Inferior extension along the pararenal spaces and the psoas compartments and towards the pelvis can also be observed (Fig. 6.11). The mesentery, mesocolon, posterior pararenal space, perirenal space, and peritoneal cavity are less commonly involved (Figs. 6.12–6.15). Rarely, upward extension occurs towards the mediastinum, subcapsular hepatic, or splenic collection (Figs. 6.16, 6.17).

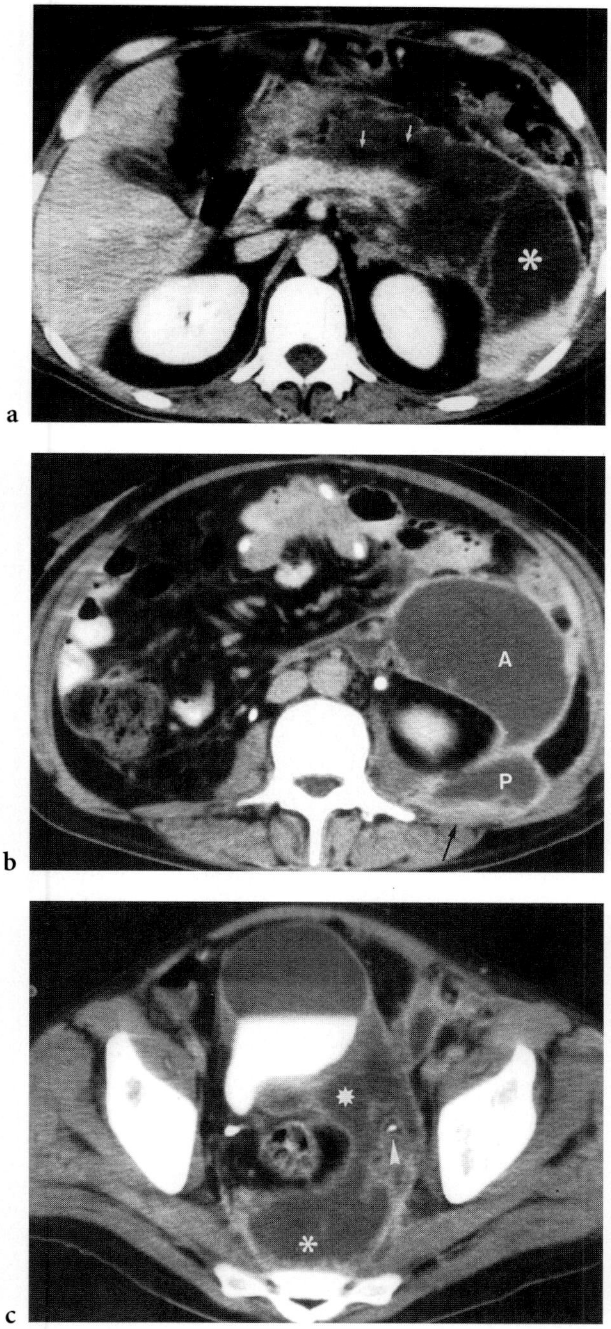

Fig. 6.11a–c. Acute pancreatitis, grade E staging. **a** Large hypodense collection (*asterisk*) with unenhanced pancreatic tail related to parenchymal necrosis. Small foci of fatty densities represent areas of cytosteatonecrosis (*arrows*). **b** Extension of the collection into the left anterior (*A*) and posterior (*P*) pararenal spaces, as well as into the posterior muscular wall (*arrow*). **c** Extension to the pelvis in the presacral and laterorectal spaces (*star*), as well as into the Douglas pouch (*asterisk*). The left ureter (*arrowhead*) is not compressed by the collection

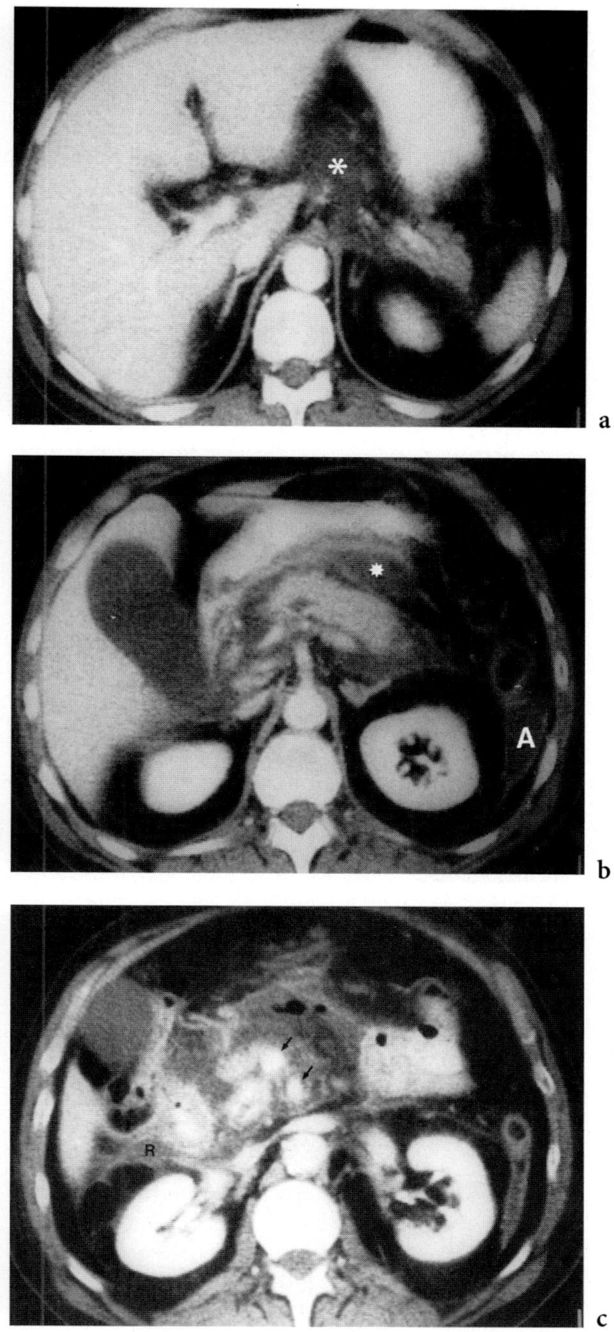

Fig. 6.12a–c. Acute pancreatitis, grade E staging. Peripancreatic collection with extension to: **a** Lesser omentum (*asterisk*); **b** peripancreatic (*star*) and anterior pararenal spaces (*A*); **c** root of the mesentery, centered by mesenteric vessels (*arrows*) and right anterior pararenal space (*R*)

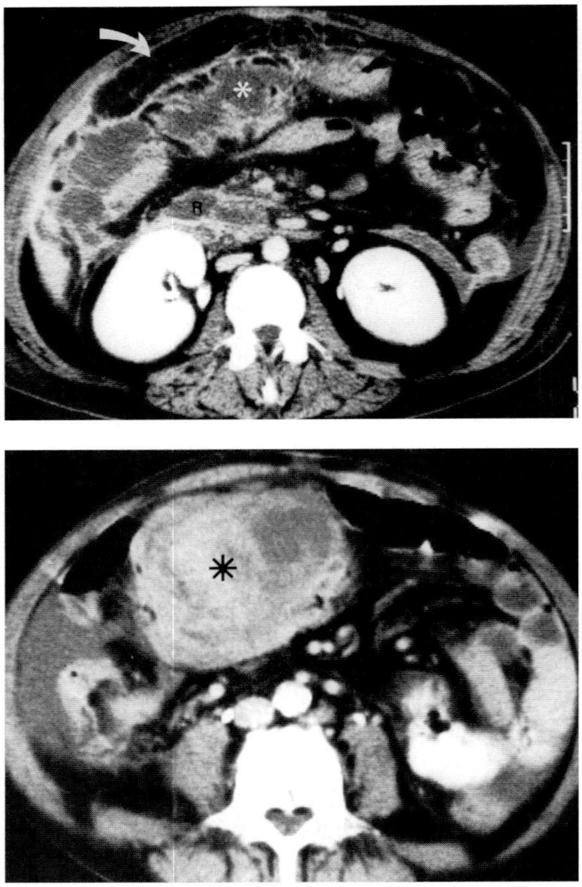

a

b

Fig. 6.13. a Acute pancreatitis. Computed tomography showing an ill-defined collection located in the mesocolon (*asterisk*) and right pararenal space (*R*). Note the streaky densities of the great omentum seen anteriorly (*curved arrow*). **b** Acute pancreatitis, grade E staging. Large heterogeneous mesenteric mass with spontaneous hyperdense areas representing a fresh hematoma (*asterisk*)

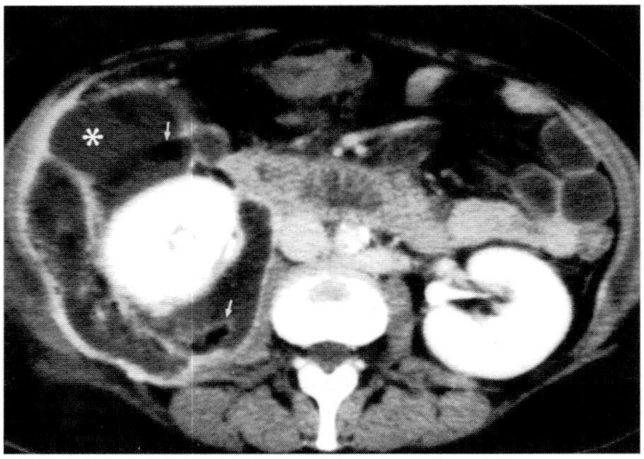

Fig. 6.14. Postsphincterotomy acute pancreatitis. Pararenal and perirenal space involvement with a large collection (*asterisk*). Small foci of hypodense areas may be related to cytosteatonecrosis (*arrows*)

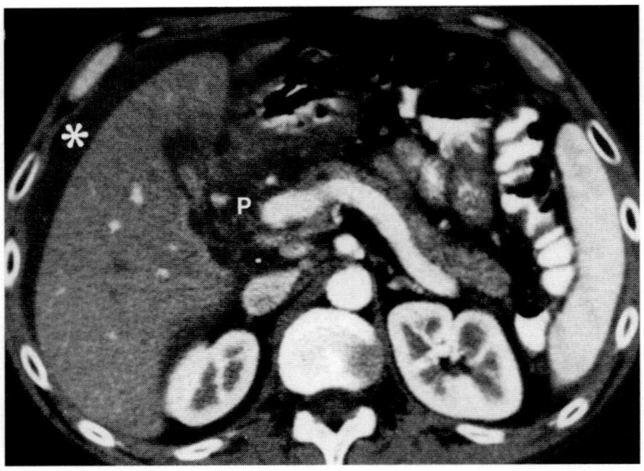

Fig. 6.15. Cephalic acute pancreatitis. Collection surrounding the head of the gland (*P*) with intraperitoneal fluid collection (*asterisk*)

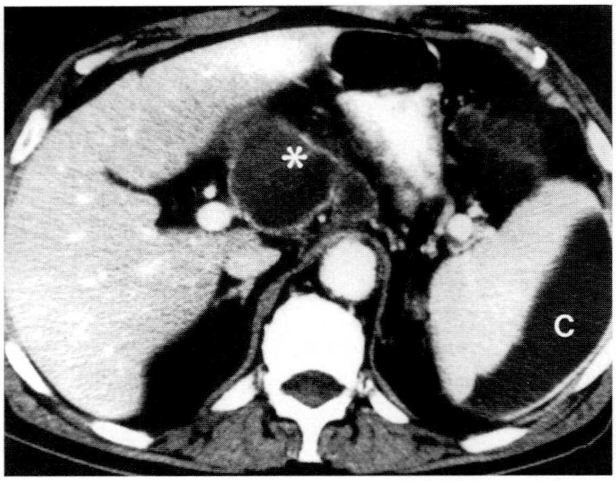

Fig. 6.16. Acute pancreatitis with lesser sac (*asterisk*) and subcapsular splenic (*C*) fluid collections

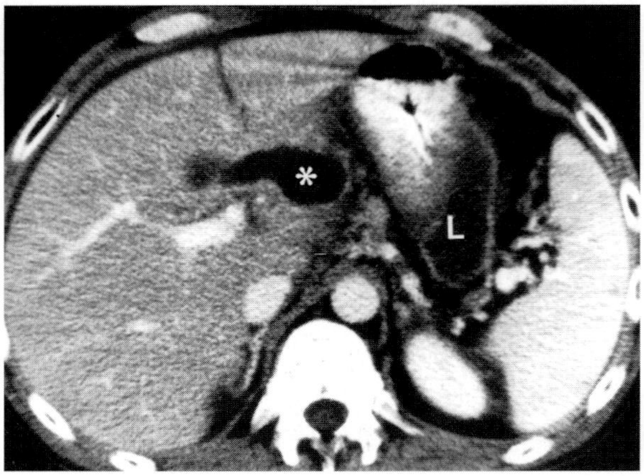

Fig. 6.17. Acute pancreatitis, grade E staging. Fluid collections are visible in the porta hepatis (*asterisk*) and lesser sac (*L*)

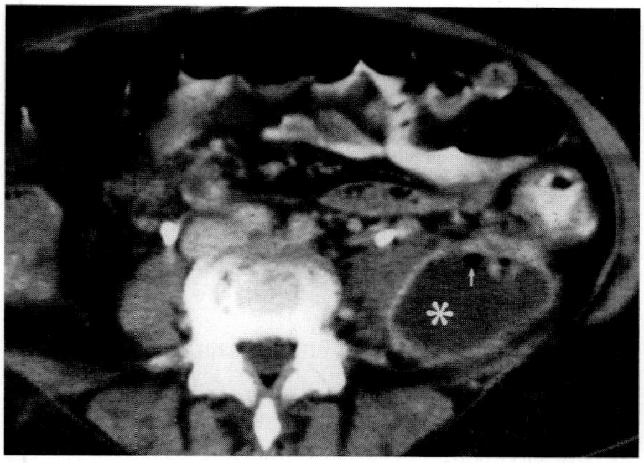

Fig. 6.18. Enhanced computed tomography of a pancreatic abscess complicating acute pancreatitis 3 weeks after onset of the attack. A bubble of gas is depicted within an acute fluid collection behind the left psoas indicating sepsis

Infection of fluid collections develops in 3%–21% of patients with acute pancreatitis (FEDERLE et al. 1981; RANSON et al. 1985). Air bubbles produced by anaerobic germs are visualized in about 22% of cases on CT and strongly suggest the diagnosis (Fig. 6.18), although they may also signify enteric or colic fistula (BALTHAZAR 1989) (Fig. 6.19).

Approximatively 80% of deaths occurring in patients with acute pancreatitis are estimated to be caused by complications arising from bacterial infection of pancreatic necrosis (BEGER et al. 1997) (Fig. 6.20).

Various other associated findings may be found:

- Streaky and fluffy soft tissue densities in the flank and gluteal regions have been reported in severe pancreatitis, being due to the extravascular movement of fluid (GHIATAS et al. 1990)
- Presence of serous fluid in the peritoneal and pleural regions has been reported in 29%–32% of cases (BALTHAZAR et al. 1985). Pleural involvement is most common on the left side, but occasionally it is bilateral
- Free intraperitoneal ascites, present in about 7% of cases, is most commonly observed in severe forms. Ascites with a normal pancreas is rarely observed and the diagnosis in such cases is by amylase determination.

Sudden and severe retroperitoneal hemorrhage is due to erosion of vessels by extravasation of proteolytic enzymes, resulting in bleeding or in the formation of pseudoaneurysm (BURKE et al. 1986). On unenhanced CT slices, a hematoma appears as a spontaneous, hyperdense mass (Fig. 6.13).

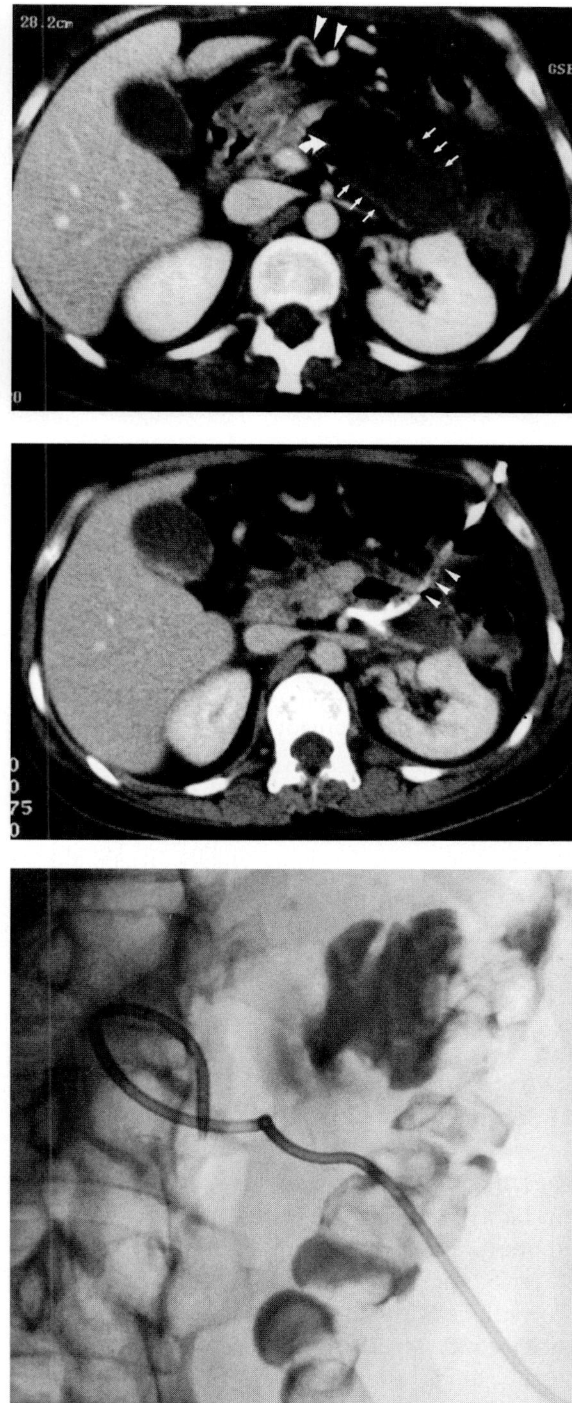

a

b

c

Fig. 6.19a–c. Enhanced computed tomography (CT) of acute pancreatitis in a patient who developed sepsis. **a** A large amount of gas observed within an acute anterior pararenal collection (*small arrows*) with air-fluid level (*curved arrows*). There is an enlarged right gastroepiploic vein (*arrowhead*) (segmental portal hypertension) due to thrombosis of the splenic vein. **b** Percutaneous drainage using an 8-F catheter (*arrowheads*) under CT guidance is performed secondarily. **c** Direct opacification through the catheter clearly evidences colic fistula

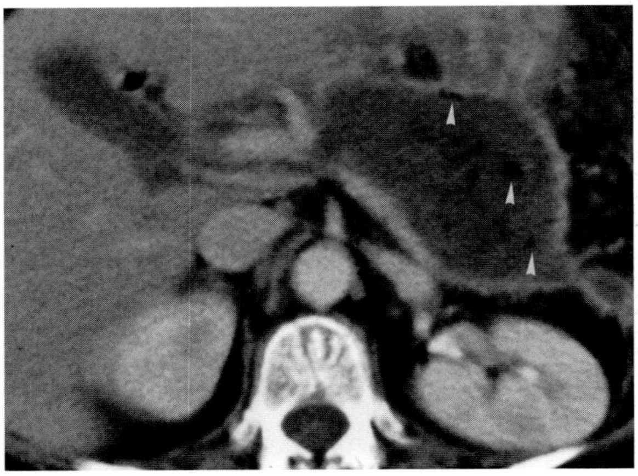

Fig. 6.20. Enhanced computed tomography of acute pancreatitis. There is a large unenhanced area of necrosis within the body and tail of the pancreas. Bubbles of gas (*arrowheads*) are depicted within this area of pancreatic necrosis, corresponding in fact to infected necrosis requiring surgical débridement

In the largest two series carried out, the sensitivities of CT were reported as 77% and 92% (Hill et al. 1982; Balthazar 1989). False-positive CT diagnoses are seldom, occurring, for example, in rare cases of acute pancreatitis on top of an underlying pancreatic tumor, or in cases of intra-abdominal abscesses of other origin. Finally, it should be stressed that, in patients presenting with acute abdomen, a normal pancreas and normal retroperitoneal structures on CT exclude a severe form of acute pancreatitis (Jeffrey et al. 1983).

6.7.3 CT Staging

The value of CT as an early predictive indicator of morbidity and mortality was first established by Siegelman et al. (1980) and Hill et al. (1982).

Various authors have assessed the significance of CT findings prospectively by correlating CT appearance with the severity of the disease, development of complications, and mortality. The correlated contrast-enhanced CT findings included the presence or absence and extent of peripancreatic inflammation and acute fluid collection (Balthazar et al. 1985; Nordestgaard et al. 1986; Vernacchia et al. 1987; Clavien et al. 1988), and the presence or absence and extent of pancreatic necrosis (Kivisaari et al. 1984; Büchler et al. 1986; Maier 1986; Balthazar et al. 1990). Ranson criteria are mainly indicative of cardiovascular, pulmonary, and renal failure, while CT demonstrates local features. A close correlation between early CT findings and Ranson criteria is not to be expected (Ranson et al. 1985). The most widely used classification was described by Balthazar et al. (1985) to assess the severity of acute inflammatory processes into five categories (Table 6.2). They showed that patients with lower grades (A–C) have a mild uncomplicated clinical cause (Fig. 6.21), while those with higher grades (D, E) often exhibit a protracted clinical illness with a higher frequency of morbidity and mortality. In patients presenting with grade D or E acute pancreatitis, Balthazar et al. (1985) observed spontaneous resolution of acute fluid collections in 54% and pancreatic abscesses in the remaining 46%. An excellent correlation has been established between contrast-enhanced CT depiction of necrosis and the development of morbidity and mortality (Balthazar et al. 1990). While patients without necrosis had no mortality and only 6% morbidity, patients with necrosis exhibited 23% mortality and 82% morbidity. The extent of pancreatic necrosis is estimated at <30%, 30%–50%, and >50% of the pancreatic gland. The combined morbidity of patients with extensive necrosis (over 30%) was 94% and the mortality was 29% (Balthazar et al. 1990). This clearly shows that necrosis and the acute inflammatory process are the two CT prognostic indicators of the severity of acute pancreatitis. Balthazar et al. (1990) have developed a grading system combining these two CT prognostic indicators called the "CT severity index" (CTSI) (Table 6.3) (Fig. 6.22). Patients with a CTSI of 0–3 showed a 3% mortality rate and an 8% morbidity rate, while patients with a CTSI of 7–10 had showed a 17% mortality rate and a 92% morbidity rate.

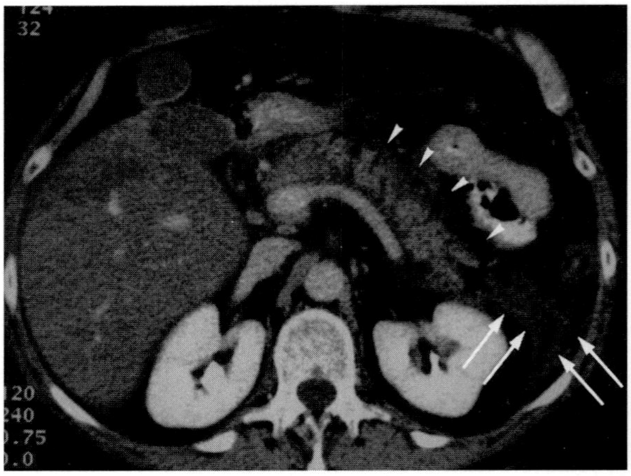

Fig. 6.21. Enhanced computed tomography of gallstone pancreatitis. There is a thickening of the left anterior pararenal fascia and left lateroconal fascia (*arrows*). Hazy and dirty appearance of mesenteric fat (*arrowheads*). Grade C staging

Table 6.2. CT classification of the severity of acute inflammatory processes. [From BALTHAZAR et al. (1985)]

Grade A	Normal pancreas
Grade B	Focal or diffuse pancreas enlargement (including contour irregularities, inhomogeneous attenuation of gland, dilatation of pancreatic duct, and foci of small fluid collections within gland with no peripancreatic disease)
Grade C	Intrinsic pancreatic abnormalities with haziness and streaky densities representing inflammatory changes in peripancreatic fat
Grade D	Single, ill defined fluid collection (low attenuation, poorly defined fluid collections with no recognizable capsule or wall)
Grade E	Two or more poorly defined fluid collections or presence of gas in or adjacent to pancreas

Table 6.3. Calculation of CT severity index. [From BALTHAZAR et al. (1990)]

a. Inflammatory process		
Grade A	Normal pancreas	0
Grade B	Focal or diffuse enlargement of pancreas	1
Grade C	Pancreatic gland abnormalities associated with peripancreatic inflammation	2
Grade D	Fluid collection in a single location	3
Grade E	Two or more fluid collections and/or the presence of gas in/or adjacent to pancreas	4
b. Gland necrosis	No	0
	Less than 30%	2
	30%--50%	4
	Greater than 50%	6
c. CT severity index		a+b

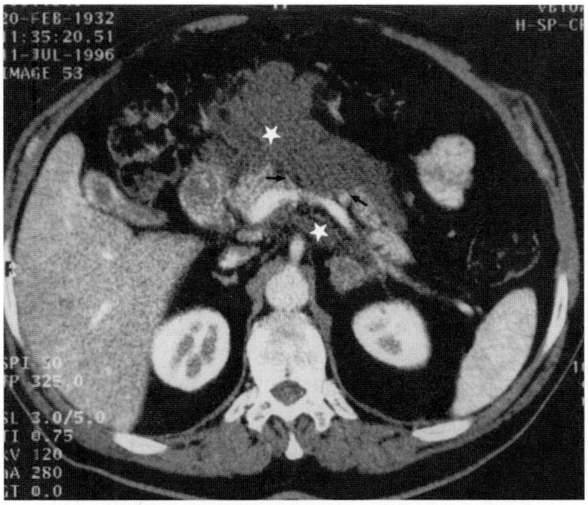
a

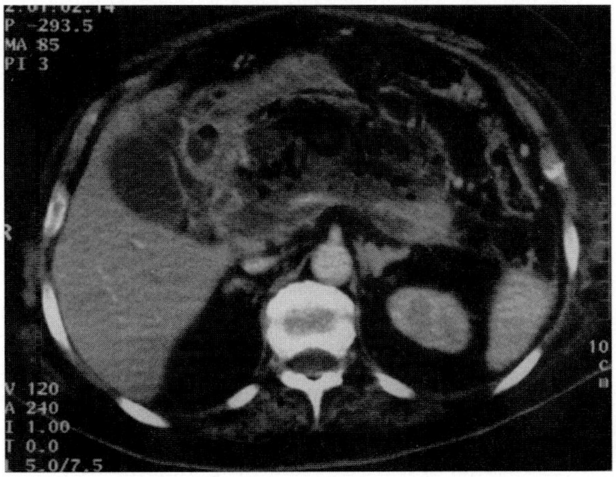
b

Fig. 6.22a,b. Contrast-enhanced computed tomography (CT) severity score. **a** Contrast-enhanced CT of drug-induced pancreatitis. Two acute fluid collections are depicted within the retropancreatic space and within the mesocolon (*stars*) (score = 4). Staging for gland necrosis (within the body) is 30% or less (score = 2) (*between arrows*). The CT severity index is equal to 6 (4+2). **b** Contrast-enhanced CT of gallstone pancreatitis. Massive infected pancreatic necrosis is depicted, score grade E (gas), and more than 50% for necrosis. The CT severity index is maximum (4+6=10) with a high risk of mortality. Surgical débridement is recommended

6.7.4 When Should CT Be Used in Patients with Acute Pancreatitis?

Not all patients with acute pancreatitis require a CT scan to establish the diagnosis and suggest the etiology. Firstly, conservative medical therapy should be initialized, and, secondly, imaging evaluation should be performed. FREENY (1993) suggests the following guidelines for efficacious use of CT in patients with acute pancreatitis. Gland perfusion is best assessed using iodinated contrast-enhanced CT.

6.7.4.1 Indications for Initial CT Examination

1. Patients in whom the clinical diagnosis is doubtful

2. Patients with severe pancreatitis (Ranson score >3; Apache score >8), including high fever, leukocytosis, and tenderness. Recent reports in both animal and human studies have questioned the safety of injecting iodinated contrast medium during the early stage of pancreatitis (Foitzik et al. 1994; McMenamin and Gates 1996). In this debated context, postponing the initial scan until 72 h after the onset of the symptoms is recommended; furthermore, studies showed that areas of necrosis were better established after this delay.
3. Patients who demonstrate clinical improvement during initial medical therapy, but then manifest an acute change in clinical status, indicating a developing complication (e.g., fever, pain, ability to tolerate oral intake, hypotension, failing hematocrit).

6.7.4.2
Indications for Follow-Up CT Examination

1. For patients with mild pancreatitis only if there is a change in clinical status that suggests a developing complication
2. For patients with severe pancreatitis, a follow-up scan is recommended at 7–10 days. Improvement in the clinical status of the patient always precede the disappearance of radiological abnormalities. Additional follow-up scanning during hospitalization is recommended only if the patient's clinical status deteriorates or fails to show continued improvement
3. A scan should be obtained at the time of hospital discharge to confirm resolution of the lesions in order to eliminate notable evolution of a fluid collection into a pseudocyst (Fig. 6.23) or development of an arterial pseudoaneurysm (Burke et al. 1986).

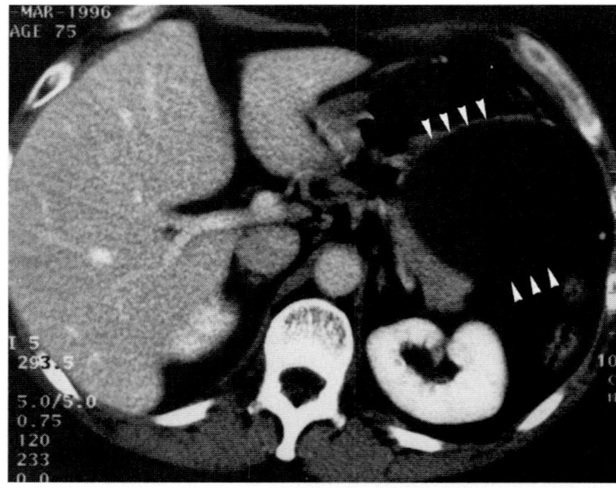

a

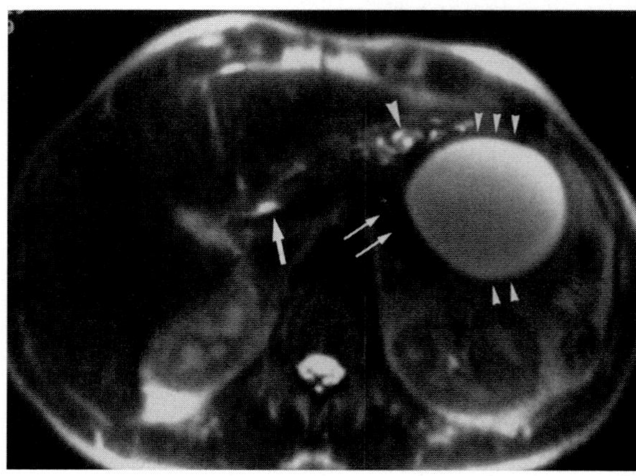

b

Fig. 6.23. a Contrast-enhanced computed tomography, performed 2 months after an attack of acute pancreatitis. A round fluid collection (*arrowheads*) is observed within the lesser sac consistent with a simple pseudocyst. **b** Magnetic resonance imaging using a single-shot T2-weighted sequence evidences a homogeneous pseudocyst (*small arrowheads*). Stomach (*large arrowhead*), main pancreatic duct (*small arrows*), and common bile duct (*large arrow*) are also well depicted

6.8
Magnetic Resonance Imaging

Magnetic resonance imaging (MRI) still plays a minor role in the routine work-up of patients with pancreatic diseases. However, recent technical improvements such as phased array multicoils, fat suppression, and gradient moment nulling allow us to obtain excellent contrast resolution of the pancreatic tissue relative to surrounding organs and of lesions with an acceptable spatial resolution (Winston et al. 1995; Saiffudin et al. 1993; Ward et al. 1997). Published results of MRI in acute pancreatitis are promising but very limited. These studies suggested that T2-weighted and gadolinium (Gd)-enhanced T1 sequences are valuable imaging techniques for the assessment of patients with severe pancreatitis, and define a semiology of inflammatory processes and necrosis in comparison with CT (Outwater and Siegelman 1996). The pancreas is classified as normal (grade A) when it is of homogeneous signal intensity and hyperintense relative to liver on fat-suppressed short TR sequences (Winston et al. 1995). Grade B is defined as a heterogeneous pancreas without peripancreatic fat involvement. Grade C is defined as the presence of strands in the peripancreatic fat (Semelka et al. 1991). Acute fluid collections (grades D and E) are defined as peripancreatic ill-defined confluent areas of homogeneous or heterogeneous intensity, but without wall or capsule (Fig. 6.24). Gas is defined as an area of hyposignal intensity on short and long TR sequences. Necrosis is considered when well marginated areas of signal intensity different from the signal of the remaining pancreas are present on unenhanced images (Fig. 6.25) (Semelka and Ascher 1993). Semiquantitative evaluation of pancreatic enhancement is possible on post-Gd images. Using a routine protocol [T2-weighted sequence fast spin echo; fat-suppressed T1-weighted spin echo sequence, and a series of T1-weighted gradient echo sequences prior to or immediately after diethylenetriaminopentoacetic acid (DTPA)-Gd intravenous injection], a recent study shows that MRI is a reproducible method for staging pancreatitis and is at least as accurate as CT in establishing the prognosis of disease (Lecesne et al. 1998) (Fig. 6.26). MRI could replace CT in patients with renal failure. Moreover, by using additional MR cholangiopancreatography (MRCP), MRI is accurate in diagnosing choledocholithiasis(Fig. 6.27) or pancreas divisum (Reinhold and Bret 1996). Evaluation of MRI compared with CT and US in patients with pancreatic fluid collections prior to drainage, shows the superiority of MRI to predict drainability. Using a T2-weighted sequence, MRI, allows a better depiction of fluid and solid components within complex collections, pro-

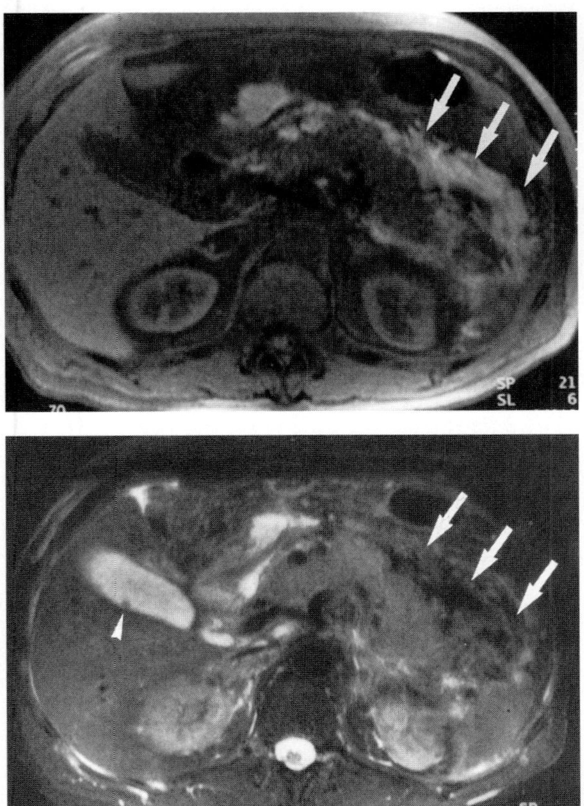

a

b

Fig. 6.24a,b. Gallstone pancreatitis. **a** On fat-saturated T1-weighted gradient echo sequence, hyperintense acute fluid collections are seen within peripancreatic spaces, but also within the left anterior pararenal space (*arrows*). **b** On fast inversion recovery sequence (T2-weighted), acute collections (*arrows*) are heterogeneous (hyper- and hypointense). The gallstone is conspicuously depicted (*arrowhead*)

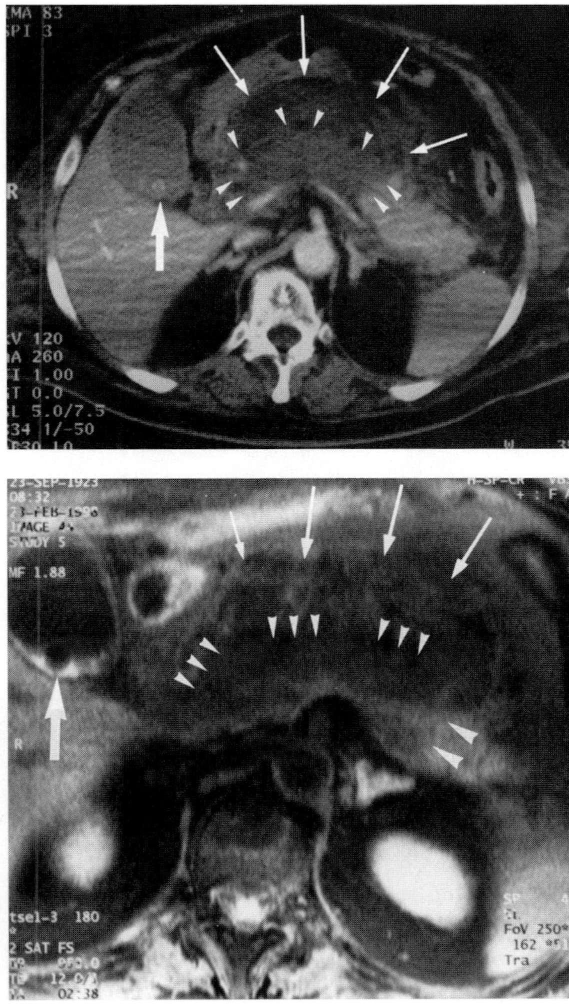

a

b

Fig. 6.25a,b. Gallstone pancreatitis. **a** Contrast-enhanced computed tomography shows a well marginated hypoattenuating area of pancreatic necrosis within the body of the pancreas (*arrowheads*). A hypodense heterogeneous acute fluid collection is evidenced within the lesser sac (*small arrows*). Hyperdense gallstone (*large arrow*). **b** Fat-saturated T1-weighted fast spin echo sequence. More than 50% of the pancreatic gland appears as a well marginated (*arrowheads*) area of signal intensity different from the signal of the tail of the pancreas (*large arrowheads*), corresponding to extensive necrosis. A hypointense heterogeneous acute fluid collection is located within the lesser sac (*small arrows*)

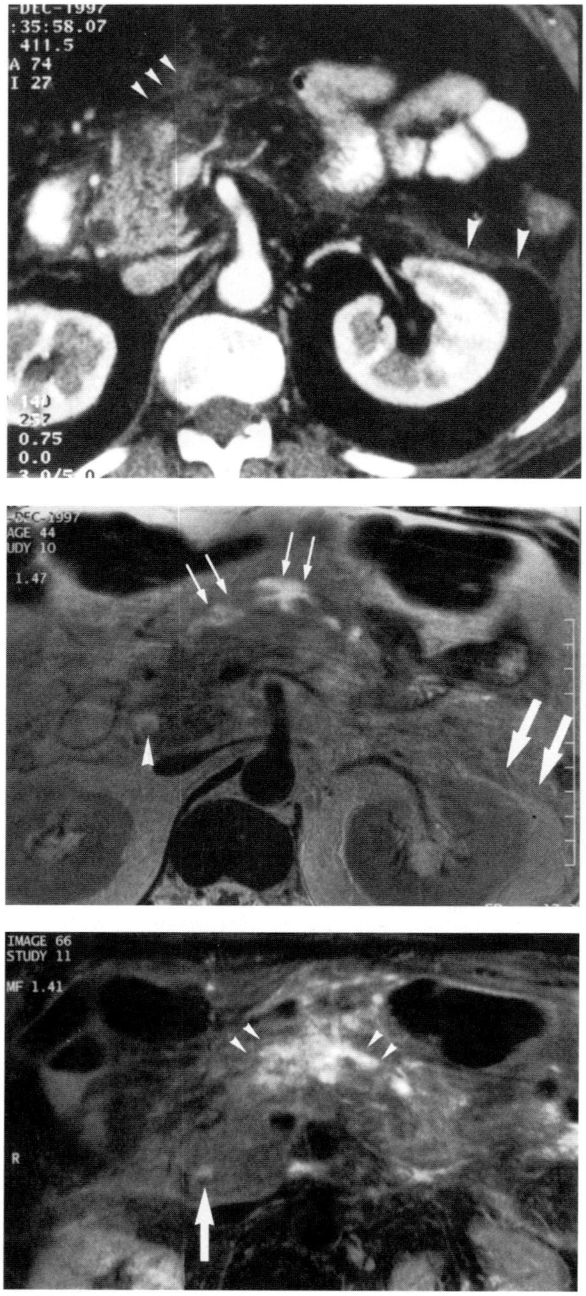

a b c

Fig. 6.26a--c. Discrepancy between contrast-enhanced computer tomography (CT) and magnetic resonance imaging scoring gallstone acute pancreatitis. a On contrast-enhanced CT, haziness and streaky densities representing inflammatory changes in the peripancreatic fat (small arrowheads) are noted and scored grade C. There is a thickened left anterior pararenal fascia (large arrowheads). b On high-resolution T2-weighted spin echo sequence, acute fluid collection (hyperintense) is shown (small arrows) at the same place and is scored grade D. Thickened left anterior pararenal fascia (large arrows) is also observed, but choledocholithiasis is better depicted (arrowhead). c On inversion recovery fat-saturated T2-weighted sequence, acute fluid collections are clearly better depicted (arrowheads). Choledocholithiasis (arrow) is also observed

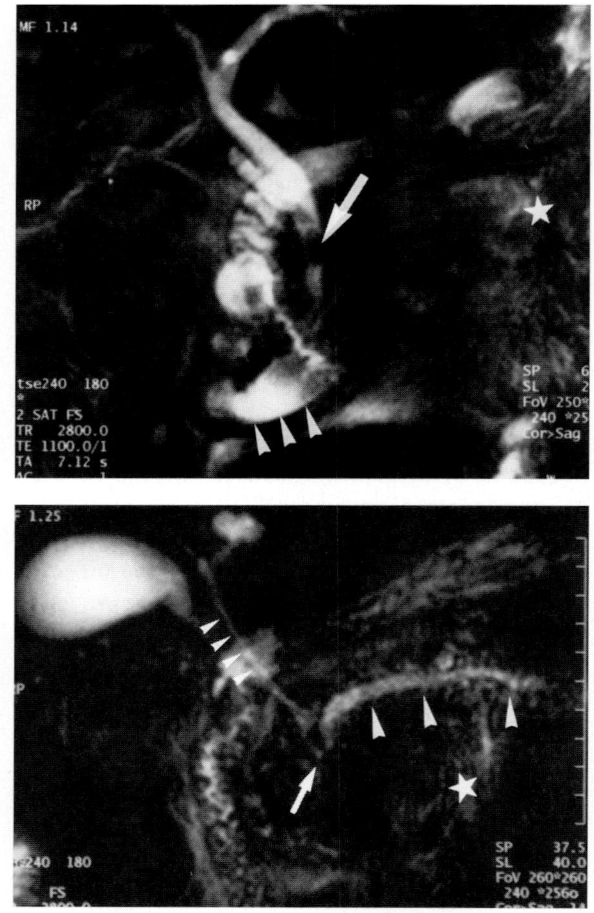

a b

Fig. 6.27a,b. Magnetic resonance cholangiopancreatography (MRCP) of acute pancreatitis. **a** On MRCP, a stone is detected within the common bile duct in this cholecystectomized patient (*arrow*). Hyperintensity of the background is due to acute fluid collection (*star*). A dilated jejunal loop is shown (*arrowheads*) corresponding to a paralytic ileus. **b** Episode of acute pancreatitis in a patient with underlying chronic pancreatitis, normal findings of the biliary tract (*small arrowheads*). There is a dilated main pancreatic duct (*large arrowheads*) and its side branches above a stenosis within the pancreatic head (*arrow*). Hyperintensity of the background is due to acute fluid collection (*star*)

viding the necessary information regarding the presence or absence of solid debris prior to drainage of pseudocyst, pancreatic abscesses, or infected necrosis (Morgan et al. 1997) (Fig. 6.28). However, because of its cost and inability to guide interventional procedures, the role of MRI in staging and management of pancreatitis needs to be confirmed by cost-efficiency analysis.

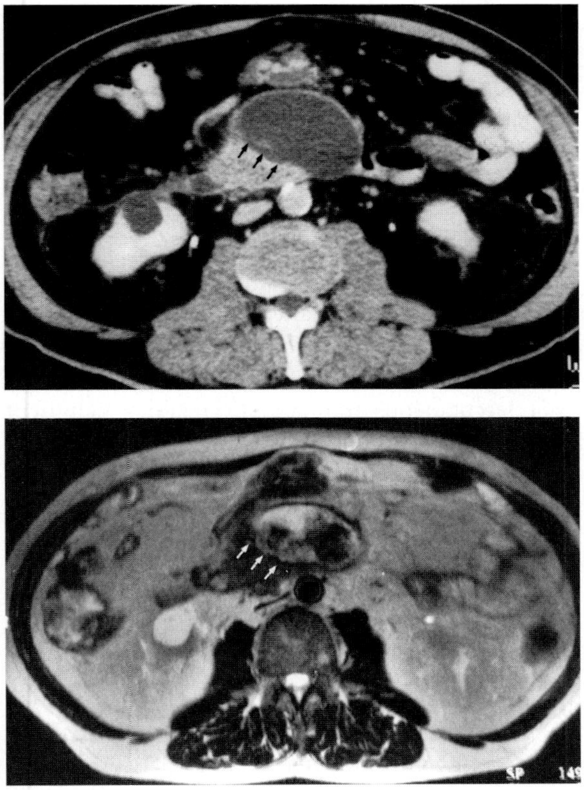

a

b

Fig. 6.28a,b. Pseudocyst following acute pancreatitis. **a** A round, homogeneous, encapsulated pseudocyst behind the uncinate process is shown on contrast-enhanced computed tomography (*arrows*). **b** On T2-weighted spin echo sequence, the pseudocyst appears as a complex collection with some clots and debris within the pseudocyst (*arrows*)

6.9 Endoscopic Retrograde Cholangiopancreatography

Endoscopic retrograde cholangiopancreatography (ERCP) can detect the etiology of pancreatitis as choledocholithiasis or pancreas divisum. However, ERCP may cause acute pancreatitis in 1.3%–7.4% of procedures (Ruppin et al. 1974). For this reason, acute pancreatitis was considered in the past as an absolute contraindication for ERCP. However, a randomized, controlled trial (Neptolemos et al. 1988) demonstrated that urgent ERCP associated with endoscopic sphincterotomy and stone extraction, where necessary, reduced complications, mortality, and hospital stays. But a recent study (Fölsch et al. 1997) demonstrated that patients with acute pancreatitis without biliary obstruction or biliary sepsis did not benefit from early ERCP and papillotomy.

Furthermore, following endoscopic sphincterotomy, complications such as hemorrhage, cholangitis, and perforation or aggravation of the existing pancreatitis can occur (Barbier et al. 1996; Ott et al. 1992).

6.10 Interventional Procedures

Currently, a more conservative attitude is being adopted towards the management of acute pancreatitis, and improvements in survival rates are mainly due to progress in intensive care units. However, drainage of infected fluid collections remains necessary. Interventional radiology can play an important role in this field.

6.10.1 Diagnostic Needle Aspiration

Needle aspiration using an 20-gauge needle is a safe, relatively straightforward procedure (Banks et al. 1995). It is used to determine the presence of infection in a critically ill patient with fever, elevated white blood cell counts, and increased fluid requirements. A positive needle aspiration helps to determine the correct antibiotic coverage, as well as the need for surgery.

The most important decision is to determine a safe access route. Most pancreatic aspiration procedures are performed with CT guidance, but when a large, superficial collection occurs, US-guided aspiration can be used. Commonly described access routes include the transhepatic, transgastric, retroperitoneal, or direct approach (Fig. 6.29). The approach should avoid the bowel, since a non-infected collection could be contaminated using a transenteric approach, or a false-positive diagnosis of abscess could be made. If fluid is withdrawn, its appearance can vary from dark (hemorrhagic debris) to yellow (purulent abscesses) or brown (necrosis). The main indication for fine needle aspiration is to diagnose infected necrosis which has been a specific indication for surgical intervention (Banks et al. 1995).

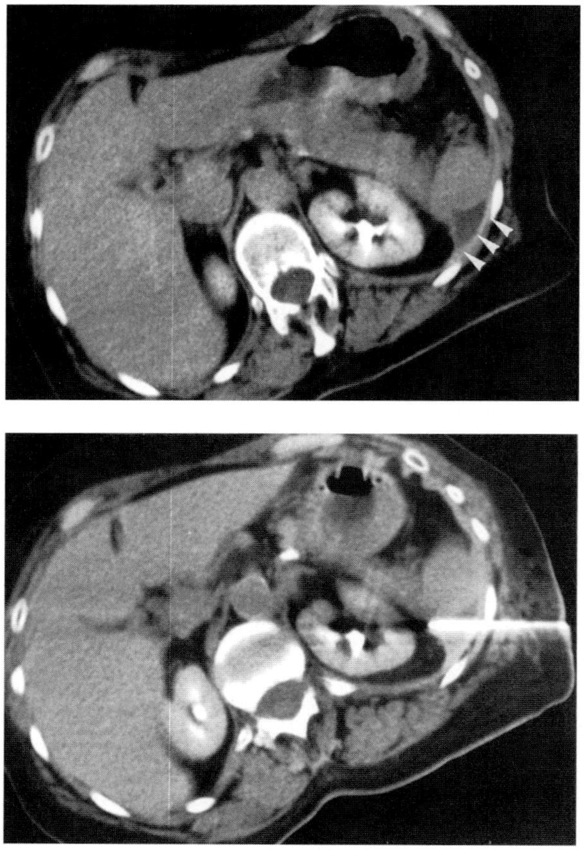

a

b

Fig. 6.29a,b. A patient with hypercalcemia-induced acute pancreatitis has high clinical and biochemical suspicion of sepsis. **a** On contrast-enhanced computed tomography, a collection is depicted within the lateroconal space with enhanced wall (*arrowheads*). **b** Diagnostic fine needle aspiration (18-gauge needle) is performed using direct left flank approach evidencing the presence of pus

6.10.2 Percutaneous Drainage

Drainage in complicated acute pancreatitis requires an extensive commitment in terms of time and labor on the part of the interventional radiologist. The choice of percutaneous drainage is to a large extent dependent on the available facilities and the experience of an institution in this procedure. The success of interventional radiology varies among series, with cure rates of between 60% and 90% having been reported (Karlson et al. 1982; Steiner et al. 1988; VanSonnenberg et al. 1989, 1992). This difference may be attributable to the type of collection drained. A high success rate is obtained with simple collections (Lee et al. 1992), but the frequently multilocular and multiple collections in acute pancreatitis cannot be drained easily via a catheter. A recent study indicates that CT-guided percutaneous drainage of infected necrosis is safe and efficacious, but requires intensive radiological involvement in catheter management (Freeny et al. 1998).

If the fluid can be drained percutaneously, the necrotic element must be grossly separated and extracted by complementary surgical débridement (Lee et al. 1992). A study of 30 patients with acute complicated pancreatitis showed completely successful drainage in 47%, a temporizing effect in 13%, a partially successful outcome in 13%, and complete failure in 27% (Lee et al. 1992). In unsuccessful cases of percutaneous drainage, MRI could be helpful in depicting solid components within complex collections (Morgan et al. 1997). The success rate could also vary with the site of collection. Drainage was more successful in peripheral areas, which were much more accessible than central areas (pancreas and lesser sac) where a success rate of only 10% was obtained (Fig. 6.30).

Therefore, the most judicious use of interventional radiology might be to drain the peripheral collections percutaneously, leaving the surgeon to treat the more central ones. Moreover, if surgical débridement is incomplete, postoperative percutaneous drainage can be performed. Percutaneous drainage can also have a temporizing effect and can be performed in association with surgery, making less aggressive surgery possible and thereby reducing surgical morbidity (Lee et al. 1992).

CT is used for guidance in most cases since it best enables visualization and avoidance of vital organs. The tandem trocar technique represents a rapid method for catheter insertion which is quite easy and not uncomfortable for the patient. Once the collection is evacuated, irrigation of the cavity with sterile saline is recommended and should be continued until a clear aspiration is obtained. Irrigation should be performed at regular intervals (every 4–12 h). Patients are followed-up by repeated CT scan in order to identify undrained collections. "Abscessography" is used to search for fistulous communications between the pancreatic duct and the gastrointestinal tract (see Fig. 6.19). A complication rate of 17% has been reported following percutaneous drainage. Complications included colonic fistulae with spontaneous remission and pneumothorax (Lee et al. 1992). The major risk is an accidental puncture of a pseudoaneurysm. One case, treated by embolization through the catheter, has been reported (Lee et al. 1991).

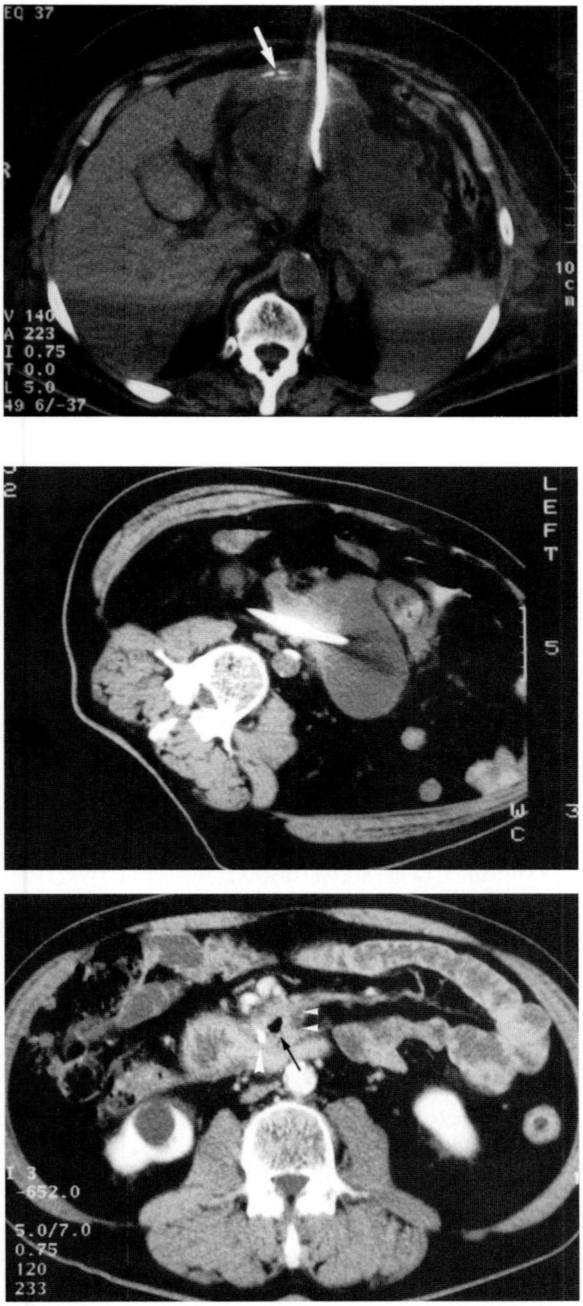

a b c

Fig. 6.30a–c. Acute pancreatitis. Access route for pancreatic abscesses located in the central areas of the abdomen. **a** A transgastric approach (16-F catheter) is performed to drain the pancreatic abscess located within the lesser sac. A gastric tube is depicted within the antrum (*arrow*). **b** A retroperitoneal approach (16-F catheter) is performed in order to drain the pancreatic abscess located within the mesentery (described also in Fig. 6.28). **c** Successful drainage of the pancreatic abscess of the mesentery. Note that the collection is almost completely drained (*small arrowheads*). Tip of the catheter (*large arrowhead*). Air bubble is due to the drainage (*arrow*)

6.11 Conclusion

Imaging studies play a primary role in the management of acute pancreatitis. US, being an easy and practical examination, is often the first procedure to be performed in a patient with acute abdomen. CT and MRI are the modality of choice to confirm the diagnosis, as well as to stage severity of the disease and to follow its course. MRI and endoscopic US are more better suited to determining the etiology of the acute pancreatitis. Combined imaging modalities including US, CT, MRI, ERCP, and the Doppler technique are useful for diagnosing complications and for road-mapping interventional procedures.

References

Amouyal P, Palazzo L, Amouyal G et al (1989) Endosonography: promising method for diagnosis of extrahepatic cholestasis. Lancet 2:1195–1198

Balthazar EJ (1989) CT diagnosis and staging of acute pancreatitis. Radiol Clin North Am 27:19–37

Balthazar EJ, Ranson JHC, Naidich DP, Megibow AJ, Caccavale R, Cooper MM (1985) Acute pancreatitis: prognostic value of CT. Radiology 156:767–772

Balthazar EJ, Robinson DL, Megibow AJ, Ranson JHC (1990) Acute pancreatitis: value of CT in establishing prognosis. Radiology 174:331–336

Balthazar EJ, Freeny PC, VanSonnenberg E (1994) Imaging and intervention in acute pancreatitis. Radiology 193:297–306

Banks P, Gerzof S, Longevin R et al (1995) CT guided aspiration of suspected pancreatic infection bacteriology and clinical outcome. Int J Pancreatol 18:265–270

Barbier C, Bazin C, Blum A, Boccaccini H, Denis B, Régent D (1996) Aspects radiologiques des complications des sphinctérotomies endoscopiques. J Radiol 77:555–562

Beger H, Bittner R, Block S et al (1986) Bacterial contamination of pancreatic necrosis: a prospective study. Gastroenterology 91:433–438

Beger H, Rau B, Mayer J et al (1997) Natural cause of acute pancreatitis. World J Surg 21:130–135

Benziane K, Azais O, Gasquet C (1992) Une nouvelle classification tomodensitométrique des pancréatites aiguës. Gastroenterol Clin Biol 16:720–721

Bittner R, Block S, Büchler M, Beger H (1987) Pancreatic abscess and infected pancreatic necrosis: different local septic complication in acute pancreatitis. Dig Dis Sci 32:1082–1087

Bradley EL III (1993) A clinically based classification system for acute pancreatitis: summary of the international symposium on acute pancreatitis. Arch Surg 128:586–590

Büchler M, Malfertheiner P, Beger HG (1986) Correlation of imaging procedures, biochemical parameters, and clinical stage in acute pancreatitis. In: Malfertheiner P, Ditschuneit H (eds) Diagnostic procedures in pancreatic disease. Springer, Berlin Heidelberg New York, pp 123–143

Büchler M, Uhl W, Beger H (1992) Acute pancreatitis: when and how to operate. Dig Dis Sci 10:354–362

Burke JW, Erickson SJ, Kellum CD, Tegtmeyer CJ, Williamson RJ, Hansen MF (1986) Pseudoaneurysms complicating pancreatitis: detection by CT. Radiology 161:447–450

Clavien PA, Hauser H, Meyer P, Rohner A (1988) Value of contrast-enhanced computerized tomography in the early diagnosis and prognosis of acute pancreatitis. A prospective study of 202 patients. Am J Surg 155:457–466

Dupuy DE, Costello P, Ecker CP (1992) Spiral CT of the pancreas. Radiology 183:815–818

Federle MP, Jeffrey RB, Crass RA, Van Dalsem V (1981) Computed tomography of pancreatic abscesses. AJR 136:879–882

Fitz R (1889) Acute pancreatitis: a consideration of pancreatic hemorrhage, hemorrhagic suppurative, and gangrenous pancreatitis and disseminated pancreatic fat necrosis. Boston Med Surg J 120:181–187, 205–207, 229–235

Foitzik T, Bassi DG, Schmidt J et al (1994) Intravenous contrast medium accentuates the severity of acute necrotizing pancreatitis in the rat. Gastroenterology 106:207–214

Fölsch UR, Nitsche R, Lüdtke R, Hilgers RA, Creutzfeldt W (1997) Early ERCP and papillotomy compared with conservative treatment for acute biliary pancreatitis. N Engl J Med 336:237–242

Freeny P (1993) Incremental dynamic bolus computed tomography of acute pancreatitis: state of the art. Int J Pancreatol 13:147–158

Freeny PC, Hauptmann E, Althaus SJ, Traverso LW, Sinanan M (1998) Percutaneous CT-guided catheter drainage of infected acute necrotizing pancreatitis: techniques and results. AJR 170:969–975

Freise J (1987) Evaluation of sonography in the diagnosis of acute pancreatitis. In: Beger HG, Büchler M (eds) Acute pancreatitis. Springer, Berlin Heidelberg New York, pp 118–138

Fujiwara T, Takehara Y, Ichijo K et al (1995) Anterior extension of acute pancreatitis: CT findings. J Comput Assist Tomogr 19:963–966

Ghiatas AA, Nguyen VD, Perusek M (1990) Subcutaneous soft tissue densities: a computed tomography indicator of severe pancreatitis. Gastrointest Radiol 15:17–21

Hashimoto BE, Laing FC, Jeffrey RB Jr, Federle MP (1984) Hemorrhagic pancreatic fluid collections examined by ultrasound. Radiology 150:803–808

Hill MC, Barkin J, Isikoff MB, Silverstein W, Kalser M (1982) Acute pancreatitis: clinical vs. CT findings. AJR 139:263–269

Isenmann R, Büchler M, Uhl W, Malfertheiner P, Martini M, Beger H (1993) Pancreatic necrosis: an early findings in severe acute pancreatitis. Pancreas 8:358–361

Isikoff MB, Hill MC, Silverstein W, Barkin J (1981) The clinical significance of acute pancreatic hemorrhage. AJR 136:679–684

Jeffrey RB Jr (1989) Sonography in acute pancreatitis. Radiol Clin North Am 27:5–17

Jeffrey RB Jr, Federle MP, Laing FC (1983) Computed tomography of mesenteric involvement in fulminant pancreatitis. Radiology 147:185–188

Jeffrey RB Jr, Laing FC, Wing VW (1986) Extrapancreatic spread of acute pancreatitis: new observations with real-time US. Radiology 159:707–711

Johnson CD, Stephens DH, Sarr MG (1991) CT of acute pancreatitis: correlation between lack of contrast enhancement and pancreatic necrosis. AJR 156:93–95

Kane NM, Korobkin M, Francis IR, Quint LE, Cascade PN (1991) Percutaneous biopsy of left adrenal masses: prevalence of pancreatitis after anterior approach. AJR 157:777–780

Karlson KB, Martin EC, Fankuchen EI, Mattern RF, Schultz RW, Casarella WJ (1982) Percutaneous drainage of pancreatic pseudocysts and abscesses. Radiology 142:619–624

Kishimoto W, Nakao A, Takagi H, Hayakawa T (1989) Acute pancreatitis after transcatheter arterial embolization (TAE) for hepatocellular carcinoma. Am J Gastroenterol 84:1396–1399

Kivisaari L, Somer K, Standertskjöld-Nordenstam CG, Schröder T, Kivilaakso E, Lempinen M (1984) A new method for the diagnosis of acute hemorrhagic-necrotizing pancreatitis using contrast-enhanced CT. Gastrointest Radiol 9:27–30

Knaus W, Draper E, Wagner D et al (1985) Apache II: a severity of disease classification system. Crit Care Med 13:818–829

Kourtesis G, Wilson S, Williams R (1990) The clinical significiance of fluid collections in acute pancreatitis. Am Surg 56:769–799

Kuhlman JE, Fishman EK, Milligan FD, Siegelman SS (1989) Complications of endoscopic retrograde sphincterotomy: computed tomographic evaluation. Gastrointest Radiol 14:127–132

Lecesne R, Taourel P, Bret PM, Atri M, Reinhold C (1998) CT and MRI in acute pancreatitis: interobserver agreement and correlation with outcome. Radiology (to be published)

Lee MJ, Saini S, Geller SC, Warshaw AL, Mueller PR (1991) Pancreatitis with pseudoaneurysm formation: a pitfall for the interventional radiologist. AJR 156:97–98

Lee MJ, Rattner DW, Legemate DA et al (1992) Acute complicated pancreatitis: redefining the role of interventional radiology. Radiology 183:171–174

Leung JWC, Mok SD, Metreweli C (1987) Ascaris-induced pancreatitis. AJR 149:511–512

Lumson A, Bradley EL (1990) Secondary pancreatic infections. Surg Gynecol Obstet 170:459–467

Maier W (1986) Grading of acute pancreatitis by computed tomography morphology. In: Malfertheiner P, Ditschuneit H (eds) Diagnostic procedures in pancreatic disease. Springer, Berlin Heidelberg New York, pp 44–64

Malfertheiner P, Büchler M (1987) Clinical symptoms and signs and diagnostic requirements in acute pancreatitis. In: Beger HG, Büchler M (eds) Acute pancreatitis. Springer, Berlin Heidelberg New York, pp 104–124

McMenamin DA, Gates LK (1996) A retrospective analysis of the effect of contrast-enhanced CT on the outcome of acute pancreatitis. Am J Gastroenterol 91:1384–1387

Medich DS, Lee TK, Melhem MF, Rowe MI, Schraut WH, Lee KK (1993) Pathogenesis of pancreatic sepsis. Am J Surg 165:46–50

Meyers MA, Evans JA (1973) Effects of pancreatitis on the small bowel and colon: spread along mesenteric planes. AJR 119:151–165

Morgan DE, Baron TH, Smith JK, Robbin ML, Kenney PJ (1997) Pancreatic fluid collections prior to intervention: evaluation with MR imaging compared with CT and US. Radiology 203:773–778

Müeller PR, Miketic LM, Simeone JF et al (1988) Severe acute pancreatitis after percutaneous biopsy of the pancreas. AJR 151:493–494

Neff CC, Simeone JF, Wittenberg J, Mueller PR, Ferrucci JT Jr (1984) Inflammatory pancreatic masses: problems in differentiating focal pancreatitis from carcinoma. Radiology 150:35–38

Neptolemos JP, Carr Locke DL, London NJ et al (1988) Controlled trial of urgent endoscopic retrograde cholangiopancreatography and endoscopic sphincterotomy versus conservative treatment for acute pancreatitis due to gallstones. Lancet 2:979–983

Nordestgaard AG, Wilson SE, Williams RA (1986) Early computerized tomography as a predictor of outcome in acute pancreatitis. Am J Surg 152:127–132

Ott DJ, Gilliam JH III, Zagoria RJ, Young GP (1992) Interventional endoscopy of the biliary and pancreatic ducts: current indications and methods. AJR 158:243–250

Outwater EK, Siegelman ES (1996) MR imaging of pancreatic disorders. Top Magn Reson Imaging 8:265–289

Pombo F, Marini M, Beraza A, Rodriguez E (1991) Aortic dissection presenting as acute pancreatitis: CT diagnosis. Computer Med Imaging Graph 15:407–409

Ranson JHC (1982) Etiological and prognostic factors in human acute pancreatitis: a review. Am J Gastroenterol 77:633–638

Ranson JHC, Balthazar E, Caccavale R, Cooper M (1985) Computed tomography and the prediction of pancreatic abscess in acute pancreatitis. Ann Surg 201:656–665

Reinhold C, Bret PM (1996) MR cholangiopancreatography: current status. AJR 166:1285–1295

Ruppin H, Aron R, Ett W et al (1974) Acute pancreatitis after endoscopic radiological pancreatography (ERCP). Endoscopy 6:94–98

Sadry F, Hauser H (1990) Fatal pancreatitis secondary to iatrogenic intramural duodenal hematoma: a case report and review of the literature. Gastrointest Radiol 15:296–298

Safrit HD, Rice RP (1989) Gastrointestinal complications of pancreatitis. Radiol Clin North Am 27:73–79

Saiffudin A, Ward J, Ridgway J, Chalmers AG (1993) Comparison of MR and CT scanning in severe acute pancreatitis: initial experience. Clin Radiol 48:111–116

Semelka RC, Ascher SM (1993) MR imaging of the pancreas. Radiology 188:593–602

Semelka RC, Kroeker MA, Shoenut JP, Kroeker R, Yaffe CS, Micflikier AB (1991) Pancreatic disease: prospective comparison of CT, ERCP, and 1.5-T MR Imaging with dynamic Gadolinium enhancement and fat suppression. Radiology 181:785–791

Siegelman SS, Copeland BE, Saba GP, Cameron JL, Sanders RC, Zerhouni EA (1980) CT of fluid collections associated with pancreatitis. AJR 134:1121–1132

Steiner E, Mueller PR, Hahn PF et al (1988) Complicated pancreatic abscesses: problems in interventional management. Radiology 167:443–446

Sugiyama M, Wada N, Atomi Y, Kuroda A, Muto T (1995) Diagnosis of acute pancreatitis: value of endoscopic sonography. AJR 165:867–872

Thoeni RF, Fell SC, Goldberg HI (1990) CT detection of asymptomatic pancreatitis following ERCP. Gastrointest Radiol 15:291–295

Topazian M (1994) Acute pancreatitis, pancreatic duct obstruction, and the secretin-ultrasound test (editorial). J Clin Gastroenterol 18:277–279

VanSonnenberg E, Casola G, Varney RR, Wittich GR (1989) Imaging and interventional radiology for pancreatitis and its complications. Radiol Clin North Am 27:65–72

VanSonnenberg E, D'Agostino HB, Sanchez RB, Casola G (1992) Percutaneous abscess drainage: editorial comments. Radiology 184:27–29

Vernacchia FS, Jeffrey RB Jr, Federle MP et al (1987) Pancreatic abscess: predictive value of early abdominal CT. Radiology 162:435–438

Vujic I (1989) Vascular complications of pancreatitis. Radiol Clin North Am 27:81–91

Ward J, Chalmers AG, Gathie AJ, Larvin M, Robinson PJ (1997) T2-weighted and dynamic MRI in acute pancreatitis: comparison with contrast enhanced CT. Clin Radiol 52:109–114

Weill F, Brun P, Rhomer P, Belloir A (1983) Migrations of fluid of pancreatic origin: ultrasonic and CT study of 28 cases. Ultrasound Med Biol 9:485–496

White EM, Wittenberg J, Mueller PR et al (1986) Pancreatic necrosis: CT manifestations. Radiology 158:343–346

Winston CB, Mitchell DG, Outwater EK, Ehrlich SM (1995) Pancreatic signal intensity on T1 weighted fat saturation MR images: clinical correlation. J Magn Reson Imaging 5:267–271

7 Chronic Pancreatitis

R. Lecesne, F. Laurent, J. Drouillard, E. Ponette, P. Brys W. Van Steenbergen, and L. Van Hoe

CONTENT

R. Lecesne, MD,
Service d'Imagerie Médicale, Radiologie Diagnostique et Thérapeutique, Université de Bordeaux II, Hôpital Haut Lévêque, USN, C.H.U. Bordeaux, Avenue de Magellan, F-33604 Pessac, France
F. Laurent, MD,
Professeur de Radiologie, Service d'Imagerie Médicale, Radiologie Diagnostique et Thérapeutique, Université de Bordeaux II, Hôpital Haut Lévêque, USN, C.H.U. Bordeaux, Avenue de Magellan, F-33604 Pessac, France
J. Drouillard, MD,
Professeur de Radiologie, Service d'Imagerie Médicale, Radiologie Diagnostique et Thérapeutique, Université de Bordeaux II, Hôpital Haut Lévêque, USN, C.H.U. Bordeaux, Avenue de Magellan, F-33604 Pessac, France
E. Ponette, MD,
Professor, Department of Radiology, University Hospital K.U.L., Herestraat 49, B-3000 Leuven, Belgium
W. Van Steenbergen, MD,
Professor, Department of Internal Medicine, Liver Unit, University Hospital K.U.L., Herestraat 49, B-3000 Leuven, Belgium
L. Van Hoe, MD, PhD,
Assistant Professor, Department of Radiology, University Hospital K.U.L., Herestraat 49, B-3000 Leuven, Belgium

7.1 Pathogenesis and Clinical Features

F. Laurent and J. Drouillard

Chronic pancreatitis is defined as a continuous inflammatory process usually characterized by a relentless and progressive loss of pancreatic parenchymal tissue (Kloppel and Maillet 1992). After a subclinical phase of variable duration, recurrent attacks of abdominal pain are noted, and exocrine or endocrine insufficiency (or both) appears (Lankisch et al. 1993). In most cases, both exocrine and endocrine functions are lost, although the loss of endocrine function appears later in the disease (Steer et al. 1995).

Morphologic changes consist of irregular sclerosis with permanent loss of exocrine parenchyma. All types of inflammatory cells can be present to varying degrees, together with edema and focal necrosis. Pseudocysts which may or may not communicate with ducts are not uncommon. The changes of chronic pancreatitis may be focal, segmental, or diffuse and may be associated with varying degrees of ductal dilatation, ductal strictures, and intraductal protein plugs or calculi. Calculi are composed of calcium carbonate in a form of calcite which represents more than 95% of the stone weight, protein, and polysaccharides. They are often preceded by relatively radiolucent protein plugs. Filling defects on endoscopic retrograde cholangiopancreatography (ERCP) not detected at computed tomography (CT) are related to protein plugs. "Obstructive chronic pancreatitis", a destructive form, is characterized by dilatation of the pancreatic duct proximal to an obstruction, atrophy of the acinar parenchyma, and uniformly diffuse fibrosis. Many of these changes may regress if the obstruction is relieved (Freeny 1988). Chronic pancreatitis has various causes, the most common being chronic alcoholism (6–12 years). Obstruction of the pancreatic duct can also lead to chronic pancreatitis, including post-traumatic ductal stricture, pseudocysts, pancreas divisum with stenosed lesser papilla, and periampullary tumor (OWYANG and LEVITT 1991). Chronic pancreatitis can occasionally occur in association with cystic fibrosis or hyperparathyroidism, or as a hereditary disease transmitted by an autosomal dominant gene with incomplete penetrance (OWYANG and LEVITT 1991). Finally, between 30% and 40% of patients with chronic pancreatitis have no apparent underlying cause and are considered to have "idiopathic" chronic pancreatitis.

The most common clinical symptom of chronic pancreatitis is pain, occurring in 95% of cases. Weight loss is also quite common. Both endocrine and exocrine insufficiency occur with progressive destruction of the gland. Few patients with chronic pancreatitis presenting malabsorption without pain, have pancreatic atrophy. Common complications include jaundice due to extrahepatic bile duct obstruction, bowel obstruction, pseudocysts, pancreatic ascites, and vascular complications, i.e., venous thrombosis or arterial aneurysms.

Approximately 15%–25% of patients die of complications associated with attacks of pancreatitis (MIYAKE et al. 1987). A study indicates that pancreatic cancer develops in roughly 4% of patients within 20 years of a diagnosis of chronic pancreatitis (LOWENFELS et al. 1993).

Non-alcoholic duct-destructive chronic pancreatitis is a newly described type of chronic pancreatitis. This form of non-alcoholic pancreatitis has fairly specific pathological features with a conspicuous periductal inflammation that apparently causes duct obstruction and focal duct destruction. The periductal infiltrate consists mainly of lymphocytes, and is associated with periductal and interlobular fibrosis (ECTORS et al. 1997). The presence of extensive fibrosis with periductal inflammation has also been described in patients with Sjögren's syndrome, primary sclerosing cholangitis, and chronic ulcerative colitis (LASZIK et al. 1988; KAWAGUSHI et al. 1991; BALL et al. 1950; SOOD et al. 1995). It appears, therefore, that previously published cases of chronic "sclerosing" pancreatitis in patients with autoimmune and related diseases had histopathologic features that were similar or even identical to those observed in non-alcoholic duct-destructive chronic pancreatitis.

On the other hand, these pancreatic changes are quite different from those classically seen in alcoholic chronic pancreatitis: in the latter, the ducts are distorted and often contain calcifications; periductal inflammation and duct destruction are not encountered (ECTORS et al. 1997).

7.2 Imaging Studies

Diagnosis of chronic pancreatitis of mild to moderate clinical severity often requires a combination of clinical evaluation, laboratory studies, function testing, and one or more imaging procedures.

The aim of radiologic imaging is firstly to aid the diagnosis, secondly to stage the severity of the disease, thirdly to detect complications, and fourthly to map out the treatment alternatives.

7.2.1 Plain Film

E. PONETTE and P. BRYS

7.2.1.1 Plain Abdominal Film

Pancreatic Calcifications

Pancreatic calcifications are a common finding in chronic panereatitis. According to MARKS and BANK (1985), in most series of alcohol-induced chronic pancreatitis they have been noted in 25%–50% of cases (alcohol abuse is the most frequent cause of panereatitis in the Western countries). In a report by PRINGOT et al. (1976) on 113 eases of chronic panereatitis, pancreatic calcifications were noted in 59% of the cases.

Pancreatic calcifications are most frequently encountered in alcohohe chronic pancreatitis; however, they also may be found in nonalcoholic tropical pancreatitis, in pancreatitis associated with hyperparathyroidism, and in hereditary pancreatitis. They are extremely rare in fibrocystic disease and in pancreatitis caused by gallstones (MARKS and BANK 1985).

Calcifications in chronic pancreatitis may be punctiform, coarse, or, in rare instances, annular. The last-mentioned form probably corresponds to calcification of the wall of a pseudocyst (PRINGOT et al. 1976). The former two forms are almost invariably intraductal stones, located either in the main pancreatic duct or in the side branches (MARKS and BANK 1985). These punctiform or coarse calcifications may have a focal, segmental, or diffuse distribution. The significance of calcifications for the diagnosis of chronic pancreatitis is maximal when they are diffuse.

The genesis of the intraductal calcifications is probably related to impaired evacuation of the inspissated pancreatic secretions, leading to intraductal protein plugs that later calcify (MARKS and BANK 1985; NODA et al. 1987; SARLES and SAHEL 1976).

The minimum interval between the onset of the symptoms of chronic pancreatitis and visualization of pancreatic calcifications in the series of PRINGOT et al. (1976) was 2 years. According to LAMMER et al. (1985), pancreatic calcifications take 1–3 years to become radiologically visible.

The finding of an obvious hiatus within an area of pancreatie calcifications is suggestive of a pseudocyst or tumor (PRINGOT et al. 1976) (Fig. 7.1). MISRA et al. (1990) reported a case in which the calcifications due to chronic pancreatitis decreased simultaneously with the development of a superimposed pancreatic adenocarcinoma.

On the anteroposterior plain film, small pancreatic calcifications may be masked by the spine; therefore additional lateral and oblique views are indicated. Calcifications are more easily visualized by plain film than by US (BAERT et al. 1981; FOLEY et al. 1980). There is, however, controversy about the comparative sensitivity of plain film and CT for the detection of pancreatic calcifications: some claim that CT is more sensitive (FOLEY et al. 1980), while others believe that there is no difference between CT and good plain films (JONES et al. 1988). In a series of 56 patients with calcifying pancreatitis in our hospital, we detected calcifications by plain film in 80%, by CT in 98%, and by US in 67%.

Pancreatic calcifications have to be differentiated from stones in the gallbladder and bile ducts. Moreover, calcifications in chronic pancreatitis have to be differentiated from pancreatic calcifications of other origin, given that a small fraction of cases with pancreatic calcifications are indeed found in conditions other than chronic pancreatitis. In a series of 72 patients with pancreatic calcifications, out of 282 patients with pancreatic pathology, 93% had chronic pancreatitis whereas in the remaining 7% pancreatic cancer was found; the latter calcifications may be due to either preexistent or secondary chronic pancreatitis or intratumoral calcifications (PRINGOT et al. 1976). Besides adenocarcinoma, other pancreatic diseases rarely responsible for pancreatic calcifications are cystic tumors, endocrine tumors, angiomas, and hydatid cysts (GUIEN 1972).

Pseudocysts

Most pancreatic pseudocysts are not visible on plain film. Sometimes a very large pseudocyst may be suspected owing to displacement of airfilled bowel loops.

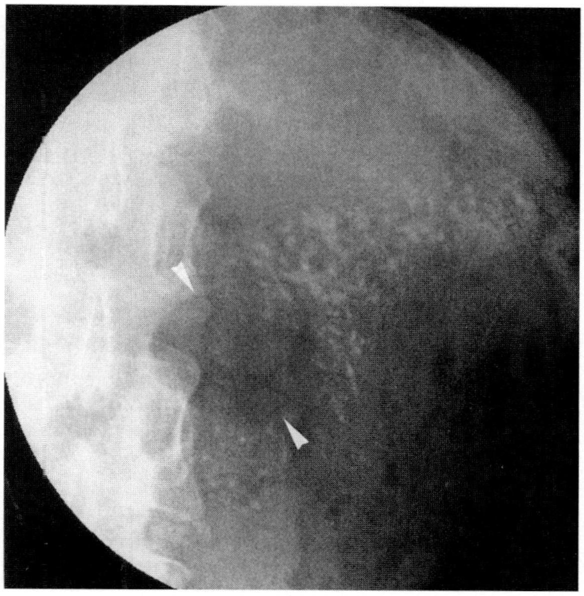

Fig. 7.1. Pseudocyst in chronic calcifying pancreatitis. The diagnosis of a pseudocyst was suggested on this pancreatic plain film on the basis of a rounded hiatus (*arrowheads*) within an area of pancreatic calcifications. The pseudocyst was proved by ultrasonography

7.2.1.2
Other Films Without Contrast

Although anomalies on conventional chest films are best known in the context of acute pancreatitis, pleural effusion may also occur rarely as a complication of chronic pancreatitis. A pancreatic pseudocyst may migrate through the diaphragmatic hiatus or even through the diaphragm and fistulize into the left or right pleural cavity (GUIEN 1972; VAN STEENBERGEN et al. 1990a) (Fig. 7.2).

In chronic pancreatitis calcified intramedullary foci or aseptic necrosis of the skeleton rarely may be seen (GUIEN 1972).

7.2.2
Ultrasonography

R. LECESNE and F. LAURENT

The development of ultrasonography (US) in the early 1970s represented a very important advance in the direct visualization of the pancreas. At that time, reproducible imaging of the gland was not achievable by other techniques. Over the last 10 years, many reports have described a wide variety of US findings

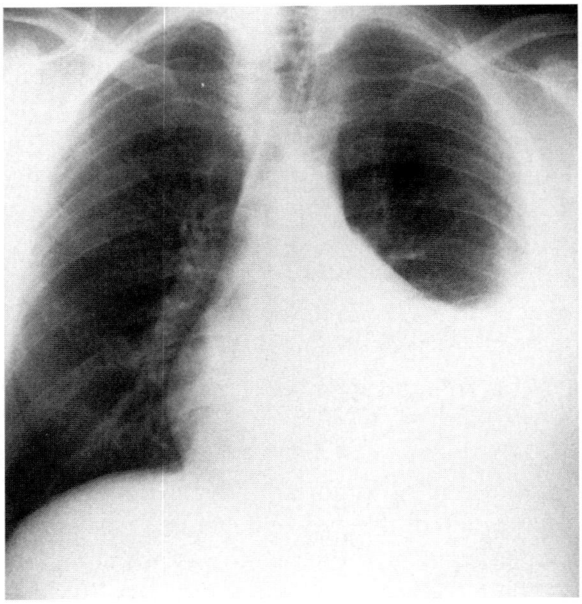
a

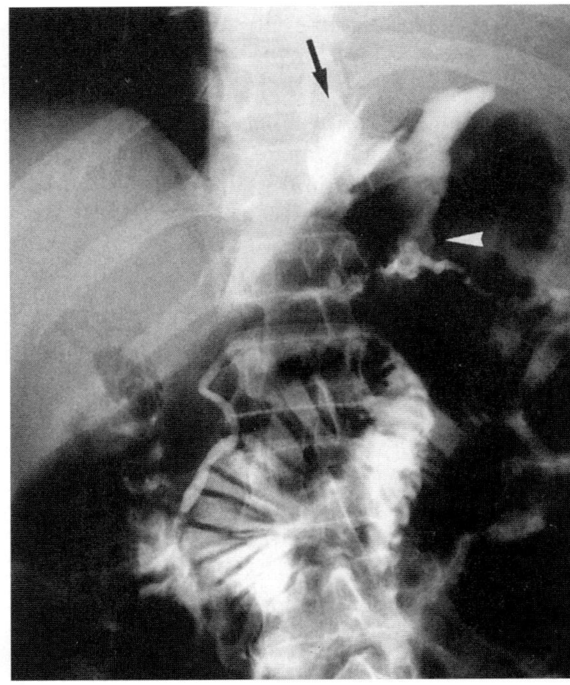
b

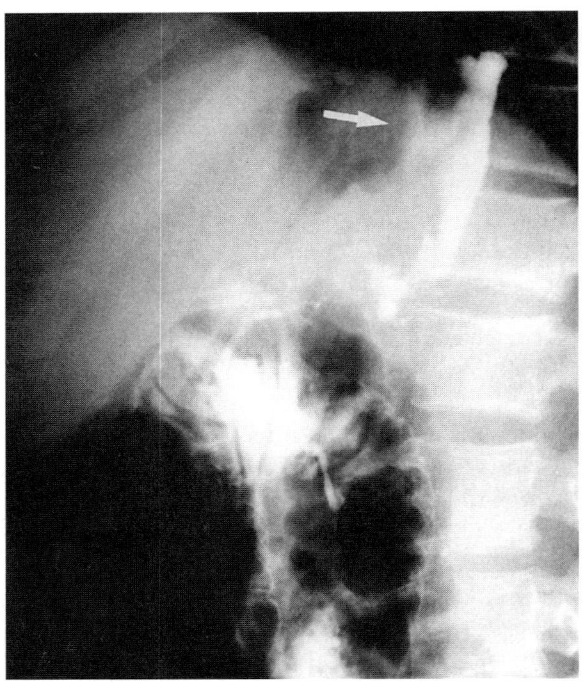
c

Fig. 7.2a–c. Chronic pancreatitis with pseudocyst fistulizing into left pleural cavity. **a** Chest film showing left pleural effusion. **b** Endoscopic retrograde cholangiopancreatography (ERCP) (anteroposterior view) demonstrating an irregularly lined pseudocyst, starting from the body segment of the main pancreatic duct (*arrowhead*) and reaching as far as the area of the diaphragmatic hiatus (*arrow*). **c** ERCP (profile view). The prevertebral course of the pseudocyst (*arrow*) is compatible with the hiatal area

occurring in chronic pancreatitis and have evaluated the diagnostic possibilities of US (Alpern et al. 1985; Bolondi et al. 1989; MacCain et al. 1984; Otte 1986; Shawker et al. 1984).

Various morphologic alterations can be detected by US: alterations in size, variations in shape and contour, changes in the parenchymal echo texture, calcifications, dilatation of the main pancreatic duct, dilatation of the biliary tree, the presence of fluid collections and obstruction of the venous portal system. These findings may occur in varying combinations and with different frequencies depending on the duration of the disease.

7.2.2.1
Alterations in Size

The pancreas may be normal, atrophic, or focally or diffusely enlarged. Alteration in size is present in 38%–55% of cases (Bolondi et al. 1989; Alpern et al. 1985; Otte 1986). Diffuse enlargement tends to be present early in the course of the disease (Fig. 7.3),

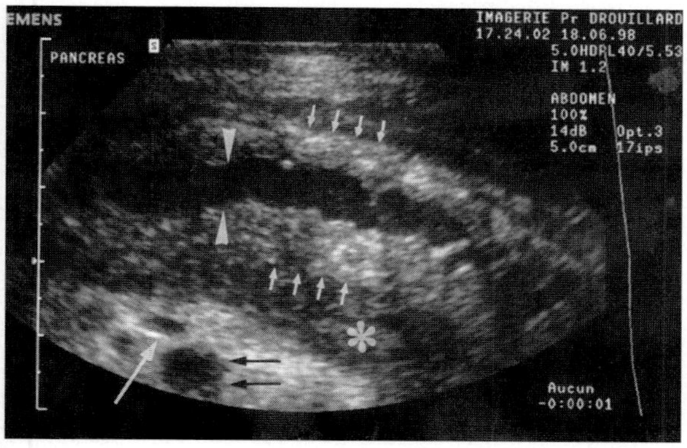

Fig. 7.3. Ultrasonography of obstructive chronic pancreatitis above a cephalic pancreatic tumor. The pancreatic gland is enlarged and heterogeneous (*small white arrows*). The tumor obstructs the main pancreatic duct, which is dilated upstream (*arrowheads*). The splenic vein appears hyperechoic (*asterisk*) and dilated due to a thrombosis. A right hepatic artery (*large white arrow*) arises from the superior mesenteric artery

whereas focal enlargement and atrophy are late features. Atrophy is the most difficult feature to detect confidently as an atrophic gland can easily be misinterpreted as normal, or may not be visualized by US. Focal enlargement is generally the result of localized inflammation and is often seen during relapses of chronic pancreatitis. The upper limit of normal size remains a critical point in the correct diagnosis of pancreatic enlargement. Measurements of the maximum anteroposterior diameter at different levels (head, body, tail) are made on transverse/oblique scans, on which the maximum length of the longitudinal axis of the gland is visualized. Most authors refer to the following maximum anteroposterior diameters: head, 2.6 cm; body, 2.2 cm; tail, 1.5 cm (Niederau et al. 1983). The tail is the most difficult part of the pancreas to examine, being visualized in only 30% of cases. In young and thin people, however, the tail may appear even larger and thicker than the head.

Changes in pancreatic size may be present in physiologic and pathologic conditions other than chronic pancreatitis. Diffuse enlargement is a typical finding in acute pancreatitis. Atrophy may be seen in many normal elderly patients.

7.2.2.2 Changes in Shape and Contour

Advanced chronic pancreatitis generally causes loss of the normal regular shape of the gland due to diffuse or partial enlargement. When the echogenicity of the parenchyma is increased, it is difficult to distinguish the diseased pancreas from retroperitoneal structures.

7.2.2.3 Alterations in Echo Texture

Both fat and fibrous tissues are important causes of increased echogenicity of the gland. Various degrees of fatty replacement of the gland occur in the obese and in the elderly. In chronic pancreatitis, the echo texture may be unevenly modified, with both echogenic foci and anechoic areas. When marked fibrosis is present, the gland appears diffusely but irregularly hyperechoic. Echo texture alterations have been observed in 57% of cases; in cases with severe exocrine insufficiency, the prevalence was 81.8% (Bolondi et al. 1989). These abnormalities are relatively sensitive but nonspecific for chronic pancreatitis; therefore, texture changes as an isolated finding are frequently of no value in its diagnosis.

7.2.2.4 Calcifications

Calcifications appear as clumps of high-level echoes within the pancreatic parenchyma or within the dilated excretory system. Only large stones cast an acoustic shadow (Fig. 7.4). Small calcifications are not detected by US (Alpern et al. 1985).

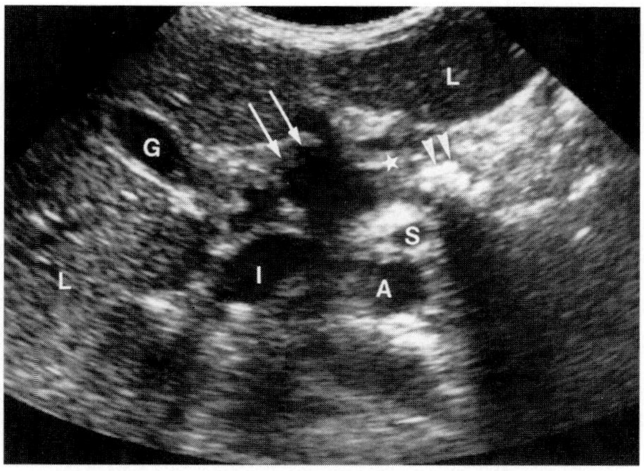

Fig. 7.4. Ultrasonography of chronic calcified pancreatitis. Axial epigastric scan shows typical findings associating a corporocaudal calculus with a posterior shadow (*arrowheads*) and a hypoechoic pseudocyst encompassing the head of the pancreas (*arrows*). Echo texture of the pancreas appears hyperechoic (*star*). *L*, liver; *G*, gallbladder; *S*, superior mesenteric artery; *I*, inferior vena cava; *A*, abdominal aorta

7.2.2.5
Dilatation of the Main Pancreatic Duct

Dilatation of the main pancreatic duct is the most reliable sign of pancreatic disease and has been reported in 11.2%–52.3% of cases (Otte 1986; Alpern et al. 1985; Bolondi et al. 1989). In early cases, the main pancreatic duct may be normal: a diameter of up to 2 mm can be considered normal. Comparison of US and endoscopic retrograde cholangiopancreatography (ERCP) measurements cannot be made because ERCP displays a duct diameter 2.5 times greater than that displayed by US owing to pressure injection and underestimation by US related to apparent thickening of duct walls. A dilated main pancreatic duct in chronic pancreatitis can be irregular, but this is difficult to appreciate (see Fig. 7.3).

7.2.2.6
Pseudocysts

These appear anechoic with posterior enhancement, sometimes with intracystic echoes related to debris. Catheter drainage is now an accepted front line form of therapy for pancreatic pseudocyst (Grosso et al. 1989). US guidance may be used with good results in 65%–90% of cases (Grosso et al. 1989). Such pseudocysts can lead to biliary obstruction (Fig. 7.5) when located within the head of the pancreas.

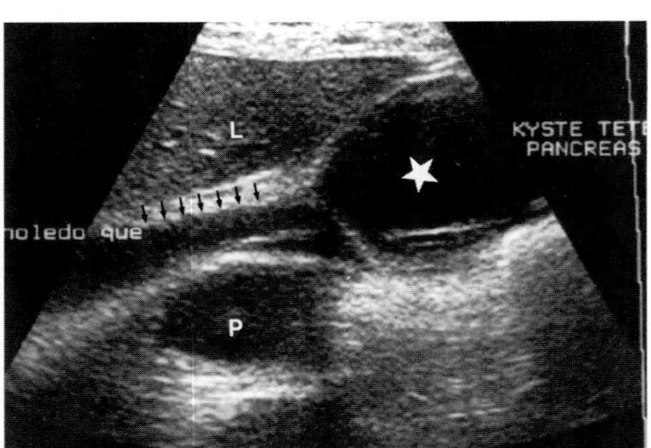

Fig. 7.5. Chronic pancreatitis. Pseudocyst: ultrasonography in a patient complaining of jaundice. Sagittal epigastric scan shows a round anechoic pseudocyst (*star*) encompassing the head of the pancreas which obstructs the distal part of the common bile duct (*small arrows*). *L*, liver; *P*, portal vein

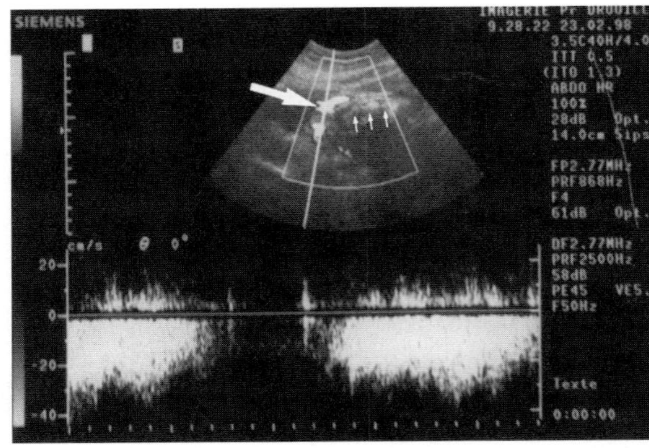

Fig. 7.6. Color Doppler ultrasound analysis of chronic pancreatitis with vascular complications. An enlarged right gastroepiploic vein (*large arrow*) is shown in front of the pancreatic head (*small arrows*). These collateral pathways are the result of splenic vein involvement (segmental portal hypertension)

7.2.3
Color Doppler US

R. Lecesne and F. Laurent

Color Doppler evaluation of chronic pancreatitis aids the depiction of vascular complications such as pseudoaneurysms or thromboses of the portal system. The splenomesenteric vein is most commonly occluded in chronic pancreatitis and collateral pathways (right or left gastroepiploic veins) may be detected (Fig. 7.6). In the case of rupture of a pseudoaneurysm, the sonographic findings are rapid enlargement of a cystic pancreatic mass and sudden change of echogenicity. Color Doppler US can establish the diagnosis by demonstrating pulsatile arterial flow within the cystic mass.

7.2.4
Endoscopic Ultrasonography

R. Lecesne and F. Laurent

Endoscopic ultrasonography (EUS) appears to be an attractive imaging procedure for the diagnosis of chronic pancreatitis. It has a high sensitivity and specificity in detecting morphological changes evocative of chronic pancreatitis such as heterogeneous patterns of pancreatic echogenicity, small cysts, dilatation of the Wirsung duct, and microcalcifications (Buscail et al. 1995) (Fig. 7.7).

In patients with early stages of chronic pancreatitis, EUS may reveal abnormalities when other imag-

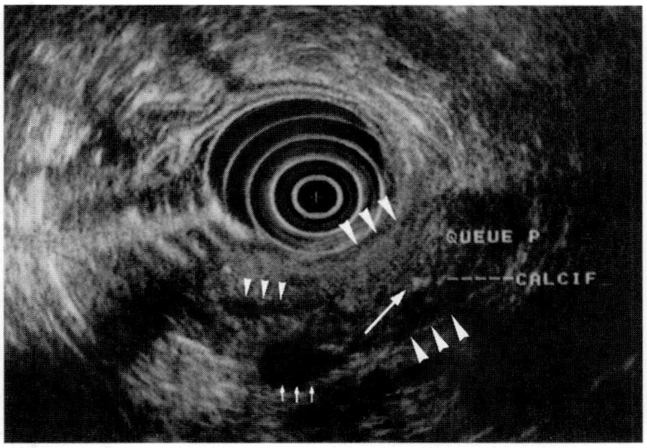

Fig. 7.7. Endoscopic ultrasonography of alcohol-induced chronic pancreatitis. Typical findings of chronic pancreatitis are observed within the body and the tail of the pancreas: heterogeneous pattern of the pancreatic gland (*large arrowheads*); calcification (*large arrow*); dilated main pancreatic duct (*small arrowheads*); pseudocyst (*small arrows*)

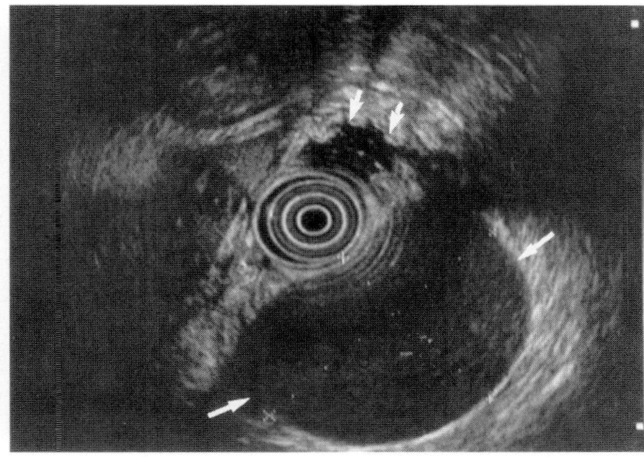

Fig. 7.8. Endoscopic ultrasonography of a compressive pseudocyst. A large pseudocyst (*large arrows*) appears very close from the gastric wall (*small arrows*). The puncture of the cyst could be performed easily with endoscopic ultrasonography guidance

ing tests, including ERCP, are normal. When fibrosis occurs, the enhanced reflectivity of collagen can be expected to generate echogenic foci or septa. With progression, the gland's smooth surface becomes replaced by lobules accentuated by intervening septa. Similarly, periductal fibrosis appears as a thickening of the duct wall and an irregular caliber of the main pancreatic duct, with areas of narrowing and dilatation (Wieserma and Wierserma 1995). In these cases, the accuracy of EUS is made difficult to determine due to the absence of an available gold standard (pathologic proof). EUS-guided fine needle aspiration biopsy may assist in this determination and may be helpful in differentiating a focal area of chronic pancreatitis from pancreatic tumor (Wieserma et al. 1994), and in performing cystogastrostomy in the case of compressive pseudocyst (Fig. 7.8).

7.2.5 Endoscopic Retrograde Cholangiopancreatography

E. Ponette, P. Brys, and W. Van Steenbergen

7.2.5.1 Technique

An early description of the ERCP technique was provided by Cotton (1972), Demling et al. (1974), and Ponette et al. (1978c). In the context of chronic pancreatitis it is important to prevent infection of pseudocysts and cholangitis when there is stenosis of the common bile duct. Therefore it is wise to stop filling a pseudocyst when it becomes apparent (Axon 1989; Silvis and Schuman 1977), to give antibiotic prophylaxis when contrast is injected proximal to a common bile duct stenosis (Van Steenbergen et al. 1990b), and if necessary to perform a drainage procedure.

7.2.5.2 ERCP Anomalies

The general ERCP features of chronic pancreatitis have been described in several publications (Axon 1986; Caletti et al. 1982; Helwig et al. 1990; Silvis and Schuman 1977) and are summarized in Table 7.1.

Anomalies of Pancreatic Ducts

The earliest signs of chronic pancreatitis are noted in the *side branches* (Figs. 7.9-7.11). Side branch changes include: dilatation without stenosis, dilatation with downstream stenosis, irregular lining and later cystic dilatation, intraluminal filling defects, and small calcified stones in dilated side branches. Dilatation of side branches without stenosis is probably caused by impaired evacuation of inspissated pancreatic secretions (Marks and Bank 1985). The intraluminal filling defects are probably due to thus formed protein plugs, which may later become calcified (Noda et al. 1987).

Table 7.1. ERCP anomalies in chronic pancreatitis

Side branches
Dilatation with or without downstream stenosis
Irregular lining
Obstruction (paucity of contrast-filled side branches)
Intraluminal filling defects or calcified stones
Main pancreatic duct
Dilatation with or without downstream stenosis
Irregular lining
Obstruction: seldom
Intraluminal filling defects or calcified stones
Pancreatic parenchyma
Pseudocyst(s) communicating with main pancreatic duct or side branches
Abscess: seldom
Common bile duct (pancreatic segment)
Long smooth stenosis (Caroli I)
Short smooth preterminal stenosis (Caroli III)
Deviation (pseudocyst)
Obstruction, asymmetric stenosis: seldom

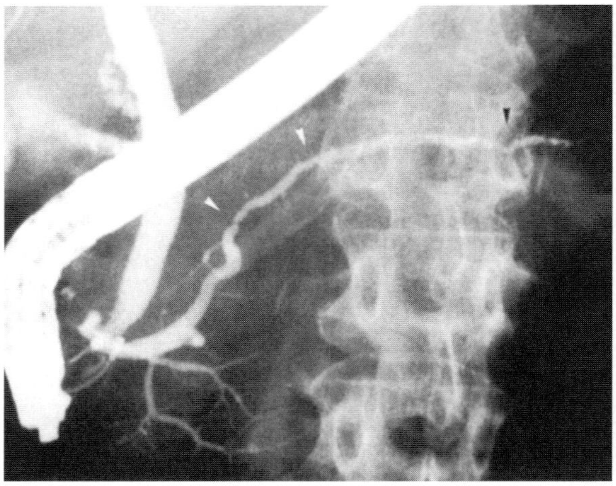

Fig. 7.10. Moderate chronic pancreatitis. Several narrowed areas are present in the main pancreatic duct (*arrowheads*). Note, moreover, the paucity of side branches in the body and tail of the pancreas

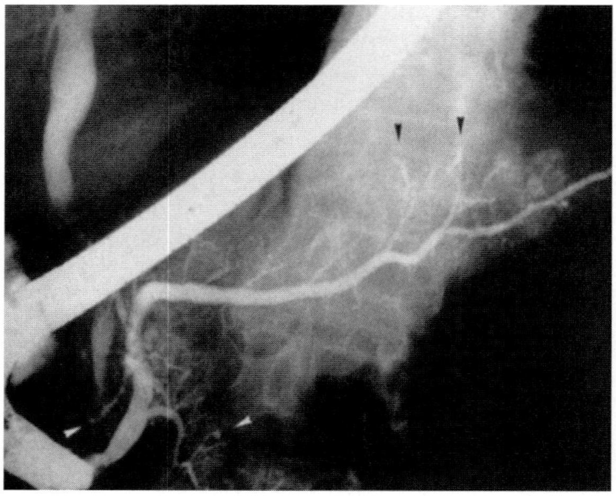

Fig. 7.9. Mild chronic pancreatitis. Note anomalies of at least four side branches (*arrowheads*)

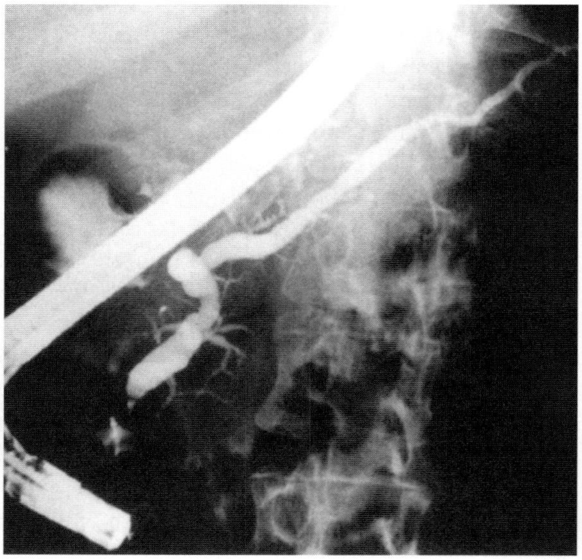

Fig. 7.11. Moderate chronic pancreatitis. There is slight diffuse dilatation of the main pancreatic duct without downstream stenosis. Furthermore, several side branches show dilatation

The number of opacified side branches may be reduced if some of them are totally obstructed. In most cases the side branch anomalies are diffusely spread over the pancreatic gland with a scattered distribution.

In a later stage the *main pancreatic duct* becomes abnormal and here too the anomalies are mostly diffuse or multisegmental, though they may be focal (Freeny 1989). They are analogous to the mentioned features in the side branches and include dilatation without stenosis, dilatation with downstream stenosis, slight segmental narrowing causing irregular lining, and, at a later stage, intraluminal radiolucent filling defects or calcified stones (Figs. 7.10-7.13). A single short stenosis may occur (Fig. 7.24) or the duct may be narrowed over a considerable length. Complete obstruction of the main pancreatic duct is rather rare in chronic pancreatitis, unless it is due to a pseudocyst (Figs. 7.20, 7.21). It is interesting that ERCP changes of chronic pancreatitis may be present

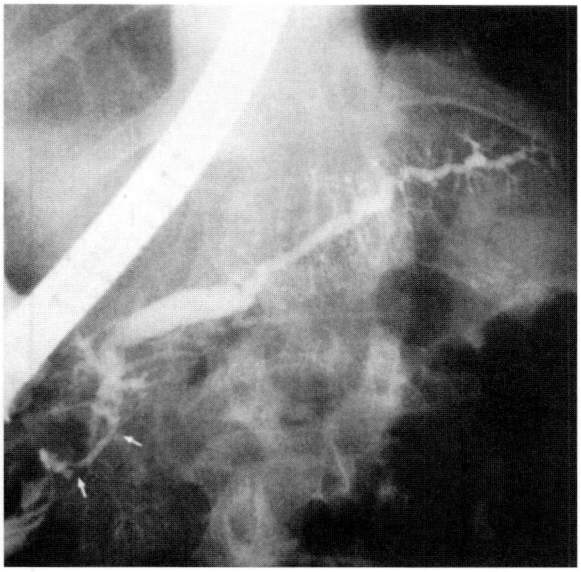

Fig. 7.12. Moderate chronic pancreatitis. There is moderate stenosis of the terminal and preterminal segment of the main pancreatic duct (*area between two arrows*) with prestenotic dilatation in the head. Note also the alternating diameter of the main pancreatic duct in the body and tail

in chronic heavy drinkers, even if symptoms of pancreatic disease are not yet apparent (Angelini et al. 1987; Elsborg et al. 1981).

Anomalies of Pancreatic Parenchyma

Regularly lined cavities filling with contrast are mostly caused by pseudocysts. They may be smaller than 1 cm or present a diameter as great as 20 cm or more (Figs. 7.14, 7.18). In general they are round, but they may be oblong or present an irregular shape. They may be uni- or multilocular and may be located in or around the pancreas. Such cavities are only filled with contrast when they communicate with the main pancreatic duct or a side branch.

A pseudocyst may, in rare instances, fistulize into a splanchnic artery and cause an arterial pseudoaneurysm; it may also fistulize into the portal vein and this complication may be visualized by ERCP (Van Steenbergen et al. 1990b). Finally, a pancreatic pseudocyst may extend in all directions and fistulize into the pleural cavity, either through the diaphragmatic hiatus or through the diaphragmatic dome; this complication, too, may be demonstrated by ERCP (Cuykx et al. 1992; Van Steenbergen et al. 1990a).

Cystic dilated side branches may not be distinguishable from small pseudocysts.

A pancreatic abscess may have a less regular internal wall than a pseudocyst.

Anomalies oft the Common Bile Duct

Since the distal part of the common bile duct presents an intrapancreatic course in 85% of the population and an immediate retropancreatic course in the remaining 15%, it is no wonder that changes of this bile duct segment may be found in chronic pancreatitis (Van Steenbergen and Ponette 1990).

Common bile duct changes have been well described by several authors (Aranha et al. 1984; Gregg et al. 1981; Plumley et al. 1982; Rohrmann and Baron 1989; Van Steenbergen and Ponette 1990) and the most frequent changes are summarized in Fig. 7.15 (Rohrmann and Baron 1989). The most frequent change of the common bile duct is a long, smooth narrowing with gradual transition,

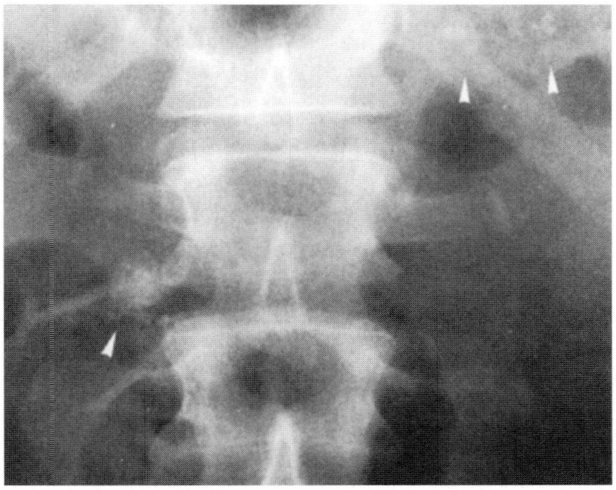

a

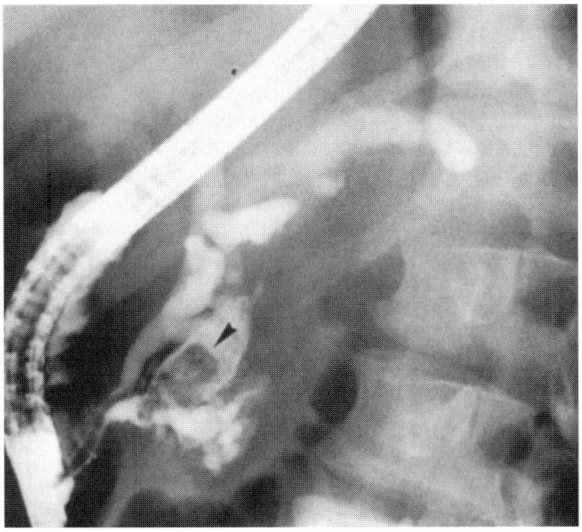

b

Fig. 7.13a,b. Chronic pancreatitis (marked degree) with lithiasis of the duct of Wirsung. **a** Several calcifications are present in the head and tail of the pancreas (*arrowheads*). **b** A calcified stone (*arrowhead*) is observed in the dilated main pancreatic duct

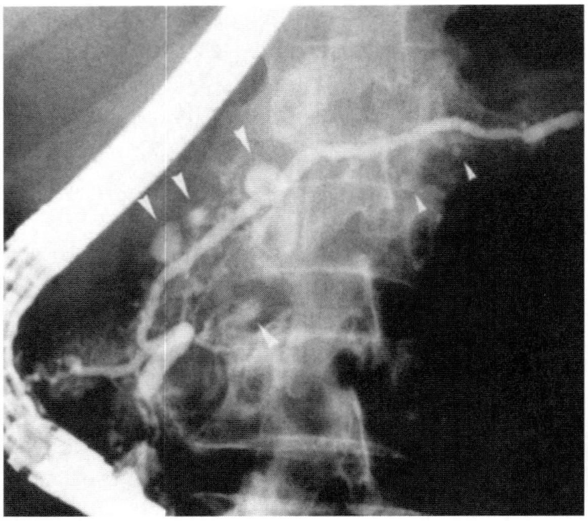

Fig. 7.14. Chronic pancreatitis with small pseudocysts. Several small, rounded contrast collections (*arrowheads*) with a greatest diameter ≤10 mm are visible in the head and body of the pancreas. Note, moreover, segmental narrowing of the main pancreatic duct in the tail (moderate degree of chronic pancreatitis)

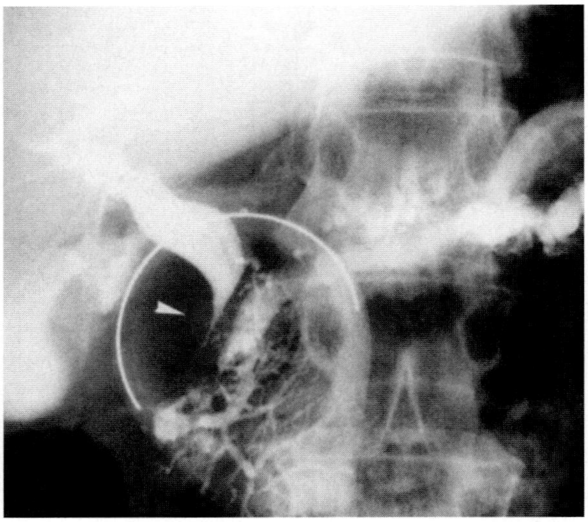

Fig. 7.16. Chronic pancreatitis with common bile duct stenosis (Caroli I lesion). There is long, gradually tapering, smooth-lined stenosis of the pancreatic segment of the common bile duct (*arrowhead*). Note also the obvious dilatation of the main pancreatic duct and side branches (marked chronic pancreatitis)

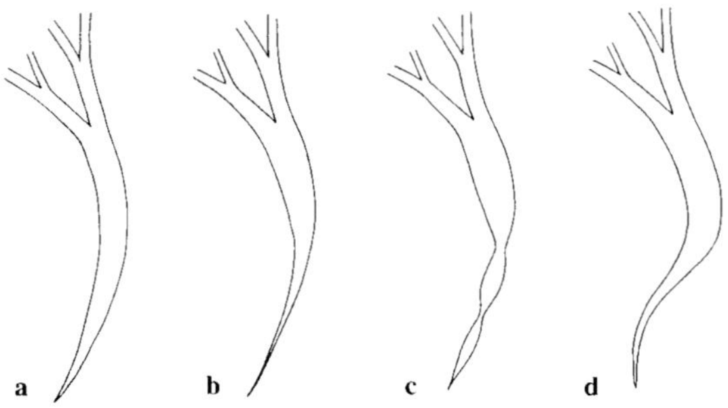

Fig. 7.15a–d. Typical configurations of the normal and stenosed common bile ducts in chronic pancreatitis and pancreatic pseudocyst. **a** The normal common bile duct traverses the area of the pancreatic head with a gentle medial bowing. Note that its caliber is constant throughout most of its course. **b** The typical configuration of the common bile duct in chronic pancreatitis is a gradual tapering of the duct as it passes through the pancreatic head. This type of stenosis occurs in approximately two thirds of chronic pancreatitis patients who have common bile duct stenosis. **c** The"hourglass" configuration of alternating stenosis and dilatation is found in approximately 25% of stenoses. **d** In less than 10% of stenoses, a laterally deflected bile duct is due to an adjacent pseudocyst

located in the pancreatic segment, which may or may not be surrounded by pancreatic calcifications; this is the earlier Caroli I lesion (Guien 1972) (Fig. 7.16). The narrowing is, however, sometimes shorter and limited to the preterminal segment; this is the earlier Caroli III lesion (Guien 1972). Just as in the first type of narrowing, the lining here is also smooth and the transition also gradual (Fig. 7.17).

A deviation of the common bile duct in the context of chronic pancreatitis is usually due to a pseudocyst (Fig. 7.18). Chronic pancreatitis only seldom causes complete obstruction of the common bile duct; it is, however, important to bear in mind that obstruction does not exclude this disease.

Stone formation may occur in the bile ducts proximal to a common bile duct stenosis in the context of chronic pancreatitis (Gregg et al. 1981).

7.2.5.3 ERCP Classification of Chronic Pancreatitis

The first ERCP classification of chronic pancreatitis was made by Kasugai et al. (1974) and was based on three categories: minimal, moderate, and advanced. The first category included changes of side branches without obvious changes of the main pancreatic duct; the second category included obvious but moderate changes of this main duct and possibly of the common bile duct; the third category included serious changes of the main pancreatic duct, such as irregular dilatation or obstruction, and possibly other anomalies such as intraductal calculi, cavities, coarse acinar filling, or changes of the common bile duct.

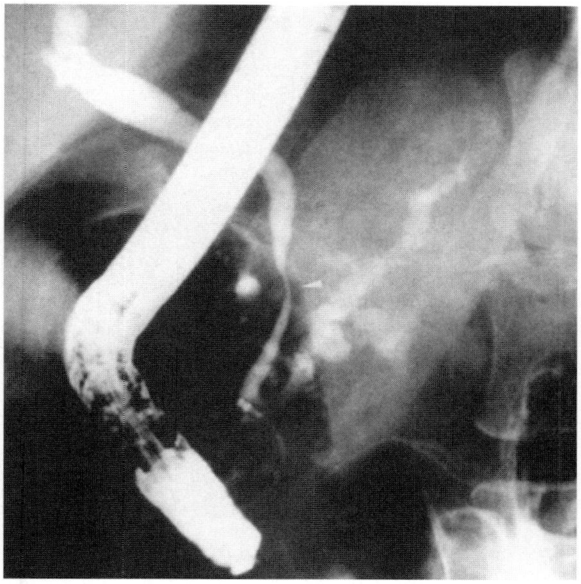

Fig. 7.17. Chronic pancreatitis with common bile duct stenosis (Caroli III lesion). There is rather short, smooth, symmetric hourglass stenosis of the pancreatic segment of the common bile duct (*arrowhead*). Observe the variations in caliber and irregularity of the main pancreatic duct; calcifications in side branches were also present (marked chronic pancreatitis)

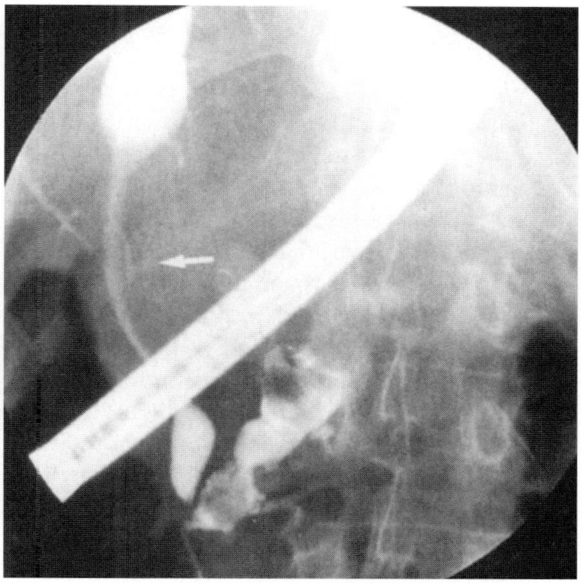

a

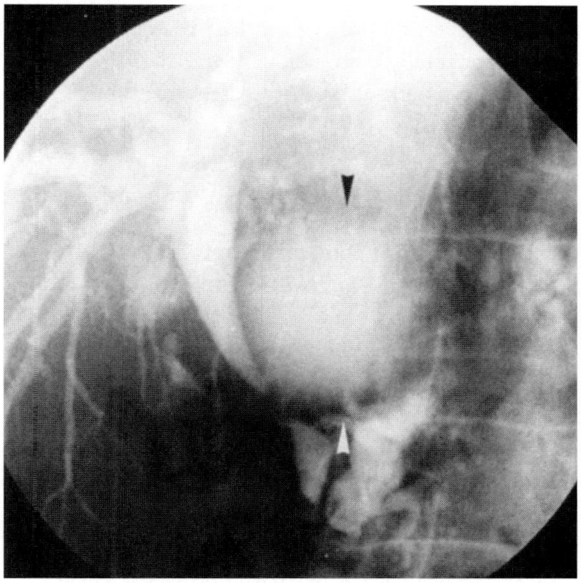

b

Fig. 7.18a,b. Narrowing and deviation of the common bile duct due to a pseudocyst. **a** Smooth narrowing and lateral deflection of the common bile duct (*arrow*) with lithiasis in the dilated main pancreatic duct. **b** Subsequent faint opacification of a large pseudocyst (*arrowheads*) in the head of the pancreas, responsible for the alterations of the common bile duct (marked chronic pancreatitis)

The inclusion of patients with relatively minor side branch changes in the first category of Kasugai's classification raised the problem of the limits of the normal pancreatogram, and apparently led to the *Cambridge classification* of 1983 (Axon 1986, 1989; Sarner and Cotton 1984). This classification (Table 7.2) also includes three "real" categories ("mid," "moderate," and "marked") preceded by the groups "normal" and "equivocal." The mild category includes cases in which at least three side branches are abnormal (Fig. 7.9); those with changes in less than three side branches are classified as equivocal. The moderate category includes, in addition to abnormal side branches, changes of the main pancreatic duct (Figs. 7.10-7.12, 7.14). The marked category includes, in addition to the anomalies of the preceding category, one or more of the following: a large cavity (wider than 10 mm), an intraductal filling defect, severe main pancreatic duct dilatation (wider than 10 mm) , and severe irregularity or obstruction

Table 7.2. Cambridge classification of chronic pancreatitis

Category	Pancreatogram
1 .Normal	Normal main pancreatic duct (MPD) and normal side branches
2. Equivocal	Normal MPD, <3 abnormal side branches
3. Mild	Normal MPD, ≥ abnormal side branches
4. Moderate	Abnormal MPD, >3 abnormal side branches
5. Marked	As in category 4, with one or more of the following: – large cavity (>10 mm) – intraductal filling defect or calculus – severe irregularity, dilatation (>10 mm) or obstruction of MPD

of the main pancreatic duct (Figs. 7.13, 7.16-7.18, 7.20, 7.21).

JONES et al. (1988) proposed some slight modifications of the Cambridge classification. On the one hand they did not retain the presence of an abnormal main duct as an essential condition for the marked category, rather judging large cavities or calculi to be indicative of marked pancreatitis in their own right. On the other hand they replaced the term "intraductal filling defects" in the marked category by the term "intraductal calculi", since they judged that protein plugs are often transitory and can be seen at any stage of chronic pancreatitis (Fig. 7.19).

The above-mentioned problem of the normal limits of the pancreatogram was again raised by later publications. In 1985 SCHMITZ-MOORMANN et al. described slight pancreatitis-like changes in postmortem ductograms of subjects without clinical or histologic signs of chronic pancreatitis. JONES et al. (1989) drew attention to the fact that this problem occurs especially in the elderly and that the criteria of chronic pancreatitis in this age group have to be more restrictive.

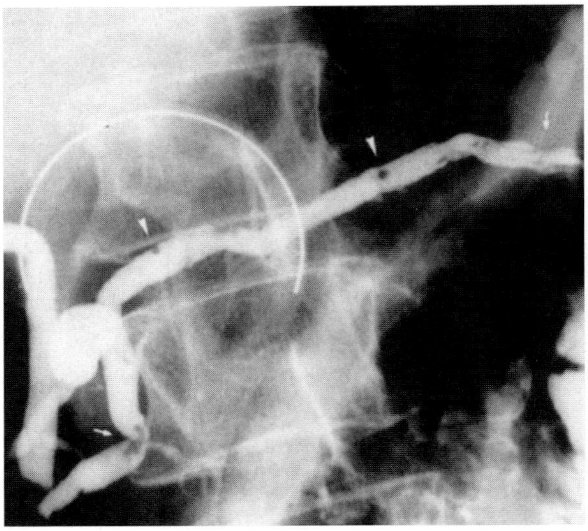

Fig. 7.19. Chronic pancreatitis with probably intraductal protein plugs. Several rounded (*arrowheads*) and amorphous (*arrows*) intraluminal filling defects are present in a dilated main pancreatic duct. Most of these disappeared or were displaced on control endoscopic retrograde cholangiopancreatography. There were no calcifications on ultrasonography or computed tomography

7.2.5.4 ERCF Differential Diagnosis Between Chronic Pancreatitis and Pancreatic Carcinoma

The ERCP features most important in the differential diagnosis between chronic pancreatitis and pancreatic carcinoma are summarized in Table 7.3.

The ERCP diagnosis of classic diffuse calcifying chronic pancreatitis naturally does not cause problems. Problems of differential diagnosis may, however, occur when pancreatic or bile duct changes atypical or less typical for pancreatitis are present, when the distribution of pancreatitis or tumoral lesions over the gland is atypical, or when there is an

Table 7.3. ERCP differential diagnois

	Chronic pancreatitis	Pancreatic carcinoma
Lesional distribution	Diffuse, multisegmental, or focal	Focal (with upstream duct dilatation)
Main pancreatic duct changes	Narrowing (regular), seldom obstruction (mostly by pseudocyst) *or* dilatation *or* alternating narrowing and dilatation	Narrowing (irregular or regular) or obstruction Upstream dilatation
Side branch changes	Inhomogeneous (funnel-shaped) or homogeneous dilatation with scattered distribution Presence of these lesions also downstream from main duct lesion	Homogeneous smooth dilatation of all side branches upstream from main duct lesion
Calcifications	Frequent (intraductal calculi)	Seldom
Cavity	Frequent: regularly lined pseudocyst (single or multiple)	Seldom: tumoral necrosis
Common bile duct changes	Long (sometimes short preterminal), smooth, mostly symmetric narrowing Deviation (pseudocyst) Seldom obstruction Double duct sign less common	Irregular or smooth rather short narrowing or obstruction (symmetric or asymmetric) Double duct sign common

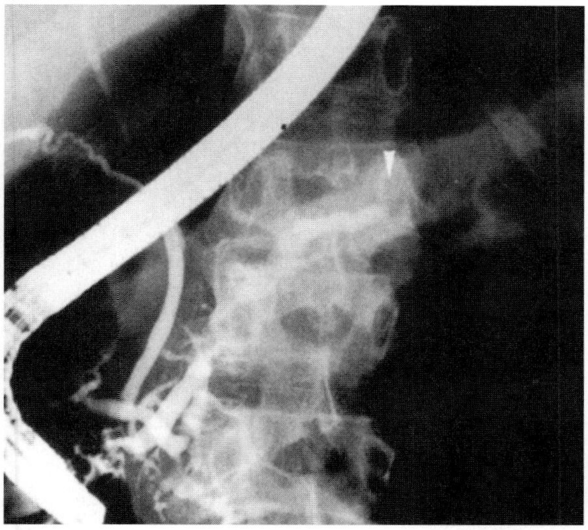

Fig. 7.20. Chronic pancreatitis with obstruction in the body segment of the main pancreatic duct (*arrowhead*). Preoperative endoscopic retrograde cholangiopancreatography suggested chronic pancreatitis rather than a tumor owing to the presence of (a) alterations in the diameter of the main pancreatic duct downstream, and (b) side branch dilatation. No pseudocyst was observed on ultrasonography or computed tomography

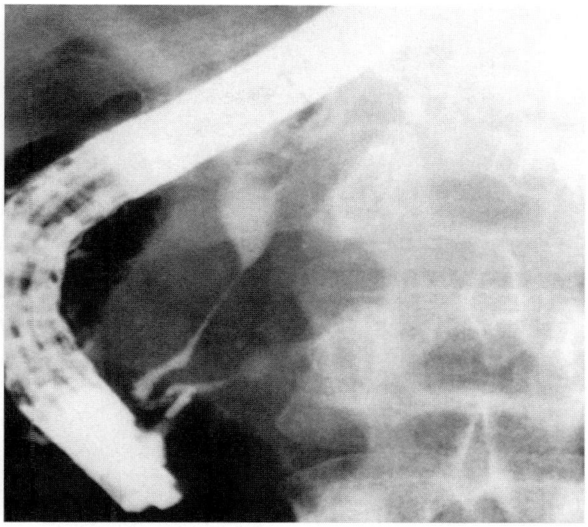

Fig. 7.22. Chronic pancreatitis with double duct sign. There is obstruction of the main pancreatic duct and long stenosis of the common bile duct in the head of the pancreas. In this case, two signs argued in favor of the preoperative endoscopic retrograde cholangiopancreatography diagnosis of chronic pancreatitis: the calcifications near the obstruction of the duct of Wirsung and the long, symmetric, smooth, gradual tapering of the bile duct stenosis

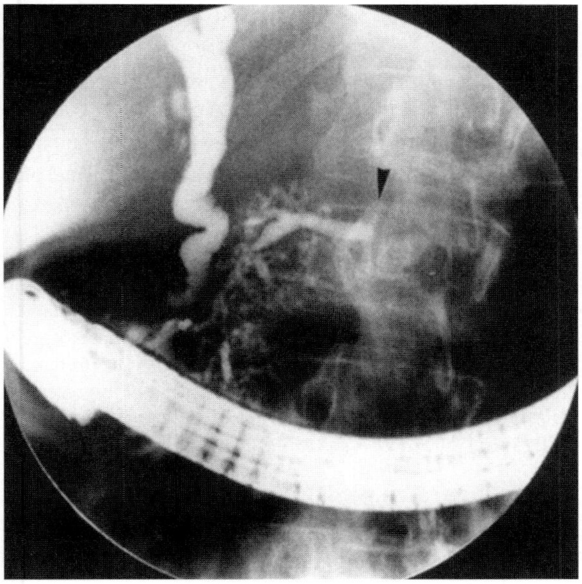

Fig. 7.21. Chronic pancreatitis with obstruction of the body segment of the main pancreatic duct (*arrowhead*). Anomalies of side branches are present downstream, suggesting the diagnosis of chronic pancreatitis. A pseudocyst was observed in the body of the pancreas on computed tomography

association of chronic pancreantis and pancreatic carcinoma. The reality of this differential diagnostic ERCP problem is reflected by the long list of reports dealing with the subject. When it has been possible to ascertain the frequency of this problem, the figure rises to at least 10% , and to much more in most publications (Anacker et al. 1981; Caletti et al. 1982; Frick et al. 1982; Helwig et al. 1990; Janus et al. 1982; Lammer et al. 1985; Mackie et al. 1979; Neff et al. 1984; Njx and Schmitz 1981; Plumley et al. 1982; Pomerri et al. 1988; Ralls et al. 1980; Thomas and Morse 1985; Tobin et al. 1987).

Statistical studies reveal that obstructions of the main pancreatic duct, obstructions of the common bile duct, and the double duct sign are more frequently encountered in pancreatic carcinoma, but it is important to realize that these signs may also occur in chronic pancreatitis (Frick et al. 1982; Neff et al. 1984; Plumley et al. 1982; Ralls et al. 1980; Van Steenbergen et al. 1990b) (Figs. 7.20-7.23).

Classic chronic pancreatitis is a diffuse or multisegmental disease, but the frequency of this presentation must not be allowed to cause focal chronic pancreatitis to be overlooked (Freeny 1989). Against this background it is readily comprehensible that this focal variant of pancreatitis may constitute a differential diagnostic problem with pancreatic carcinoma (Lammer et al. 1985; Neff et al. 1984) (Fig. 7.24). On the other hand it is important to bear in mind the fact that while pancreatic carcinoma is

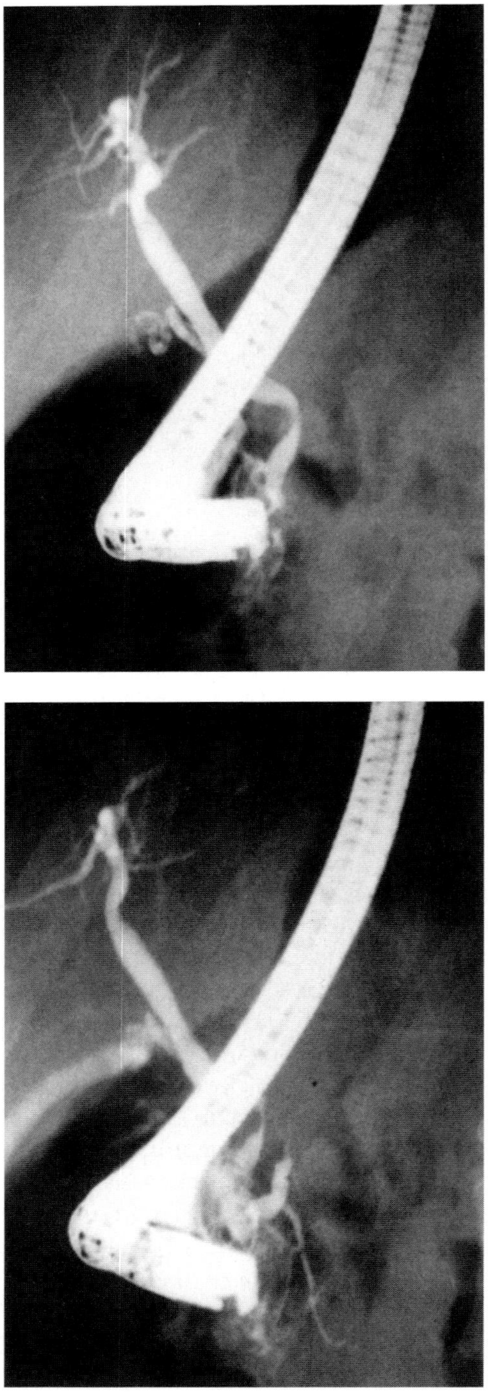

a

b

Fig. 7.23a,b. Chronic pancreatitis with double duct sign. **a** Rather short, smooth, but asymmetric narrowing of the preterminal common bile duct segment. **b** Obstruction of the main pancreatic duct in the head of the pancreas without calcifications. The preferential preoperative endoscopic retrograde cholangiopancreatography diagnosis was pancreatic tumor, but anatomopathologic examination of the operative specimen showed only chronic pancreatitis

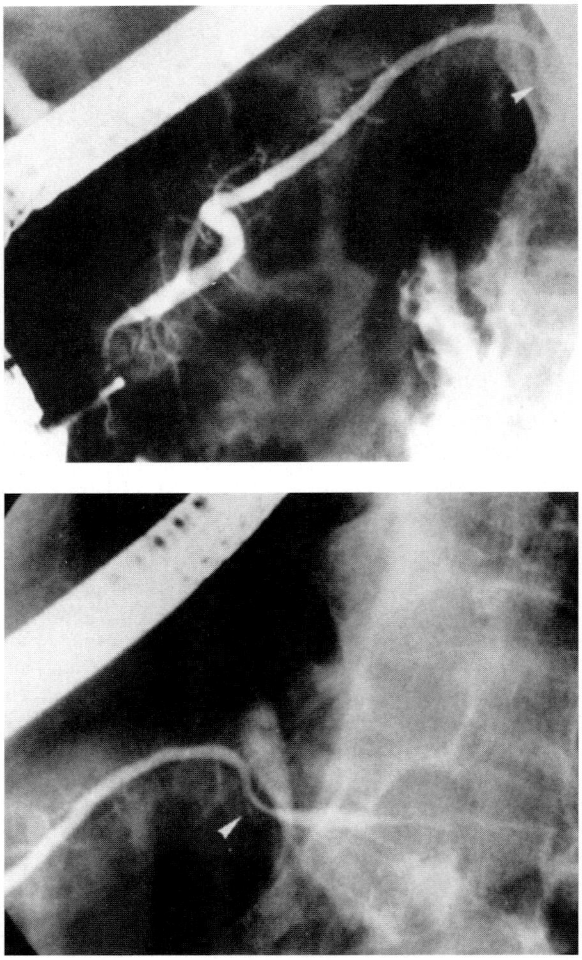

a

b

Fig. 7.24a,b. Focal chronic pancreatitis. **a** Nearly normal pancreatogram except for slight segmental narrowing of the main pancreatic duct in the tail (*arrowhead*). **b** Spot film of the tail of the pancreas. The slight narrowing is now better visible (*arrowhead*), as is slight prestenotic duct dilatation. Differential diagnosis between tumor and chronic pancreatitis was difficult on the basis of preoperative endoscopic retrograde cholangiopancreatography, but there was a slight preference for a tumor. Anatomopathologic examination of the resection specimen revealed chronic pancreatitis

in principle restricted to a small part of the pancreas, it may invade a larger part of the gland and so mimic chronic pancreatitis (Conley et al. 1987; Rigauts et al. 1992; Tracey et al. 1984).

Finally, when chronic pancreatitis and pancreatic carcinoma occur together in the same patient, it is very difficult in our opinion and in that of others (Frick et al. 1982; Ralls et al. 1980) to make the correct diagnosis (Fig. 7.25), although some are much more optimistic on this point (Shemesh et al. 1990). Regression of calcifications in previously identified chronic pancreatitis may be a sign of superimposed carcinoma (Misra et al. 1990; Pringot et al. 1976).

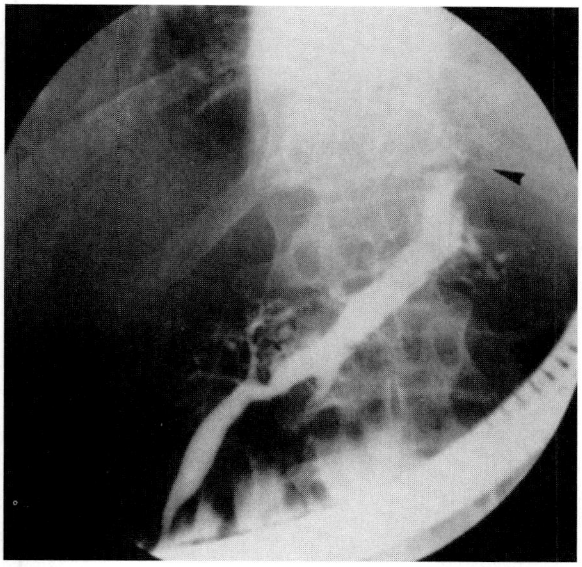

Fig. 7.25. Combination of chronic pancreatitis and pancreatic adenocarcinoma. Classic signs of severe chronic pancreatitis are present in the main duct and side branches, and there is obstruction of the main pancreatic duct in the tail (*arrowhead*). The preoperative preferential endoscopic retrograde cholangiopancreatography (ERCP) diagnosis was chronic pancreatitis. Computed tomography demonstrated a large tumoral mass in the tail of the pancreas, as well as liver metastases. Cytologic examination of pleural effusion revealed class 5, compatible with adenocarcinoma. In this case, the correct ERCP differential diagnosis is as good as impossible: compare Figs. 7.20 and 7.21

7.2.5.5 Diagnostic Value of ERCP in Comparison with Other Imaging Techniques

In a number of studies an attempt has been made to evaluate quantitatively the diagnostic possibilities of ERCP and other techniques in chronic pancreatitis (Anacker et al. 1981; Caletti et al. 1982; Foley et al. 1980; Frick et al. 1982; Gmelin et al. 1981; Gowland et al. 1981; Helwig et al. 1990; Mackie et al. 1979; Pomerri et al. 1988; Ralls et al. 1980; Swobodnik et al. 1983; Tobin et al. 1987; Triller et al. 1980). A good comparison is often hindered by several problems: many studies mention figures for sensitivity but not specificity (Phillips et al. 1983), it is not always clear how the selection of patients is made for the calculation of "sensitivity," there is no uniformity in relation to the clearance of the failures of a technique, some series are rather small, and many studies are retrospective. Moreover, the performance of a technique is dependent on various factors: the ability of the operator, the operator's experience, and the state of technical evolution.

Sensitivity and Specificity of ERCP

Bearing in mind the above limitations, the sensitivity of ERCP in chronic pancreatitis in the larger series is about 80%–85% , with the extreme values being 93% and 35%. The specificity of ERCP varies in these studies between 100% and 65%. The study that yielded the latter figure (Gowland et al. 1981), however, also included some cases of pancreatic cancer.

In our experience the differential diagnostic score of ERCP in respect of chronic pancreatitis and pancreatic carcinoma, and consequently its sensitivity, shows an obvious increase when not only the pancreatic ducts but also the common bile duct is opacified.

Comparison of ERCP with US and CT

Comparing ERCP, CT, and US, it appears that US is the least sensitive diagnostic test for chronic pancreatitis; however, its specificity seems to be as high as that of the other two techniques and, according to some publications, is even higher than that of ERCP. Most studies report ERCP to be more sensitive than CT in the diagnosis of chronic pancreatitis, though in some publications CT is the most sensitive test.

In regard to chronic pancreatitis, all three techniques have their strong points. ERCP is the best technique for the fine assessment of pancreatic and bile duct changes, but it bears the risk of overdiagnosis and consequently of reduced specificity (Gowland et al. 1981; Jones et al. 1989; Schmitz-Moormann et al. 1985). US and CT are more successful than ERCP in demonstrating pseudocysts (Baert et al. 1981; Cotton et al. 1980; Frederic 1983; Kolars et al. 1989; Laxson et al. 1985; Pinson et al. 1990; Pringot et al. 1979; Triller et al. 1980). Moreover US is the least invasive technique (Swobodnik et al. 1983) and thus the most suitable for the follow-up of pseudocysts (Gmelin et al. 1981). CT is the best technique for the evaluation of the pancreatic contours and surroundings (Foley et al. 1980; Gmelin et al. 1981; Pringot et al. 1979). For all these reasons the highest diagnostic score in respect of chronic pancreatitis is achieved by the combination of ERCP and other imaging techniques (Swobodnik et al. 1983).

7.2.5.6 Indications for ERCP

The indications for ERCP in chronic pancreatitis are diagnosis, preoperative staging, and sometimes endoscopic therapy (Axon 1989; Helwig et al. 1990; Schuman 1990).

Diagnosis
One group of patients referred for ERCP are those with unexplained abdominal pain in whom other investigations have failed to establish a diagnosis (Axon 1986). Furthermore ERCP is a valuable method in the sometimes difficult differential diagnosis between chronic pancreatitis and pancreatic carcinoma.

Preoperative Staging
Before deciding on pancreatic surgery in chronic pancreatitis, exact anatomic information is required (Aranha et al. 1984; Axon 1986; Frick et al. 1982; Laxson et al. 1985; Pringot et al. 1979). The surgical possibilities in the management of chronic pancreatitis are: cholecystectomy and choledochotomy to remove calculi, drainage procedures between a markedly dilated main pancreatic duct or pseudocyst and the gastrointestinal tract, partial or total pancreatectomy, and surgical decompression of dilated bile ducts.

The following anomalies may be considered for, or have to be identified prior to, surgical intervention: a stricture or obstruction of the main pancreatic duct with prestenotic dilatation, whether or not in combination with intraductal lithiasis, a stricture or obstruction of the common bile duct, a pseudocyst and its relation with the main pancreatic duct, and lithiasis of the gallbladder and biliary tract.

Finally, it is important to identify the developmental anomaly pancreas divisum before surgical intervention in chronic pancreatitis. Earlier reports suggested a relationship between pancreas divisum and chronic pancreatitis (Cotton 1980; Richter et al. 1981). This hypothesis was not, however, confirmed in later, larger series (Delhaye et al. 1985; Ott and Rösch 1983). Chronic pancreatitis usually occurs in the dorsal part of the pancreas divisum but sometimes occurs in its ventral part (Brinberg et al. 1988) (Fig. 7.26).

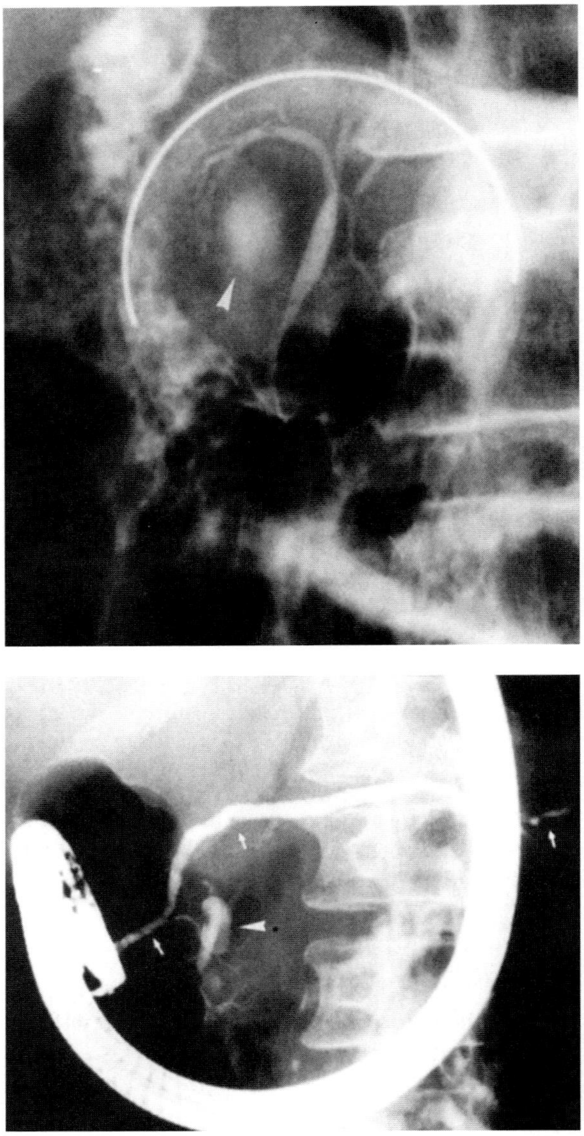
a
b

Fig. 7.26a,b. Chronic pancreatitis in pancreas divisum. **a** Ventral pancreas. Note the partial opacification of a pseudocyst (*arrowhead*). **b** Opacification of the main duct of the dorsal pancreas via Santorini's duct. Slightly irregular lining of this main duct (*small arrows*) is suggestive of chronic pancreatitis. Note also the residual contrast in the small pseudocyst (*arrowhead*) in superposition with the branches of the ventral pancreas, visualized in (**a**)

Endoscopic Therapy
Several endoscopic techniques can be used for the treatment of chronic pancreatitis (Axon 1986; Rohrmann and Baron 1989). The most frequently performed endoscopic therapy, used in acute rather than in chronic pancreatitis, is ampullary sphincterotomy followed by bile duct stone extraction. Other hitherto less frequent therapeutic procedures are sphincterotomy followed by pancreatic duct stone extraction, stent placement in the main pancreatic duct for important stenosis or lithiasis, stent placement in the common bile duct for important stenosis, and endoscopic drainage of pseudocysts into the stomach or duodenum.

7.2.6
Other Pancreatography Techniques

If ERCP is impossible, unsuccessful, or incomplete, and if simultaneously the duct of Wirsung appears dilated, an attempt may be made to perform US-guided percutaneous pancreatography with the patient under local anesthesia (Chong et al. 1992; Lees and Heron 1987) (Fig. 7.27). If this technique also fails, peroperative pancreatography is still possible (Guien 1972).

7.2.7 Percutaneous Transhepatic Cholangiography

7.2.7.1 Technique

The technique, indications, contraindications, results, and complications of percutaneous transhepatic cholangiography (PTC) have been reported previously (Okuda et al. 1974; Ponette et al. 1978d). Within the context of chronic pancreatitis, antibiotic prophylaxis may be indicated when performing PTC in cases of common bile duct stenosis (Van Steenbergen et al. 1990b).

7.2.7.2 Bile Duct Changes

The possible bile duct changes of chronic pancreatitis that are visualized by PTC have been described in several reports (Aranha et al. 1984; Neff et al. 1984; Rohrmann and Baron 1989; Van Steenbergen et al. 1990b) and have already largely been dealt with in Sect. 7.2.5. They include a smooth symmetric stricture of the pancreatic portion of the common bile duct (Caroli I or III lesions), a deviation of the common bile duct, and, rarely, complete obstruction. In PTC the obstruction is visualized from upstream and generally appears smoothly lined. In our experience, an irregular lining of a common bile duct stenosis or obstruction, an abrupt transition of this stenosis or obstruction, or a concomitant asymmetric impression of small radius on the duct are suggestive of pancreatic cancer.

Especially in cases of complete obstruction of the common bile duct by chronic pancreatitis; the differential diagnosis with pancreatic carcinoma is difficult (Figs. 7.28, 7.29). The degree of prestenotic bile duct dilatation in general seems less important in chronic pancreatitis than in pancreatic carcinoma. Moreover, in our experience correct differential diagnosis between chronic pancreatitis and pancreatic cancer is enhanced by combination of the results of ERCP without bile duct opacification and PTC.

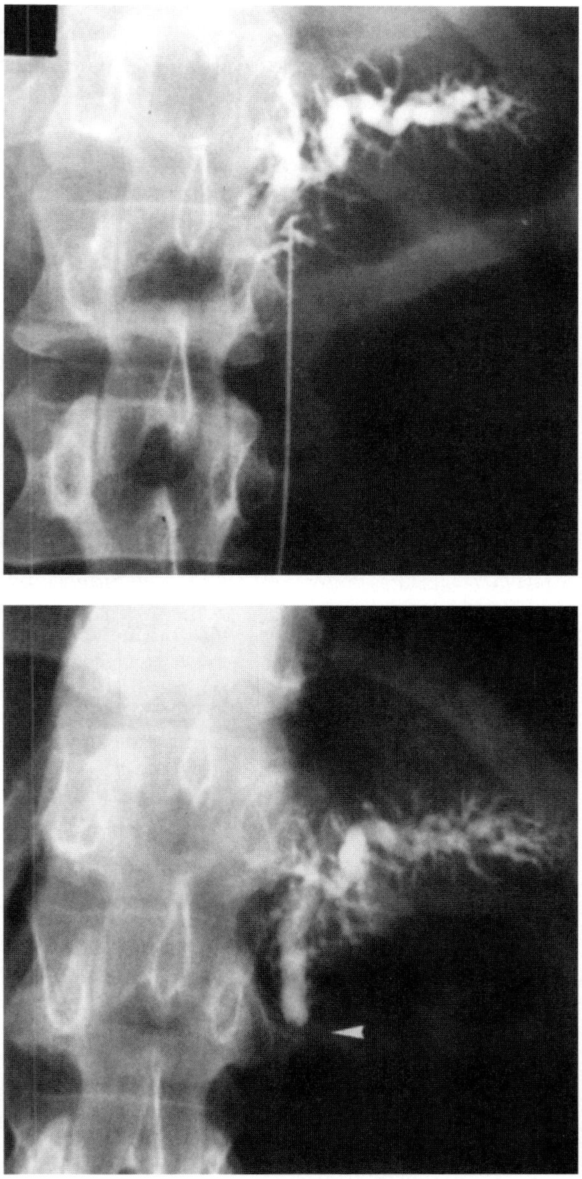

a

b

Fig. 7.27a,b. Percutaneous pancreatography. Previously, a partial pancreatic resection had been performed for a duct of Wirsung stenosis in the head–body transition area, terminoterminal pancreatojejunostomy at the pancreatic body side. Anatomopathologic examination revealed chronic pancreatitis. The patient subsequently suffered recurrent attacks of acute pancreatitis. **a** Injection of contrast into the main pancreatic duct via a Chiba needle. **b** Obstruction of the body segment of the main pancreatic duct in the pancreatojejunostomy area, confirmed by reoperation. (Anatomopathologic examination: chronic pancreatitis)

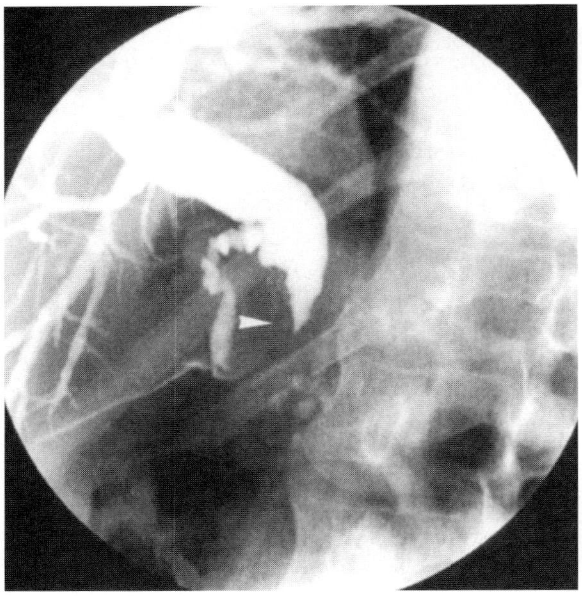

Fig. 7.28. Chronic pancreatitis with common bile duct obstruction. Opacification of bile ducts by percutaneous transhepatic cholangiography. Note the symmetric and gradually tapering obstruction of the intrapancreatic segment of the common bile duct (*arrowhead*). The calcifications around the obstruction suggest chronic pancreatitis, and this was confirmed at operation

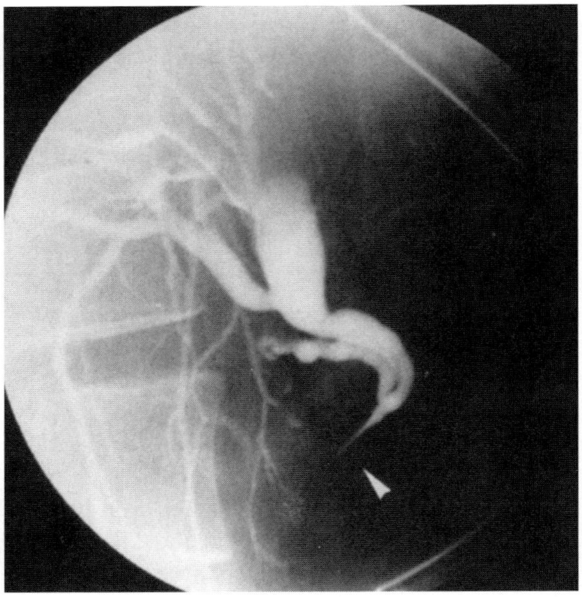

Fig. 7.29. Chronic pancreatitis with common bile duct obstruction. Opacification of bile ducts by percutaneous transhepatic cholangiography (PTC). Note a rather long and smooth, gradually tapering obstruction in the pancreatic part of the common bile duct (*arrowhead*). The absence of calcifications hindered the correct preoperative PTC diagnosis of chronic pancreatitis

7.2.7.3 Indications

Like ERCP, PTC has three main indications in chronic pancreatitis: diagnosis, preoperative assessment, and therapeutic management. The common diagnostic indication for PTC in chronic pancreatitis is the partial failure of ERCP, resulting in a pancreatogram without a cholangiogram in patients in whom bile duct stenosis is suspected. The second indication for PTC in chronic pancreatitis is the need to gather anatomic information on the biliary tract so that a decision can be made on whether to perform a surgical bilidigestive anastomosis (Aranha et al. 1984; Van Steenbergen et al. 1990b). Lastly, in some cases of common bile duct stenosis, percutaneous external or internal drainage may be indicated as an alternative to endoscopic stent placement (Rohrmann and Baron 1989), or as an intermediate step prior to such placement.

7.2.8 Other Direct Cholangiography Techniques

Besides ERCP and PTC, two other techniques have to be mentioned in the context of direct cholangiography. Peroperative cholangiography is performed when preoperative ERCP and PTC have failed in the opacification ofbile ducts. Transjugular cholangiography (Kadell and Weiner 1973; Ponette et al. 1977), has now been abandoned because of the relative advantages of the newer techniques.

7.2.9 Intravenous Cholangiography

Prior to the advent of ERCP, intravenous cholangiography (IVC), was an essential technique in the exploration of chronic pancreatitis (Guien 1972; Pringot et al. 1976). In recent years it has been applied far less often in this disease for several reasons: the image contrast is poorer than in direct cholangiography, the image quality is still worse in cases of impaired bile evacuation, and ERCP is able to provide not only a cholangiogram but also a pancreatogram. IVC is, however, still indicated in cases of chronic pancreatitis where ERCP has resulted in a pancreatogram without a cholangiogram and where the liver function tests are normal.

The appearance of the common bile duct changes on IVC in chronic pancreatitis is the same as that on direct cholangiography and was reported in earlier publications (GUIEN 1972; PRINGOT et al. 1976).

7.2.10
Alimentary Tract Opacification

In the era prior to the application of the modern imaging methods for visualization of the pancreas, gastrointestinal tract opacification (and especially hypotonic duodenography) was an important technique in the diagnosis of chronic pancreatitis (GUIEN 1972; PRINGOT et al. 1976; PONETTE et al. 1978a). However, the study of the alimentary tract remains important for two reasons. First, many patients with chronic pancreatitis present atypical abdominal complaints and a barium examination may be ordered by the clinician before US or CT (BAERT et al. 1981). Second, complications of chronic pancreatitis, such as acute exacerbation, a large pseudocyst, or abscess formation, may cause obvious alimentary tract changes. Thus the current importance of alimentary tract study in chronic pancreatitis lies in the staging rather than the diagnosis of the disease.

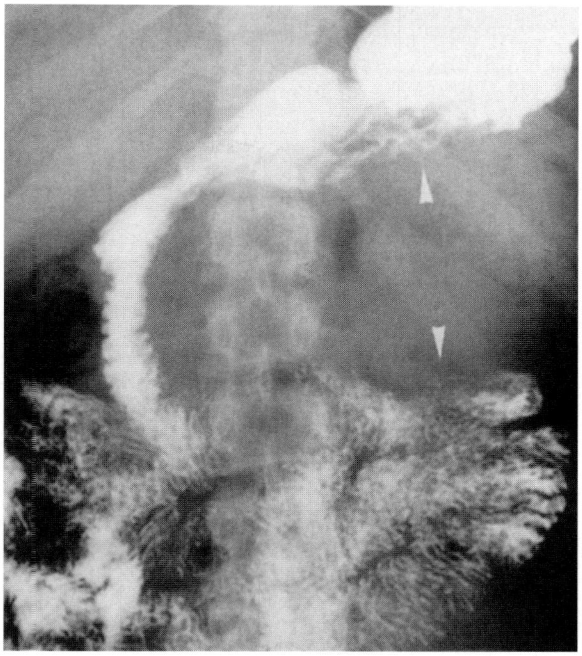

Fig. 7.30. Large pancreatic pseudocyst with gastric and jejunal alterations. Note extrinsic impression on greater gastric curve and caudal displacement of the duodeno-jejunal transition (*arrowheads*) due to an ultrasonography-proven pseudocyst of the body and tail of the pancreas

7.2.10.1
Stomach

Very large pancreatic pseudocysts may produce an extrinsic impression on the posterior gastric wall (PONETTE et al. 1978b) (Fig. 7.30). Pen-gastritis and gastric fistula, resulting from exacerbation of pancreatitis or infected pancreatic pseudocyst, ; are rare.

7.2.10.2
Duodenum

Duodenal impression due to a pseudocyst in the head of the pancreas is generally located at the internal border (PONETTE et al. 1978b) (Fig. 7.31). Deformity of this border may also occur in chronic pancreatitis without pseudocyst, either by attraction due to pancreatic fibrosis or by impression due to an inflammatory pancreatic mass effect (PONETTE et al. 1978a). Attraction causes spiculation of the mucosal folds of the internal duodenal border (Fig. 7.31); the epsilon or inverted "3" sign of Frostberg is probably due to impression. Other possible alterations of the internal duodenal border are flattening and, in rare instances, slight nodularity. All of these alterations are, however, nonspecific and also may be encoun-

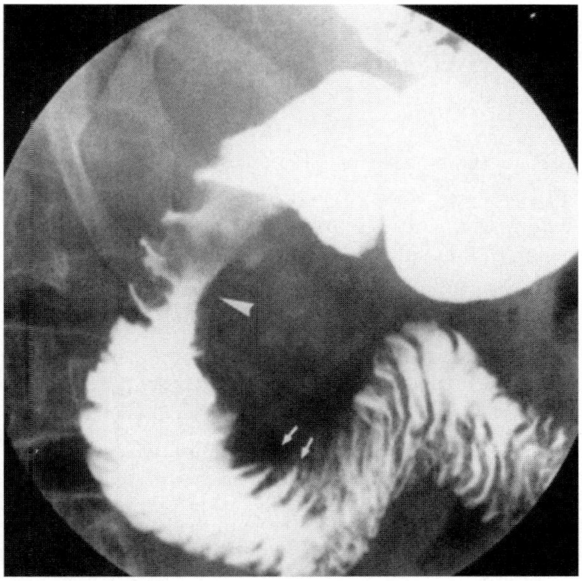

Fig. 7.31. Chronic pancreatitis with duodenal alterations. Note the extrinsic impression on the inner border of the proximal half of the descending part of the duodenum (*arrowhead*) due to an ultrasonography-proven pseudocyst with surrounding calcifications. Note also the spiculation of mucosal folds in the distal half of the descending duodenum (*arrows*), probably caused by attraction due to pancreatic fibrosis

tered in cancer of the head of the pancreas (PRINGOT et al. 1976).

Concentric duodenal narrowing is rather seldom in chronic pancreatitis and also may be found in pancreatic cancer (PONETTE et al. 1978e) (Fig. 7.32). Duodenal fistula due to pancreatitis is very rare.

7.2.10.3 Small Intestine

Changes of the duodenojejunal transition area due to chronic pancreatitis may occur in the same circumstances as duodenal lesions (Fig. 7.30). Small bowel lesions distal to the duodenojejunal transition area, however, are exceedingly rare.

7.2.10.4 Colon

Possible colonic abnormalities indirectly due to chronic pancreatitis are impression by a pseudocyst and narrowing or fistula formation following pericolitis. These lesions result from complications of chronic pancreatitis (MARKS and BANK 1985). The splenic flexure and transverse colon are most frequently affected but lesions of the ascending and descending colon may also occur (L'HERMINÉ et al. 1980) (Fig. 7.33). Association of chronic pancreatitis

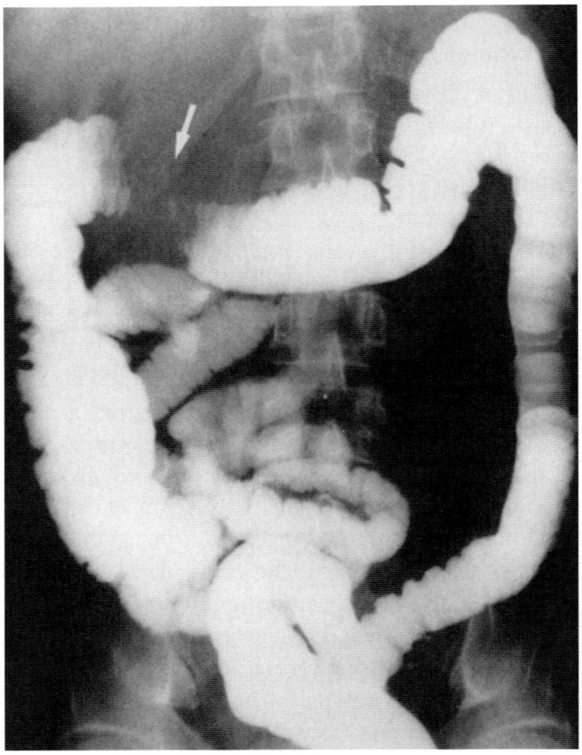

Fig. 7.33. Large pancreatic pseudocyst with colonic impression. Note narrowing of the right transverse colon with conserved mucosal folds (*arrow*), caused by extrinsic impression due to a large ultrasonography-proven pseudocyst of the head of the pancreas

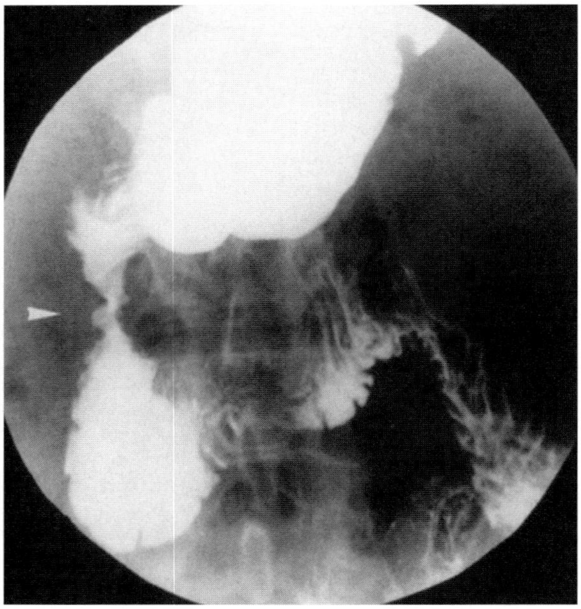

Fig. 7.32. Chronic pancreatitis with concentric duodenal narrowing. Thickened mucosal folds are observed (*arrowhead*). This type of duodenal alteration is less common in chronic pancreatitis than those illustrated in Fig. 7.31

and ulcerative colitis is rarely reported (VAN STEENBERGEN et al. 1986).

7.2.11 Computed Tomography

Helical (spiral) CT is the technique of choice for the evaluation of suspected pancreatic abnormalities. Helical CT permits scanning of the entire pancreas during a single breath hold, during the optimal temporal window of contrast medium administration (RICHTER et al. 1996). This ability of helical CT to acquire motion free, thin section images of the pancreas precisely tuned to peak parenchymal and vascular enhancement, renders this form of imaging ideally suited to the evaluation of vascular structures and vascular complications (thrombosis, pseudoaneurysms) in cases of chronic pancreatitis. To evaluate vascular structure, image analysis should begin with a careful review of reconstructed axial images. Multiplanar reformatted images generally are the next step and often clarify confusing anatomy promptly. True three-dimensional (3D) rendering (maximum intensity projection, shaded surface display), although often not necessary for diagnostic purposes and always time consuming, provides an excellent demonstration of pancreatic vascular anatomy.

Our protocol includes a prior bowel opacification in order to differentiate acute fluid collections from small bowel and stomach. The scan volume is chosen to include the entire abdomen. Unenhanced slices are necessary to eliminate recent hemorrhage. Contrast-enhanced acquisition is performed after intravenous injection of 2 ml/kg of body weight of iodinated contrast agent (300 mg of iodine per milliliter) using a power injector. Dual phase helical acquisition was obtained 30 s (collimation, 3 mm; table speed, 4.5 mm/s; pitch, 1.5) and 60 s (collimation, 5 mm; table speed, 7.5 mm/s; pitch, 1.5) after injection of contrast medium with a rate of 3–4 ml/s. Vascularization of the pancreas is best evaluated at the peak of pancreatic perfusion (initial phase). The whole abdominal cavity from the diaphragm down to the pelvis is surveyed during the other phase.

A normal CT appearance does not exclude the diagnosis of chronic pancreatitis (LUETMER et al. 1989). Morphologic changes observed are identical to those previously described.

7.2.11.1 Dilatation of the Main Pancreatic Duct

According to recent series, dilatation of the main pancreatic duct (MPD) is present in up to 68% of cases of chronic pancreatitis (LUETMER et al. 1989). The maximal normal MPD diameter is usually considered to be 5 mm in the head and 2 mm in the body and tail. These findings are nonspecific since such dilatation can also be found in pancreatic and ampullary carcinoma (Fig. 7.34). Although a beaded appearance is more typical, smooth and irregular patterns can be found, and none of these presentations can characterize the cause of the dilatation. Associated intraductal calcification within a dilated main pancreatic duct is more in favor of chronic pancreatitis, but even a dilated main duct followed up to the level of the ampulla does not exclude ampullary carcinoma (Fig. 7.35).

7.2.11.2 Pancreatic Calcifications

Pancreatic calcifications are more easily detected with CT than with US. They have been reported in up to 50% of cases (LUETMER et al. 1989). They vary widely in size and distribution (Figs. 7.36, 7.37). Tiny stippled to large coarse calcifications can be observed, the latter most usually being found in patients with hereditary chronic pancreatitis. Although their intraductal location is not always evident on CT, they are most often located in the ductal system. Regression of calcifications may be observed despite progression of the disease.

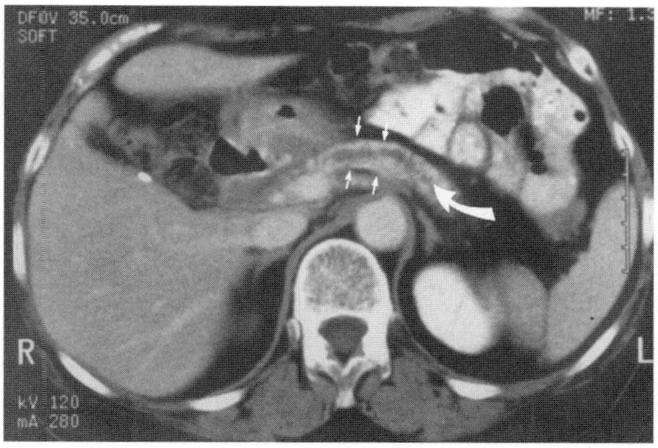

Fig. 7.34. Enhanced computed tomography of chronic pancreatitis. Typical dilatation of the main pancreatic duct (*curved arrow*) associated with thinning of the pancreatic gland (*small arrows*)

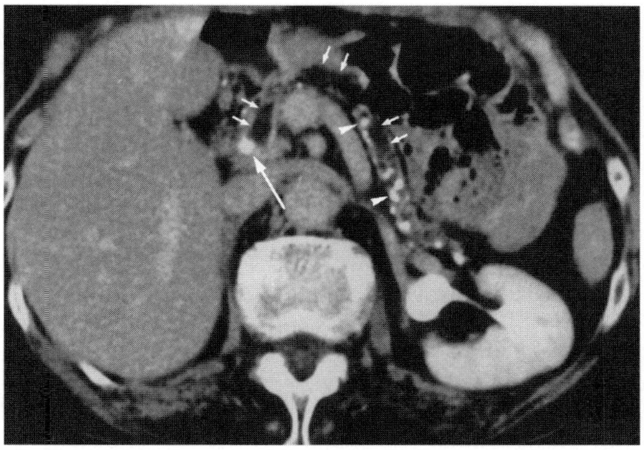

Fig. 7.35. Enhanced computed tomography of calcified chronic pancreatitis. Small intraductal calcifications are depicted in the body and tail of the pancreas (*arrowheads*). The pancreatic gland is atrophic. A calculus (*large arrow*) is shown in the main pancreatic duct within the head of the gland, just below the dilated duct segment (*small arrows*)

7.2.11.3 Modification of Size, Shape, and Contour

While diffuse enlargement is common in acute pancreatitis, it is a less common finding in chronic pancreatitis. Pancreatic atrophy, a subjective finding

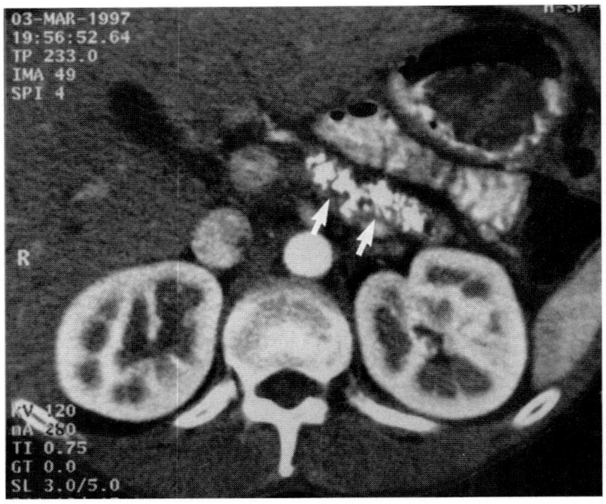

Fig. 7.36. Helical enhanced computed tomography (arterial phase) of calcified chronic pancreatitis. Extensive small intraductal calcifications (*arrows*) are shown involving the body of the pancreas

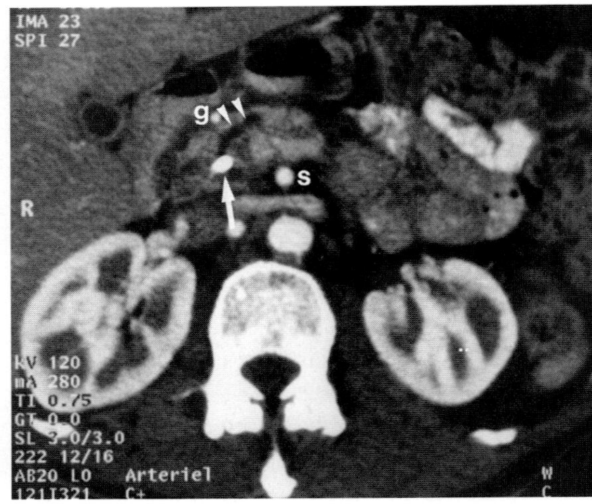

Fig. 7.37. Helical enhanced computed tomography (arterial phase) of chronic pancreatitis. A large coarse calcification (*arrow*) of the pancreatic head associated with upstream dilated pancreatic duct (*arrowheads*). *g*, Gastroduodenal artery; *s*, superior mesenteric artery

judged as the thinning of the gland, together with the ductal dilatation, has been reported in 10%–54% of cases (LUETMER et al. 1989).

Focal pancreatic enlargement can be due to extensive interlobular and periductal fibrous tissue proliferation as well as chronic infiltration by inflammatory cells. Enlargement can occur to varying degrees, with or without calcifications throughout the mass or at its periphery (Fig. 7.38). Visualization of dilated ductal branches within the mass is difficult to differentiate from pseudocysts (LUETMER et al. 1989).

Differentiation from a malignant process is extremely difficult, although the presence of ductal calculi within the mass is more suggestive of a benign lesion. Obliteration of the peripancreatic fat, giving an ill-defined contour, is usually seen in acute episodes. Although obliteration of fat and encasement of the mesenteric artery or celiac trunk have been described in patients with pancreatic ductal carcinomas, these findings have been found in a large retrospective series to be nonspecific, and also to occur in chronic pancreatitis with or without acute episodes (SCHULTE et al. 1991).

In the differentiation between chronic pancreatitis and adenocarcinomas, DEL MASCHIO et al. (1991) found a sensitivity for US and CT of 98% and 94% and a specificity of 90% and 95%, respectively. Both techniques were superior to serum CA 19-9 assay (sensitivity and specificity of 81%), but inferior to CT-guided fine needle aspiration biopsy, which proved to be the most reliable diagnostic technique with sensitivity, specificity, and positive and negative predictive values of 100% (DEL MASCHIO et al. 1991). However, US and CT should often be considered as complementary techniques in the diagnosis of pancreatic mass.

7.2.11.4 Pseudocysts

Pseudocysts can occur in chronic pancreatitis with or without superimposed acute pancreatitis. Their reported incidence is about 25%–40%. Although

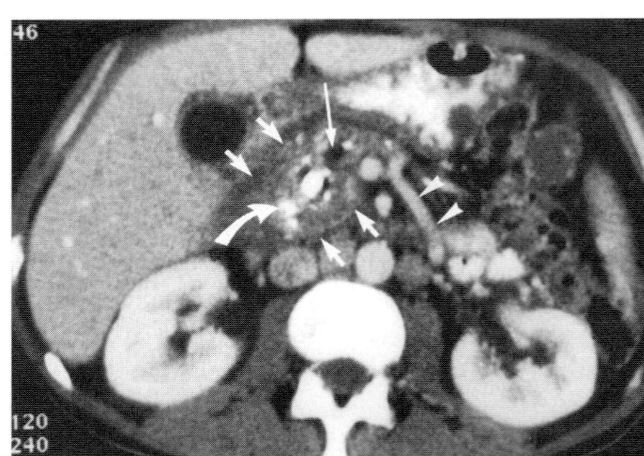

Fig. 7.38. Helical enhanced computed tomography (portal phase) of calcified chronic pancreatitis. The head of the pancreas is enlarged (*small arrows*) associated with calcifications (*curved arrow*) and a dilatation of the pancreatic duct branch (*thin arrow*). Dilatation of the inferior mesenteric vein (*arrowheads*) is due to compression of the portal vein by the pseudomass of the head of the pancreas

often detectable by US, they are best evaluated with CT. They vary in shape and size and can be located in intra- (Fig. 7.39) or extrapancreatic sites, namely greater and lesser sac (Fig. 7.40), perirenal spaces, psoas sheath, and within the liver or spleen. On CT, they appear encapsulated, containing low attenuation fluid. Presence of intracystic gas bubbles may indicate infection or gastrointestinal tract fistulae.

US and CT are efficient methods of guiding percutaneous drainage. In large series, their efficiency has been reported as up to 90% with a low complication rate (FREENY 1988; VAN SONNENBERG et al. 1989; GROSSO et al. 1989). It is presently acknowledged that treatment of pancreatic pseudocyst solely by needle aspiration is ineffective. A sufficiently long percutaneous drainage is required until closure of existing fistulae with the main pancreatic duct. The choice of drainage route is controversial. The most direct route avoiding the bowel is recommended. Retroperitoneal, transperitoneal, transhepatic, and transgastric approaches have also been reported with success.

Complications of pseudocyst include infection, hemorrhage, rupture, and obstruction of biliary tract or bowel. Infected cysts should be drained on an emergency basis. Other therapeutic indications are controversial. Symptomatic, obstructive lesions and large cysts prone to serious complications are usually drained (VAN SONNENBERG et al. 1989).

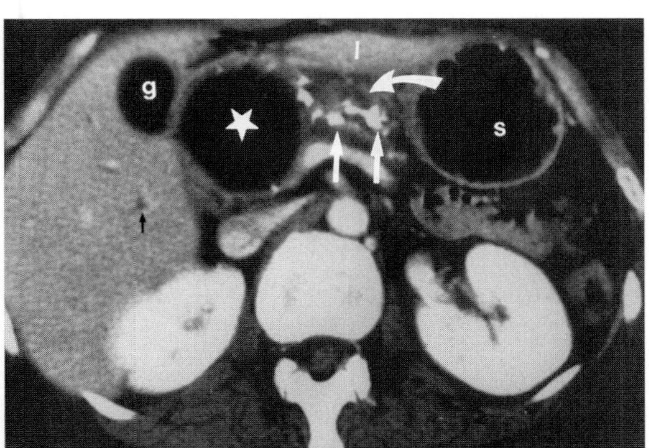

Fig. 7.39. Helical enhanced computed tomography of calcified chronic pancreatitis. A mild intrahepatic biliary dilatation is depicted (*black arrows*) secondary to a compressive pseudocyst of the head of the pancreas (*star*). A dilated main pancreatic duct (*curved arrow*) and calcifications (*arrows*) are also shown. *s*, Stomach; *g*, gallbladder; *l*, liver

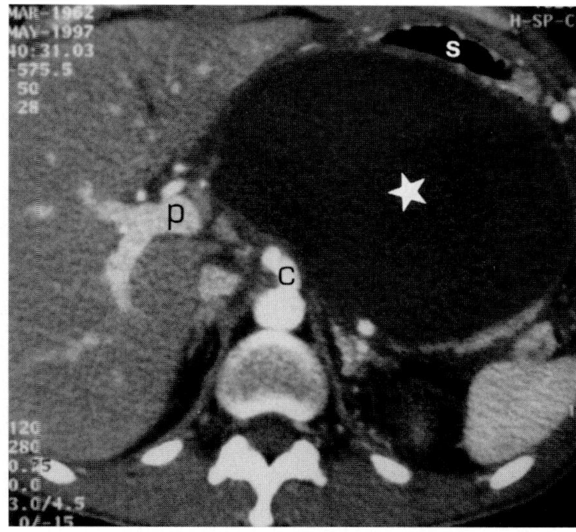

Fig. 7.40. Helical enhanced computed tomography of pseudocyst. A large pseudocyst (*star*) has developed within the lesser sac displacing anteriorly the stomach (*s*), celiac trunk (*c*), and portal vein (*p*)

7.2.11.5 Biliary Complications

Biliary complications include cholestasis, cholangitis, fistulization affecting the hepatobiliary system, and secondary biliary cirrhosis (ROHRMAN and BARON 1989).

Cholestasis is present in two thirds of patients with chronic pancreatitis, most commonly being due to inflammatory stricture. The most common US and CT finding is a dilated common bile duct (CBD) proximal to a tapered stricture. On CT, the typical finding of smooth gradual tapering of the intrapancreatic portion of CBD can be seen as serial circles of progressively decreasing diameter (HUNTINGTON et al. 1989). However, focal masses can cause abrupt termination similar to pancreatic carcinoma. Clinical and ERCP/magnetic resonance cholangiopancreatography (MRCP) correlations, serial examinations, and fine needle percutaneous biopsy may be required to exclude malignancy.

Choledocholithiasis can be the consequence of pancreatic inflammation. In cases with bile tree dilatation, US sensitivity for detection proved to be 45%–80%, while that of CT was up to 75%–90%. One third of cases of choledocholithiasis do not involve dilatation and hence are more difficult to detect (ROHRMAN and BARON 1989).

Pancreaticobiliary fistulae can be evidenced by contrast injection in the draining tube or by retrograde or percutaneous cholangiography. Management of biliary complications is also possible with interventional techniques (van Sonnenberg et al. 1989).

7.2.11.6 Vascular Complications

Arterial bleeding should be considered in patients with repeated episodes of gastrointestinal bleeding and in patients with increasing abdominal pain or an enlarging pulsatile abdominal mass. Mortality in these cases approaches 50%, so emergency imaging studies are required (Vujic 1989). Because of their contiguity with the pancreas, the splenic and hepatic arteries are the vessels most commonly involved, but all peripancreatic or pancreatic vessels can be equally implicated. Erosion of arteries can result in free hemorrhage from the erosion site or in the formation of a pseudoaneurysm. Pseudoaneurysms may develop in pancreatic pseudocyst, or a pseudocyst may erode into an adjacent artery. The end result of both processes is the formation of total or partial vascular cystic mass. On rare occasions, the vascular mass may rupture into the pancreatic duct producing "hemosuccus pancreaticus". Rupture into the aorta, portal vein, and venous tributaries has also been reported (van Steenbergen and Ponette 1990).

Enhanced CT can diagnose the presence of hemorrhage within a fluid collection by displaying increased attenuation on plain CT, and identify a pseudoaneurysm by displaying transient vascular enhancement of the cystic mass (Fig. 7.41). A diagnosis of arterial complication is nowadays usually made prior to angiography (Pantongrag-Brown et al. 1991).

Venous complications are being increasingly recognized, with splenic occlusion seen in 45% of patients in some studies (Vujic 1989). Segmented or total portal vein thrombosis with cavernous transformation is diagnosed by many noninvasive tests; color Doppler US and enhanced CT are the most efficient (Zalcman et al. 1987). Multiple collateral pathways, including left and right gastroepiploic veins, tend to develop. Visualization of a dilated (>6 mm) left gastroepiploic vein on CT has been shown to be an early response to splenic vein disease in patients with chronic pancreatitis (Moody and Poon 1992).

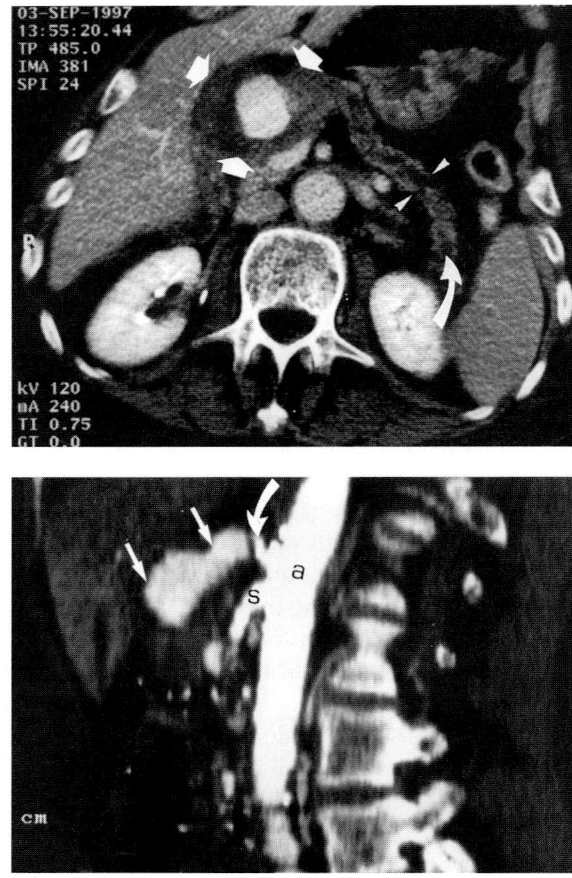

a

b

Fig. 7.41a,b. Helical enhanced computed tomography of chronic pancreatitis. **a** Detection of a partially thrombosed pseudoaneurysm (*arrows*) within the head of the pancreas in a patient complaining of abdominal pain associated with gastrointestinal bleeding. The pancreatic gland is thin (*arrowhead*) and the pancreatic duct is dilated (*curved arrow*). **b** On sagittal oblique reformatted reconstruction (arterial phase), the pseudoaneurysm (*arrows*) seems to be connected with the hepatic artery (*curved arrow*). Surgery was performed. *a*, Aorta; *s*, superior mesenteric artery

7.2.11.7 Postoperative Imaging

CT is valuable in detecting surgical complications and recurrence or progression of the primary disease. Complications occurring shortly after surgery include anastomotic leak, fluid collection, and abscess. They are best evaluated by a combination of contrast studies and CT.

7.2.12
Magnetic Resonance Imaging

L Van Hoe, R. Lecesne

7.2.12.1
Introduction

Until recently, ERCP and percutaneous transhepatic cholangiography (PTC) were the only techniques capable of providing continuity images of the pancreatic duct. The invasive nature of both techniques, however, carries inherent mortality and morbidity of 1% and 7%, respectively (Lenriot et al. 1993). Acute pancreatitis is one of the most frequently encountered complications of ERCP (Sherman and Lehman 1991). Magnetic resonance imaging (MRI) combines the advantages of cross-sectional imaging techniques such as US and CT, with the ability to visualize the pancreatic duct as in ERCP and PTC.

7.2.12.2
Technique

A pancreatic MR examination should always include T1- and T2-weighted images and projective MR cholangiograms. Obtaining dynamic contrast-enhanced images may be helpful, particularly if clinical data or initial imaging findings suggest the presence of a pancreatic neoplasm. A variety of imaging techniques has been proposed by different authors (Mitchell et al. 1995; Semelka et al. 1996; Miyazaki et al. 1996; Ichikawa et al. 1996; Laubenberger et al. 1995; Reuther et al. 1996; Wallner et al. 1991; Reinhold and Bret 1996; Reinhold et al. 1996; Soto et al. 1995a,b). With the introduction of snapshot T1- and T2-weighted MRI, breath-hold dynamic contrast-enhanced imaging, and breath-hold rapid acquisition with relaxation-enhanced (RARE) cholangiography, a large number of images each displaying a different aspect of the same organ can be obtained within 30–40 min (Van Hoe et al. 1998b). Our standard protocol consists of double echo half-Fourier single-shot turbo spin echo (HASTE) (images obtained in axial and coronal planes) and turbo fast low-angle shot (FLASH) (axial plane) images. All images are obtained during quiet breathing. As a next step, continuity images of the pancreatic duct are generated using a breath-hold RARE sequence with an effective TE of 1100 ms and 3-cm slice thickness. After real-time evaluation of all these images on the console, the radiologist decides on the next step. This can be to perform a contrast-enhanced study, to perform a dynamic study of the sphincter of Oddi, to give specific contrast media or drugs, or to let the patient leave the examination room.

For a more detailed discussion of technical advances in pancreatic MRI-MRCP, see Chap. 8.

Usually, no drugs are administered in pancreatic MRI. However, administration of secretin has been recommended to improve the visualization of subtle ductal abnormalities (Matos et al. 1997).

7.2.12.3
Findings

7.2.12.3.1
Chronic Pancreatitis

Microscopically, the main features of obstructive and alcoholic chronic pancreatitis include dilatation of ducts and acini, and perilobular and intralobular sclerosis. MRI strategies in patients with suspected chronic pancreatitis are thus directed at evaluating fibrosis, calcifications, and secondary ductal changes, as well as carcinoma or intraductal stones. Although very small calcifications are usually not seen on MRI (Fig. 7.42), larger calcifications are seen as small signal-void foci. Fibrosis results in a diminished proteinaceous fluid content of the glandular elements and diminished vascularity of the pancreas. These changes explain the diminished signal intensity of the pancreas on T1-weighted images (Fig. 7.43), and a diminished capillary blush immediately after contrast agent injection. These MRI features may be seen both in patients with and without pancreatic calcifications on CT scans (Semelka et al. 1993). It has been suggested that MRI might detect changes associated with chronic pancreatitis earlier than CT (Semelka and Ascher 1993).

The features of ductal changes in chronic pancreatitis are well known from ERCP studies (Figs. 7.44–7.49). It should be stressed that the MRCP appearance of ductal abnormalities may be quite different from their ERCP appearance. The main reason for this is the fact that during ERCP there is slight overdistension of the pancreatic ducts due to the direct injection of contrast material, while in MRCP the ducts are imaged in their"physiologic" state. As a result, MRCP may be less sensitive in the detection of subtle ductal abnormalities and, in comparison with ERCP, may over- or underestimate the length and severity of stenoses (Soto et al. 1995b; Macauley et al. 1995; Takehara et al. 1994; Van Hoe et al. 1998b).

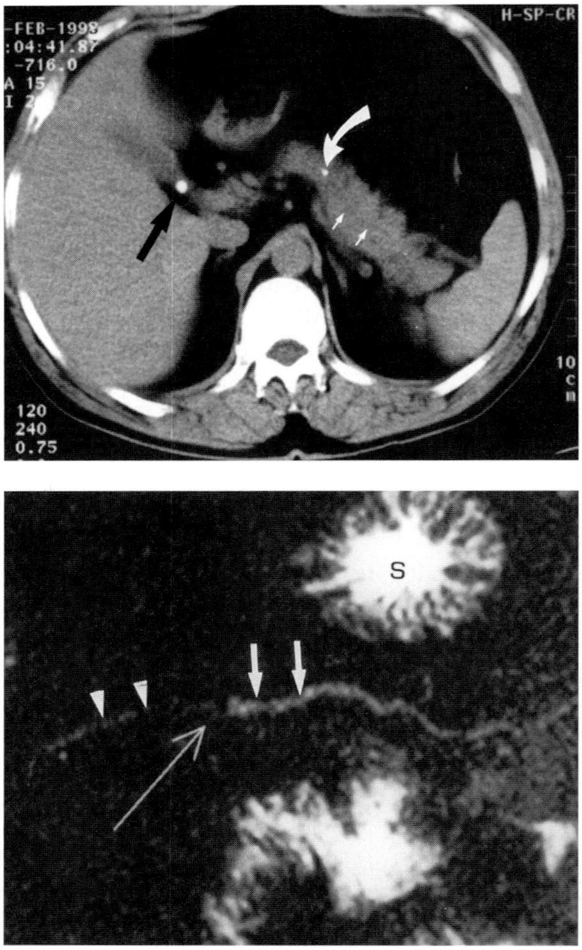

Fig. 7.42a,b. Discrepancy between computed tomography (CT) and magnetic resonance imaging (MRI) in detecting chronic calcified pancreatitis. **a** Plain CT of chronic pancreatitis. A tiny calcification is depicted within the body of the pancreas (*curved arrow*) with an upstream dilated pancreatic duct (*small arrows*). Gallstone (*black arrow*). **b** MR pancreatogram. The stone is not visualized as well as on CT, but suspected (*thin arrow*) at the junction between the upstream dilated (*arrows*) and downstream nondilated pancreatic duct (*arrowheads*). *S*, stomach

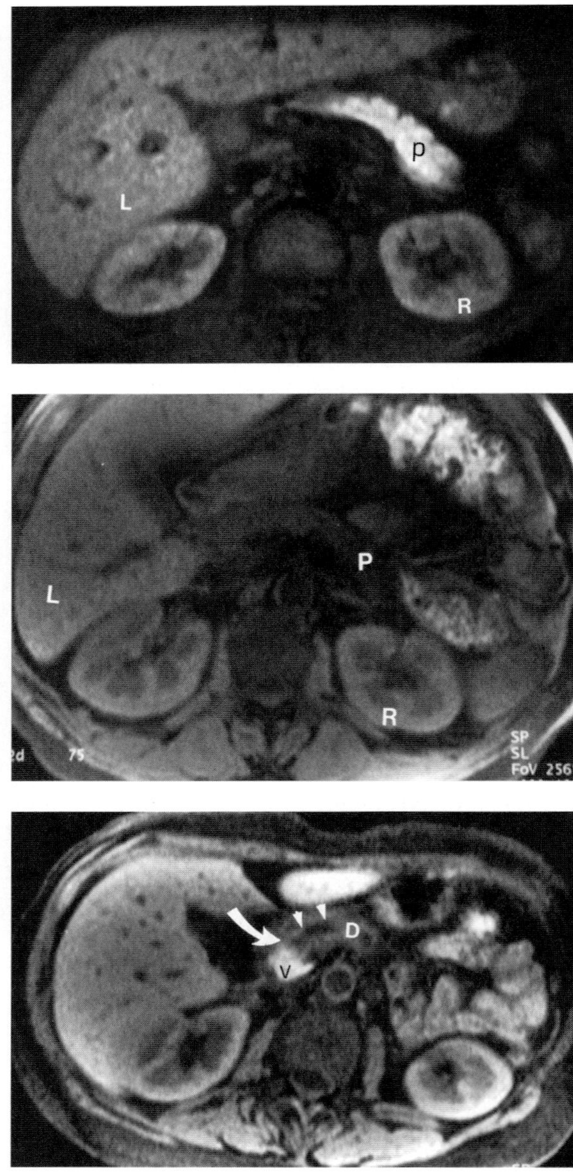

Fig. 7.43a–c. Magnetic resonance imaging of chronic pancreatitis. **a** On fat-saturated T1-weighted sequence. The normal pancreas (*P*) appears lobulated and hyperintense relative to liver (*L*) and renal cortex (*R*). **b** In this case of alcohol-induced chronic pancreatitis on fat-saturated T1-weighted sequence, the pancreas (*P*) appears hypointense relative to liver (*L*) and renal cortex (*R*). **c** A case of obstructive chronic pancreatitis (pancreas divisum associated with stenosis of the minor papilla). A sharp delineation (*curved arrow*) is observed between normal ventral pancreas (*V*) and inflamed dorsal pancreas (*D*) associated with upstream dilated main pancreatic duct (*arrowheads*)

MRCP has been shown to be an excellent modality for the evaluation of main pancreatic duct stones, with reported sensitivities close to 100% (Soto et al. 1995b; Macauley et al. 1995; Takehara et al. 1994).

In non-alcoholic duct-destructive chronic pancreatitis periductal inflammation and duct destruction are prominent features (Ectors et al. 1997). On MRI, this entity commonly presents as a focal mass (see Chap. 8, Fig. 8.52). Fibrosis results in a hypointense aspect of the affected parenchyma on T1-weighted images, and absence of normal blush on dynamic enhanced FLASH images. The periductal inflammatory changes may result in a hyperintense aspect of the pancreatic parenchyma on T2-weighted images; however, a hypointense aspect has also been observed (Van Hoe et al. 1998a). MR cholan-

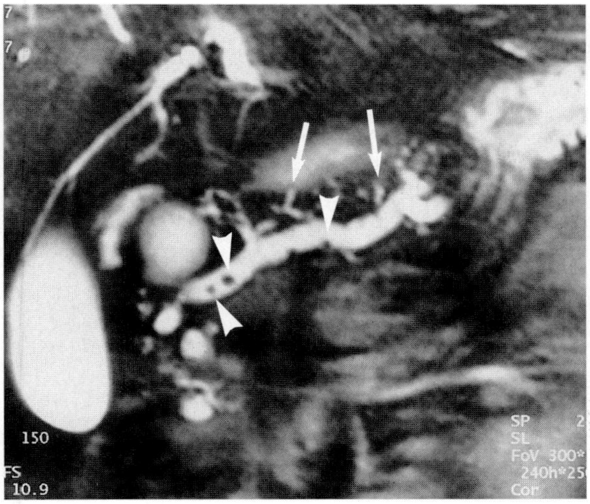

Fig. 7.44. Chronic pancreatitis. Typical ductal changes at magnetic resonance cholangiopancreatography. T2-weighted image obtained in coronal plane shows several dilated side branches of pancreatic duct (*arrows*), together with the presence of intraductal stones (*arrowheads*)

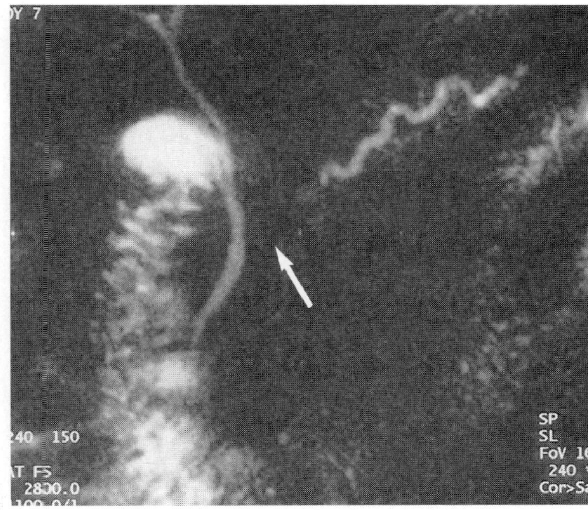

Fig. 7.45. Chronic pancreatitis. Atypical ductal changes. Projective magnetic resonance image shows long stenosis of main pancreatic duct (*arrow*). Although the length of the stenosis suggested tumor rather than pancreatitis as the underlying disorder, no tumor was found

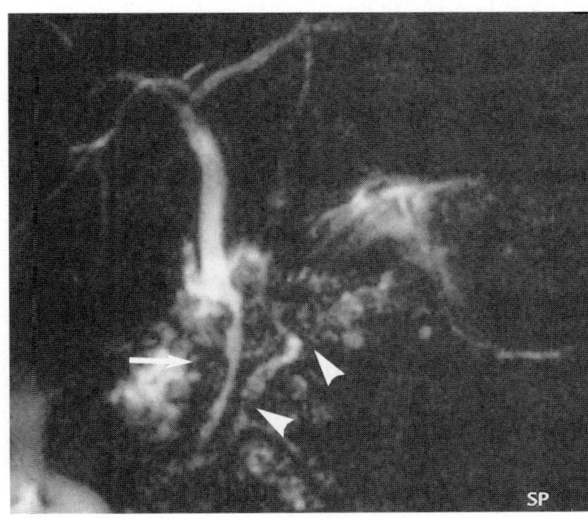

Fig. 7.46. Chronic pancreatitis. Narrowing of common bile duct. Projective magnetic resonance image shows irregular global narrowing of intrapancreatic portion of common bile duct (*arrow*). Also note severe destruction of duct of Wirsung with the presence of pseudocysts and intraductal stones (*arrowheads*)

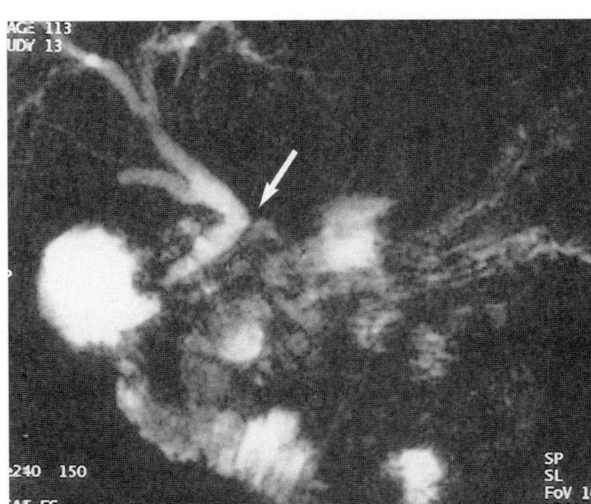

Fig. 7.47. Chronic pancreatitis. Attraction of common bile duct. Projective magnetic resonance image shows attraction of common bile duct (*arrow*), probably resulting from fibrosis. Also note severe destruction of duct of Wirsung with the presence of pseudocysts and intraductal stones

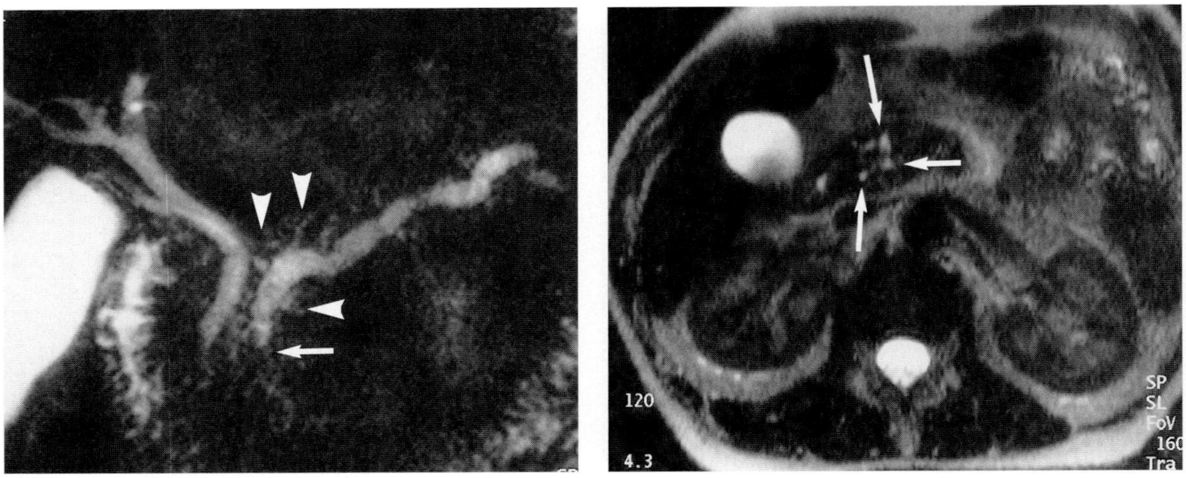

a b

Fig. 7.48a,b. Chronic pancreatitis. Double duct sign. **a** Projective magnetic resonance image shows sudden narrowing of common bile duct and pancreatic duct (*arrow*): double duct sign. Note presence of multiple dilated side branches (*arrowheads*). **b** Cross-sectional T2-weighted image confirms presence of multiple dilated side branches in pancreatic head (*arrows*). No focal mass was seen

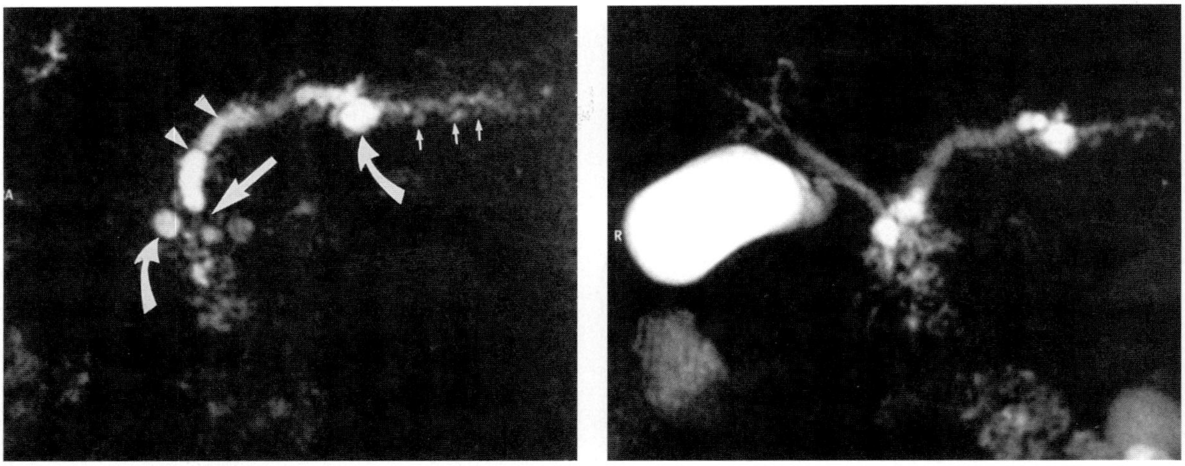

a b

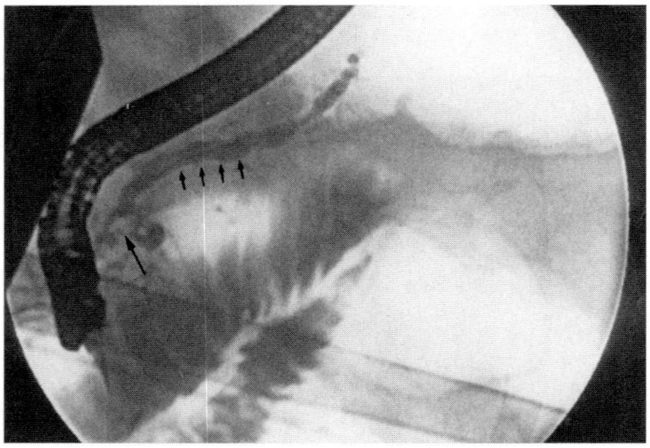

c

Fig. 7.49a–c. Diagnostic value of magnetic resonance cholangiopancreatography (MRCP) in comparison with endoscopic retrograde cholangiopancreatography (ERCP). **a** MRCP focused on the pancreatic duct system (MR pancreatogram). Pseudocyst (*curved arrows*), dilatation of both the main pancreatic duct (*arrowheads*) and its side branches (*small arrows*), and stenosis (*large arrow*) are well shown. **b** MRCP using 6-cm thick slice displays an excellent overview of gallbladder, biliary, and pancreatic duct system. **c** ERCP. Stenosis (*long arrow*) is well detected as the beaded and enlarged main pancreatic duct (*small arrows*). However, noncommunicating pseudocysts are not shown, conversely to MRCP giography typically shows narrowing of the pancreatic duct. Pancreatic carcinoma is the main differential diagnosis (see Chap. 8).

7.2.12.3.2
COMPLICATIONS

Cholestasis, cholangitis, fistulization affecting the hepatobiliary system, and secondary biliary cirrhosis constitute the spectrum of biliary complications that may (uncommonly) be encountered in the setting of chronic pancreatitis (ROHRMANN and BARON 1989). MRCP demonstrates equally as well as ERCP the well-known typical changes in the CBD seen in chronic pancreatitis. These may include gradual tapering, alternating stenosis and dilatation („hourglass“ configuration) (Fig. 7.46), focal lateral or medial deflection, which may be caused by the presence of a pseudocyst (ROHRMANN and BARON 1989), or by fibrosis (Fig. 7.47). The“double duct sign“, which was once considered pathognomonic for pancreatic carcinoma, may also be observed (Fig. 7.48).

Arterial bleeding, pseudoaneurysms, and venous thrombosis are well demonstrated on contrast-enhanced MR images (Figs. 7.50, 7.51).

Pseudocysts are nicely displayed with MRCP (SOTO et al. 1996) (Fig. 7.52). MRCP is also well suited to visualizing pancreatic pleural effusion, which is defined as a massive fluid accumulation in the tho-

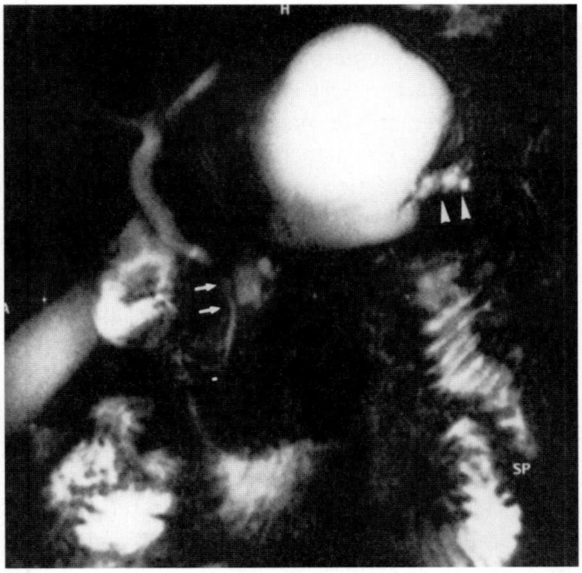

a

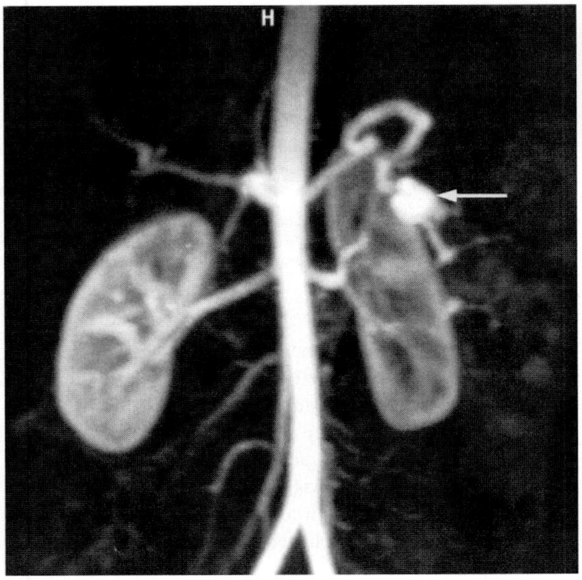

b

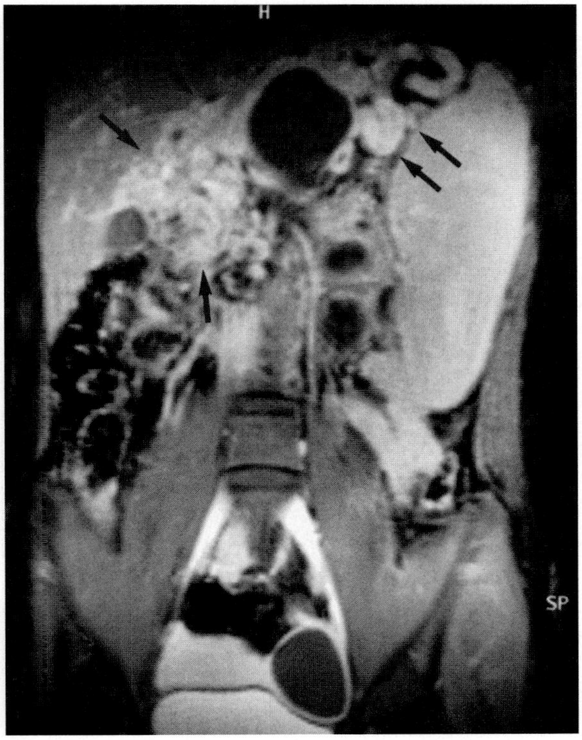

c

Fig. 7.50a–c. Chronic pancreatitis with vascular complications. **a** Projective magnetic resonance (MR) image shows narrowing of common bile duct (*arrows*), dilatation of pancreatic duct in pancreatic tail (*arrowheads*), and presence of a pancreatic pseudocyst. **b** Maximum-intensity projection image obtained in arterial phase shows aneurysm of the splenic artery as an incidental finding (*arrow*). **c** Image obtained in venous phase shows multiple collaterals around the pseudocyst and in the liver hilum (*arrows*) This case illustrates how MRI can be used for "all-in-one" evaluation of complicated pancreatitis

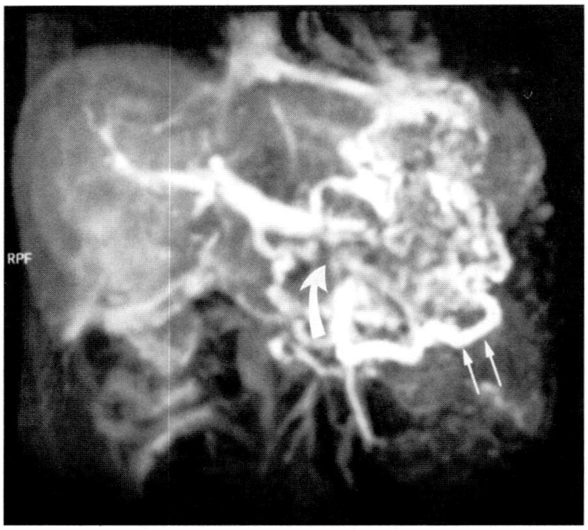

Fig. 7.51. Vascular complication of chronic pancreatitis. Magnetic resonance angiography using three-dimensional gradient echo sequence and diethylenetriaminopentoacetic acid gadolinium intravenous injection (maximum-intensity projection). On this coronal view, thrombosis of the mesentericoportal system secondary to cephalic mass of the pancreas (pseudomass of chronic pancreatitis) is shown (*curved arrow*). Enlarged right gastroepiploic vein is well depicted (*arrows*)

a

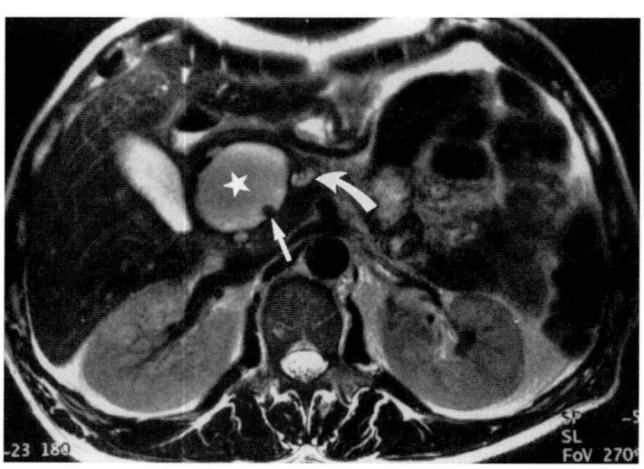

b

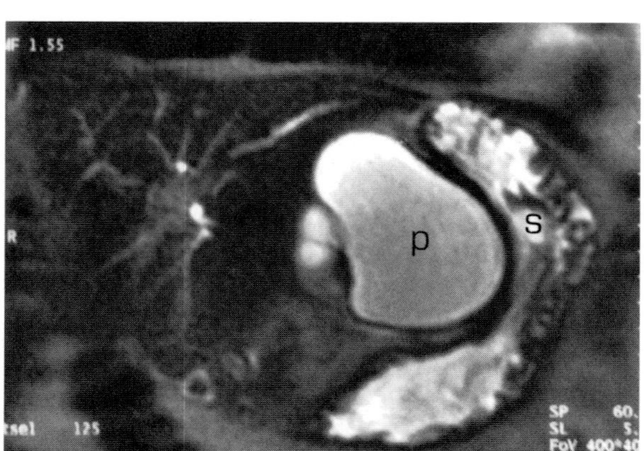

Fig. 7.52a,b. Magnetic resonance imaging of pseudocyst. **a** High resolution T2-weighted turbo spin echo sequence. A hyperintense pseudocyst (*star*) is well depicted within the head of the pancreas. A stone is shown within the pseudocyst. An upstream dilated main pancreatic duct is also observed (*curved arrow*). **b** Coronal view using single-shot turbo spin echo. The relationships between the pseudocyst (*P*) and the stomach (*S*) are well established prior to performing endoscopic cystogastrostomy

rax with a high amylase content resulting from a disrupted pancreatic duct (Uchiyama et al. 1992). Heavily T2-weighted MR images obtained in the coronal plane nicely demonstrate the rupture of the pancreatic duct, as well as the connection of the peripancreatic fluid collection with the pleural space (Gryspeerdt et al. 1998). MRI-MRCP is less reliable than ERCP or cystography for assessing whether or not pseudocysts are connected to the pancreatic ductal system (Fig. 7.53)

7.2.12.3.3 Role of MRCP in Differentiation Between Chronic Pancreatitis and Pancreatic Carcinoma

The differentiation between pancreatic carcinoma and "atypical" chronic pancreatitis (focal chronic pancreatitis, chronic pancreatitis with superimposed focal or diffuse acute pancreatitis, chronic pancreatitis with inflammatory enlargement of the pancreatic head) remains a major challenge. Moreover, chronic obstructive pancreatitis may develop secondary to pancreatic carcinoma, which may cause diagnostic problems. MRCP is a unique modality because it shows not only ductal changes that may be helpful in the differential diagnosis (like ERCP; Table 7.3), but, in addition, enables the evaluation of focal or diffuse changes in signal intensity and contrast uptake pattern. MRI signs suggesting chronic pancreatitis include the presence of dilated side branches within a focal"mass" and the absence of a hypointense mass on T1-weighted turbo FLASH images (see Chap. 8, Sect. 8.7.3). Even in the presence of typical changes of chronic pancreatitis, the presence of a focal hypointense mass on turbo FLASH images should be considered as diagnostic of pancreatic carcinoma until proved otherwise (Fig. 7.54).

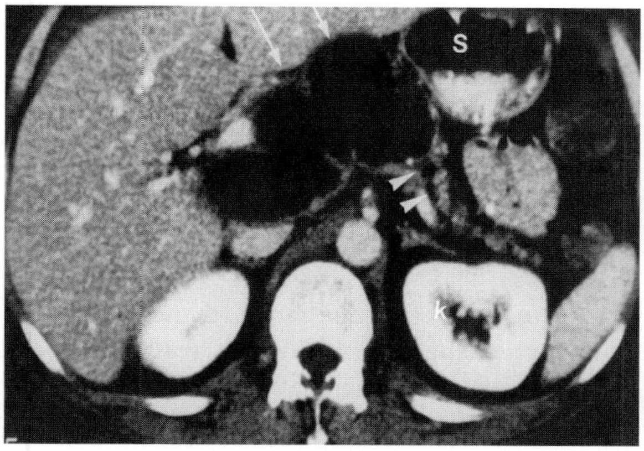

a

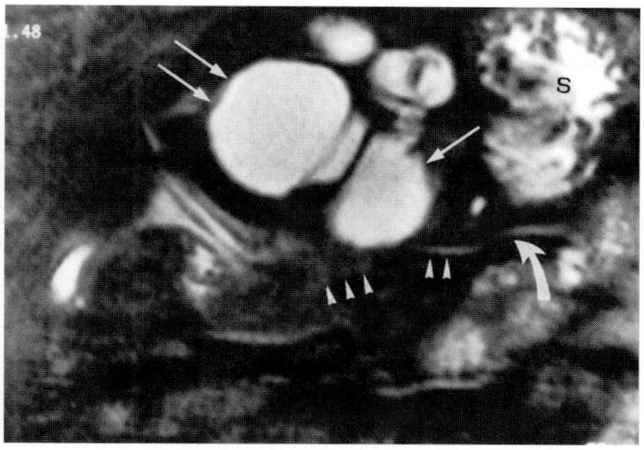

b

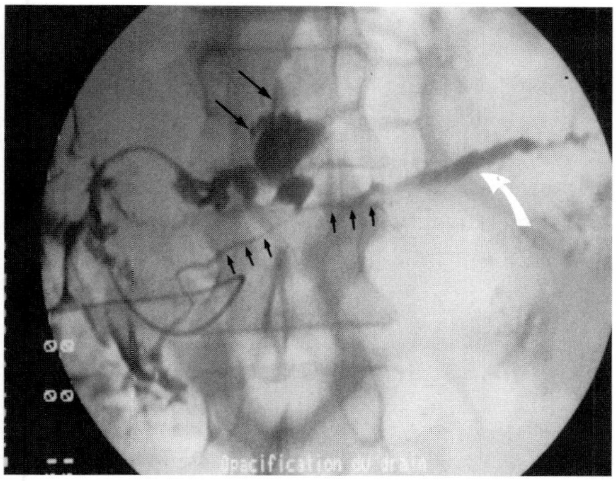

c

Fig. 7.53a–c. Chronic pancreatitis. Communicating pseudocyst with dilated main pancreatic duct. **a** Contrast-enhanced computed tomography (CT) of chronic pancreatitis. A huge pseudocyst (*arrows*) is shown developed beside the lesser curvature of the stomach (*S*). The upstream pancreatic duct is dilated (*arrowheads*) and the pancreatic gland is thin. **b** Single-shot magnetic resonance cholangiopancreatography (MRCP) on coronal view depicts the relationship between the pseudocyst (*arrows*) and the pancreatic duct (*arrowheads*), which appears upstream dilated (*curved arrow*). *S*, stomach. MRCP cannot evidence communication between the pseudocyst and the main pancreatic duct. **c** Opacification after percutaneous drainage of the pseudocyst under CT guidance. After draining off the pseudocyst, opacification through the catheter shows evidence of communication between the pseudocyst (*large arrows*) and the pancreatic duct (*small arrows*), which appears more dilated above the fistula (*curved arrow*)

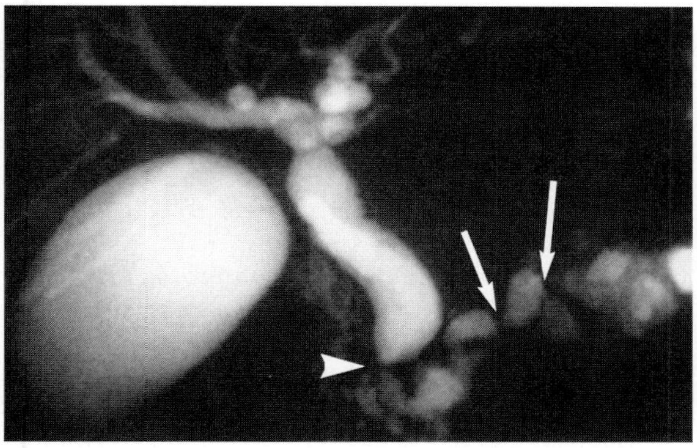
a

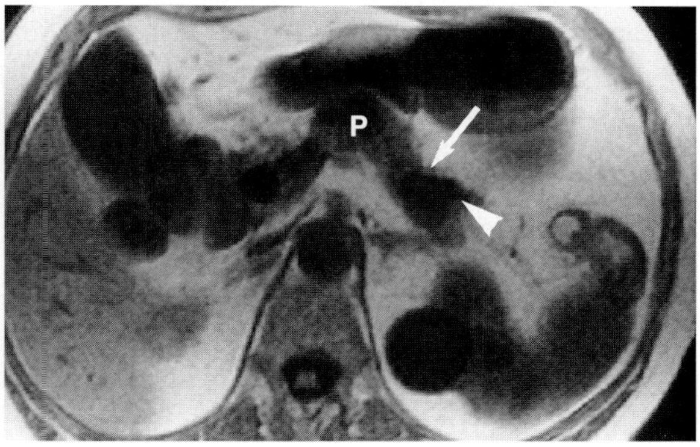

b

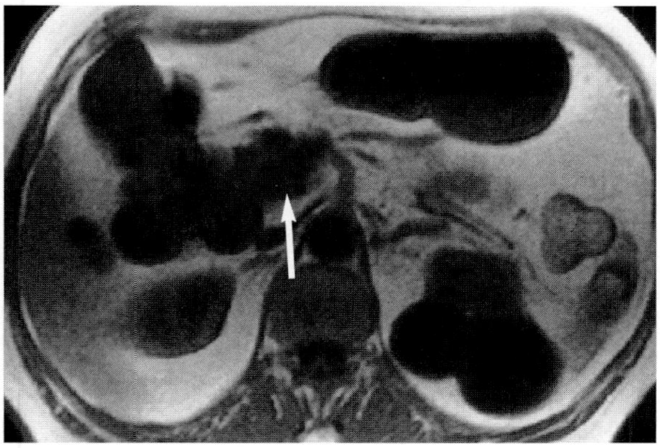
c

Fig. 7.54a–c. Chronic pancreatitis associated with pancreatic carcinoma. **a** Projective magnetic resonance (MR) image shows typical ductal features seen in chronic pancreatitis with the presence of multiple stenoses of pancreatic duct (*arrows*). Also note sudden narrowing of the common bile duct (*arrowhead*). **b** Cross-sectional T1-weighted image obtained at the level of the pancreatic body shows relatively normal (hyperintense) signal intensity of pancreatic parenchyma (*arrow*). The pseudocysts (*P*) have a low signal intensity. **c** Cross-sectional T1-weighted image obtained at level of the pancreatic head shows focal hypointense mass in the pancreatic head (*arrow*): adenocarcinoma

7.2.12.4
Value

MRCP is particularly useful in the evaluation of the pancreatic duct in patients in which ERCP is unsuccessful or incomplete. In the study by Soto and colleagues (1996), chronic pancreatitis was found to be a major cause of unsuccessful or incomplete ERCP: chronic pancreatitis was found in seven of 20 patients in which ERCP was unsuccessful, and in five of seven patients in which ERCP showed complete pancreatic duct obstruction. In this particular group of patients, a two-fold role of MRCP can be distinguished: MRCP may help to determine whether antegrade or retrograde cannulation should be attempted, and, by depicting the obstructed segment as well as the obstruction itself, MRCP might be helpful in differentiating tumoral from nontumoral (e.g., inflammatory) obstruction.

Because of its noninvasive nature and unique diagnostic capabilities, it is likely that the role of MRI-MRCP will progressively increase in the future. Indications could include: (a) the detection of congenital anomalies that predispose to chronic or relapsing acute pancreatitis (pancreas divisum, annular pancreas); (b) the diagnosis of (advanced) chronic pancreatitis; (c) follow-up in patients with known chronic pancreatitis; (d) detection of complications; and (e) differential diagnosis with pancreatic cancer. There is a tendency to use MRCP as a first imaging modality in patients with known chronic pancreatitis, and to reserve ERCP for those patients requiring some intervention (e.g., stent placement) or tissue sampling. MRCP images can also be used as a"roadmap", i.e., as a guide in the planning of endoscopic, percutaneous, or surgical interventions.

As stated above, MRCP is not as sensitive as ERCP for the detection of early ductal changes. This technique, therefore, has a limited potential in the diagnosis of early (beginning) chronic pancreatitis.

7.2.13
Angiography

Although arterial, parenchymal, and venous findings have been described in chronic pancreatitis, angiography is no longer used as a screening test. However, it provides the most detailed evaluation of vascular complications, especially when performed at the time of active hemorrhage or when other tests are equivocal. The use of therapeutic angiography contributed to the reduction in the mortality rate from arterial involvement in chronic pancreatitis (Vujic 1989).

7.3
Conclusion

Many imaging tests can be used to demonstrate morphological changes in chronic pancreatitis. EUS and MRI are sufficiently sensitive to replace diagnostic ERCP. Enhanced helical CT seems to be the most exhaustive and readily available technique to carry out patient follow-up, to detect complications such as pseudocysts, and to roadmap prior to the intervention. MRI using MRCP seems to be the best alternative modality to CT. However, differentiating pancreatic neoplasms from a benign pseudomass of chronic pancreatitis may remain difficult for each imaging modality and may require serial imaging studies and percutaneous fine needle biopsies.

References

Alpern MB, Sandler MA, Kellman GM, Madrazo BL (1985) Chronic pancreatitis: ultrasonic features. Radiology 155:215–219

Ammann RW, Muench R, Otto R, Buehler H, Freiburghaus A, Siegenthaler W (1988) Evolution and regression of pancreatic calcification in chronic pancreatitis. Gastroenterology 95:1018–1028

Amouyal G (1992) Pathologie pancréatique. In: Amouyal G, Amouyal P (eds) Echo-endoscopie digestive pratique. Merck Sharp Dohme-Chribet, Paris, pp 95–104

Anacker H, Weiss HD, Kramann B, Gmelin E (1981) Die Treffsicherheit der endoskopischen retrograden Pancreatiko-Cholangiographie in der Diagnostik der Pankreaskrankheiten. Ene Analyse von 3000 Untersuchungen. Dtsch Med Wochenschr 106:230–233

Angelini G, Antolini G, Bovo P, et al. (1987) Frequency of pancreatographic changes in subjects with upper abdominal symptoms and its relationship with alcohol intake. Int J Pancreatol 2:305–310

Aranha GV, Prinz RA, Freeark RJ, Greenlee HB (1984) The spectrum of biliary tract obstruction from chronic pancreatitis. Arch Surg 119:595–600

Axon ATR (1986) Endoscopy in the diagnosis and therapy of panreatic disorders. Clin Gastroenterol 15:279-303

Axon ATR (1989) Endoscopy in the diagnosis cholangiopancreatography in chronic pancreatitis. Cambridge classification. Radiol Clin North Am 27:39–50

Baert AL, Ponette E, Marchal G (1981) Radiology of the pancreas: overview. In: Dommer MW, Heuck FHW (eds) Radiology today I. Springer, Berlin Heidelberg New York, pp 178–185

Baker ME, Cohan RH, Nadel SN, Leder RA, Dunnick NR (1990) Obliteration of the fat surrounding the celiac axis and superior mesenteric artery is not a specific CT finding of carcinoma of the pancreas. AJR 155:991-994

Ball WP, Baggenstoss AH, Bargen JA (1950) Pancreatic lesions associated with chronic ulcerative colitis. Arch Pathol 50:347–358

Bolondi L, Li Bassi S, Gaiani S, Barbara L (1989) Sonography of chronic pancreatitis. Radiol Clin North Am 27:815

Brinberg DE, Carr MF Jr, Premkumar A, Stein J, Green PHR (1988) Isolated ventral pancreatitis in an alcoholic with pancreas divisum. Gastrointest Radiol 13:323-326

Buscail L, Escourrou J, Moreau J et al (1995) Endoscopic ultrasonography in chronic pancreatitis: a comparative prospective study with conventional ultrasonography, computed tomography and ERCP. Pancreas 10:251–257

Caletti G, Brocchi E, Agostini D, Balduzzi A, Bolondi L, Labo G (1982) Sensitivity of endoscopic retrograde pancreatography in chronic pancreatitis. Br J Surg 69:507–509

Chezmar JL, Nelson RC, Small WC, Bernardino ME (1991) Magnetic resonance imaging of the pancreas with gadolinium-DTPA. Gastrointest Radiol 16:139–142

Chong WK, Theis B, Russell RCG, Lees (1992) US-guided percutaneous pancreatography: an essential tool for imaging pancreatitis. Radiographics 12:79–90

Conley CR, Scheithauer BW, Weiland LH, Van Heerden JA (1987) Diffuse intraductal papillary adenocarcinoma of the pancreas. Ann Surg 205: 246–249

Cotton PB (1972) Progress report. Cannulation of the papilla of Vater by endoscopy and retrograde cholangiopancreatography (ERCP). Gut 13:1014–1025

Cotton PB (1980) Congenital anomaly of pancreas divisum as cause of obstructive pain and pancreatitis. Gut 13:105-114

Cotton PB, Lees WR, Vallon AG, Cottone M, Croker JR, Chapman M (1980) Gray-scale ultrasonography and endoscopic pancreatography in pancreatic diagnosis. Radiology 134:453–459

Cuykx H, Theunissen P, Leyssens G, Deraemaeker C, Valgaeren F (1992) Pancreaticopleural fistula. J Belge Radiol-Belg Tijdschr Radiol 75:115–118

Delhaye M, Engelholm L, Cremer M (1985) Pancreas divisum: congentical anatomic variant or anomaly? Gastroenterology 89:951–958

Del Maschio A, Vanzulli A, Sirunis et al (1991) Pancreatic cancer versus chronic pancreatitis: diagnosis with CA 19.9 assessment, US, CT and CT-guided fine needle biopsy. Radiology 178:95–99

Demling L, Classen M, Frühmorgen P (1974) Atlas der Enderoskopie - Endoskopie des Dünndarms und des Dickdarms, retrograde Cholangio-pancreaticographie. Springer, Berlin Heidelberg New York, pp 1–46, 78-161

Dupuy DE, Costello P. Ecker CP (1992) Spiral CT of the pancreas. Radiology 183-815–818

Ectors N, Maillet B, Aerts R et al Non alcoholic duct destructive chronic pancreatitis. Gut (in press)

Elsborg L, Bruusgaard A, Strandgaard, Reinicke V (1981) Endoscopic retrograde pancreatography and the exocrine pancreatic function in chronik alcoholism. Scand J Gastroenterol 16:941–944

Foley WD, Stewart ET, Lawson TL, Greenan J, Loguidice J, Maher L, Unger GF (1980) Computed tomography, ultrasonography, and endoscopic retrograde cholangiopancreatography in the diagnosis of pancreatic disease: a comparative study. Gastrointest Radiol 5:29–35

Frederic N, Deltenre M, d'Hondt M, de Reuck M, Hermanus A, Potvliege R (1983) Comparative study of ultrasound and ERCP in the diagnosis of hepatic, biliary and pancreatic diseases: a prospective study based on a continuous series of 424 patients. Eur J Radiol 3:208–211

Freeny PC (1982) Chronic pancreatitis. In: Freeny PC, Lawson TL (eds) Radiology of the pancreas. Springer, Berlin Heidelberg New York, pp 223–294

Freeny PC (1988) Radiology of the pancreas: two decades of progress in imaging and intervention. AJR 150:975–981

Freeny PC (1989) Classification of pancreatitis. Radiol Clin North Am 27:1–3

Frick MP, O'Learn JF, Walker HC, Goodale RL (1982) Accuracy of endoscopic retrograde cholangiopancreatography (ERCP) in differentiating benign and malignant pancreatic disease. Gastrointest Radiol 7:241–244

Gehl HB, Vorwerk D, Klose KC, Gunther RW (1991) Pancreatic enhancement after low-dose infusion of Mn-DPDP. Radiology 180:337–339

Gmelin E. Weiss HD, Fuchs HD, Raiser M (1981) Vergleich der diagnostischen Treffsicherheit von Ultraschall Computertomographie und ERCP bei der chronischen Pankreatitis und beim Pancreaskarzinom. Fortschr Röntgenstr 134:136–141

Gowland M, Warwick F, Kalantzis N, Braganza J (1981) Relative efficiency and predictive value of ultrasonography and endoscopic retrograde pancreatography in diagnosis of pancreatic disease. Lancet II:190–193

Gregg JA, Carr-Locke DL, Gallagher MM (1981) Importance of common bile duct stricture associated with pancreatitis. Am J Surg 141:199–203

Grosso M, Gandini G, Cassinis MC, Regge D, Righi D, Rossi P (1989) Percutaneous treatment (including pseudocystogastrostomy) of 74 pancreatic pseudocysts. Radiology 173:493–497

Guien C (1972) General radiology of the pancreas. In Howat HT (ed) Clinics in gastroenterology - the exocrine pancreas. W.B. Saunders, London, pp 61–83

Gryspeerdt S, Van Hoe L, Baert AL (1998) Acute and chronic pancreatitis. In: Heuck A, Reiser M (eds) Abdominal and pelvic MRI. Springer, Berlin Heidelberg New York, pp 91–108

Hahn PF, Stark DD, Lewis JM, et al. (1990) First clinical trial of a new superparamagnetic iron oxide for use as an oral gastrointestinal contrast agent in MR imaging. Radiology 175:695–700

Hamed MM, Hamm B, Ibrahim ME, Taupitz M, Mahfouz AE (1992) Dynamic MR imaging of the abdomen with gadopenetate dimeglumin: normal enhancement patterns of the liver, spleen, stomach, and pancreas. AJR 158: 303–307

Helwig A, Dinkel E, Mundinger A, Biebl S. Buscher HP, Rückauer K (1990) Stellenwert der ERCP in der Pankreasdiagnostik. Radiologe 30:413-419

Huntington DK, Hill MC, Steinberg W (1989) Biliary tract dilatation in chronic pancreatitis: CT and sonographic findings. Radiology 172:47–50

Ichikawa T, Nitatori T, Hachiya J, Mizutani Y (1996) Breath-held MR cholangiopancreatography with half-averaged single shot hybrid rapid acquisition with relaxation enhancement sequence: comparison of fast GRE and SE sequences. J Comput Assisted Tomogr 20:798–802

Janus C, Hertz I, Horner N, Waye J (1982) Diagnostic retrospective in pancreaticobiliary imaging: ultrasound and ERCP. Gastrointest Radiol 7:363-365

Jones SN, Lees WR, Frost RA (1988) Diagnosis and grading of chronic pancreatitis by morphological criteria derived by ultrasound and pancreatography. Clin Radio. 39:43–48

Jones SN, McNeil NI, Lees WR (1989) The interpretation of retrograde pancreatography in the elderly. Clin Radiol 40:393–396

Kadell BM, Weiner M (1973) Current status of the transjugular approach for direct cholangiography. Surg Clin North Am 53:1019–1042

Kasugai T, Kuno N, Kizu M (1974) Manometric endoscopic retrograde pancreatocholangiography. Dig Dis 19:485–502

Kawagushi K, Koike M, Tsuruta K, Okamoto A, Tabata I, Fukita N (1991) Lymphoplasmacytic sclerosing pancreatitis with cholangitis: a variant of primary sclerosing cholangitis extensively involving the pancreas. Hum Pathol 22:387–395

Kloppel G, Maillet B (1992) The morphological basis for the evolution of acute pancreatitis into chronic pancreatitis. Virchows Arch [A] Pathol Anat Histopathol 420:1–4

Kolars JC, Allen MO, Ansel H, Silvis SE, Vennes JA (1989) Pancreatic pseudocysts: clinical and endoscopic experience. Am J Gastroenterol 84:259–264

Lammer J, Herlinger H, Zalaudek G, Hofler H (1985) Pseudotumorous pancreatitis. Gastrointest Radiol 10:59–67

Lankisch PG, Lohr-Happe A, Otto J, Creutzfeldt W (1993) Natural course in chronic pancreatitis: pain, exocrine and endocrine insufficiency and prognosis of the disease. Digestion 54:148–155

Laszik GZ, Pap A, Farkas G (1988) A case of primary sclerosing cholangitis mimicking chronic pancreatitis. Int J Pancreatol 3:503–508

Laubenberger J, Buchert M, Schneider B, Blum U, Hennig J, Langer M (1995) Breath-hold projection magnetic resonance-cholangio-pancreaticography (MRCP): a new method for the examination of the bile and pancreatic ducts. Magn Reson Med 33:18–23

Laxon LC, Fromkes JJ, Cooperman M (1985) Endoscopic retrograde cholangiopancreatography in the management of pancreatic pseudocysts. Am J Surg 150:683–686

Lees WR (1986) Endoscopic ultrasonography of chronic pancreatitis and pancreatic pseudocysts. Scand J Gastroenterol 21 (Suppl 123):123–129

Lees WR, Heron CW (1987) US-guided percutaneous pancreatography: experience in 75 patients. Radiology 165:809–813

Lenriot JP, Le-Neel JC, Hay JM, Jaeck D, Millat B, Fagniez PL (1993) Cholangio-pancreatographie retrograde et sphincterotomie endoscopique pour lithiase biliare. Gastroenterol Clin Biol 17:244–250

L'Herminé C, Pringot J, Monnier JP, et al. (1980) Le retentissement colique des pancretites. A propos de 39 oberservations. J. Radiol 61:27–34

Lowenfels AB, Maisonneuve P, Cavallini G et al (1993) Pancreatitis and the risk of pancreatic cancer. N Engl J Med 328:1433–1437

Luetmer PH, Stephens DH, Ward EM (1989) Chronic pancreatitis: reassesment with current CT. Radiology 171:353–357

Macauley SE, Schulte SJ, Sekijima JH, Obregon RG, Simon HE, Rohrmann CA, Freeny PC, Schmiedl UP (1995) Evaluation of a non-breath-hold MR cholangiography technique. Radiology 196:227–232

MacCain AH, Berkman WA, Bernardino ME (1984) Pancreatic sonography: past and present. J Clin Ultrasound 12:325

Mackie CR, Cooper MJ, Lewis MH, Moossa AR (1979) Non-operative differentiation between pancreatic cancer and chronic pancreatitis. Ann Surg 189:480–487

Malfertheiner P, Buchler M (1989) Correlation of imaging and function in chronic apncreatitis. Radiol Clin North Am 27:51

Marks IN, Bank S (1985) Etiology, clinical aspects and medical management of chronic pancreatitis. In: Berk JE (ed) Bockus' gastro-enterology. W.B. Saunders, Philadelphia, pp 4020–4040

Matos C, Metens T, Devière J et al (997)Pancreatic duct: morphologic and functional evaluation with dynamic MR pancreatography after secretin stimulation. Radiology 203:435–41

Misra SP, Thorat VK, Vij JC, Amand BS (1990) Development of carcinoma in chronic calcific pancreatitis. Int J Pancreatol 6:307–312

Mitchell DG, Vinitski S, Saporano S, Tasciyan T, Bruk DL Jr, Rifkin MD (1991) Liver and pancreas: improved spin-echo T1 contrast by shorter echo time and fat supression at 1.5T. Radiology 178:67–71

Mitchell DG (1995) MR imaging of the pancreas. MRI Clin North Am 3:51–71

Miyake H, Harada H, Kunichika K, Ochi K, Kimur I (1987) Clinical course and prognosis of chronic pancreatitis. Pancreas 2:378–385

Miyazaki T, Yamashita Y, Tsuchigame T, Yamamoto H, Urata J, Takahashi M (1996) MR cholangiopancreatography using HASTE (half-Fourier acquisition single-shot turbo spin-echo) sequences. AJR 166:1297–1303

Moody AR, Poon PY (1992) Gastroepiploic veins: CT appearance in pancreatic disease. AJR 158:779–783

Neff CC, Simeone JF, Wittenberg J, Mueller PR, Ferrucci JT (1984) Inflammatory pancreatic masses. Problems in differentiating focal pancreatitis from carcinoma. Radiology 150:35–38

Niederau C, Sonnenberg A, Müller JE, Erkenbrecht JF, Scholten T, Fritsch WP (1983) Sonographic measurements of the normal liver, spleen, pancreas and portal vein. Radiology 149:537

Nix GA, Schmitz PI (1981) Diagnostic features of chronic pancreatitis distal to benign and to malignant pancreatic duct obstruction. Diagn Imaging 50:130–137

Noda A, Hamano H, Shibata T, Hayakawa T, Tsuchie K, Nimura Y, Nakanishi Y (1987) Chronic pancreatitis at early age of onset presenting interesting findings throug endoscopic retrograde panceratography and chemical analysis of nonpaque pancreatic concretion. Dig Dis Sci 32:433–440

Noguchi T, Aibe T, Amano H, Fuji T, Takemoto T (1986) The diagnosis of chronic pancreatitis and pancreatic cancer by endoscopic ultrasonography. Dig Dis Sci 30:62S

Okuda K, Tanikawa K, Emura T, et al. (1974) Nonsurgical, percutaneous transphepatic cholangiography – diagnostic significance in medical problems of the liver. Dig Dis 19:21–36

Ormson MJ, Charboneau JW, Stephens DH (1987) Sonography in patients with a possible pancreatic mass shown on CT. AJR 148:551–555

Ott H, Rösch W (1983) Pankreas divisum – Ursache einer Pankreatitis? Med Welt 34:466–468

Otte M (1986) Ultrasound in chronic pancreatitis. In: Malfertheiner P, Ditschuneit II (eds) Diagnostic procedures in pancreatic disease. Springer, Berlin Heidelberg New York, p 143

Owyang C, Levitt M (1991) Chronic pancreatitis. In: Yamada Talpers DH, Owyang C, Powell DW, Silverstein EE (eds) Textbook of gastroenterology, vol 2. Lipincott, New York, pp 1874–1893

Pantongrag-Brown L, Suwanwela N, Arjhansiri K, Chetpukdeechit V, Kitisin P (1991) Demonstration on computed tomography of two pseudo-aneurysms complicating chronic pancreatitis. Br J Radiol 64:754–757

Philips WC, Scott JA, Blasczcynski G (1983) How sensitive is "sensitivity"; how specific is "specificity"?Am J Roentgenol 140:1265–1270

Pinson CW, Munson JL, Deveney CW (1990) Endoscopic retrograde cholangiopancreatography in the preoperative diagnosis of pancreatic neoplasms associated with cysts. Am J Surg 159:510–513

Plumley TF, Rohrmann CA, Freeny PC, Silverstein FE, Bail TJ (1982) Double duct sign: reassessed significance in ERCP. Am J Radiol 138:31–35

Pomerri F, Pittarello F, Muzzio PC (1988) Pancreatic carcinoma, diagnostic ERCP. Int J Pancreatol 3:131-136

Ponette E, de Peneranda M, Collette JM, Fevery J, Ponette S. Van Steen AS (1977) Biligrafie door punktietechnieken. J Belge Radiol 50:215

Ponette E, Aerts A, Baert A-L (1978a) Tecnica di indagine radiologica del duodeno. In: Bertoncello Artigrafiche (ed) La Radiologia dell'Esofago, dello Stomaco e del Duodeno. Atti del II corso die Aggiornamento Post-Universitario in Radiologia "P. Perona", 13-16 ottobre 1977. Cittadella, Padova, pp 293–301

Ponette E, Baert AL, Coenen Y, Brugman E, Pringot J (1978b) Le impronte sullo stomaca e sul duodeno. In: Bertoncello Artigrafiche (ed) La Radiologia dell'Esofago, dello Stomaco e del Duodeno. Atti del II corso die Aggiornamento Post-Universitario in Radiologia "P. Perona", 13-16 ottobre 1977. Cittadella, Padova, pp 427–439

Ponette E, Broeckaert L, Ponette S, Vandevoorde P, Baert AL (1978c) Endoscopische retrograde cholangioen pancreaticografie (ERCP). In: Vandenbroucke J (ed) Aanwinsten in de inwendige Geneeskunde 5. European Press, Ghent, pp 313–326

Ponette E, Fevery J, Vandevoorde P, Ponette S, Kerremans R, Baert AL (1978d) Percutane transhepatische cholangiografie (PTC). In: Vandenbroucke J (ed) Aanwinsten in de inwendige Geneeskunde 5. European Press, Ghent, pp 293–306

Ponette E, Pringot J, Baert AL, Goncette L, Coenen Y, De Groote J (1978e) Konventionele radiologische methoden bij het pancreasonderzoek. In: Vandenbroucke J (ed) Aanwinsten in de inwendige Geneeskunde 5. European Press, Ghent, pp 263–287

Pringot J, Ponette E, Goncette, Baert A, Dautreband J (1976) Contribution des examens radiologiques classiques et angiographiques au diagnostic de la pancréatite chronique. Acta Gastroenterol Belg 39:426–457

Pringot J, Dardenne AN, Henrion J, et al. (1979) Diagnostic adduracy of computeriz of tomography by comparison with ultrasonography and endoscopic pancreatography. In: Gerhardt P, Van Kaick G (eds) Total body computerized tomography – International Symbosium Heidelberg 1977. Thieme, Stuttgart, pp 95–103

Ralls PW, Halls J, Renner I, Juttner H (1980) Endoscopic retrograde cholangiopancreatography (ERCP) in pancreatic disease. Radiology 134:347–352

Reimer P, Saini S, Hahn PF, Mueller PR, Brady TJ, Cohen MS (1992) Techniques for high-resolution echoplanar MR imaging of the pancreas. Radiology 182:175–179

Reinhold C, Bret PM (1996) Current status of MR cholangiopancreatography. AJR 166:1285–1295

Reinhold C, Bret PM, Guibaud L, Barkun ANG, Genin G, Atri M (1996) MR cholangiopancreatography: potential clinical applications. Radiographics 16:309–320

Reuther G, Kiefer B, Tuchmann A (1996) Cholangiography before biliary surgery: single-shot MR cholangiography versus intravenous cholangiography. Radiology 198:561–566

Richter JM, Schapiro RH, Mulley AG, Warshaw AL (1981) Association of pancreas diversum and pancreatitis, and its treatment by sphincteroplasty of the accessory ampulla. Gastroenterology 81:1104–1110

Richter GM, Simon C, Hoffmann V et al (1996) Hydrohelical CT of the pancreas in thin section technique. Radiology 36:397–405

Rigauts H, Delanote J, Verhilfe R, Marchal G, Schillebeeckz (1992) Chronic focal fibrosing pancreatitis: detection by MRI. Bel Tijdschr voor Geneesk 75:489–491

Rohrmann CA, Baron RL (1989) Biliary complications of pancreatitis. Radiol Clin North Am 27:93–104

Sarles H, Sahel J (1976) Pathology of chronic calcifying pancreatitis. Am J Gastroenterol 66:117–139

Sarner M, Cotton PB (1984) Classification of pancreatitis. Gut 25:756–759

Schmitz-Moormann P, Himmelmann GW, Brandes JW, et al. (1985) Comparative radiological and morphological study of human pancreas. Pancreatitis like changes in postmortem ductograms and their morphological pattern. Possible implication fpr ERCP. Gut 26:406–414

Schulte SJ, Baron RL, Freeny PC, Patten RM, Gorel HA, Maclin ML (1991) Root of the superior mesentery in pancreatitis and pancreatic carcinoma: evaluation with CT. Radiology 180:659–662

Schuman BM (1990) The evolution of diagnostic ERCP. Gastrointest Endosc 36:155–156

Semelka RC, Kroeker MA, Shoenut JP, Kroeker R, Yaffe CS, Micflikier AB (1991) Pancreatic disease: prospective comparison of CT, ERCp and 1,5 T MR imaging with dynamic gadolinium enhancement and fat suppression. Radiology 181:785–791

Semelka RC, Ascher SM (1993) MR Imaging of the pancreas. Radiology 188:593–602

Semelka RC, Shoenut JP, Kroeker MA, Micflikier AB (1993) Chronic pancreatitis: MR imaging features before and after administration of gadopentate dimeglumine. J Magn Reson Imaging 3:79–82

Semelka RC, Kelekis NL, Thomasson D, Brown MA, Laub GA (1996) HASTE MR imaging – description of technique and preliminary results in the abdomen. J Magn Reson Imaging 6:698–699

Shawker T et al (1984) Chronic pancreatitis: the diagnostic significance of pancreatic size and echo amplitude. J Ultrasound Med 3:267

Shawker T, et al. (1984) Chronic pancreatitis: the diagnostic significance of pancratic siz e and echo amplitude. J Ultrasound Med 3:267

Shemesh E, Czerniak A, Nass S, Klein E (1990) Role of the endoscopic retrograde cholangiopancratography in differentiating pancreatic cancer coexisting with chronic pancreatitis. Cancer 65:893-896

Sherman S, Lehman GA (1991) ERCP- and endoscopic sphincterotomy-induced pancreatitis. Pancreas 6:350–367

Silvis SE, Schuman BM (1977) Benign conditions of the pancreas. In: Stewart ET, Vennes JA, Geenen JE (eds) Atlas of endoscopic retrograde cholangiopancreatography. C.V. Mosby, Saint Louis, pp 124–180

Sood S, Fossard DP, Shorrock K (1995) Chronic sclerosing pancreatitis in Sjogren's syndrome: a case report. Pancreas 10:419–421

Soto JA, Barish MA, Yucel EK, Ferrucci JT (1995a) MR cholangiopancreatography: findings on 3D fast spin-echo imaging. AJR 165:1397–1401

Soto JA, Barish MA, Yucel EK, Clarke P, Siegenberg D, Chuttani R, Ferrucci JT (1995b) Pancreatic duct MR cholangiopancreatography with a three-dimensional fast spin-echo technique. Radiology 196:459–464

Soto JA, Yucel EK, Barish MA, Chuttani R, Ferrucci JT (1996) MR cholangiopancreatography after unsuccessful or incomplete ERCP. Radiology 199:91–98

Steer ML, Waxman I, Freedman S (1995) Chronic pancreatitis. N Engl J Med 332:1482–1490

Swobodnik W, Meyer W, Brecht-Kraus D, et al. (1983) Ultrasound computed tomography and endoscopic retrograde cholangiopancreatography in the morphologic diagnosis of pancreatic disease. Klin Wochenschr 61:291–296

Takehara Y, Ichiko K, Tooyama N et al (1994) Breath-hold MR cholangiopancreatography with a long echo train fast spin echo sequence on a surface coil in chronic pancreatitis. Radiology 192:73–78

Thomas E, Morse J (1985) Evaluation of the pancreas by endoscopic retrograde cholangiopancreatography and computerized tomography. South Med J 78:1102–1110

Tobin RS, Vogelzang RL, Gore RM, Keighley B (1987) A comparative study of computed tomography and ERCP in pancreaticobiliary disease. J Comput Assist Tomogr 11:261-266

Tracey KJ, O'Brien MJ, Williams LF, Klibaner M, George PK, Saravis CA, Zamcheck N (1984) Signet ring carcinoma of the pancreas, a rare variant with very high CEA values. Dig Dis Sci 29:573-576

Triller J, Fischedick AR, Haertel M, Scheurer U (1980) Sonographie und endoskopisch retrograde Cholangio-Pakreatikographie zur Diagnostik von Pankreas- und Gallenwegserkrankungen. Fortschr Röntgenstr 132:255–261

Uchiyama T, Suzuki T, Adachi A, Hiraki S, Iizuka N (1992) Pancreatic pleural effusion: case report and review of 113 cases in Japan. Am J Gastroenterol 87:387–391

Van Hoe L, Gryspeerdt S, Ectors N et al (1998a) Nonalcoholic duct-destructive chronic pancreatitis: imaging findings. AJR 170: 643–647

Van Hoe L, Vanbeckevoort D, Van Steenbergen W (1998b) Atlas of cross-sectional and projective magnetic resonance cholangio-pancreatography. Springer, Berlin Heidelberg New York

Van Sonnenberg E, Casola G, Varney RR, Wittich GR (1989) Imaging and interventional radiology for pancreatitis and its complications. Radiol Clin North Am 27:65–72

Van Sonnenberg E, Wittich GR, Casola G et al. (1989a) Percutaneous drainage of infected and non-infected pancreatic pseudycysts: experience in 101 cases. Radiology 170:757–761

Van Sonnenberg E, Casola G, Varney RR, Wittich GR (1989b) Imaging and interventional radiology for pancreatitis and its complications. Radiol Clin North Am 27:65–72

Van Steenbergen W, Ponette E (1990) Pancreaticoportal fistula: a rare complication of chronic pancreatitis. Gastrointest Radiol 15:299–300

Van Steenbergen Verdamme M, W, Ponette E et al. (1986) Primary sclerosing pancreatistis: chronic pancreatitis associated with inflammatory bowel disease, a distinct entity.Tijdschrift voor Gastro-enterologie 14:101–112

Van Steenbergen W, Daels J, Ponette E, Rigatus H, Kerremans R, Fevery J, De Groote J (1990a) Pancreaticoppleurale fistel als verwikkeling van chronische pancreatitis. Tijdschr voor Geneeskunde 46:117–122

Van Steenbergen W,Ponette E, Fevery J, De Groote J (1990b) Galwegproblemen bij chronische pancreatitis. Tijdschr voor Geneeskunde 46:123–128

Vujic I (1989) Vascular complications of pancreatitis. Radiol Clin North Am 27:81–91

Warshaw AL, Ottinger LW (1987) Mesenteric and portal vein obstruction in chronic pancreatitis. Arch Surg 122:410-415

Wallner BK, Schumacher KA, Weidenmaier W, Friedrich JM (1991) Dilated biliary tract: evaluation with MR cholangiography with a T2-weighted contrast-enhanced fast sequence. Radiology 181:805–808

Wieserma MJ, Kochman ML, Cramer HM et al (1994) Endosonography-guided real-time fine needle aspiration biopsy. Gastrointest Endosc 40:700–707

Wieserma MJ, Wierserma LM (1995) Endosonography of the pancreas: normal variation versus changes of early chronic pancreatitis. Gastrointest Endosc Clin North Am 5:487–496

Zalcman M, Van Gansbeke D, Matos C, Engelholm L, Struyven J (1987) Sonographic demonstration of portal venous system thromboses secondary to inflammatory diseases of the pancreas. Gastrointest Radiol 12:114–116

8 Ductal Adenocarcinoma

L. Van Hoe, A.L Baert, H. Rigauts, J.W.A.J. Reeders, N.J. Smits, O.M. Van Delden, and G. Marchal

CONTENTS

L. Van Hoe, MD, PhD, Assistant Professor, Department of Radiology, University Hospital K.U.L., Herestraat 49, B-3000 Leuven, Belgium
A.L Baert, MD, Professor, Department of Radiology, University Hospital K.U.L., Herestraat 49, B-3000 Leuven, Belgium
H. Rigauts, MD, Resident, Department of Radiology, University Hospital K.U.L., Herestraat 49, B-3000 Leuven, Belgium
J.W.A.J. Reeders, MD, Dept. of Diagnostic Radiology, Academic Medical Center, Mei-bergdreef 9, 1105-AZ Amsterdam Zuidoost, The Netherlands
N.J. Smits, MD, Department of Gastrointestinal Radiology and Hepato-Pancreatic-Biliary Imaging, Academic Medical Center, Amsterdam, The Netherlands
O.M. Van Delden, MD, Department of Gastrointestinal Radiology and Hepato-Pancreatic-Biliary Imaging, Academic Medical Center, Amsterdam, The Netherlands
G. Marchal, MD, Professor and Chairman, Department of Radiology, University Hospital K.U.L., Herestraat 49, B-3000 Leuven, Belgium

8.1 Introduction

8.1.1 General Comments

Currently, a single "correct" approach to the diagnosis and staging of patients with suspected pancreatic cancer does not exist. In this chapter, the strong and weak points of the different modalities are compared, keeping in mind that local expertise and interest will determine the strategy chosen for work-up of these patients in different centers. In the final paragraph, an attempt is made to put the different techniques in perspective.

The marked differences between strategies proposed by different authors (see, for example, Figs. 8.14, 8.44) indicate the need to find a more "evidence-based" approach to a rational and cost-effective use of imaging modalities in this patient group.

8.1.2 Incidence and Location

Pancreatic carcinoma accounts for 22% of deaths due to gastrointestinal carcinoma in Western countries (Catalano et al. 1998). Ductal adenocarcinoma is the most frequent type (82%) (Chen and Baithun 1985). The peak incidence of occurrence lies between the sixth and seventh decade. Men predominate over women by a ratio varying between 2:1 and 1:1 (Klöppel and Maillet 1989). Symptoms and signs may include epigastric pain radiating to the back, obstructive jaundice, and new onset diabetes (resulting from endocrine dysfunction) or steatorrhea (resulting from exocrine dysfunction). CA 19.9 values are increased in 80%–90% of cases.

Ductal adenocarcinoma of the pancreas predominantly occurs in the head of the pancreas (60%–70%). A total of 45% of the tumors arise in close contact with the intrapancreatic part of the common bile duct, in the upper dorsal region of the head. The remaining tumors in the head of the pancreas are located in the uncinate process or in the central area of the head. Whereas the first group mainly results in symptoms related to bile duct obstruction, the second group frequently results in obstruction of the main pancreatic duct or side branches, which causes retro-obstructive pancreatitis. At the time of diagnosis, the average size of tumors in the head of the pancreas is 2–3 cm. Neoplasms in the head of the gland are detected sooner than those in the tail (Nix et al. 1991). Ductal adenocarcinomas of the body and tail of the pancreas are generally larger at the time of diagnosis, their size averaging between 5 and 7 cm. Some of them may occupy the entire body or tail region (Nix et al. 1991).

With modern imaging techniques, tumors with a diameter of 5–10 mm can be diagnosed (Freeny 1991; Ormson et al. 1987). Unfortunately, many patients have advanced disease once clinical symptoms arise: Of all common forms of cancer, ductal adenocarcinoma of the pancreas remains the neoplasm most likely to have spread beyond the organ of origin by the time of diagnosis (Stephens 1996).

8.1.3 Staging and Treatment

Direct extension beyond the pancreas primarily involves the retroperitoneal space. The duodenum is the organ most often invaded by cancer of the head of the pancreas. The stomach, peritoneum, and gallbladder may also be involved. In carcinoma of the body and tail, local extrapancreatic extension and metastatic involvement of the liver, peritoneum, and left adrenal gland is more common, which is related to delayed tumor detection. Microscopically, the large majority of carcinomas have infiltrated the peripancreatic fatty tissues by invasion of perineural spaces and/or lymphatic channels. Invasion of the veins occurs in more advanced cases. The lymph nodes most commonly involved in pancreatic head carcinoma are the retroduodenal and superior pancreatic head groups. Carcinomas of the body and tail metastasize preferentially to the superior body and head groups. Patients with lymph node metastases have significantly lower 5-year survival. Hematogenous metastases occur in descending order of frequency in the liver, lungs, adrenals, kidneys, and bones. In only 5%–15% of autopsies are no hematogenous metastases found. Warshaw et al. (1990) found liver metastases in 13 of 55 patients (24%) with carcinoma of the pancreatic head. Most liver metastases measured 1–3 mm in diameter. Arterial encasement involves the superior mesenteric, splenic, celiac, hepatic, gastroduodenal, and left renal artery in descending order of frequency. TNM staging of carcinoma of the endocrine pancreas is being used increasingly. This staging scheme assigns an independent score for the primary tumor (T), nodal disease (N), and distant metastases (M) (Table 8.1) (Zeman et al. 1997).

Table 8.1. TNM staging of pancreatic cancer

State	Definition
Primary tumor stage	
T0	No tumor visible
T1	Tumor limited to pancreas
T2	Tumor extends into peripancreatic tissue or duodenum
T3	Tumor involves major arteries (celiac, mesenteric, splenic), veins (mesenteric, portal), stomach, colon, or spleen
Tx	Unknown
Regional nodes	
N0	No regional adenopathy
N1	Regional adenopathy
Nx	Unknown
Distant metastases	
M0	No distant metastases
M1	Distant metastases present
Mx	Unknown

Complete surgical resection of the tumor is the only curative treatment. Unfortunately, fewer than 20% of patients have surgically resectable tumors at the clinical onset of symptoms and the 5-year survival rates following surgery are less than 5% (usually 2%–3%) in most series, regardless of the type of resection employed (pancreatoduodenectomy, Whipple resection, or total pancreatectomy)

(Coombs et al. 1990). The complications of duodenopancreatectomy remain a factor of concern, although mortality has decreased to less than 5% in many centers (Crist et al. 1987; Choi et al. 1997). Morbidity has been reduced by pylorus-preserving surgery to avoid postgastrectomy symptoms. In any case, accurate selection of those patients with resectable disease is of major importance. Ideally, this should be done by using noninvasive imaging techniques.

While the indications for surgical management are still controversial (Ichikawa et al. 1997), it is clear that the degree of local tumor extension and vascular involvement are important factors in determining the prognosis and the likelihood of benefit from surgery. The following criteria can be used to define a tumor as irresectable based on imaging findings (Diehl et al. 1998):

- Tumor diameter of 5 cm or larger
- Extrapancreatic invasion of adjacent tissues and organs other than the duodenum
- Occlusion, stenosis, or semicircular encasement of major peripancreatic vessels, including the portal venous system, superior mesenteric artery, and major branches of the celiac trunk
- Hematogenous or distant lymph node metastases (other than the peripancreatic nodes) or signs of peritoneal carcinomatosis.

While the presence of liver metastases, marked vascular encasement, and extrapancreatic extension can be considered as absolute criteria for nonresectability, the significance of lymph node enlargement is less clear: Since inflammation rather than invasion by tumor may be the cause, it is wise to consider these patients as "probably unresectable" and to confirm this diagnosis by surgical exploration (Trede et al. 1997). However, because survival correlates with nodal status (Martin et al. 1990), identification of lymph node metastases is important. Some surgeons consider limited infiltration of the portal venous wall not as an absolute contraindication to surgical resection and advocate vascular wall resection or complete portal vein resection with vascular graft interposition (Warshaw and Fernandez del Castillo 1992).

8.2 Ultrasonography

Transabdominal ultrasonography (US) is the classic ultrasonographic approach. More recently, endoscopic US (EUS) and laparoscopic US (LUS) have been proposed (Müller et al. 1994; Hann et al.)

8.2.1 Transabdominal and Endoscopic Ultrasonography

J.W.A.J. Reeders, N.J. Smits, O.M. van Delden, H. Rigauts, L. Van Hoe

8.2.1.1 Technique

8.2.1.1.1 Transabdominal Ultrasonography

Transabdominal US of the pancreas can be performed with or without distention of the stomach. If gastric distention is chosen, the patient should be given a drink such as orange juice, which yields relatively homogeneous echoes (Op den Orth 1987). While distention of the stomach may improve pancreatic visualization in some patients, it does not eliminate pancreatic obscuration caused by air in the transverse colon or jejunum. It is often necessary to examine patients in different positions. Most frequently used are the supine, right lateral, and upright positions. Use of intercostal access with the patient in the right lateral position frequently permits better appreciation of the distal portion of the main bile duct than can be achieved by direct suprapancreatic access in the supine position. Disturbing air superposition may be overcome by examining the patient in the upright position. A 3.5-MHz convex probe is most commonly used. In thin patients, a 5-MHz transducer may be applied.

Duplex Doppler sonography combines real-time and pulsed Doppler sonography. There have been several reports about the applicability of duplex Doppler sonography to the portal venous system in portal hypertension (Angeli et al. 1997). Pulsed Doppler sonography can also be used to stage malignant pancreatic tumors. Narrowing of the portal venous system caused by tumor compression or ingrowth results in changes in blood flow velocities that pulsed Doppler sonography can detect (Garber and Lees 1992). Pulsed Doppler sonography in portal hypertension examines the mean velocity, but in pancreatic malignant tumors only the maximal velocity is important. Because low velocities are to be examined, the wall filter that eliminates low-velocity signals is as low as possible. The sample is taken from the middle of the vessel, and the portal venous system can be traced from the caudal part of the superior mesenteric vein upward to the cranial part of the portal vein.

8.2.1.1.2
Endoscopic US

Echoendoscopes for the upper gastrointestinal tract are side-viewing endoscopes with a small ultrasonic transducer incorporated into their rigid tip (Rösch et al. 1991; Faigel et al. 1997). The sonographic frequency typically ranges from 7.5 to 12 MHz. The examination is performed as a conventional endoscopic study, after local oropharyngeal anesthesia and under endoscopic guidance. The contact between the surface of the transducer and the tissues is assured by the mucous secretions or by the injection of a fluid through the aspiration system of the endoscope. The pancreas is studied through the posterior wall of the stomach and medial wall of the duodenum. It can be visualized by sagittal or transverse slices. Transverse slices may allow the visualization of larger portions of the pancreatic duct. Conscious sedation is required.

Recently, EUS-guided fine-needle aspiration cytology (FNAC) was introduced. As yet, only cytologic specimens can be obtained. Instruments with larger instrumentation channels and larger needles are currently under development (Rösch 1998).

8.2.1.2 Findings

Most adenocarcinomas are hypoechoic as compared to the normal pancreatic parenchyma (Fig. 8.1). The difference between the hypoechoic pattern of neoplastic tissue and the more hyperechoic pattern of normal pancreatic tissue increases with increasing degree of pancreatic lipomatosis (Marchal et al. 1989).

An important secondary sign is pancreatic ductal dilatation. Sonographically, abnormal dilatation of the pancreatic duct is considered to be present when the duct measures more than 2.5 mm in the head and more than 2 mm in the tail (Cotton et al. 1980) (Fig. 8.2). In tumors located in the pancreatic head, common bile duct dilatation may be another associated finding (Fig. 8.3). As a simplifying rule, an inner diameter of the common bile duct of more than 8 mm is considered to be abnormal (Laing et al. 1986; Robledo et al. 1988). More precisely, 5 mm is considered as the upper normal value for patients aged up to 50, plus 1 mm per decade aged over 50.

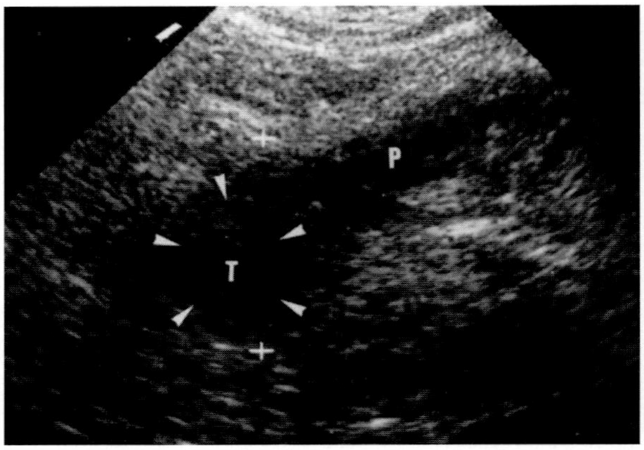

Fig. 8.1. Ductal adenocarcinoma of the pancreatic head. Ultrasonography, transverse section. The head of the gland is seen to be enlarged (*arrowheads*), with a central hypoechoic area representing tumor (*T*). *P*, body and tail of the pancreas

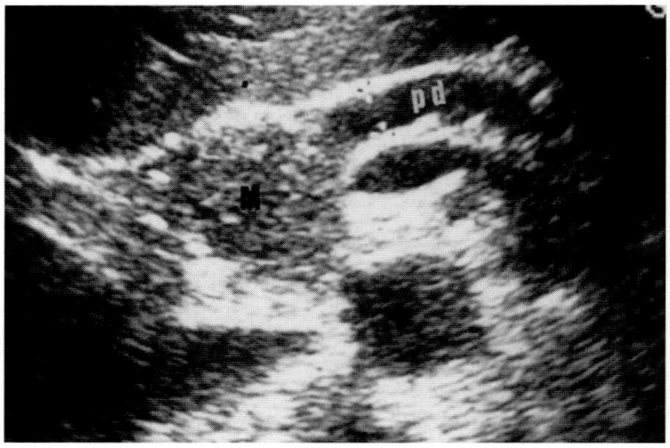

Fig. 8.2. Ductal adenocarcinoma of the pancreatic head. Ultrasonography; transverse section. There is marked dilatation (diameter, 7.4 mm) of the pancreatic duct (*pd*), abruptly ending in a hypoechoic mass (*M*)

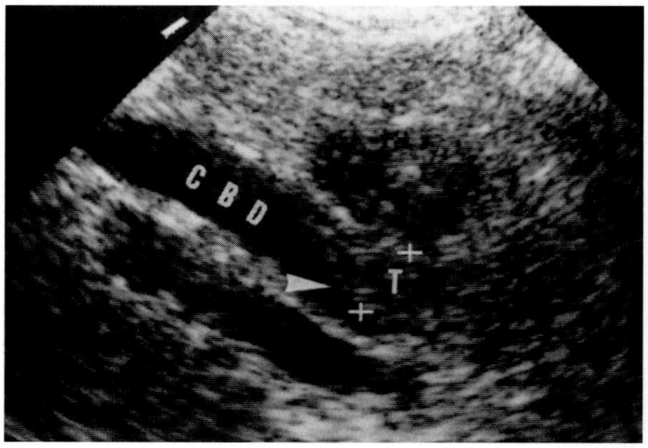

Fig. 8.3. Ductal adenocarcinoma of the pancreatic head. Ultrasonography in a plane along the common bile duct (*CBD*) shows marked dilatation of the latter, ending abruptly (*arrowhead*) at the level of obstruction by tumor (*T*)

The gradual increase in diameter of the normal bile duct is related to the fact that duct walls are composed of elastic fibers; loss of elasticity may occur with age. It should be stressed, however, that diameters of up to 10 mm may be observed in individuals <50 years, even in the absence of disease. Another problem is that a normal bile duct diameter does not rule out obstructive disease. After cholecystectomy, slight dilatation of the common bile duct occurs; however, the increase in diameter is usually small (<1 mm) (Feng and Song 1995).

Carcinomas of the pancreatic head often present with dilatation of both the common bile duct and pancreatic duct. Typically, there is sudden narrowing of both ducts at the level of the tumor ("double duct sign"). However, there are some exceptions to this general rule. Firstly, if the lesion is located in the uncinate process, one or both ducts might have a normal diameter. Secondly, if the lesion infiltrates the duct of Wirsung, drainage of the pancreatic duct may be effected via a normal duct of Santorini draining into the minor papilla. The double duct sign may be helpful in the differential diagnosis between pancreatic cancer and chronic pancreatitis: In patients with pancreatitis involving the pancreatic head, the presence of a typical double duct sign is less common. Moreover, in chronic calcifying pancreatitis, the pancreatic duct typically terminates in a hyperreflective area due to fibrosis and calcium deposits, in contrast to the hypoechoic lesion seen in pancreatic cancer (Smits and Reeders 1995). In the case of obstructive pancreatitis proximal to the tumor mass, no difference in echogenicity may be seen between the tumor and the pancreatic body or tail. Calcifications and pseudocysts suggest chronic pancreatitis. In chronic pancreatitis, a discrepancy can be expected between the size of the mass and the involvement of the portal venous system. If a large hypoechoic mass is seen in the head of the pancreas and pulsed Doppler sonography yields normal blood flow velocities, pancreatic cancer is unlikely. Enlarged lymph nodes are not a major diagnostic parameter in either carcinoma or pancreatitis. Irregular dilatation of the pancreatic duct suggests pancreatitis.

Peripancreatic extension is frequently hard to diagnose on transabdominal US (Fig. 8.4). Moreover, it may be difficult to differentiate tumor extension from peripancreatic inflammation (DelMaschio et al. 1991).

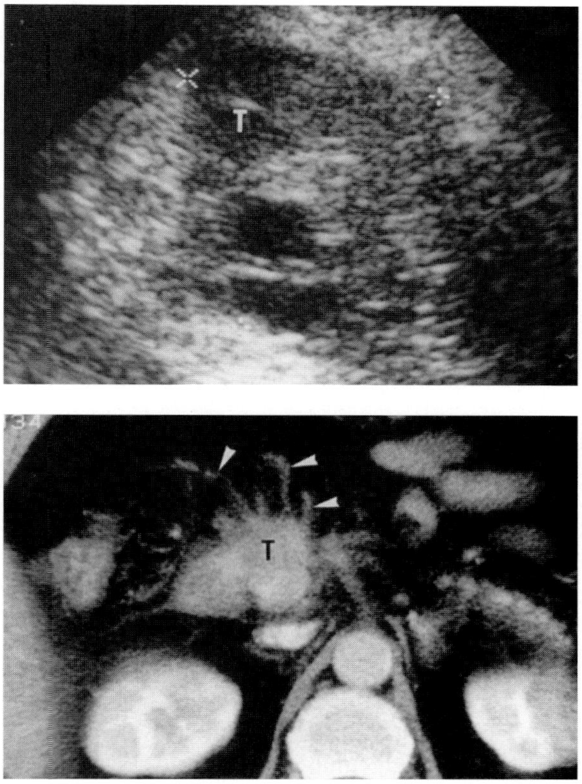

a

b

Fig. 8.4a,b. Pancreatic adenocarcinoma with infiltration of the peripancreatic fat. **a** Ultrasonography. The tumor in the pancreatic head can be recognized as a hypoechoic zone (*T*), but no changes are detected in the peripancreatic fat. **b** Contrast-enhanced computed tomography image shows streaky linear structures (*arrowheads*) surrounding the tumor (*T*) in the pancreatic head and representing tumoral infiltration within the peripancreatic fat

8.2.1.3 Staging

8.2.1.3.1 Regional Lymph Node Metastases

Transabdominal US is able to detect retroperitoneal and mesenteric metastatic adenopathies (Fig. 8.5). Lymph nodes that are confluent with the tumor mass cannot be detected by sonography. In pancreatic head carcinoma, more remote lymph nodes can be identified in 54% of cases, regardless of location, size, shape, or texture of the lymph nodes (Martin et al. 1990). Campbell and Wilson (1988) reported lymphadenopathy in 16 of 50 patients (32%) with pancreatic neoplasms (adenocarcinoma, $n=30$; other malignant tumor, $n=10$; unknown, $n=10$). A typically benign lymph node is long with a small short axis and a hyperechoic center. Such lymph nodes can

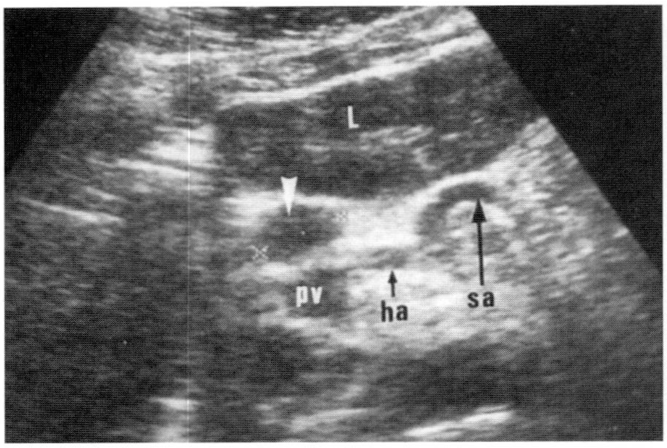

Fig. 8.5. Pancreatic adenocarcinoma with metastatic adenopathies. Ultrasonography; transverse section. A hypoechoic adenopathy (*arrowhead*) is detected in the hepatogastric ligament. *L*, left liver lobe; *pv*, portal vein; *ha*, hepatic artery; *sa*, splenic artery

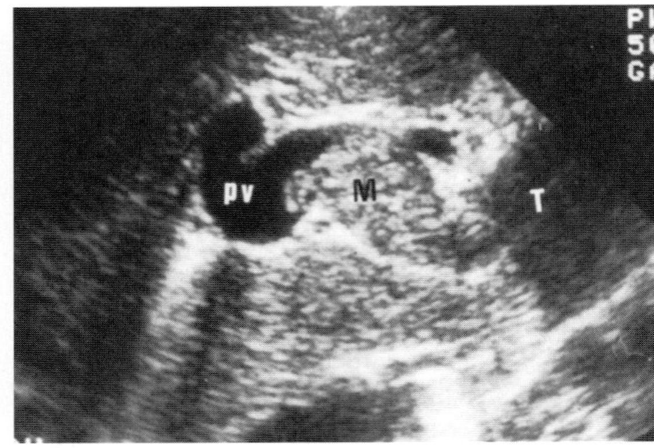

Fig. 8.6. Tumoral invasion of the portal vein in ductal adenocarcinoma of the pancreas. Ultrasonography. The pancreatic head is enlarged by tumor (*T*), seen as a hypoechoic area. A metastatic tumoral thrombus (*M*) is seen protruding into the lumen of the main branch of the portal vein (*pv*)

often be seen in the region of the hepatic artery. Large oval-shaped hypoechoic lymph nodes can indicate both inflammation and malignancy. Reliable morphologic differentiation between reactive lymph nodes and lymph node metastases is generally not possible. This is even difficult with EUS (Tio et al. 1990). Therefore, lymph node enlargement is not a reliable sign of unresectability. On the other hand, small lymph nodes that are missed by sonography may contain tumor.

8.2.1.3.2
Liver and Peritoneal Metastases

Metastatic liver lesions of approximately 1 cm in size or larger can be detected by sonography, depending on location and echogenicity relative to the adjacent liver parenchyma. Liver metastases are usually hypoechoic. Special attention is required for the near field because most liver metastases are superficial. For this purpose, additional scanning with a 7.5-MHz linear-array or curved-array probe is recommended. Peritoneal metastases are also usually tiny and only detectable during laparoscopy or open surgery.

8.2.1.3.3
Vascular Involvement

Involvement of the *portal venous system* commonly precedes encasement of the major peripancreatic arteries. Invasion and/or obstruction of the portal venous system is usually well seen (Fig. 8.6) and may be excluded when a clear tumor-free margin is observed (Fig. 8.7). The pulsed Doppler signal is considered normal if blood flow is not impaired and a low-velocity signal is seen with periodicity corresponding to cardiac activity (Fig. 8.8). On inspiration, mechanical compression of the liver results in increased pressure in the portal venous system with a diminished flow velocity. On expiration, the situation is reversed and the blood flow velocity increases. During tracing of the portal venous system, an abrupt increase in Doppler shift indicates narrowing caused by compression or tumor ingrowth. While the presence of a fat plane between tumor and vessels virtually excludes (macroscopic) vessel involvement by tumor, tumor recurrence may be observed if complete resection of the mass is technically not possible (Fig. 8.10). Special attention is required for the venous confluence – the region where the superior mesenteric, splenic, and portal veins merge – because this is the most commonly involved part (Fig. 8.10). Compared with the late phase of angiography, a 50% stenosis of the portal venous system corresponds to a blood flow velocity of approximately 1 m/s with pulsed Doppler sonography, provided that the Doppler angle is <60%. Beyond such a significant stenosis, blood turbulence creates spectral broadening, a feature referring to the presence of a large and increased range of flow velocities at a given point in the pulse cycle. In occlusion, no Doppler signal can be detected. In severe stenosis or occlusion anywhere in the portal venous system, collaterals can be shown with US and color Doppler.

Tumor involvement of the *superior mesenteric artery or the celiac trunk* results in unresectability. Pulsed Doppler examination of these vessels is of little importance because narrowing of the lumen, resulting in an abnormal Doppler signal, occurs only

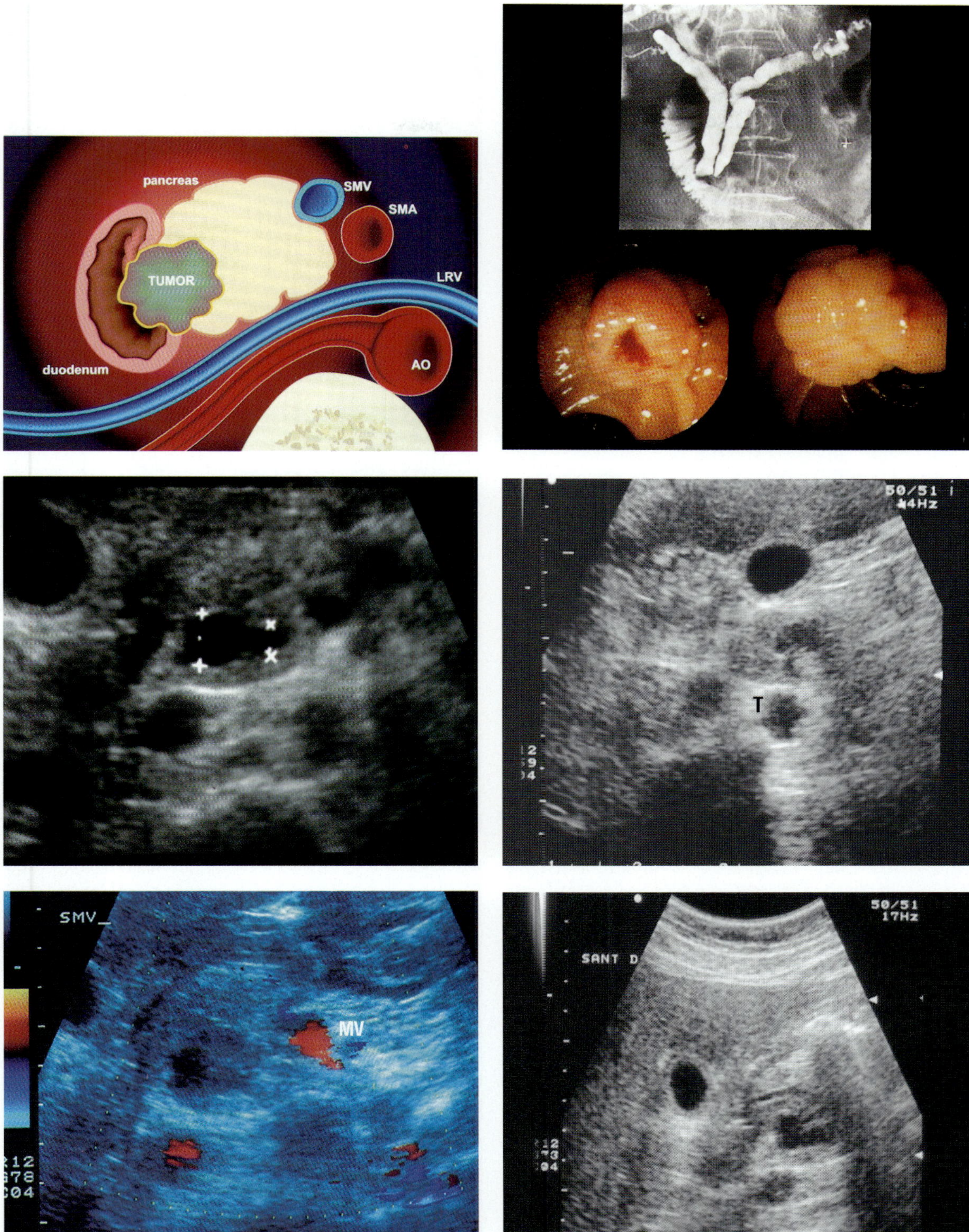

Fig. 8.7a–h. Resectable (peri-) ampullary tumor. **a** (Peri-) ampullary tumor mass, not adjacent to the surrounding peripancreatic vessels. *SMV*, superior mesenteric vein; *SMA*, superior mesenteric artery; *LRV*, left renal vein; *AO*, aorta. **b** Endoscopic retrograde cholangiopancreatography demonstrates a dilatated common bile duct and pancreatic duct with short distal obstruction (double duct sign). **c,d** Endoscopy demonstrates a cauliflower tumorous mass at the major ampulla. **e,f** Ultrasonography (US) (transverse view) shows a hypoechoic mass at the ampulla; normal pancreatic tissue between tumor and the superior mesenteric vein (*SMV*), better visualized on color Doppler (**f**). **g** US (right anterior oblique view) shows the tumor process (*T*) at the ampulla. **h.** US (transverse view) shows normal pancreatic duct

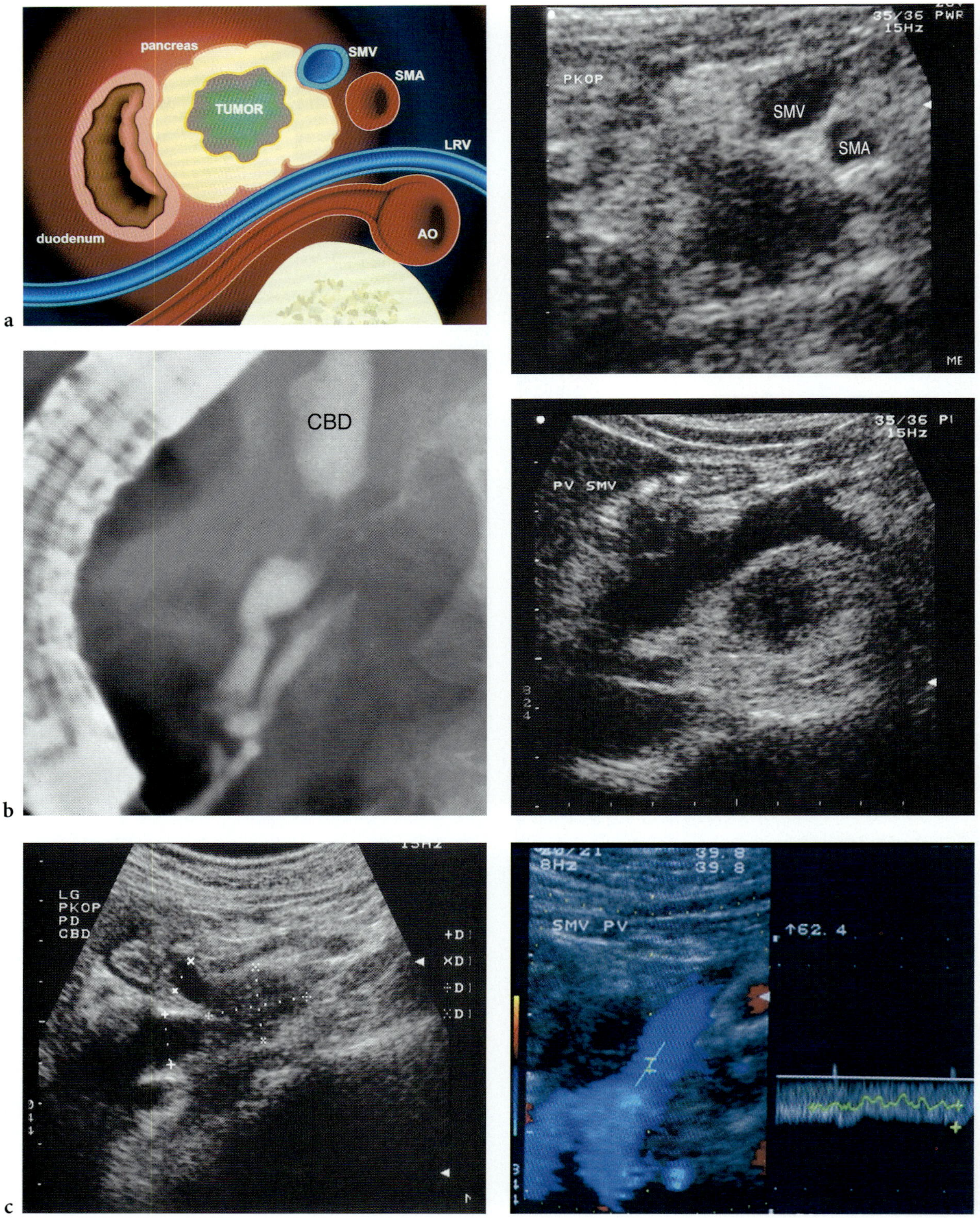

Fig. 8.8a–f. Resectable pancreatic head carcinoma. **a** Tumor at the pancreatic head free from the surrounding vessels. *SMV*, superior mesenteric vein; *SMA*, superior mesenteric artery; *LRV*, left renal vein; *AO*, aorta. **b** Endoscopic retrograde cholangiopancreatography demonstrates typical double duct sign; distal stenoses of the common bile duct (*CBD*) and a stop at the distal pancreatic duct (*PD*). **c** Ultrasonography (oblique view) shows dilatation of the common bile duct (*CBD*) and the pancreatic duct (*PD*), both bluntly obstructed by a sharply delineated hypoechoic mass at the pancreatic head. **d,e** Hypoechoic mass centrally located at the uncinate process; a clear uninterrupted fat plane is visible between the process and the superior mesenteric vein (*SMV*) and superior mesenteric artery (*SMA*); transverse view (**d**); longitudinal view (**e**). **f** Color Doppler. Normal Doppler signal at the portal venous level beyond the confluence region

in advanced disease. However, real-time color Doppler-assisted sonography can show encasement if the hyperechoic interface between tumor and vessel is lost (ANGELI et al. 1997) (Figs. 8.11, 8.12). KOSUGE et al. (1991) described thickening of the area around the superior mesenteric artery with or without decreased echogenicity (the cuff sign) as a reliable sign of tumor infiltration in patients with pancreatic carcinoma. Using an upper limit of 7 mm for normal, the sensitivity, specificity, and accuracy were 91%, 100%, and 96%, respectively.

ANGELI et al. developed a grading system describing the spatial relationship of vessels and tumor: grade 0, absence of contact; grade 1, short contiguity (≤2 cm); grade 2, long contiguity (>2 cm); grade 3, encasement or thrombosis. By using grade 2–3 as a criterion for vascular involvement, sensitivity of 79% and specificity of 89% were obtained by these authors (ANGELI et al. 1997). It should be noted that, in their series, of a total of 66 patients, five patients were excluded because bowel gas obscured the sonographic visualization of the pancreas. In five of the remaining 61 patients, the tumor could not be identified by US.

8.2.1.4
Value

Transabdominal US is commonly used as a primary screening method for tumor detection (DELMASCHIO et al. 1991). Detection of large tumors is usually easy. Small tumors may be difficult to visualize directly. In some patients, only indirect signs of pancreatic malignancy (i.e., ductal dilatation) may be seen. Major differences in sensitivity of tumor detection with US are reported in the literature. Figures range from 60% to 98% (FREENY 1991; ANGELI et al. 1997; PICHLER et al. 1989; HYOTY 1991; NIEDERAU and GRENDELL 1992). The sensitivity of transabdominal US depends on patient-dependent factors such as overlying bowel gas, cooperation, and obesity (all of which may cause incomplete visualization of the pancreas), as well as on the operator's degree of training and experience, the technical quality of the US equipment used, and the size and location of the tumor.

The addition of color and pulsed Doppler sonography has contributed much to assessing tumor involvement of the portal venous system, which is the main cause of unresectability (WREN et al. 1996; ANGELI et al. 1997).

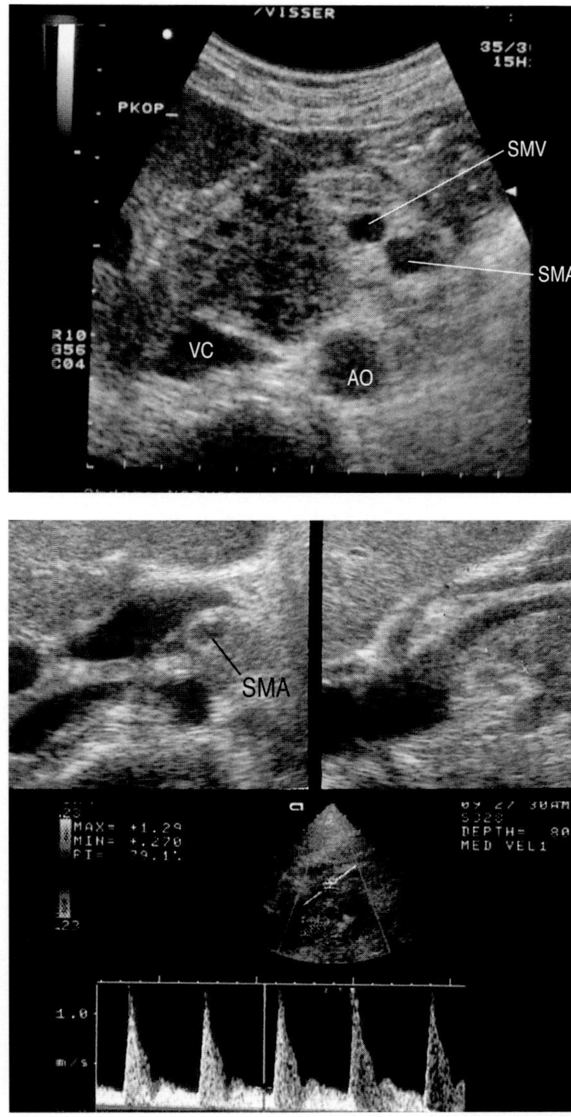

Fig. 8.9. a A 42-year-old male patient with obstructive jaundice. Ultrasonography demonstrates a hypoechoic mass at the pancreatic head region with a clear fat plane between the tumorous process, superior mesenteric vein (*SMV*), and superior mesenteric artery (*SMA*). *AO*, aorta; *VC*, vena cava. **b,c** The patient underwent subtotal pancreaticoduodenectomy. Ultrasonography 6 months later: recurrent malignant infiltration into the superior mesenteric artery. **b** Oblique/transverse view showing that almost three fourths of the superior mesenteric artery (*SMA*) circumference is involved. **c** Longitudinal view. **d** Normal Doppler signal in the superior mesenteric artery (*SMA*)

Table 8.2 summarizes the sensitivity, specificity, positive predictive value, and negative predictive value of duplex sonography and LUS (see Sect. 8.2.2) in diagnosing vascular ingrowth in pancreatic cancer, as reported by VAN DELDEN et al. (1996).

In our experience, an abnormal pulsed Doppler study is highly suspicious for major involvement of the portal venous system and unresectability of the tumor. On the other hand, because an abnormal pulsed Doppler sonogram can only be expected with >50% stenoses, a normal pulsed Doppler sonogram does not exclude infiltration of the portal venous system.

Table 8.2. Results of sonographic techniques for assessing portal venous involvement. [From VAN DELDEN et al. (1996)]

Involvement of PVS	Duplex US % (n=47)	LUS % (n=48)
Sensitivity	53 (10/19)	58 (11/19)
Specificity	89 (25/28)	97 (28/29)
Positive predictive value	77 (10/13)	92 (11/12)
Negative predictive value	74 (25/34)	78 (29/37)
Accuracy	74 (35/47)	81 (39/48)

PVS, portal venous system; US, ultrasonography; LUS, laparoscopic ultrasonography.

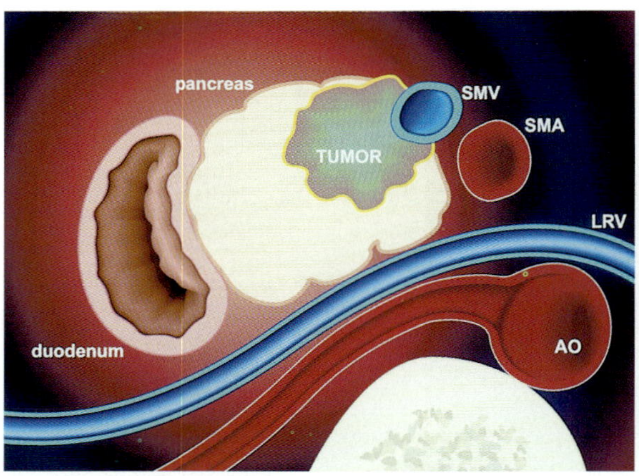

a

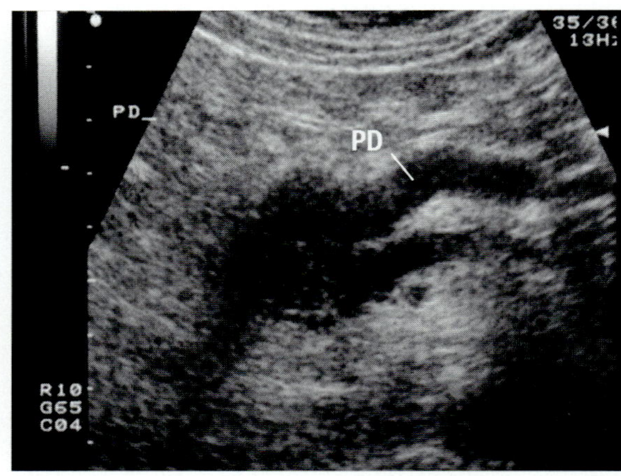

d

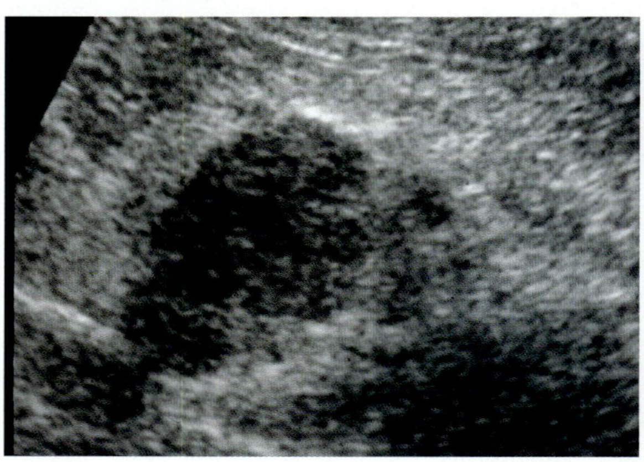
b

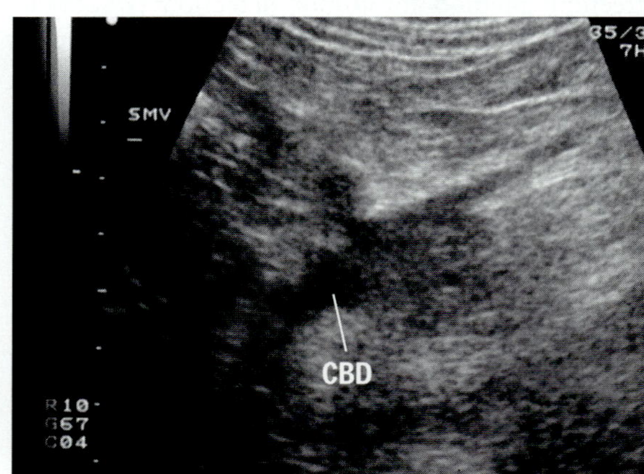

e

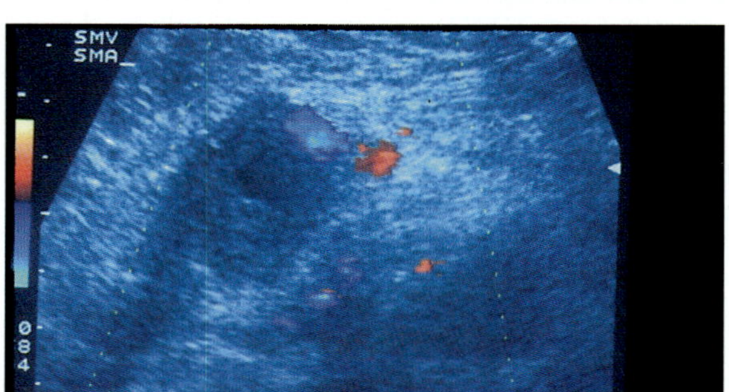

c

Fig. 8.10a–e. Dubious resectable pancreatic head carcinoma. **a** A mass in the pancreatic head adjacent to the portal venous system with normal Doppler signal. *SMV*, superior mesenteric vein; *SMA*, superior mesenteric artery; *LRV*, left renal vein; *AO*, aorta. **b,c** Ultrasonography (US) (transverse view) shows large hypoechoic mass in the pancreatic head adjacent to the confluens. **d** US (transverse view) shows dilatation of the pancreatic duct (*PD*), which abruptly stops at the tumor mass. **e** US (oblique view) shows dilatation of the common bile duct (*CBD*), which abruptly stops at the mass

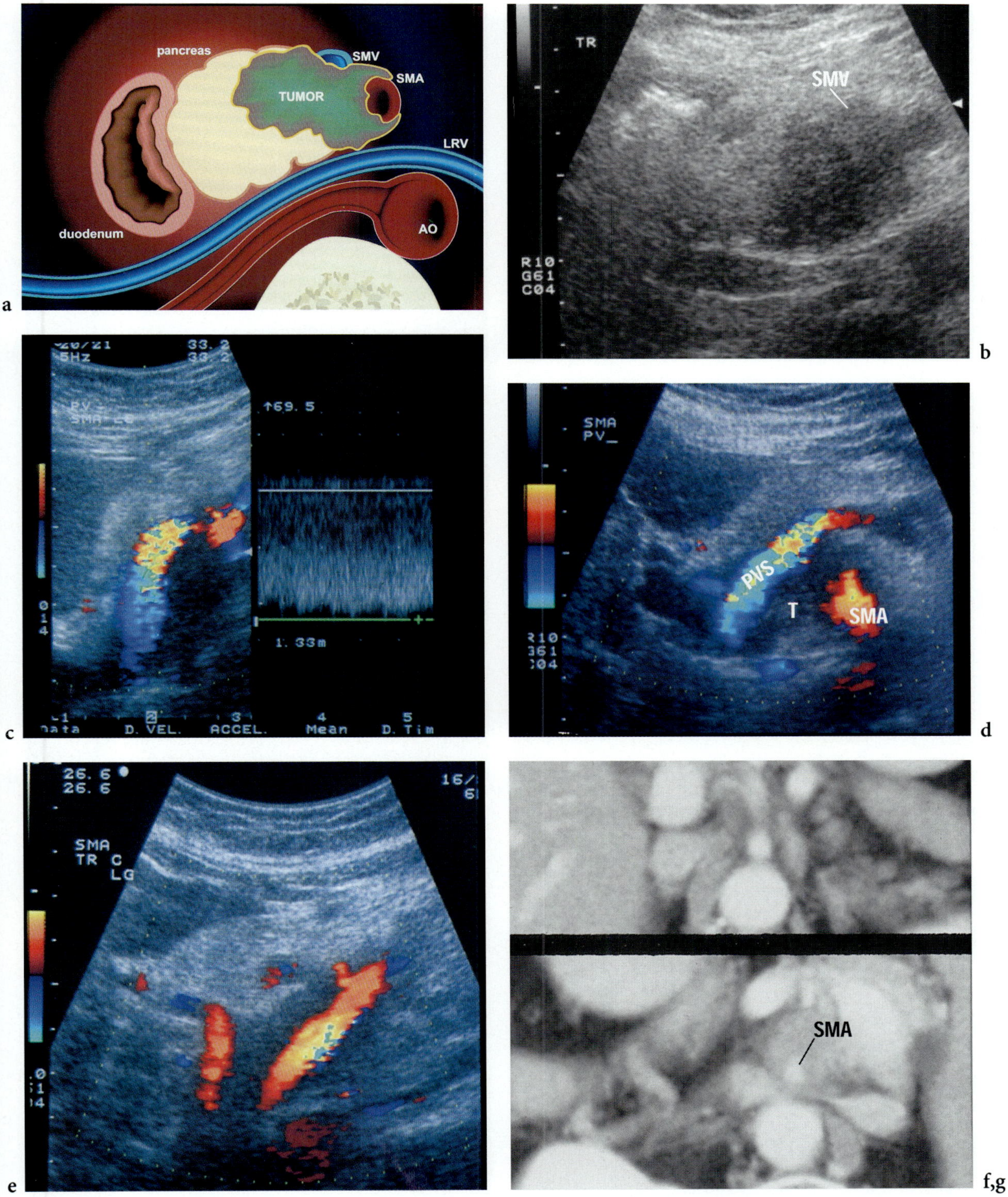

Fig. 8.11a–g. Irresectable pancreatic head carcinoma. **a** Pancreatic head carcinoma showing encasement of the major peripancreatic vessels. *SMV*, superior mesenteric vein; *SMA*, superior mesenteric artery; *LRV*, left renal vein; *AO*, aorta. **b** Ultrasonography (US) (transverse view). Large well delineated hypoechoic mass with almost 180° circumferential involvement/narrowing of the superior mesenteric vein (*SMV*). **c** US (longitudinal view). Narrowing of the portal venous system with a high velocity shift on Doppler US. **d,e** US (longitudinal view). Circumferential encasement of the superior mesenteric artery (*SMA*) and the portal venous system (*PVS*) by the tumor mass, which reaches towards the celiac trunk (*CT*). *T*, tumor. **f,g** Twin helical dynamic computed tomography. Circumferential involvement of the superior mesenteric artery (*SMA*), the superior mesenteric vein (*SMV*), and the celiac axis

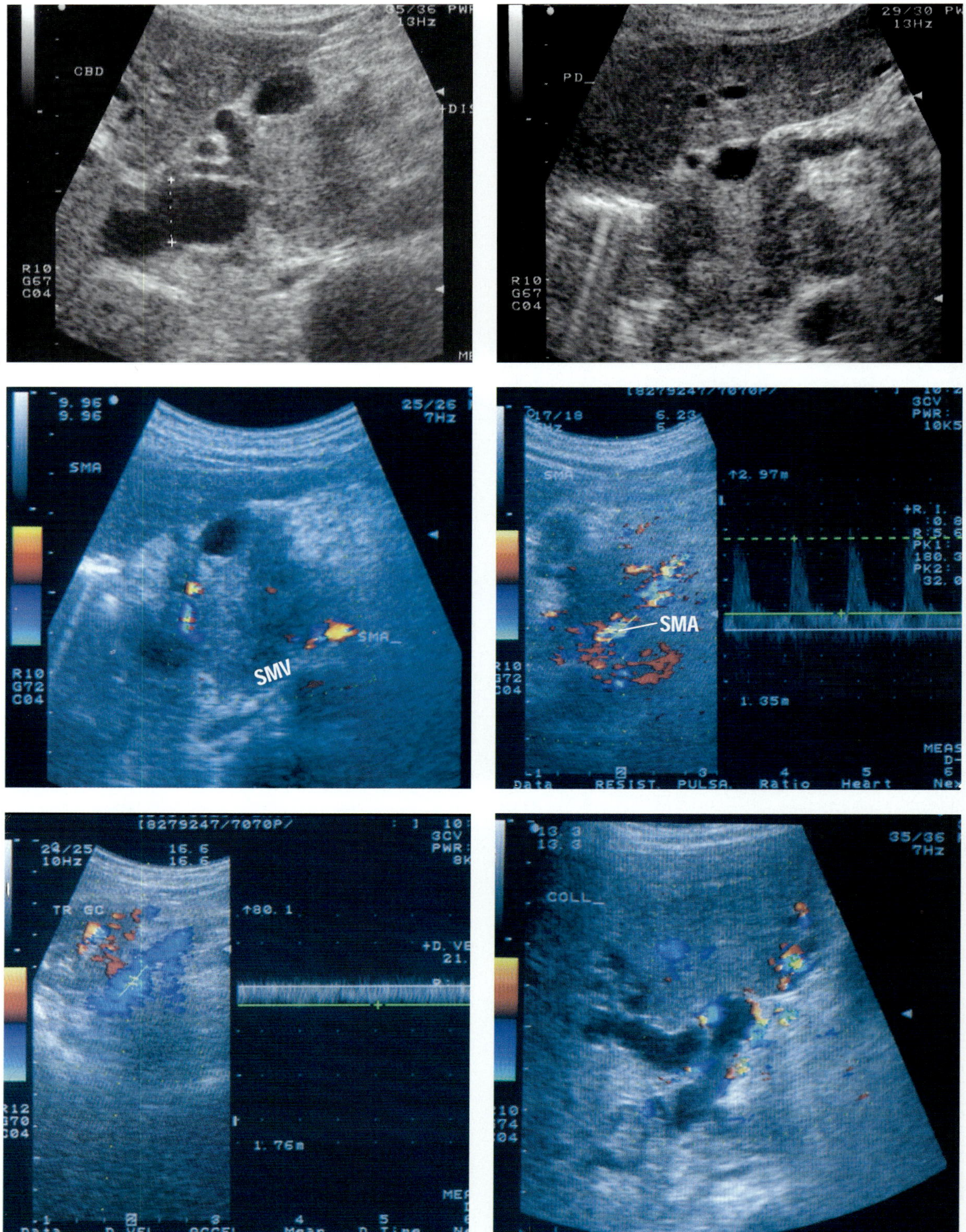

Fig. 8.12a–f. Irresectable pancreatic head carcinoma with vascular involvement. **a** Ultrasonography (US) (right oblique view). Large hypoechoic tumor mass at the pancreatic head; blunt obstruction of dilated common bile duct (*CBD*). **b,c** US (transverse view). Large hypoechoic tumor mass at the pancreatic head with a small cyst cranial to the head. Note that the superior mesenteric vein (*SMV*) is occluded; encasement of the superior mesenteric artery (*SMA*). *C*, cyst. **d** Doppler US (longitudinal view). Circumferential encasement of the superior mesenteric artery (*SMA*); however, normal Doppler signal. **e** Encasement of the gastrocolic trunk with a reversed flow. **f** Collateral circulation at the liver hilum due to portal venous occlusion

EUS eliminates the problem of overlying bowel gas and allows for focussed high-resolution imaging. However, EUS cannot always differentiate malignant from inflammatory processes of the pancreas or lymph nodes. In one large series, EUS was only 76% and 46% accurate in the diagnosis of malignancy and focal inflammation, respectively (Rösch et al. 1991). EUS-guided fine-needle aspiration biopsy (FNAB) has been proposed to increase the diagnostic accuracy in pancreatic cancer (Rösch et al. 1997). A remaining limitation is that a negative result does not enable malignancy to be ruled out. Therefore, a negative study cannot be the sole determinant of subsequent management (Cahn et al. 1996). While EUS may be limited in its ability to accurately diagnose pancreatic cancer, this technique is well suited to detect vascular invasion. Limitations of EUS are the need for patient sedation, operator dependency, and the inability to examine the entire liver and to detect peritoneal metastases. These limitations are important since many patients with pancreatic cancer have hepatic and/or peritoneal metastatic disease. In one recent study, no significant differences were found between EUS and dual-phase helical CT in the detection and staging of pancreatic tumors (Legmann et al. 1998). Helical CT was found to be slightly superior in the prediction of unresectability, which is related to its ability to detect liver metastases (Legmann et al. 1998). In another comparative study, EUS was the best technique for diagnosing lymph node involvement, while helical CT was significantly superior in diagnosing malignancy and assessing vascular involvement (Dufour et al. 1997). Others have reported disappointing results with EUS, even with the addition of US-guided FNAB (Rösch et al. 1997).

8.2.2 Laparoscopic Ultrasonography

J. W. A. J. Reeders, N. J. Smits, O. M. Van Delden

8.2.2.1 Technique

In LUS, high-frequency probes can be placed directly on the organs to be examined during diagnostic laparoscopy (Fukuda et al. 1984, 1992; Frank et al. 1985). Therefore, high-resolution US images can be obtained, without the disturbance of overlying bowel gas or thick abdominal wall (Van Delden et al. 1996). Although some studies have been published about the possibilities of LUS, few studies have investigated its use in staging pancreatic carcinoma (Okita et al. 1984; Cuesta et al. 1993; Murugiah et al. 1993; Bemelman et al. 1995; John et al. 1995).

Laparoscopy, in our institute, is performed by a surgeon under general anesthesia (Van Delden et al. 1996; Bemelman et al. 1995). Three 10-/11-mm trocars at umbilical and bilateral subcostal positions are used. The peritoneal cavity and liver surface are inspected for peritoneal metastases and subcapsular liver metastases. The transverse mesocolon and the ligament of Treitz are inspected to assess local ingrowth of the pancreatic tumor. Suspected superficial metastatic lesions and local tumor ingrowth are biopsied under laparoscopic observation using biopsy forceps. LUS is performed with a 7.5-MHz linear-array rigid LUS probe (UST-5522–7.5, Aloka, Tokyo, Japan) and the Aloka SSD 650CL US equipment. Prior to performing LUS, 1500 ml of isotonic saline solution is instilled into the right subphrenic space, to obtain a proper acoustic window. This allows ultrasonographic visualization of the whole liver, including the dome. A radiologist is present during each investigation for the interpretation of the LUS images. The liver is scanned for metastases. Intrahepatic lesions are biopsied percutaneously under LUS guidance with a screw-tip needle (Rotex, Ursus Konsult AB, Stockholm, Sweden) or core biopsy needle (Cook, Bjaeverskov, Denmark). The hepatoduodenal ligament and celiac axis are scanned for enlarged lymph nodes. The presence of a tumor in the pancreatic head region and ingrowth into the portal venous system is assessed.

8.2.2.2 Findings and Value

LUS criteria for vascular tumor involvement are:

1. No ingrowth: No contact between tumor and vessel, or contact between tumor and vessel without interruption of the echogenic interface
2. Ingrowth: contact between tumor and vessel, with interruption of the echogenic interface between tumor and vessel (Fig. 8.13).

LUS combined with diagnostic laparoscopy has a major additional role in the preoperative staging of patients with malignant pancreatic head tumors. The development of high-frequency LUS probes (7.5 MHz) enables the evaluation of solid organs and the retroperitoneal space for small intrahepatic metastases, lymph node metastases, small metastatic deposits in the peritoneal cavity, and malignant

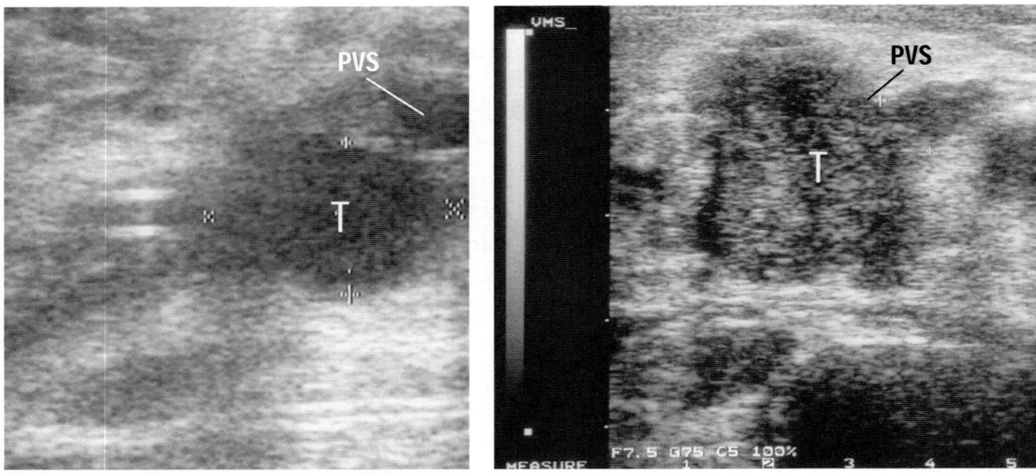

a b

Fig. 8.13. a Laparoscopic ultrasound. Large hypoechoic tumor mass at the pancreatic head at the region of the confluens. Note normal fat plane between tumor (*T*) and the portal venous system (*PVS*). **b** Large hypoechoic tumor mass with clear encasement of >90% of the portal venous system (*PVS*), therefore considered as being an irresectable tumor mass. *T*, tumor

infiltration of the portal and superior mesenteric vessels with a higher resolution and without disturbance from overlying bowel gas (Cuesta et al. 1993; Murugiah et al. 1993; John et al. 1993).

About 30% of liver metastases due to pancreatic carcinoma cannot be detected by CT if they are <2 cm in size. CT arterial portography (CTAP) is considered to be one of the most sensitive techniques for metastases detection, but is more invasive than conventional imaging, is also nonspecific, and may yield false-positive results (Heiken et al. 1989; Nelson et al. 1989; Freeny and Marks 1986).

Peritoneal and omental metastases are usually 1–2 mm in diameter and can be detected easily with laparoscopy. LUS enables lesion characterization in many cases, and small liver cysts can easily be distinguished from solid lesions. Small hyperechogenic solid lesions can be diagnosed as hemangiomas by compressing them with the LUS probe. This finding has been described using intraoperative sonography of the liver and can also be used with LUS (Paul et al. 1994). The initial results of staging of pancreatic head carcinoma by laparoscopy with LUS have been encouraging (Van Delden et al. 1996).

LUS appears to be the most accurate technique to predict unresectability of tumors of the pancreatic head. Using a combination of CT, angiography, and laparoscopy, the positive predictive value in determining unresectability can be as high as 89% (Warshaw et al. 1990). In a study by Bemelman et al. (1995), laparoscopy combined with LUS as a single diagnostic technique showed a positive predictive value of 97% for unresectability. The value of LUS in staging cancer of the pancreatic head region was compared to transabdominal US in a prospective study in our institution (Van Delden et al. 1996). A total of 80 patients who underwent LUS after transabdominal US had shown normal Doppler findings of portal vessels and no signs of metastatic disease. The detection rates for hepatic or lymph node metastases and vascular tumor infiltration were evaluated in 74 and 48 patients, respectively. LUS showed liver metastases in 10 patients (14%), and LUS combined with laparoscopy detected metastases in 17 (23%) of 74 patients. The specificity and positive predictive value of LUS in determining vascular ingrowth were 97% and 92%, respectively, compared with 89% and 77% by sonography in patients with normal Doppler findings. LUS offers the possibility of puncturing lesions as small as 3 mm, under LUS guidance, to obtain histology. However, in several patients in our studies, histologic results of punctures were inconclusive and biopsy techniques need to be refined, preferably by designing special puncture probes (Van Delden et al. 1996).

Peritoneal washings can be collected during laparoscopy and analyzed for malignant cells.

In a recent study by van Delden (1997), LUS showed slightly (statistically not significant) higher sensitivity, specificity, PPV, NPV and accuracy than contrast enhanced spiral CT in assessing vascular tumor ingrowth. the results are summarized in Table 8.3.

The same studies did not show a significant difference in the sensitivity, specificity, positive predictive value, negative predictive value, and accura-

Table 8.3. Results of laparoscopic ultrasonography (LUS) and spiral computed tomography (CT) for the prediction of portal venous tumor ingrowth compared with trial dissection and laparotomy in 44 patients. [From van Delden (1997)]

N=44	LUS (%)	Spiral CT (%)
Sensitivity	68 (13/19)	53 (10/19)
Specificity	96 (24/25)	88 (22/25)
Positive predictive value	93 (13/14)	77(10/13)
Negative predictive value	80 (24/30)	71 (22/31)
Accuracy	84 (37/44)	73 (32/44)

Table 8.4. Results of laparoscopy and laparoscopic ultrasonography (LUS) versus spiral computed tomography (CT) for the overall prediction of unresectability (metastatic disease and vascular ingrowth) compared with surgical findings and pathology results in 55 patients. [From van Delden (1997)]

N=55	Laparoscopy + LUS (%)	Spiral CT (%)
Sensitivity	77 (24/31)	64 (20/31)
Specificity	96 (23/24)	88 (21/24)
Positive predictive value	96 (24/25)	87 (20/23)
Negative predictive value	77 (23/30)	66 (21/32)
Accuracy	85 (47/55)	75 (41/55)

cy of spiral CT, and the combination of laparoscopy and LUS for overall prediction of unresectability (Table 8.4).

Unnecessary laparotomy can be prevented in at least 40% of patients with LUS (van Delden 1997). However, visualization of a local tumor extension in major vessels by LUS is technically demanding, and sonographically-guided biopsies are difficult to obtain. A learning curve must be anticipated. Surgical exploration must always be carried out if histologic proof of metastatic disease is not obtained. Trial dissection should be performed to confirm the findings of LUS on local unresectability, until sufficient experience has been obtained with this new diagnostic technique. Further studies are required to determine whether LUS significantly improves detection of metastases and local staging of potentially resectable tumors of the pancreas, compared to less invasive imaging techniques.

The referral pattern at our institution includes a diagnostic work-up starting with an adequate assessment of the level of obstruction with US as the initial examination. In some cases, the sonographic findings may obviate more invasive radiologic examinations. In malignant distal common bile duct obstruction, we use the approach shown in Fig. 8.14. When US [combined with endoscopic retrograde cholangiopancreatography (ERCP)] indicates that surgical resection of a pancreatic head mass is feasible, duplex Doppler US, helical CT, and, in doubtful cases (no metastases, no convincing local vascular ingrowth), laparoscopy combined with LUS are performed as adequate procedures for preoperative TNM staging; endoscopic ultrasonography (EUS) is recommended as a problem-solver in a limited group of patients where there is suspicion of small tumors. When surgical resection does not seem feasible (ingrowth into the mesenteric, splenic, or portal venous system; presence of liver, peritoneal, or lymph node metastases), the insertion of an endoprosthesis (polyethylene or metallic expandable stent) during ERCP is the only possible palliative treatment. Although in the 1970s and 1980s the diagnosis of obstructive jaundice by sonography was a reason either to abandon further treatment or to refer the patient to a surgeon to confirm unresectability by an exploratory laparotomy and a bypass, in the 1990s it is a reason for the hepatopancreaticobiliary team – radiologist, gastroenterologist, hepatologist, and surgeon – to discuss how to proceed with diagnostic and therapeutic steps.

8.3 Computed Tomography

8.3.1 Technique

8.3.1.1 Dynamic Incremental CT

With the dynamic incremental scanning technique, the pancreas should be examined using a slice thickness of 5–10 mm. Decreasing the slice thickness requires an increased X-ray dose in order to obtain an acceptable noise level. The drawback of using thin slices is the prolonged examination time; this may result in suboptimal contrast in the images obtained at the end of the study.

Non-contrast-enhanced images are commonly used to detect pancreatic calcification and to define the level of pancreatic and/or biliary duct obstruction. Injection of an antiperistaltic drug allows a better distention of the stomach and duodenum, and reduces streak artifacts caused by peristalsis. The

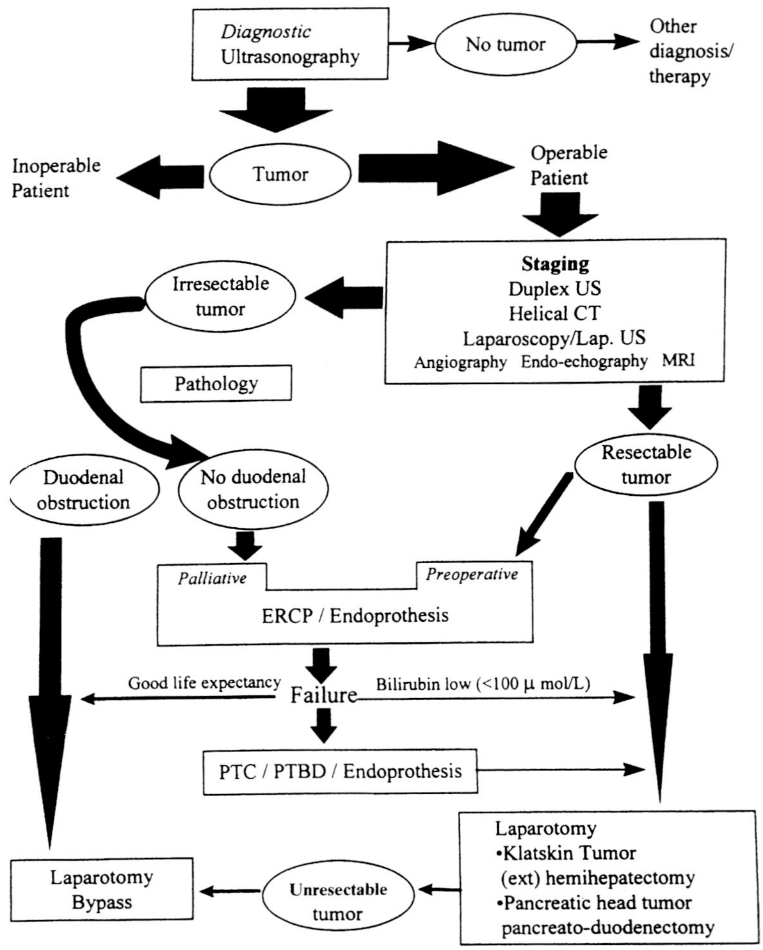

Fig. 8.14. Algorithm for the staging of pancreatic tumors. *PTBD,* percutaneous transtrepatic biliary drainage; *US,* ultrasonography; *CT,* computed tomography; *Lap. US,* laparoscopic US; *MRI,* magnetic resonance imaging; *ERCP,* endoscopic retrograde cholangiopancreatography; *PTC,* percutaneous transhepatic cholangiography (Figure courtesy J. Reeders)

administration of an oral contrast agent is mandatory for delineating the stomach and duodenum from the pancreas (Fig. 8.15). The oral contrast medium used may be a positive or a negative one. Pure tap water (500–600 ml) is preferred as a negative oral contrast agent (WINTER et al. 1996). One advantage of using a negative oral contrast agent is the improved visualization of the different layers of the wall of the stomach and duodenum. This may be a critical factor in the detection of mural invasion by pancreatic adenocarcinoma. Furthermore, intraluminal protrusions, which are commonly found in patients with periampullary carcinoma, are better seen when a negative contrast agent is used (Fig. 8.16).

While some tumors may be visible on non-contrast-enhanced scans (Fig. 8.17), tumor detection usually requires use of intravenous (IV) contrast media. Different modalities for injecting the contrast medium have been proposed including slow infusion or uniphasic and biphasic bolus injection (RIGAUTS et al. 1990).

Scanning is generally started 15–20 s after the start of the injection. Successive slices may be obtained either in the craniocaudal or caudocranial direction. In cases where previous imaging studies or unenhanced scans suggest the presence of a mass in the pancreatic head, scanning in a caudocranial direction will result in optimal differential enhancement between tumor and normal pancreatic tissue. If, on the other hand, these studies suggest the presence of a mass in the pancreatic tail, scanning in a craniocaudal direction may be preferred. In any case, an attempt should be made to include the tumor in

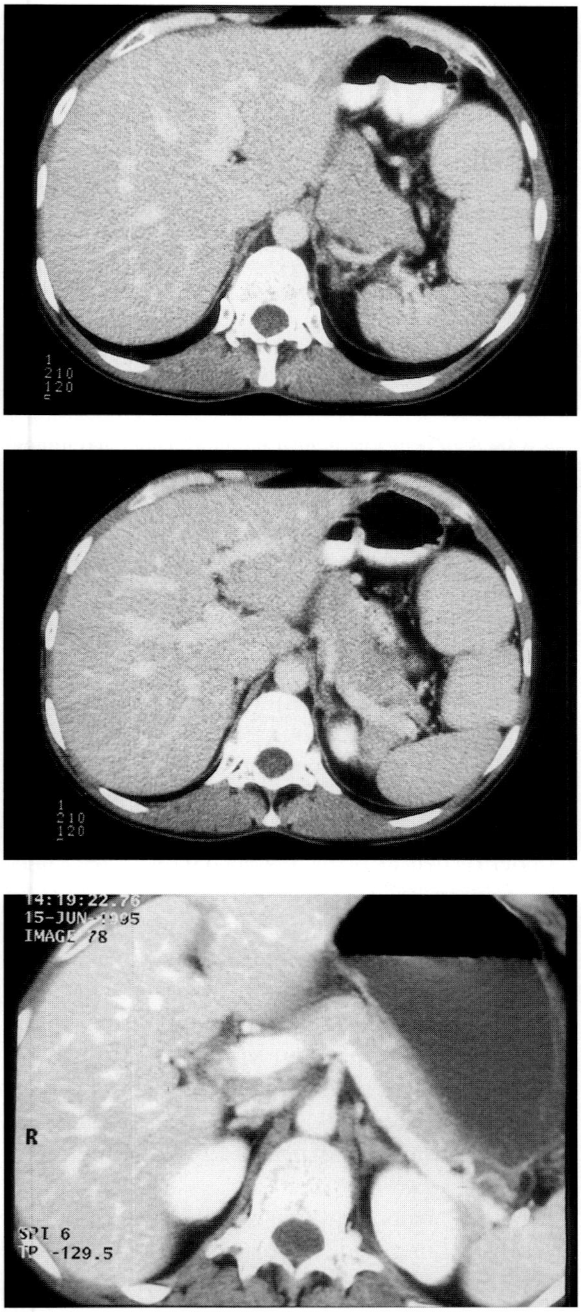

Fig. 8.15a–c. Importance of gastric distention. **a,b** Images obtained with conventional computed tomography (CT) and without the administration of oral contrast medium show an apparently enlarged pancreatic tail (*asterisk*): tumor? **c** Image obtained with helical CT in the pancreatic phase and with the use of water as an oral contrast medium in combination with a spasmolytic agent reveals normal aspect of pancreatic tail

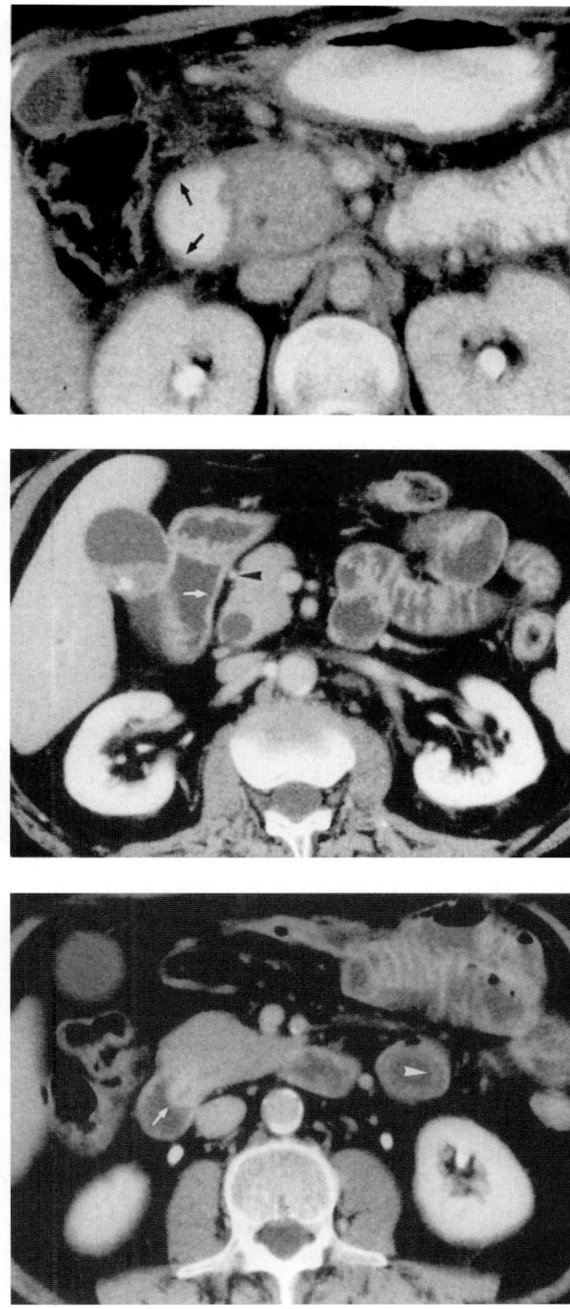

Fig. 8.16. Computed tomography technique for imaging of the pancreas: positive versus negative oral contrast medium. **a** Positive intraluminal contrast agent (diluted gastrografin). Notice the blurring of the interface between the intraluminal contrast agent and the wall of the duodenum itself (*arrows*). **b,c** Negative intraluminal contrast agent in the duodenum (pure tap water). **b** Differentiation between the wall of the duodenum (*arrow*) and the lumen is better appreciated as compared with (**a**). The gastroduodenal artery (*arrowhead*) is perfectly visualized as a structure separated from the duodenal wall and pancreatic head. **c** A section 20 mm caudad to (**b**). The distal portion of the main bile duct (*arrow*) is seen protruding into the duodenal lumen. Note apparent thickening of the jejunal wall (*arrowhead*), probably caused by motion

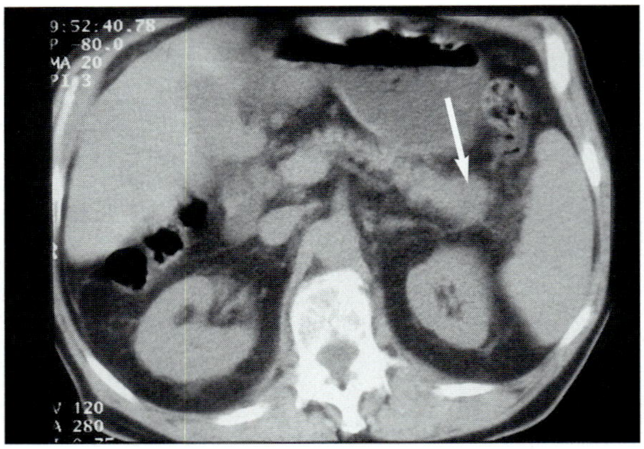

Fig. 8.17. Pancreatic mass visible on unenhanced images. Unenhanced image shows a mass in the pancreatic tail (*arrow*). This mass is visible mainly because it has a homogeneous density rather than the heterogeneous lipomatous texture of the normal pancreatic tissue

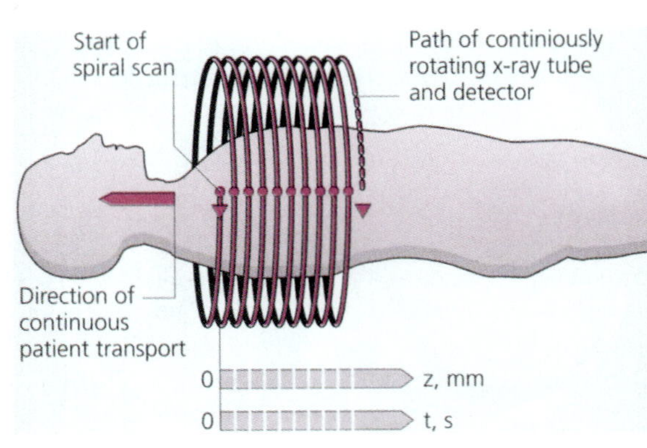

Fig. 8.18. Scan principle in helical (spiral) computed tomography. Continuous patient transport is associated with continuous rotation of the X-ray tube and detector. [Reprinted from Kalender (1995))

the first few slices. Indeed, marked enhancement of the pancreatic parenchyma occurs during the capillary phase. Peak enhancement occurs during a relatively short period of time (Marchal et al. 1979). This means that careful selection of the area of maximal diagnostic interest is necessary in order to obtain the maximum benefit of the bolus IV contrast medium injection. The liver should always be investigated within the same session, in order to allow for the detection of liver metastases.

8.3.1.2
Helical (Spiral) CT

8.3.1.2.1
General

The introduction of helical, or spiral, CT has opened new perspectives in the evaluation of pancreatic carcinoma, not only because this technique improves the conspicuity of small lesions, but also because it facilitates the detection of vascular invasion, metastatic lymph node disease, and metastatic involvement of the liver (Fuji et al. 1993). Helical CT shares some important characteristics with conventional incremental CT, particularly the high in-plane spatial resolution (pixel size typically ±0.3 mm), and the relative independence of image quality from patient-related factors. In helical CT, continuous translation of the patient (and examination table) is combined with continuous rotation of the X-ray tube and detector elements, thus leading to a spiral or helical movement of the latter components relative to the patient (Fig. 8.18) (Rigauts et al. 1990; Kalender et al. 1990; Heiken et al. 1993). In other words, slice-by-slice scanning is replaced by volumetric data acquisition: A single data set is obtained which represents the volume covered in the given number of helical turns. Planar data sets are calculated from the volume data sets for each image to be reconstructed. This intermediate calculation step demands appreciable computational efforts, but it provides a significant advantage inherent to the technique of volumetric data acquisition: Images can be constructed at any position within the scanned volume, with arbitrary fine spacing and in an overlapping way if desired. This constitutes one of the most important advantages of helical CT (Kalender et al. 1994).

Another major advantage of helical CT is the increased scan speed. In conventional incremental CT, successive slices are obtained during successive periods of breath-holding. The interscan interval, i.e., the time interval between the acquisition of two consecutive images, is used not only to translate the patient relative to the measurement system, but also to give the patient the opportunity to breathe. The length of the interscan interval can be adjusted as a function of the physical condition of the patient and the purpose of the study, and typically varies between 5 and 8 s. In helical CT, the interscan interval is eliminated since patient translation and data acquisition both occur in a continuous way. As a result, the time required to investigate an organ or body part can be reduced significantly. Typical examination times for studies of the upper abdomen (including the pancreas) with helical CT range between 15 and 30 s. If clinically indicated, the lower abdomen can be examined with a second helical scan performed approximately 2 min after the start of contrast injection. Another particular feature in helical CT is that periodic motion with a low temporal frequency (e.g., respiration) does not degrade the quality of native axial images. Indeed, since rotation times currently used in helical CT vary between 0.75 and 1 s, little motion occurs during this short acquisition window. In other words, helical CT offers the ability to obtain high-quality images in very sick patients or anyone unable to cope with the breath-hold requirements. This feature, of course, significantly improves the value of CT as a first-line examination technique. While respiration does not significantly reduce the quality of individual images, it has a potentially negative effect because it induces spatial misregistration along the longitudinal body axis (z-axis). Therefore, respiration potentially decreases the sensitivity of the technique to detect small lesions and reduces the quality of reformatted or three-dimensional images. For these reasons, helical CT imaging is performed during breath-holding unless impossible.

The spatial resolution along the longitudinal axis of the body (longitudinal resolution) and the in-plane contrast resolution are primarily determined by the following parameters: collimation (or nominal slice thickness, in millimeters), table feed (i.e., the speed of the examination table, in millimeters per second), and image reconstruction interval (i.e., the distance along the longitudinal axis between two consecutively reconstructed axial images, in millimeters). The ratio of table feed:collimation is commonly referred to as pitch. In order to obtain an optimal in-plane contrast resolution, it is mandatory to use overlapping image reconstruction (Kalender et al. 1994). In other words, the reconstruction interval (RI) should always be smaller than the nominal slice thickness (ST). It has been shown that the pitch may be increased up to 1.5 and even 2, provided that the degree of overlap between consecutively reconstructed images is large enough (Wang et al. 1994). In helical CT of (suspected) pancreatic carcinoma, the following parameters are preferred at our institution: ST, 5 mm; pitch, 1.5; RI, 3–4 mm. Using these parameters, reformatted images of diagnostic quality can be obtained in routine studies. Alternatively, thinner (2.5–3 mm) slices can be used (Lu et al. 1997). In any case, the tube current and voltage should be sufficiently high to avoid a noisy appearance of the images and to enable the detection of subtle differences in density. Typical values are 210 mAS and 120 kV, respectively.

8.3.1.2.2 Use of Intravenous Contrast Media

As in incremental CT, it is mandatory to use iodinated IV contrast media in helical CT of the pancreas. Two injection parameters are of critical importance: the contrast injection rate and the time delay between the start of contrast injection and the start of the helical scan (injection–scan interval). These parameters should be adjusted in order to maximize the difference in attenuation between the structures of interest (in this case, tumor) and the surrounding tissue. Because pancreatic adenocarcinoma is a relatively poorly vascularized neoplasm and the normal pancreas has a rich arterial blood supply, the goal is to obtain maximum enhancement of normal pancreatic tissue. While the optimum value for injection rate remains to be determined, there is no doubt that fast injection of contrast media is one of the major prerequisites of obtaining optimal tumor-to-pancreas contrast. In dedicated helical CT studies of the pancreas, injection rates typically vary between 3 and 5 ml/s. In comparison with conventional CT, the total dose of contrast medium can be reduced by 25% (Rigauts et al. 1992). A mechanical power injector is always used and contrast is injected through a 20-gauge catheter placed in a cubital vein. In order to obtain images during the phase of peak parenchymal (pancreatic) enhancement, a relatively short injection–scan interval is used (Kim et al. 1996). The optimal scan delay time is inversely related to the injection rate: the faster the injection rate, the shorter the optimal delay time (Bonaldi et al. 1996). A delay time of 30–40 s is commonly used (Lu et al. 1996). In this phase of perfusion, not only the pancreas but also all vascular structures, including the portal vein, are usually adequately enhanced (Lu et al. 1996). When dual- or double-phase helical CT is available, a second helical scan of the entire upper abdomen can be obtained in the hepatic phase of perfusion, i.e., at 70–80 s (Figs. 8.19, 8.20) (Legmann et al. 1998; Van Hoe and Baert 1997). In our practical set-up, the first helical scan focuses on the pancreas and is performed using a ST/TF/RI of 5/8/3 mm and a delay of approximately 40 s. A second helical scan is initiated at 80 s, and covers the entire upper abdomen. Scan parameters are: 8/12/6 mm. Besides enabling an optimal detection of focal liver lesions, images obtained in the hepatic phase may occasionally show a higher degree of

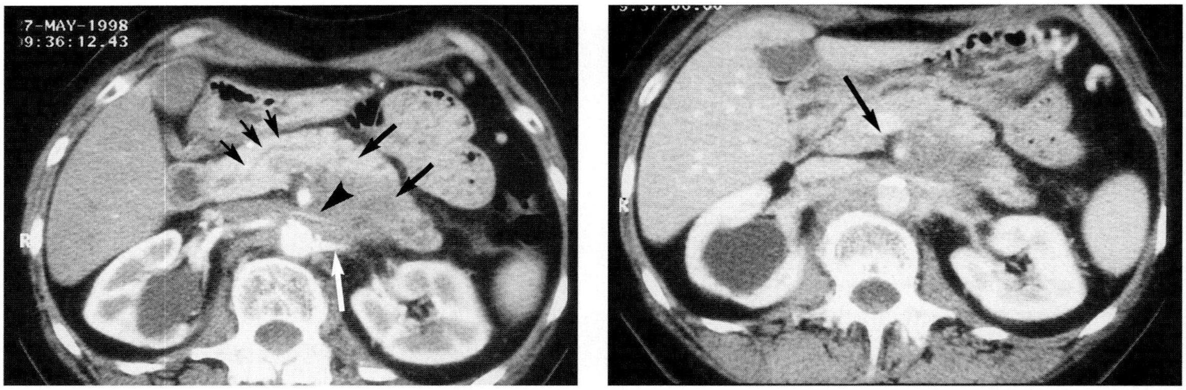

Fig. 8.19a,b. Adenocarcinoma. Comparison of images obtained in the pancreatic and hepatic phases of perfusion. **a** Image obtained in the pancreatic phase shows marked enhancement of the pancreas. The pancreatic duct is well seen (*small arrows*). A large tumor is seen as a hypoenhancing area extending into the retroperitoneum (*arrows*). Note enhancement of the left renal vein (*arrowhead*), but absence of enhancement of the splenic vein. **b** On this image obtained in the hepatic phase, the contrast between normal pancreatic tissue and tumor is somewhat less optimal. On the other hand, adequate enhancement of the splenic vein is observed (*arrow*)

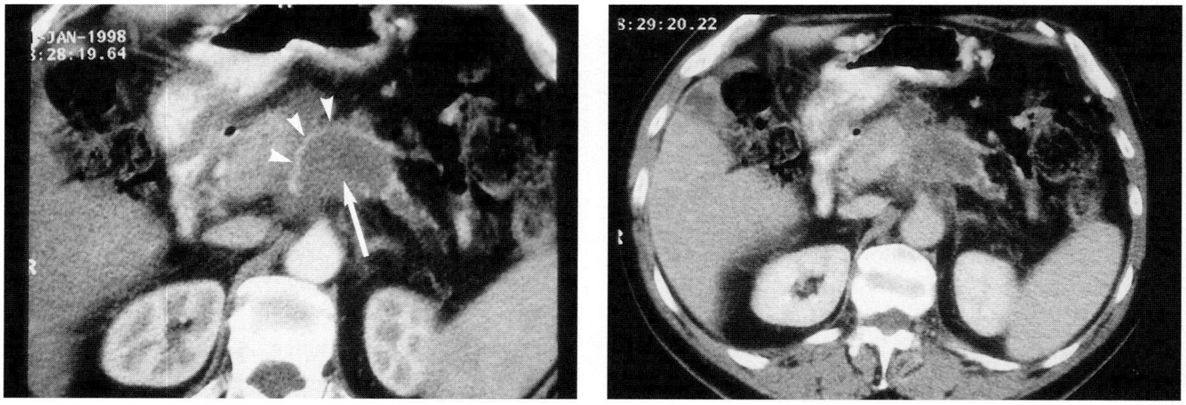

Fig. 8.20a,b. Adenocarcinoma. Comparison of images obtained in the pancreatic and hepatic phases of perfusion. **a** Image obtained in pancreatic phase at level of pancreatic body shows large mass in pancreatic body, representing adenocarcinoma (*arrow*). Note marked atrophy of pancreatic parenchyma in the pancreatic tail (*small arrow*) and narrowing of the splenic artery (tumor invasion) (*arrowheads*). **b** Image obtained in the hepatic phase shows similar features. However, the anatomy of the splenic artery cannot be assessed adequately. An additional finding is the apparent absence of the splenic vein, caused by occlusion of this vessel. Note that in this patient, the normal pancreatic parenchyma is more enhanced in (**b**) than in (**a**)

enhancement of the pancreas and peripancreatic veins, particularly in patients with poor cardiac function and long circulation times (Fig. 8.20). This constitutes another benefit of dual-phase scanning: inter-individual variability in cardiac output may be partially compensated for by obtaining images in two different phases of perfusion. In patients with previously detected focal liver lesions of undetermined nature, inclusion of the liver in the early-phase scan may be helpful. Indeed, dual-phase CT of the liver not only improves the detection of hypervascular tumors (like metastases of endocrine pancreatic tumors), but may also be helpful in the differential diagnosis between benign and malignant liver lesions (Van Hoe et al. 1997).

8.3.1.2.3 Calculation of Reformatted and Projective Images and Cine Display Evaluation

By virtue of its ability to construct overlapping images at arbitrary increments, helical CT offers the opportunity to create reformatted images (Fig. 8.21) and projective images [e.g., maximum intensity projections, MIP (Figs. 8.22, 8.23)] not affected by breathing artifacts. More recently, volume rendering has been proposed for three-dimensional visualiza-

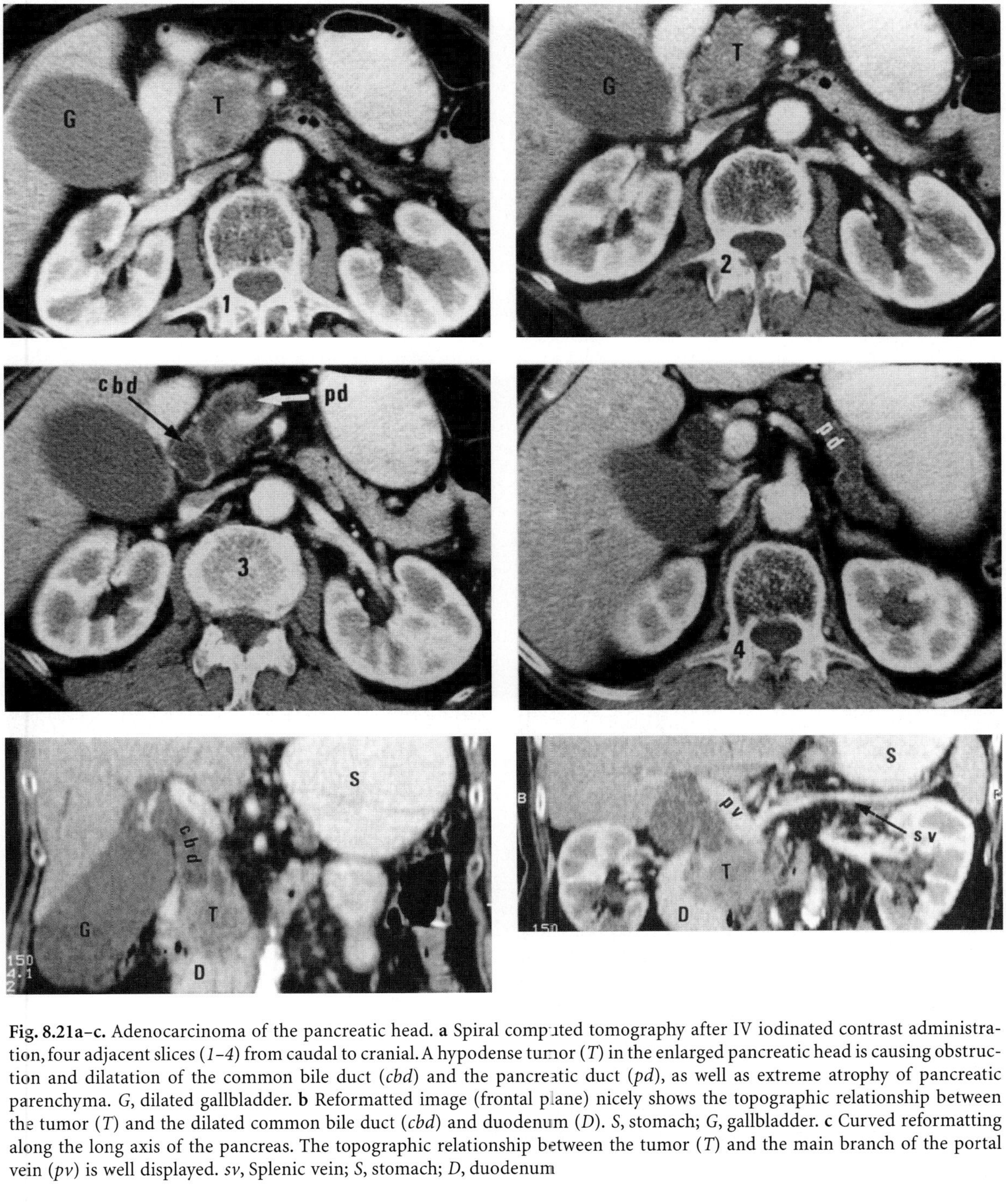

Fig. 8.21a–c. Adenocarcinoma of the pancreatic head. **a** Spiral computed tomography after IV iodinated contrast administration, four adjacent slices (*1–4*) from caudal to cranial. A hypodense tumor (*T*) in the enlarged pancreatic head is causing obstruction and dilatation of the common bile duct (*cbd*) and the pancreatic duct (*pd*), as well as extreme atrophy of pancreatic parenchyma. *G*, dilated gallbladder. **b** Reformatted image (frontal plane) nicely shows the topographic relationship between the tumor (*T*) and the dilated common bile duct (*cbd*) and duodenum (*D*). *S*, stomach; *G*, gallbladder. **c** Curved reformatting along the long axis of the pancreas. The topographic relationship between the tumor (*T*) and the main branch of the portal vein (*pv*) is well displayed. *sv*, Splenic vein; *S*, stomach; *D*, duodenum

tion (Novick and Fishman 1998). Although these images do not contain additional information when compared to axial scans, they may occasionally provide a better overview of complex anatomic relationships and/or vascular lesions. It should be kept in mind, however, that, because of the anisotropic voxel size in helical CT, representation of small structures on these types of images may be suboptimal.

While the evaluation of printed hard-copy films is still the standard procedure in diagnostic radiology, cine display evaluation of overlapping images on the computer console and use of the mouse offers major advantages. There is no doubt that subtle vascular, ductal, or parenchymal abnormalities are better seen using this technique (Bonaldi et al. 1998). With the introduction of PACS (picture archiving and com-

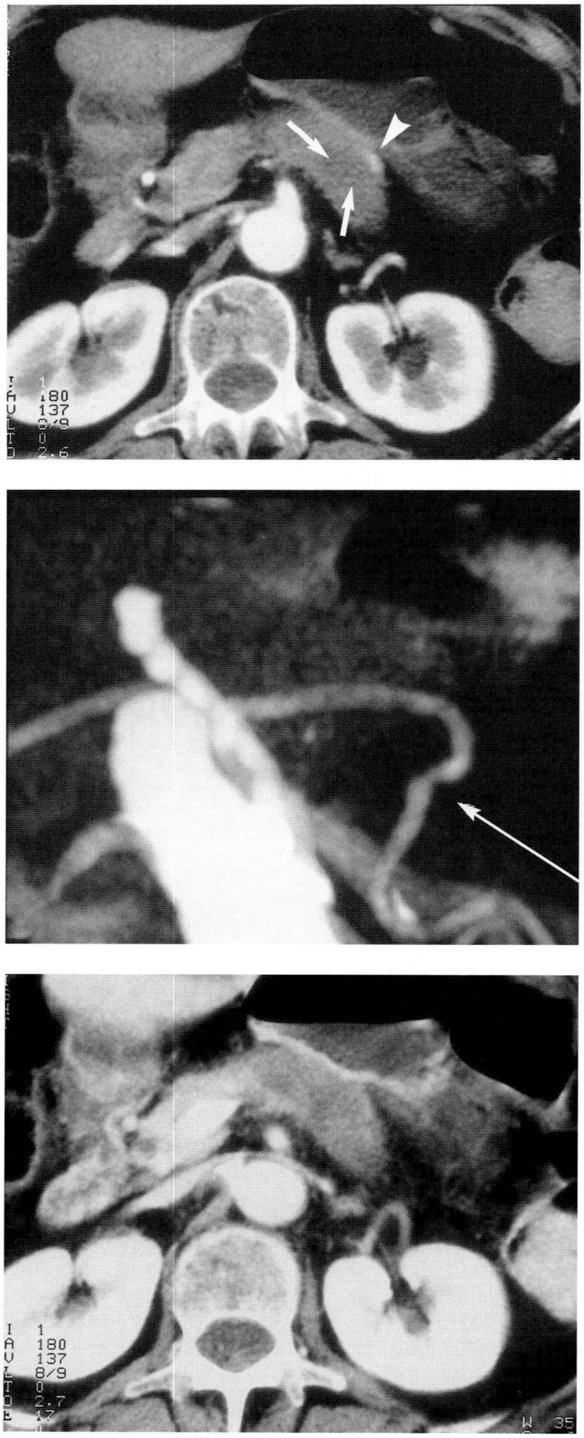

Fig. 8.22a–c. Adenocarcinoma invading the splenic artery. Scanning in the arterial phase and the pancreatic phase. **a** Image obtained in the early arterial phase shows a slightly hypodense pancreatic tumor (*white arrows*). Note part of splenic artery (*white arrowhead*). **b** Maximum intensity projection image calculated from (**a**) shows focal narrowing of the splenic artery, diagnostic of tumor invasion (*white arrow*). **c** Image obtained in the pancreatic phase shows the tumor as a mass that is markedly hypodense relative to normal pancreatic tissue

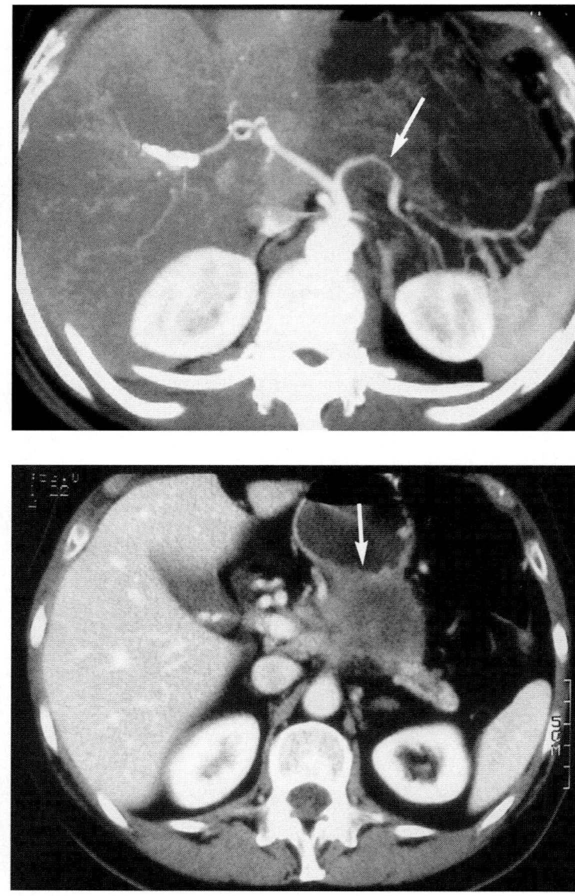

Fig. 8.23a,b. Adenocarcinoma invading the splenic artery and stomach. **a** Maximum intensity projection image calculated from images obtained in the arterial phase shows narrowing of the splenic artery (*white arrow*). **b** Image obtained in the pancreatic phase shows large tumor clearly invading the dorsal wall of the stomach (*white arrow*)

munication systems), cine display evaluation at the computer console could become the standard procedure.

8.3.2 Findings

8.3.2.1 Direct signs

Large adenocarcinomas are visible on CT as focal and abrupt changes in size or contour of the organ. Segmental or diffuse enlargement is less common (Freeny et al. 1988). The detectability of smaller tumors depends on the size of the tumor and the contrast with surrounding tissue.

In many cases, adenocarcinomas are isodense to normal pancreatic tissue at non-contrast-enhanced scans. A slight decrease in density may occasionally be seen, which may be due to tumor necrosis (PÄIVÄNSALO et al. 1988). In patients with pancreatic lipomatosis, ductal adenocarcinomas are commonly seen as relatively hyperdense masses. Another important diagnostic feature is the focal disappearance of the normal lipomatous pancreatic texture ("marbling") (see Fig. 8.17).

Adenocarcinomas are nearly invariably hypovascular relative to normal pancreatic tissue and are seen as hypoenhancing masses (see Figs 8.19, 8.20). Rarely, small tumors may be isoenhancing and thus invisible at CT.

In ductal adenocarcinoma, focal narrowing or apparent disappearance of the pancreatic duct is typical ("missing duct sign"). In tumors located in the pancreatic head, associated narrowing of the common bile duct may be observed, corresponding to the double duct sign that is well-known from ERCP studies (Figs. 8.24, 8.25). Abrupt rather than gradual narrowing of both ducts is suggestive of pancreatic carcinoma (Fig. 8.26). Small areas of necrosis are seen as hypodense foci located within the mass. Occasionally, adenocarcinomas may contain large cystic or necrotic areas (see Sect. 8.7.5).

8.3.2.2
Indirect signs

Indirect CT signs are secondary to ductal obstruction (MURANAKA 1990).

Pancreatic duct dilatation is an important feature in ductal adenocarcinoma (Fig. 8.27). Associated dilatation of side branches is also a common finding. Chronic obstruction of the pancreatic duct leads to atrophy of the parenchyma distal to the obstruction, which may be more or less pronounced. Sometimes, only a small rim of pancreatic parenchyma remains, surrounding the dilated pancreatic duct (MURANAKA 1990). The combined CT findings of a focal mass causing narrowing or obliteration of the pancreatic duct, proximal pancreatic duct dilatation, and proximal parenchymal atrophy are highly suggestive of ductal adenocarcinoma and are only rarely observed in other tumors. Chronic ductal obstruction by ductal adenocarcinoma can also lead to small intrapancreatic pseudocyst formation proximal to the tumor site (Fig. 8.28). These post-obstructive pseudocysts are seen in about 10% of patients (LIN 1988). Rarely, larger extrapancreatic fluid collections secondary to pancreatic duct obstruction by tumor may occur (Fig. 8.29). Obstructed side branches and pseudocysts should be differentiated from tumor necrosis. This is usually possible because areas of necrosis have a more irregular contour and are located within the tumor rather than upstream.

Biliary duct dilatation: Biliary dilatation is frequently present in ductal carcinoma of the pancreatic head due to direct involvement of the intrapancreatic portion of the common bile duct. In the case of minimal dilatation, the common bile duct will be seen on CT as a small, round, hypodense structure in the liver hilum, located ventrally to the portal vein and medially to the hepatic artery. It can then be traced caudally on successive slices down to the level of the obstruction. In the case of advanced dilatation, the suprapancreatic portion of the common bile duct can assume a tortuous course and may have a more elongated appearance on axial slices. If a ductal adenocarcinoma of the head of the pancreas causes contiguous involvement of both the common bile duct and the pancreatic duct, two adjacent dilated structures are visible ("double duct sign").

Isolated dilatation of the biliary and/or pancreatic duct without mass lesion is present in a small minority of patients with ductal adenocarcinoma of the pancreas and is most commonly observed in patients with small (peri-) papillary tumors. Adjunctive procedures such as ERCP, magnetic resonance cholangiopancreatography (MRCP), or EUS are indicated in these cases (SEMELKA et al. 1991). As stated above, use of helical scanning together with fast injection of contrast medium and scanning in the pancreatic phase is critical for tumor detection; many tumors are hardly visible if one of these criteria is not fulfilled. It should be stressed that severe biliary dilatation is common in patients with common bile duct stones and malignant tumors, but rare in chronic pancreatitis. Thus, CT depiction of severe biliary dilatation without detectable cause always warrants further investigation.

Intrahepatic duct dilatation is considered to be present when the intrahepatic ducts are visible in the peripheral portion of the liver, or if the diameter exceeds 4 mm in the region of the liver hilum. Intrahepatic biliary dilatation may be more pronounced in patients with enlarged metastatic lymph nodes in the liver hilum.

Dilatation of the gallbladder is most often associated with bile duct dilatation if the level of the biliary obstruction is distal to the junction of the cystic duct and the common hepatic duct. Gallbladder dilatation may be absent in the case of chronic cholecystitis (fibrosis) or cystic duct obstruction.

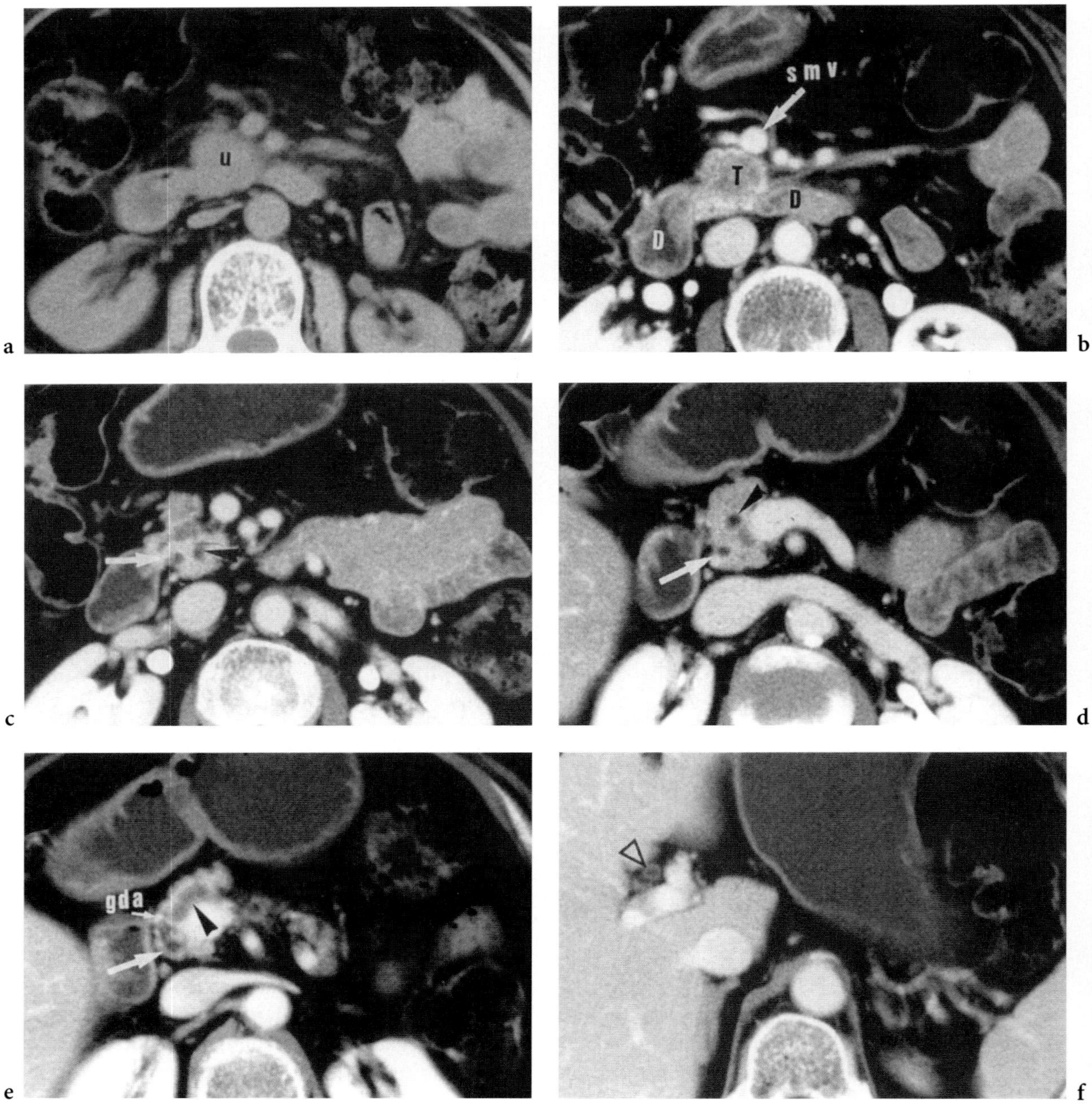

Fig. 8.24a–f. Ductal adenocarcinoma of the pancreatic head (uncinate process); double duct sign. **a** Unenhanced computed tomography (CT) image shows enlargement and loss of the triangular shape of uncinate process (*U*). **b–f** Contrast-enhanced CT images; incremental slices from caudal (**b**) to cranial (**f**). Normal enhancement of pancreatic parenchyma is seen in peripheral areas of the uncinate process only, while the central portion has a lower degree of enhancement due to the presence of tumor (*T*). There is preservation of the fat plane with the superior mesenteric vein (*smv*). On more cranial slices (**c–e**), the common bile duct (*arrow*) and pancreatic duct (*arrowhead*) are dilated, indicating obstruction. In the liver hilum, the moderately dilated hepatic duct (*open arrowhead*) is visible, but there are no signs of intrahepatic bile duct dilatation. *D*, duodenum; *gda*, gastroduodenal artery

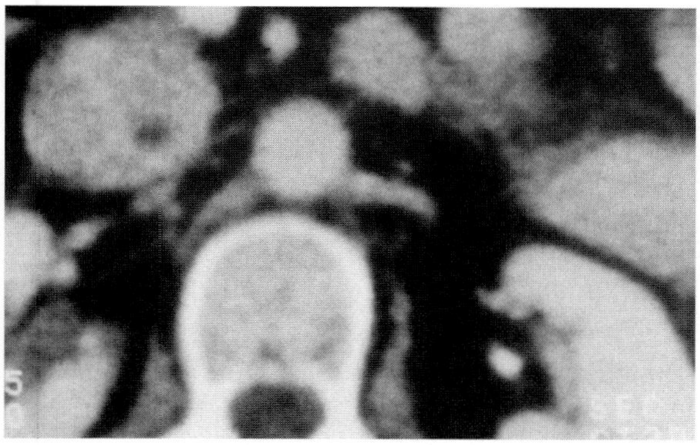

a

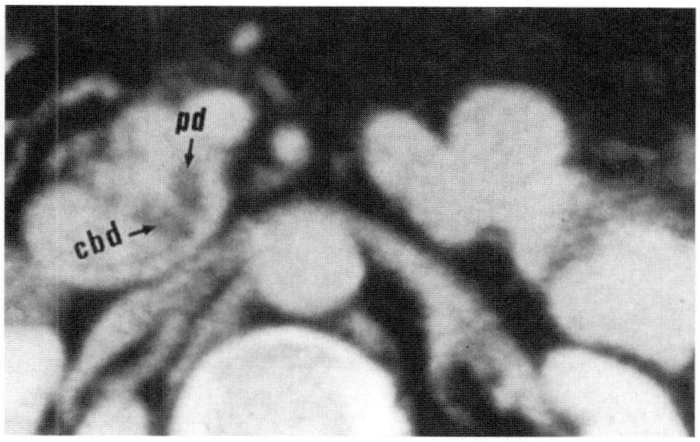

b

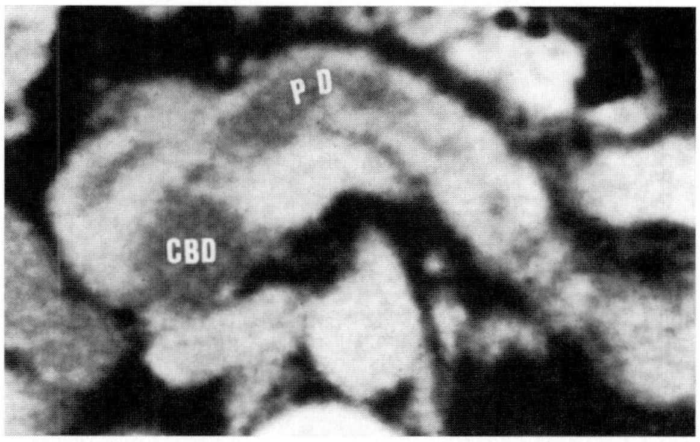

c

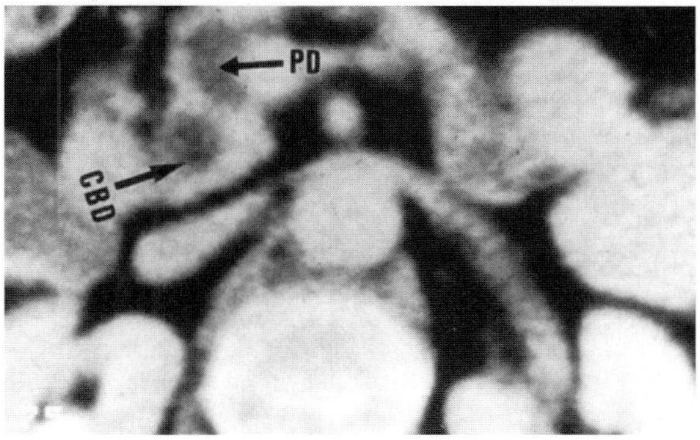

d

Fig. 8.25a–d. Nearly isodense adenocarcinoma of the pancreatic head. Computed tomography (CT) slices from caudal (**a**) to cranial (**d**) after IV iodinated contrast administration (dynamic incremental CT). **a** There is homogeneous enhancement of the slightly enlarged head of the pancreas. The lesion is not directly visualized. **b** There is evident dilatation of the common bile duct (*cbd*) and the pancreatic duct (*pd*). **c,d** The dilatation of the common bile duct (*CBD*) and the pancreatic duct (*PD*) becomes even more pronounced. Note atrophy of the pancreatic parenchyma in the body and tail

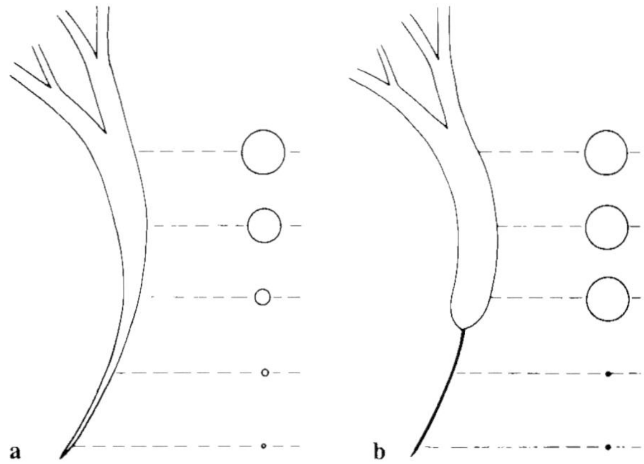

Fig. 8.26a,b. Differential diagnosis between ductal adenocarcinoma of the pancreas and chronic pancreatitis. The correlation between cholangiography and serial transaxial images of the common bile duct in chronic pancreatitis (**a**) and ductal adenocarcinoma (**b**). [From ROHRMANN and BARON (1989)]

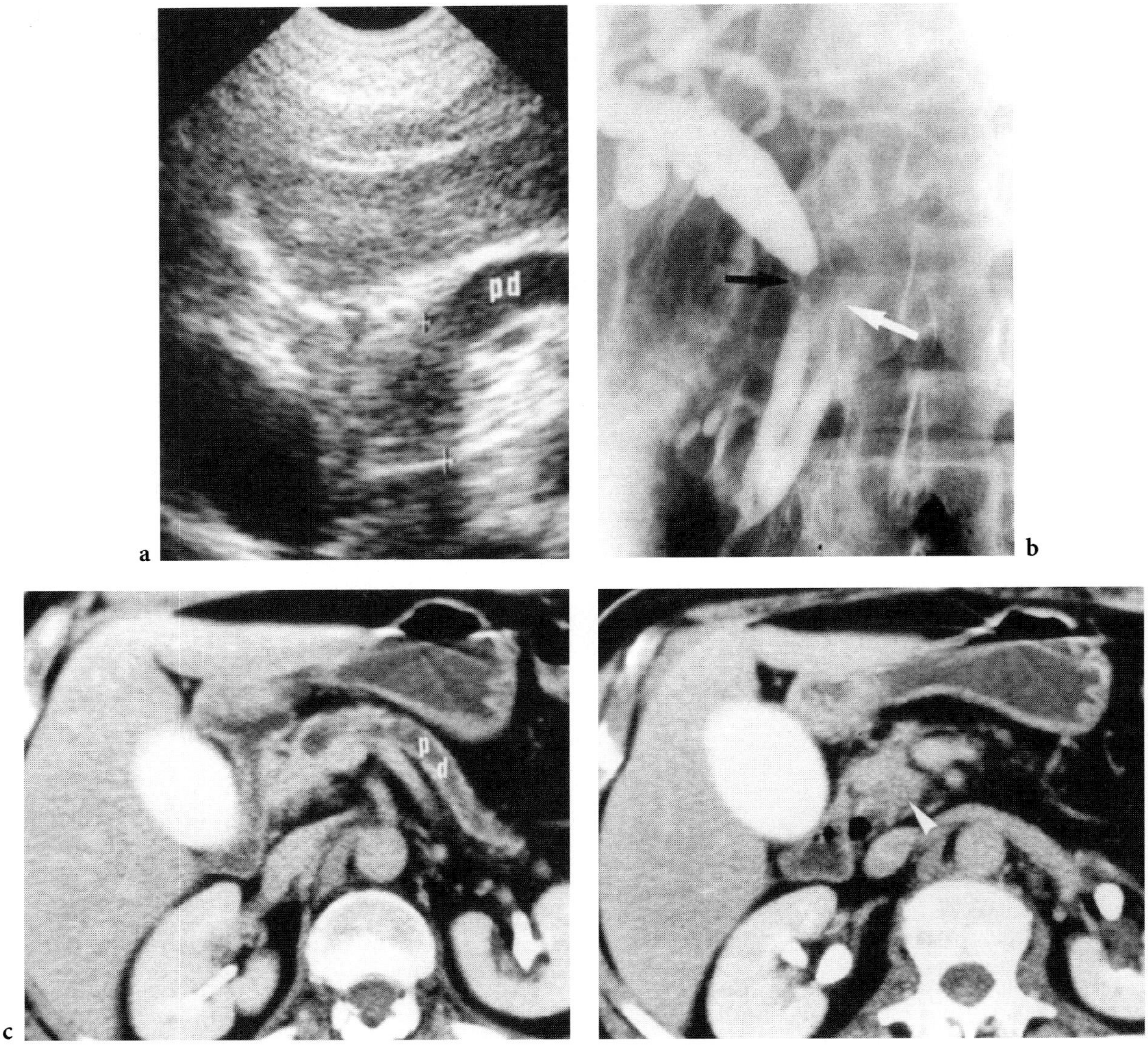

Fig. 8.27a–d. Ductal adenocarcinoma, indirect tumor signs. **a** Ultrasonography of pancreatic head and body, transverse section. Note the clear dilatation of the pancreatic duct (*pd*) in the body and neck of the pancreas. No tumoral mass could be visualized on this or other ultrasonography slices. **b** Endoscopic retrograde cholangiopancreatography demonstrating a high-grade short stenotic segment in the suprapancreatic portion of the main bile duct (*black arrow*), as well as in the pancreatic duct (*white arrow*) at the head–body transition. **c,d** Transverse computed tomography sections at adjacent levels after iodinated contrast administration. **c** Visualization of the dilated pancreatic duct (*pd*). **d** At a level immediately below the previous slice, no changes in contour or volume, but only a slight difference in enhancement is visualized in the pancreatic head (*arrowhead*). Note that the gallbladder was opacified from a previous contrast study

8.3.3 Staging

Varying CT criteria have been used for determining unresectability. Those proposed by Diehl et al. include extrapancreatic invasion of adjacent tissues and organs other than the duodenum, occlusion, stenosis, or semicircular encasement of major peripancreatic vessels, hematogenous or distant lymph node metastases, and signs of peritoneal carcinomatosis (Diehl et al. 1998) (see also Sect. 8.1). Peripancreatic extension into the retroperitoneal space is indicated by loss of the normal fat planes. Soft density streaks and strands in the retroperitoneal fat (Fig. 8.30) and thickening of the renal fascia may also be seen. While the presence of a focal mass extending into the extrapancreatic space is typical for tumor, more diffuse peripancreatic infiltration may

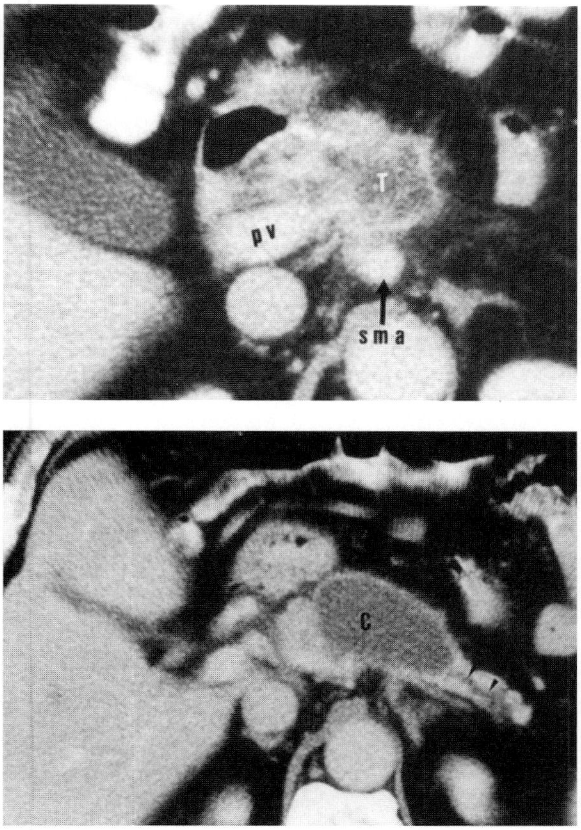

a b

Fig. 8.28a,b. Ductal adenocarcinoma with retro-obstructive pseudocyst. **a** Contrast-enhanced computed tomography (CT) image shows enlargement of the pancreatic neck and body with poorly defined and irregular borders. The tumor (*T*) is visible as an area of lower density The tumor is invading the perivascular space ventrally to the superior mesenteric artery (*sma*). *pv*, Portal vein. **b** Contrast-enhanced CT image obtained 3 cm more cranially shows fusiform enlargement of the pancreatic tail due to a lesion with fluid attenuation representing a retro-obstructive pseudocyst (*C*). Also note parenchymal atrophy and dilatation of the pancreatic duct in the tail (*arrowheads*)

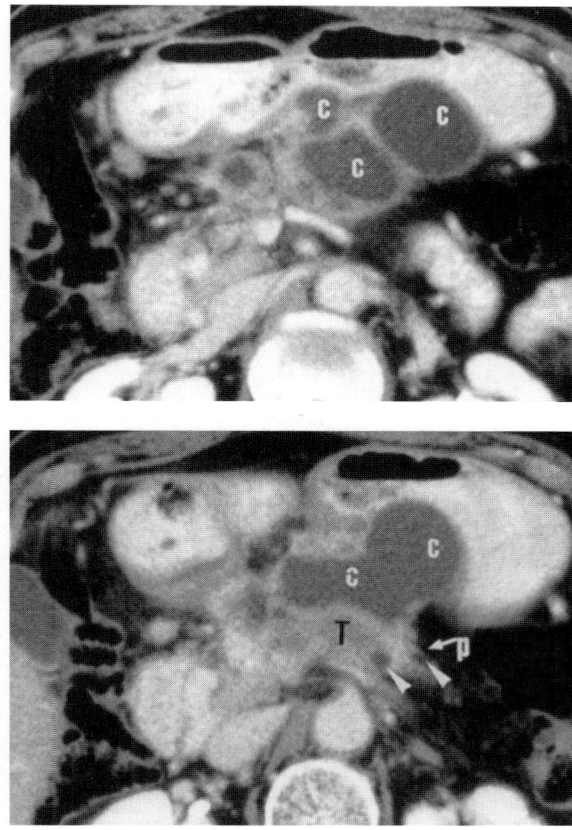

a b

Fig. 8.29. Ductal adenocarcinoma with retro-obstructive pseudocyst. **a,b** Computed tomography after IV iodinated contrast administration. Large multilocular thick-walled pseudocyst (*C*) in the lesser sac is due to ductal adenocarcinoma of the body of the pancreas (*T*) with pancreatic ductal obstruction. Note the retro-obstructive atrophy of the pancreatic tail (*P*) with a dilatated pancreatic duct (*arrowhead*) in (**b**)

be caused by pancreatitis, peritumoral desmoplastic extension, and/or tumor spread (Megibow et al. 1981; Mitchell 1987; Baker et al. 1990; Schulte et al. 1991). The absence of clinical and laboratory signs of pancreatitis may be helpful and points to tumor extension. CT signs of mesenteric extension are abnormal, streaky, soft tissue densities extending from the tumor into the small bowel mesentery in a radial fashion (see Fig. 8.4).

Helical CT is well suited to detecting vascular invasion (Figs. 8.30–8.34). Recently, criteria for assessing resectability based on evaluation of morphologic patterns of vascular involvement were proposed. Loyer et al. found that the majority of tumors

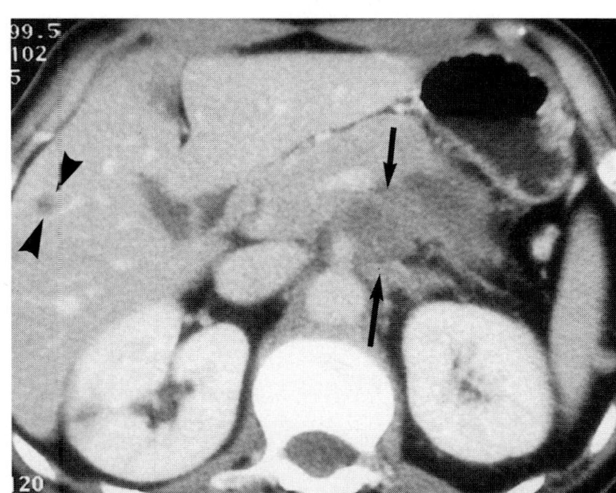

Fig. 8.30. Retroperitoneal extension of adenocarcinoma. Image obtained in hepatic phase shows hypodense tumor mass extending around the aorta (*arrows*). Note also liver metastasis (*arrowhead*)

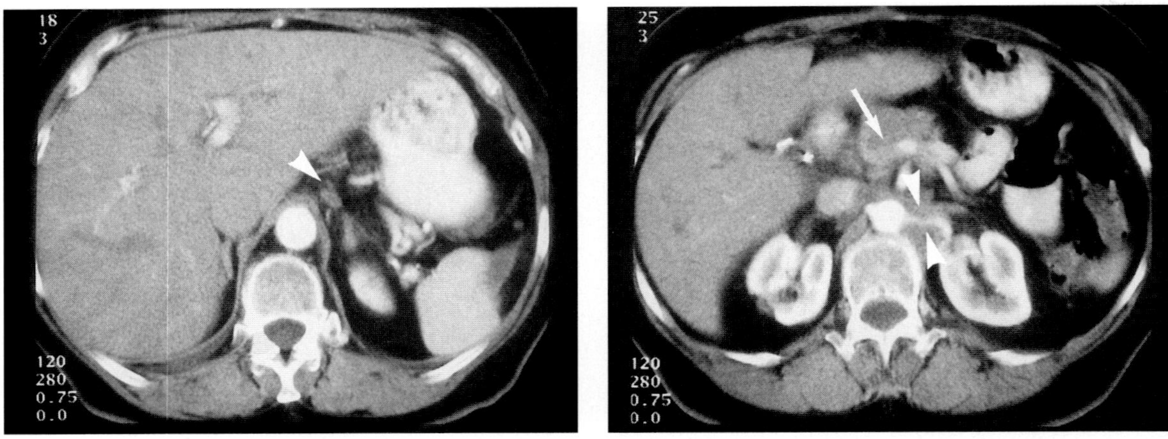

Fig. 8.31a,b. Pancreatic adenocarcinoma with metastatic lymph nodes and invasion of the left renal artery. **a** Computed tomography (CT) image obtained in the late arterial phase shows an enlarged lymph node close to the celiac trunk (*white arrowhead*). **b** CT image at the level of the pancreatic neck shows a hypodense lesion corresponding to adenocarcinoma (*arrow*). Note also a para-aortic metastatic mass with narrowing (invasion) of the left renal artery (*arrowheads*)

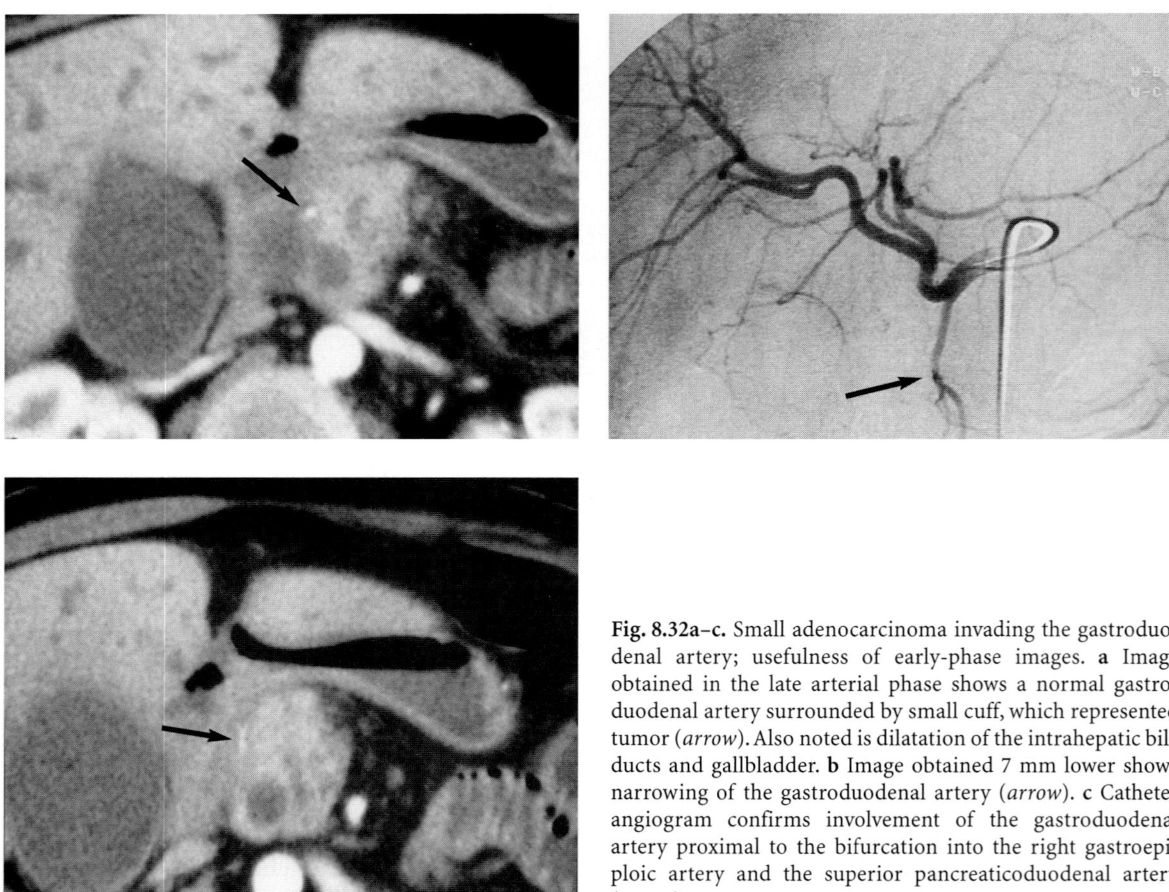

Fig. 8.32a–c. Small adenocarcinoma invading the gastroduodenal artery; usefulness of early-phase images. **a** Image obtained in the late arterial phase shows a normal gastroduodenal artery surrounded by small cuff, which represented tumor (*arrow*). Also noted is dilatation of the intrahepatic bile ducts and gallbladder. **b** Image obtained 7 mm lower shows narrowing of the gastroduodenal artery (*arrow*). **c** Catheter angiogram confirms involvement of the gastroduodenal artery proximal to the bifurcation into the right gastroepiploic artery and the superior pancreaticoduodenal artery (*arrow*)

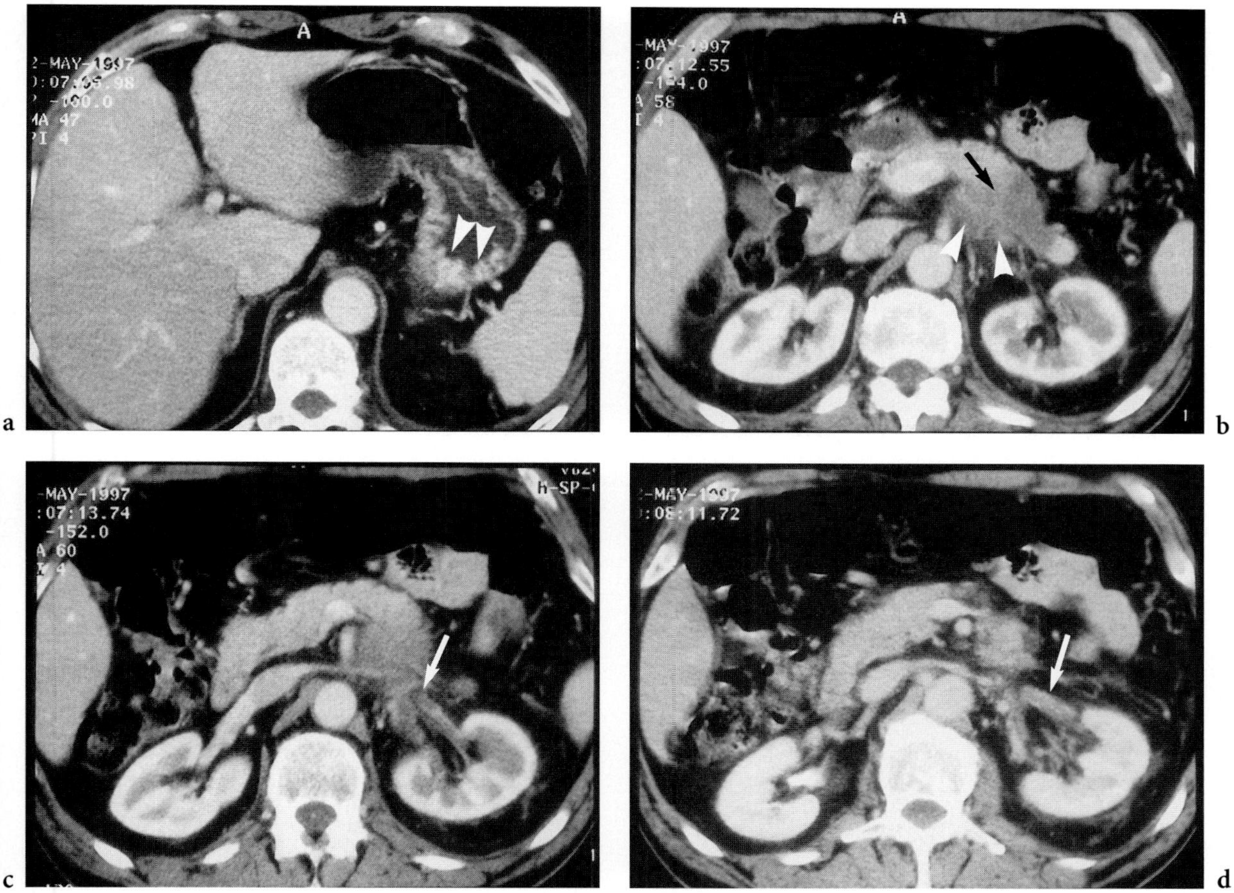

Fig. 8.33a–d. Pancreatic carcinoma with invasion of the splenic artery and vein and the left renal vein; direct and indirect helical computed tomography (CT) signs. **a** CT image at the level of the stomach obtained in the pancreatic phase shows arterial collaterals in the gastric wall and gastrosplenic ligament (*white arrowheads*). **b** CT image at the level of the pancreas obtained in the pancreatic phase shows adenocarcinoma (*arrow*) with extrapancreatic extension and invasion of the splenic artery (*arrowheads*). **c** CT image at the level of the renal veins obtained in the pancreatic phase shows tumor extension into the left renal vein, with thrombosis of the vein (*arrow*). **d** CT image at the level of the renal veins obtained in the hepatic phase shows signs of perirenal edema (*white arrowheads*) and delayed excretion of contrast material (compared to the right side), both secondary to the thrombosis of the left renal vein. The thrombus in the left renal vein is still visible (*arrow*)

partially or completely encircling or occluding adjacent vessels were unresectable (Loyer et al. 1996). Lu et al. found that a threshold corresponding to tumor involvement of one-half circumference of the vessel yielded the lowest number of false negatives and an acceptable number of false positives for unresectability (Lu et al. 1997). Some technical parameters used in this study deserve mention: a 2.5–3-mm collimation was used, images were obtained in the pancreatic phase of perfusion, and contrast medium was injected at a rate of 3 ml/s.

Hommeyer et al. showed that dilatation of small peripancreatic veins (gastrocolic trunk, anterior superior pancreaticoduodenal vein, posterior superior pancreaticoduodenal vein) may be a reliable sign of unresectability in cancer of the pancreatic head (Hommeyer et al. 1995; Mori et al. 1991) (Fig. 8.35).

Presence of venous collaterals is common in patients with occlusion or narrowing of the splenic vein or superior mesenteric vein. Even small venous collaterals are well seen on CT images obtained in the hepatic phase. They are commonly detected in the spleno- or hepatogastric ligaments and/or retroperitoneum.

It should be mentioned that invasion of the gastroduodenal artery, which is common in carcinomas of the pancreatic head (see Fig. 8.32), is not a criterion for irresectability.

Peritoneal metastatic spread is not rare (Aquino et al. 1989). CT will depict even small amounts of ascites, while the peritoneal metastatic implants

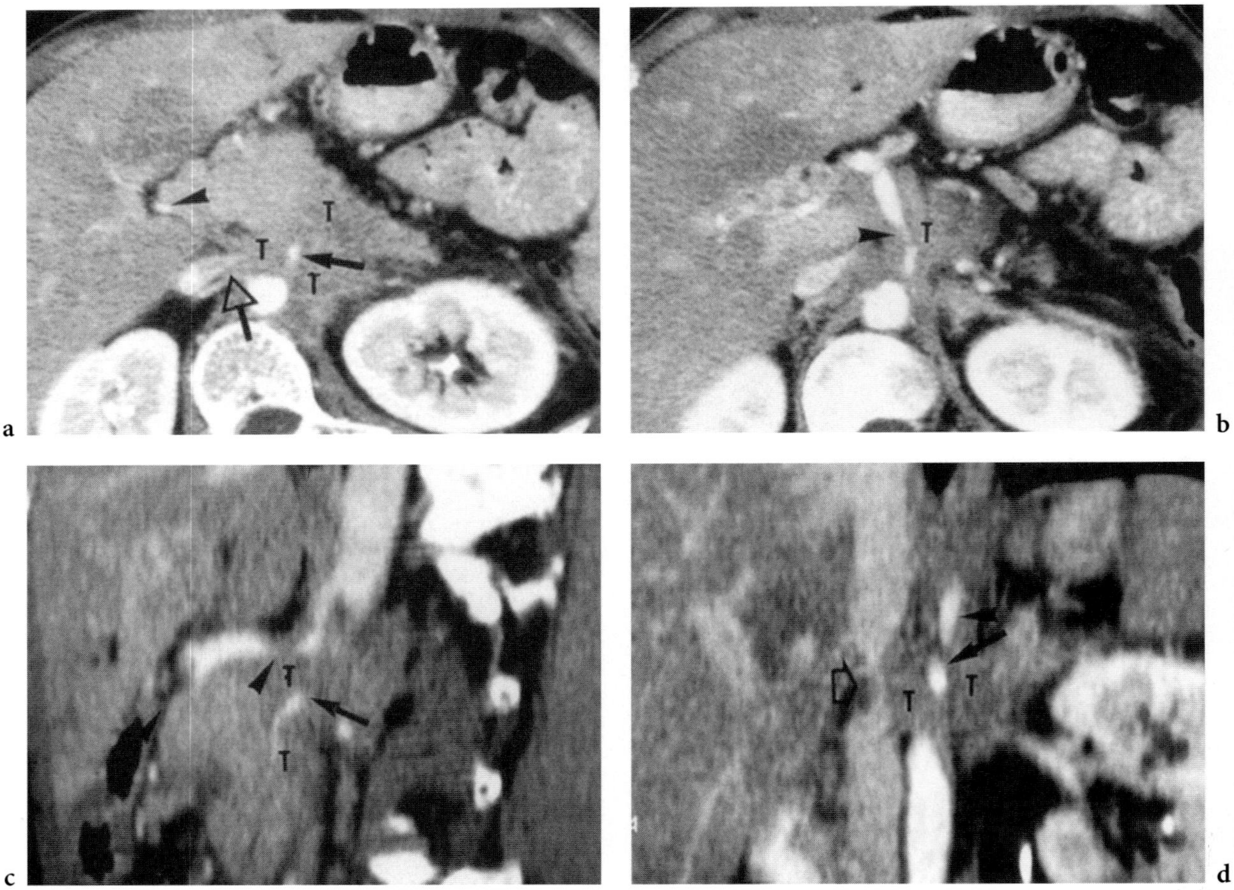

Fig. 8.34. Unresectable adenocarcinoma of the pancreatic body. **a,b** Contrast-enhanced helical computed tomography images showing a large tumor mass (*T*) invading and surrounding the superior mesenteric artery (*closed arrow*) and the common hepatic artery (*closed arrowhead*). The superior mesenteric vein is occluded. The tumor is extending toward the ventral border of the abdominal aorta and the inferior vena cava (*open arrow*). **c** Reformatting in the sagittal plane. **d** Reformatting in the frontal plane provides a better topographic depiction of perivascular tumor growth. More specifically, the narrowing of the inferior vena cava by the tumor is better displayed on the reformatted images

themselves are only rarely visualized (Fig. 8.36). Ascites may also be caused by severe narrowing or occlusion of the portal vein.

Invasion by the tumor of the vascular splenic hilum may result in segmental infarction of the spleen (Fig. 8.37).

Enlarged lymph nodes are well seen on thin-section helical scans, except in very thin patients.

Normally, the gastrointestinal wall (stomach, duodenum, colon) shows a tri-layered aspect with a maximum diameter of 3 mm (Baert et al. 1989). The peripheral layers (internal = mucosa, external = serosa) show a marked enhancement after IV injection of a contrast agent, while the middle layer (submucosa, muscularis mucosa) is relatively hypoenhancing as compared to the other layers (Minami et al. 1992). A disturbance of this tri-layered aspect may be a sign of invasion by tumor.

Invasion of the colon is seen as focal mural thickening.

Liver metastases are seen as hypoenhancing lesions on scans obtained in the hepatic phase of perfusion and are usually not as well seen on early-phase scans. In the case of multiple focal liver lesions, the diagnosis is usually straightforward. If only one lesion is present, the diagnosis of metastases may be suggested if the lesion shows faint peripheral rim enhancement in the arterial phase and is hypodense in the hepatic phase. "Late-delayed' (1 h) images may also be helpful: The presence of a peripheral hypodense halo ("peripheral washout sign") strongly suggests metastasis.

After the Whipple procedure or total pancreatectomy, local tumoral recurrence is typically seen in the retroperitoneum in close proximity to the mesenteric vessels and/or celiac trunk (Fig. 8.38). Ascites may also be present.

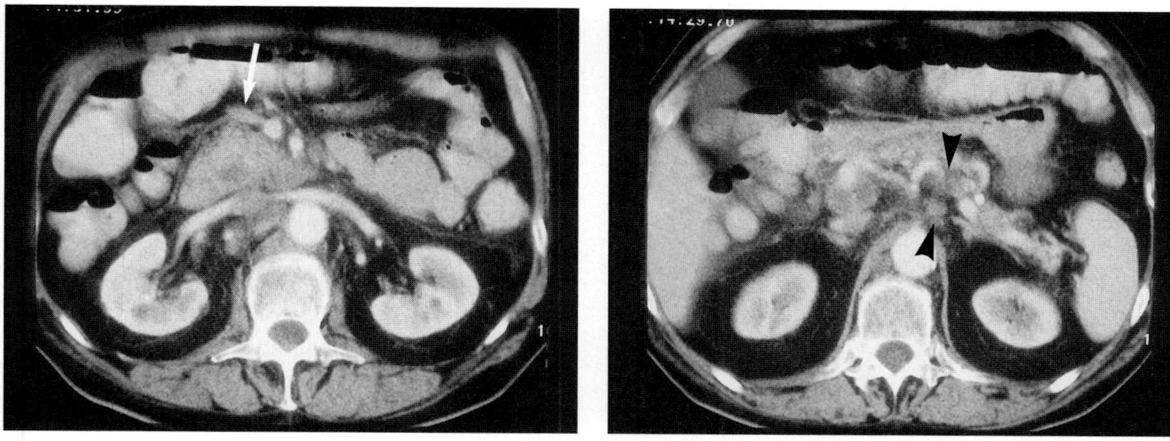

Fig. 8.35a,b. Carcinoma of the pancreatic head. Evaluation of the gastrocolic trunk. a Computed tomography image shows dilated gastrocolic trunk which drains into the superior mesenteric vein (*white arrow*). b At a more cranial level, several enlarged lymph nodes are seen (*arrowheads*)

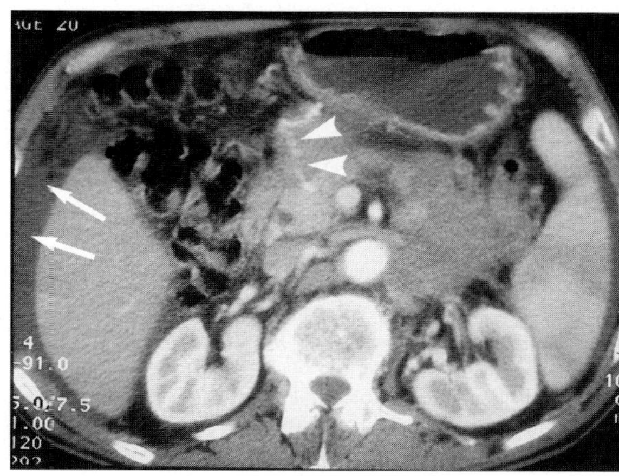

Fig. 8.36. Pancreatic cancer with peritoneal metastases. Contrast-enhanced computed tomography (CT) image shows large mass in pancreatic body and tail with marked extrapancreatic extension. Note invasion of gastroepiploic artery (*arrowheads*) and presence of ascites (*arrows*). As peritoneal implants are usually too small to be visualized, ascites may be the only CT sign suggestive of peritoneal metastatic disease

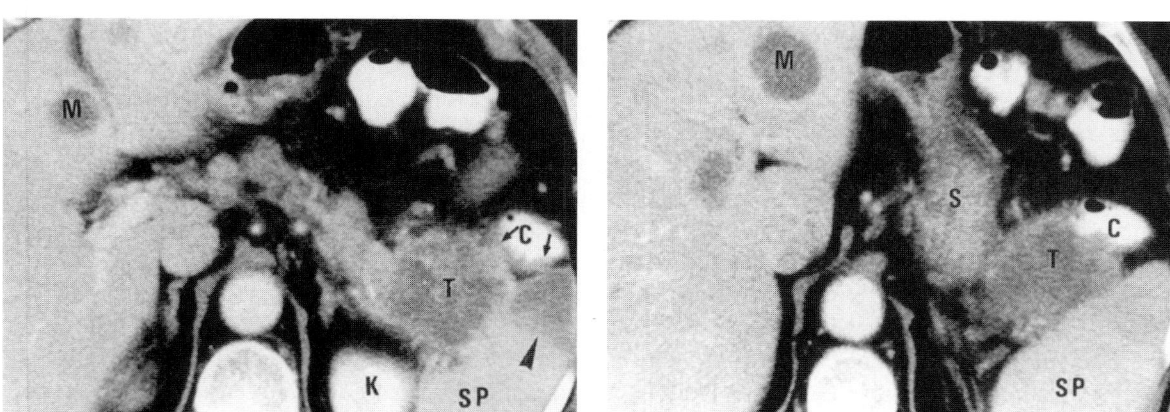

Fig. 8.37a,b. Ductal adenocarcinoma of the pancreatic tail with invasion of the spleen and colon. Contrast-enhanced computed tomography images showing a large (diameter 6 cm), weakly enhancing tumor (*T*) in the pancreatic tail. The tumor has invaded the spleen, resulting in segmental splenic infarction (*arrowhead*). The wall of the descending colon (*C*) is thickened due to tumoral invasion (*arrows*). The tumor is also in close contact with the stomach (*S*). *M*, liver metastases; *SP*, spleen; *S*, stomach; *K*, left kidney

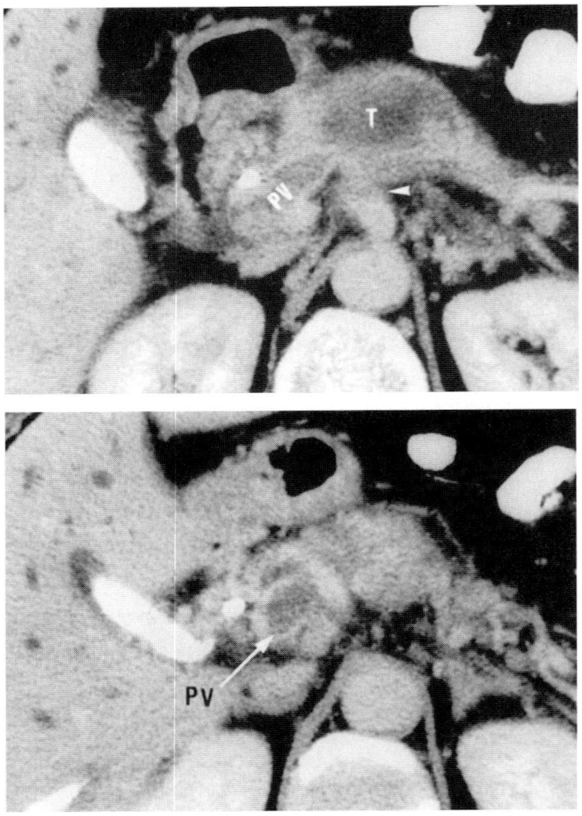

Fig. 8.38. Recurrent ductal adenocarcinoma of the pancreas after Whipple's procedure. Contrast-enhanced computed tomography images show tumor mass (*T*) surrounding and narrowing the splenic vein (*sv*) and infiltrating caudally around the superior mesenteric artery (*sma*), superior mesenteric vein (*smv*), and left renal vein (*lrv*). Massive ascites is present. *P*, remaining tail of the pancreas

8.3.4 Value

When compared to US, the performance of helical CT is less operator- and patient-dependent. Furthermore, CT provides documents showing all relevant anatomical information. Re-evaluation can be done at any moment without additional discomfort to the patient. Because of these advantages, CT is currently well established as the primary imaging modality for diagnosis and staging of pancreatic cancer (Bluemke et al. 1995; Gloor et al. 1997). Freeny et al. prospectively assessed the accuracy of dynamic CT in 213 patients with pancreatic carcinoma. A correct diagnosis was made in 97% of cases. CT correctly predicted unresectability in 100% of cases, but predicted resectability in only 67% of cases (Freeny et al. 1993). There is no doubt that helical CT offers an important improvement over conventional dynamic CT. Recent studies have revealed an improved positive predictive value for resectability when compared with conventional dynamic CT. The variable results obtained in different studies may be partially or mainly related to technical factors (slice thickness, single- versus double-phase CT, injection rate, timing, etc.). Kobayashi et al. investigated the value of helical CT in the diagnosis and staging of pancreatic carcinoma, in comparison with surgery and conventional angiography (Kobayashi et al. 1994). These authors found that helical CT correctly diagnosed pancreatic carcinoma in 78% of cases. Furthermore, accuracy in the detection of involvement of the major arteries around the pancreas and the portal vein was 100% and 71.4%, respectively. In the study of Bluemke et al., 57 of 64 carcinomas (89%) were detected with helical CT. The overall accuracy for assessing resectability was 70% (Bluemke et al. 1995). In the study by Diehl et al., overall accuracy for predicting unresectability with dual-phase helical CT was 91% (Diehl et al. 1998). Gmeinwieser et al. found helical CT to be 92.8% and 100% accurate in the detection of portal venous and arterial involvement in patients with pancreatic carcinoma (Gmeinwieser et al. 1995). Lentschig et al. (1996) reported a sensitivity of 94% and specificity of 80% for diagnosis of resectability with helical CT. In the study by Zeman et al., CT images were independently assessed by two observers with different levels of experience (10 years and 1 year of experience beyond residency, respectively). The corresponding overall accuracy in determining unresectability was 96% and 84%, respectively (Zeman et al. 1997). In the study by Legmann et al., dual-phase helical CT had a diagnostic sensitivity of 92%, an accuracy for predicting resectability of 90%, and an accuracy for predicting unresectability of 100% (Legmann et al. 1998). Lu et al. reported a positive predictive value and a negative predictive value for unresectability of 95% and 93%, respectively (Lu et al. 1997).

A remaining problem is the detection of lymph node metastases: While helical CT allows for an earlier detection of enlarged lymph nodes, it does not allow differentiation between benign and malignant causes of lymph node enlargement with certainty. Both false-positive and false-negative diagnoses of lymph node involvement are not rare (Megibow et al. 1995; Zeman et al. 1997). Because of this limitation, visualization of enlarged lymph nodes is usually not considered a contraindication to surgery. It is possible that thin-section helical CT, with assessment of the three-dimensional shape of the enlarged lymph node, will improve differentiation between benign and malignant lymph nodes (FUKUYA et al. 1995). Another limitation of helical CT in the staging of pancreatic adenocarcinoma is its poor sensitivity for detecting small metastatic peritoneal implants. If peritoneal metastatic disease is not accompanied by ascites, helical CT is usually false negative. On the other hand, the presence of ascites commonly indicates unresectable peritoneal carcinomatosis in patients with pancreatic carcinoma.

It should be stressed that technical factors are of uppermost importance: rapid bolus injection of contrast medium, use of thin-section helical scanning and overlapping image calculation, and adequate distention and opacification of gastrointestinal structures are critical requirements for a successful CT study. The suboptimal results obtained with CT in some studies could be related to non-fulfillment of these technical criteria.

8.4 Magnetic Resonance Imaging

8.4.1 Technique

8.4.1.1 Introduction: Interactive Pancreatic MRI

GAA et al. first described the "all-in-one" concept in magnetic resonance imaging (MRI) of pancreatic tumors, including cross-sectional T1- and T2-weighted imaging, MRCP, and breath-hold gadolinium-enhanced three-dimensional MR angiography (MRA) (GAA et al. 1997a,b). A similar concept has also been proposed by CATALANO et al. (1998).

With current advances in scan speed, an "all-in-one" MRI study of the pancreas can be completed in less than 30–40 min. This new examination method is unique because it provides an impressive amount of relevant information without the need for catheterization or sedation, or any other type of intervention. In our institution, pancreatic MRI is an *interactive "staged" MRI examination*. After evaluation of T1- and T2-weighted images, the radiologist decides on the next stage. This may be to perform a dynamic study of the sphincter of Oddi, to inject IV contrast media to improve the detection of focal lesions, to use specific contrast media, or to obtain angiographic images, etc.

8.4.1.2 Cross-Sectional Imaging

Accurate detection of pancreatic tumors requires an optimized MRI technique. Crucial prerequisites are high-resolution imaging and fast imaging. High-resolution imaging requires the use of body-phased array coils (ENGELHARD and HOLLENBACH 1997). While it was initially believed that fast MRI would be impossible, several solutions were proposed in the mid-1980s. Two major independent approaches to reducing acquisition times in MRI are:

1. Replacement of the classic 90° excitation pulses by lower flip angles (gradient echo MRI) (HAASE et al. 1986)
2. Generation of multiple echoes after a single excitation pulse [rapid acquisition with relaxation enhancement (RARE), fast spin echo (FSE)] (HENNIG et al. 1986).

Currently, high-resolution T1-weighted images can be obtained within a very short time interval by using a multislice breath-hold spoiled gradient echo sequence [e.g., fast low angle shot (FLASH), magnetization prepared gradient echo (MPGR)] (HAASE 1990). With currently available high-end equipment, individual non-fat-suppressed T1-weighted images can be obtained in less than 1 s ("single-shot" MRI, "turbo FLASH" technique). Excellent T1-weighting can be obtained by using an inversion recovery prepulse. The major advantage of this technique is that artifacts caused by patient motion or respiration are completely avoided. Thus, high-quality images can be obtained in every patient, irrespective of the patient's condition. The technical quality of these "snapshot" images depends on several factors, mainly the field strength (preferably 1.5 T) and the gradient performance. Alternatively, spoiled gradient images can be obtained during breath-holding (SEMELKA and MARCOS 1998). With this technique, images can be obtained with or without fat suppression. It has been demonstrated that the conspicuity of pancreatic tumors and the delineation of the pancreas from surrounding fat is best on fat-suppressed images (SEMELKA et al. 1993; MITCHELL et al. 1991). Fat suppression on T1-weighted images renders the normal pancreas high in signal intensity due to the presence of aqueous protein in the acini of the pancreas.

Since the introduction of new MRI systems equipped with stronger gradients and faster gradient switching capability, it has become possible to fully exploit the intrinsic advantages of the RARE sequence and to obtain T2-weighted images during breath-holding. This technique is called breath-hold

FSE or turbo spin echo (TSE). A more recently introduced evolution of RARE is called HASTE (half-Fourier acquisition single-shot turbo spin echo) (Kiefer et al. 1994). In this technique, single-shot T2-weighted images can be obtained in less than 1 s (±0.4 s). As in single-shot gradient echo, artifacts caused by respiration or patient motion are eliminated. A particularly interesting variant of HASTE is the double echo HASTE sequence, first proposed by Bosmans et al. (1997). With this technique, two images are calculated per anatomical slice position: one with a relatively short TE (60 ms) and one with a long TE (378 ms). The total acquisition time per slice is 700 ms, which means that images can be obtained during quiet breathing. Applications include the detection of subtle ductal abnormalities, small amounts of fluid, characterization of focal lesions, etc. (Bosmans et al. 1997; Van Hoe 1998c). As in snapshot T1-weighted imaging, the results obtained with HASTE depend on the gradient strength and the field strength. If snapshot imaging is technically impossible, FSE is a valuable alternative.

Several reports about the IV use of gadolinium diethylenetriaminopentoacetic acid (DTPA) in MRI of the pancreas have been published (Chezmar et al. 1991; Freeny 1991; Semelka et al. 1991). Theoretically, the IV administration of this paramagnetic contrast agent should increase the differences in signal intensity between the normal pancreatic tissue and the less vascularized neoplastic tissue. The normal pancreas shows a marked increase in signal intensity immediately following the IV injection of gadolinium DTPA. Preferably, postgadolinium images are obtained with spoiled gradient echo imaging (Semelka et al. 1991). As in helical CT, images can be obtained in different phases of perfusion (e.g., in the "pancreatic" and "hepatic" phases).

More specific MR contrast media are currently under evaluation. Manganese dipyridoxyl diphosphate (DPDP) has been used as a specific hepatic and pancreatic agent. The question of whether use of this agent really improves the detection rate of pancreatic tumors remains unanswered (Gehl et al. 1991; Kettritz et al. 1996). Target specific MRI of pancreatic receptors probably represents a more promising approach. It has recently been shown that administration of monocrystalline iron oxide labeled with cholecystokinin results in a significant reduction in relaxation times in normal pancreas, but not in tumor (Reimer and Rummeny 1998).

In practical terms, tumor can be ruled out if the entire pancreas has a normal high signal intensity on non-contrast-enhanced T1-weighted images. In such cases, there is *no need* for IV administration of contrast media. Many pancreatic adenocarcinomas are well seen on non-contrast-enhanced T1-weighted images as hypointense focal masses. In these patients too, contrast-enhanced scans are *not required* for diagnosis (Fig. 8.39). Problems may arise if a large part of the pancreas shows an abnormal signal inten-

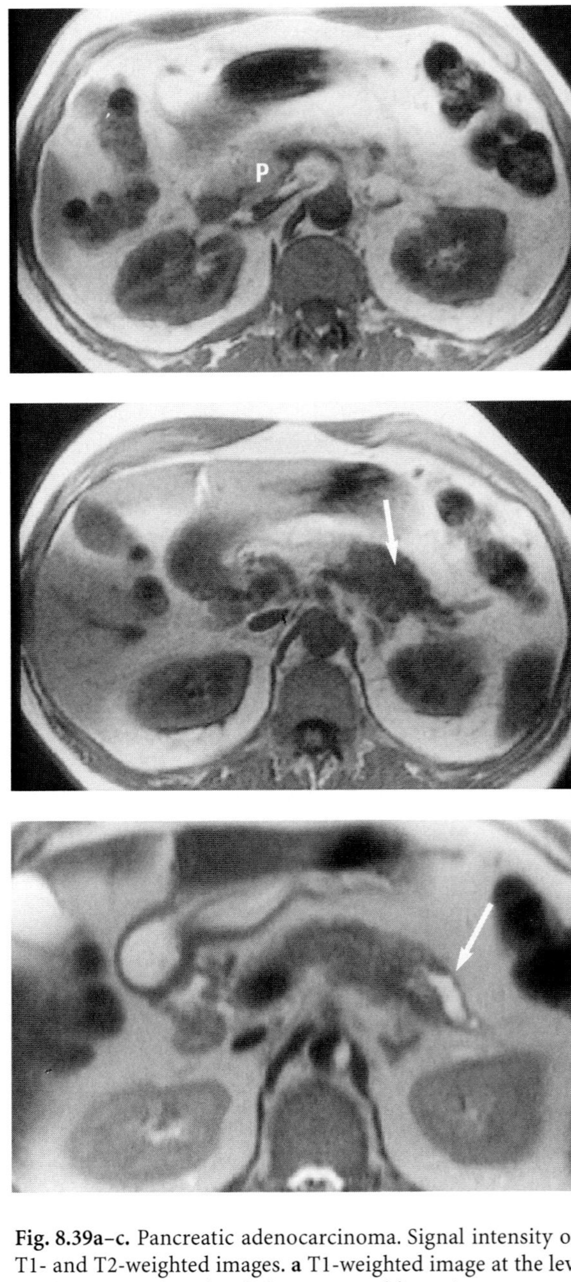

a

b

c

Fig. 8.39a–c. Pancreatic adenocarcinoma. Signal intensity on T1- and T2-weighted images. **a** T1-weighted image at the level of the pancreatic head shows normal hyperintense aspect of pancreatic parenchyma (*P*). **b** T1-weighted image at the level of the pancreatic body shows tumor that is markedly hypointense relative to normal parenchyma (*arrow*). **c** On this T2-weighted image, the tumor is nearly invisible (isointense). However, ductal narrowing with retro-obstructive dilatation is seen as a secondary sign (*arrow*) sity, which is a common finding in patients with retro-obstructive pancreatitis. In these cases, contrast-enhanced scans are helpful in defining the exact location and size of the tumor (Fig. 8.40).

Oral contrast agents may be helpful in pancreatic MRI. As in CT, administration of tap water and injection of an antiperistaltic drug is simple and effective. While use of positive contrast media such as water may be detrimental for image quality if older (spin echo) techniques are used (ghosting), they afford an excellent visualization of the stomach and duodenum in T2-weighted images obtained with snapshot techniques such as HASTE.

8.4.1.3 Magnetic Resonance Cholangiopancreatography

With MRCP techniques, "continuity images" of the bile duct and pancreatic ducts can be obtained during an MR study of the pancreas. These images may offer extremely valuable additional information. Firstly, the detection of small tumors may be facilitated by taking into account ductal abnormalities. Secondly, and most importantly, MR pancreatograms are often quite helpful in the differentiation between tumors and chronic pancreatitis.

Different techniques have been used to obtain continuity images showing ductal anatomy (Van Hoe et al. 1998c). A fast and reliable technique is to obtain a projective image through the structure of interest with a relatively large slice thickness (2–4 cm). In order to obtain sufficiently high contrast, the signal obtained from the structure of interest should be much higher than the signal of background tissue. This condition is fulfilled when fluid-containing lesions or structures are imaged with heavily T2-weighted images ("MR hydrography"). A sequence commonly used is RARE (Matos et al. 1997; Van Hoe et al. 1998b). In this technique, all echoes are obtained after a single excitation pulse and a very long echo train is used (usually ±250 echoes); the resulting image has an extremely long effective TE (e.g., 1100 ms). Acquisition times range between 3 and 5 s. Breath-holding is therefore required. Many other methods have been proposed

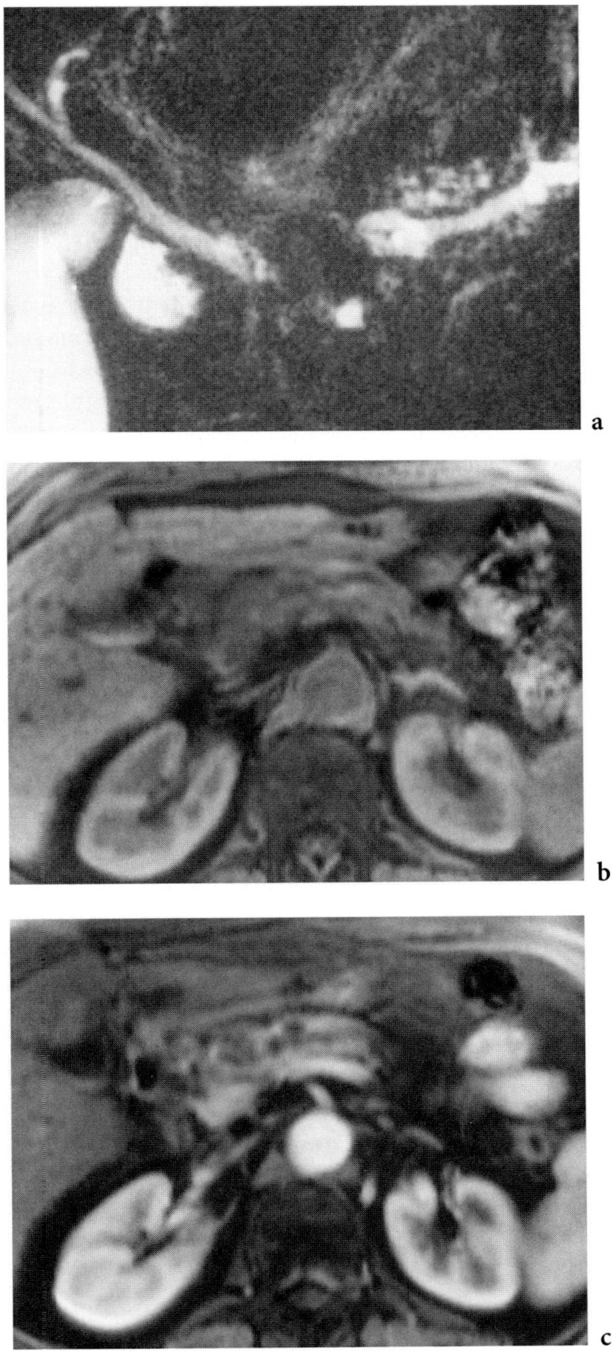

Fig. 8.40a–c. Magnetic resonance imaging (MRI) of pancreatic carcinoma; use of IV contrast media. **a** Projective MR image shows abrupt narrowing of the common bile duct (*CBD*) and pancreatic duct (double duct sign). Note presence of peripancreatic fluid, related to retro-obstructive pancreatitis. **b** Non-contrast-enhanced fat-suppressed T1-weighted image shows the pancreatic parenchyma as hypointense. Ductal dilatation is also evident. **c** Contrast-enhanced image shows focal hypoenhancing lesion in the pancreatic neck (*arrow*) corresponding to ductal adenocarcinoma. In comparison with (**b**), the parenchyma in the body shows clear uptake of contrast medium. This case illustrates one of the major indications for injecting IV contrast media in pancreaticobiliary MRI. In patients with adenocarcinoma, the spared portion of the pancreas may be hypointense on T1-weighted images because of pre-existing chronic pancreatitis or retro-obstructive pancreatitis. This portion of the gland usually shows clear enhancement, while the tumor remains hypointense after injection of contrast media

to obtain cholangiographic images. Several investigators still rely on the calculation of MIPs to obtain continuity images of biliary and pancreatic duct anatomy. These images are usually somewhat less sharp than those obtained with direct single-slice cholangiography, however, which is inherent to the algorithm used. Moreover, their calculation requires additional time. The only disadvantage of projective cholangiographic images is the dependence of the information content on the experience of the investigator: The exact location of the slice, as well as slice thickness, are critical parameters that should be selected during the MR study. Therefore, pancreatic MRI-MRCP is not a standardized procedure, but a flexible one that needs to be steered by an experienced radiologist.

As in cross-sectional MRI, administration of an oral contrast agent may be helpful, although it is usually not a crucial requirement. Besides tap water, several other types of T1 and T2 agents have been proposed. In specific situations where the purpose is to eliminate signal originating from duodenal contents, negative T2 agents, such as oral suspensions containing small iron oxide particles, may be useful. One such indication may be the evaluation of pancreatic juice secretion after IV administration of secretin (Matos et al. 1997).

8.4.1.4
Magnetic Resonance Angiography

As stated above, complementing a "classic" cross-sectional and ductal MR study of the pancreas with an MRA study may be indicated. In a preoperative setting, MRA may be required: (1) for detection of subtle signs of vascular invasion, and (2) to display the arterial and venous anatomy of this body area. The latter is important because some congenital variants (e.g., replaced right hepatic artery) may have surgical relevance.

Technically, three-dimensional contrast-enhanced MRA is the MR technique best suited to investigating (peri-) pancreatic vessels. Importantly, the MRA signal is determined by the local concentration of contrast medium rather than by in-flow phenomena. At the time of the first clinical implementation of this technique, obtaining a three-dimensional contrast-enhanced MR angiogram required several minutes (Prince et al. 1993). More recently, the development of stronger and faster gradients has made it possible to collect three-dimensional data volumes within 20–40 s or less. While breath-hold three-dimensional contrast-enhanced MRA has proved clinically useful, the technique has some limitations. Firstly, in order to optimize image quality and contrast, the use of dedicated timing studies ("test bolus") is usually required (Earls et al. 1997). Performing a bolus-timing acquisition and calculating the optimal time delay constitutes an additional step that requires some expertise and a few calculations. Automated triggering is a more elegant approach that is, at present, available only on a few MR imagers. Besides the dependence of image quality on accurate bolus timing, another limitation of breath-hold three-dimensional contrast-enhanced MRA is its inability to obtain selective visualization of *venous* anatomy, without superimposition of arterial structures. Furthermore, early enhancing veins may superimpose on pathologic segments of the arteries of interest.

Time-resolved MRA is a novel approach that could overcome these limitations (Korosec et al. 1996). In this technique, emphasis is primarily on temporal resolution. The idea is to collect sets of three-dimensional image data so rapidly that at least one data acquisition lines up with the arterial phase of the gadolinium bolus. Time-resolved imaging not only eliminates the timing problem, but also provides unique temporal information about relative rates of enhancement of arteries, parenchymal tissue, and veins. Furthermore, time-resolved imaging within a single breath-hold eliminates spatial misregistration among data sets. This feature enables the calculation of subtraction images highlighting normal anatomy or disease in body areas subject to respiratory motion. Digital subtraction MRA (MR-DSA) can be applied to visualize venous anatomy selectively, to assess flow patterns or organ perfusion, or to remove undesired high-intensity background tissue from the image. Indeed, with the use of state-of-the-art technology, either precontrast and arterial-phase scans or arterial-phase and portal venous-phase scans can be obtained within one single prolonged breath-hold. By subtracting nonenhanced images from arterial-phase images or arterial-phase images from images obtained in the portal venous phase, selective arteriograms or venograms can be obtained (Fig. 8.41) (Van Hoe et al., in press).

8.4.2
Findings

On T1-weighted images, the normal pancreas has a relatively high signal intensity. Pancreatic ductal adenocarcinomas are visible as areas of low signal

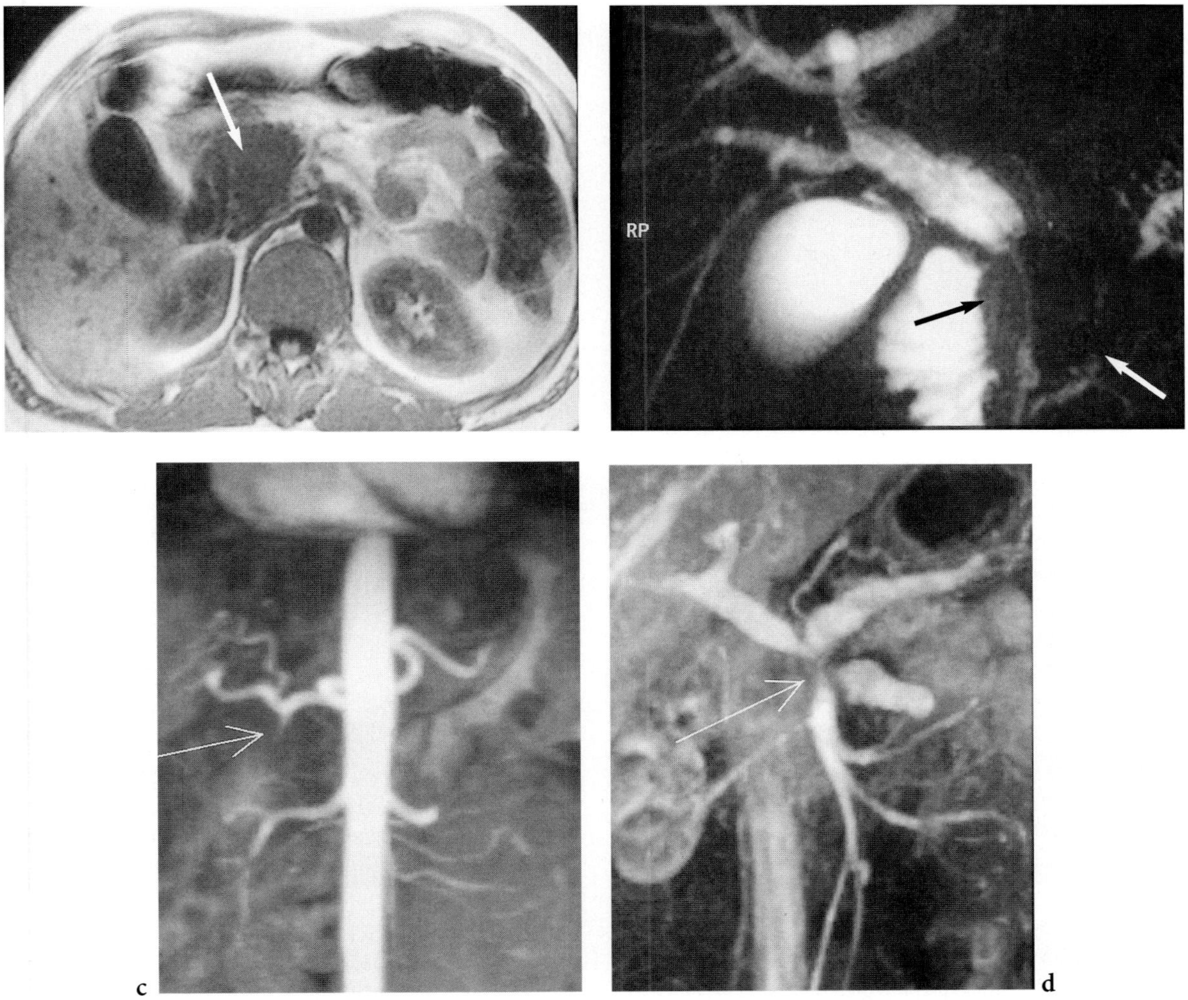

a b c d

Fig. 8.41a–d. "All-in-one" pancreatic magnetic resonance imaging (MRI). **a** Cross-sectional T1-weighted image shows large tumor in the pancreatic head (*arrow*). **b** Cholangiographic image shows severe narrowing of the common bile duct and pancreatic duct (double duct sign) (*arrows*). **c** Angiographic MR image obtained in the arterial phase shows narrowing of the gastroduodenal artery (*arrow*); invasion by tumor. **d** Subtraction MR venogram shows severe narrowing at the portosplenic venous confluence (*arrow*)

intensity on T1-weighted images (Figs. 8.39, 8.41–8.43). The only exception to the rule that adenocarcinomas are hypointense is the case of inflammatory pancreatic disease (acute or chronic pancreatitis) or fibrosis. If parenchyma adjacent to the tumor is affected by one of these conditions, it appears more hypointense, and tumor-background contrast is lower (see Fig. 40). After IV administration of gadolinium, adenocarcinomas are typically hypointense relative to normal pancreatic parenchyma (see Fig. 8.40). The intensity of neoplastic tissue relative to abnormal (inflamed or fibrotic) pancreatic tissue varies. Most commonly, pancreatic adenocarcinomas enhance less than inflamed parenchyma, particularly at the center of the tumor (Semelka and Marcos 1998). It should be mentioned that in some patients pancreatic cancers are best seen on non-contrast-enhanced T1-weighted images (Van Hoe et al. 1998c). Even relatively hypovascular tumors such as pancreatic adenocarcinomas may show visually detectable uptake of MR contrast media. Significant enhancement of both normal pancreatic tissue and tumor may lead to decreased rather than increased tumor conspicuity when compared to non-contrast-enhanced scans.

On T2-weighted sequences, pancreatic ductal adenocarcinoma may be visible as an area of higher signal intensity (Fig. 8.42). However, not uncommonly, tumors are T2-isointense.

Cholangiography is a critical part of a comprehensive MR study. Since pancreatic adenocarcinoma usually originates in the pancreatic duct, ductal

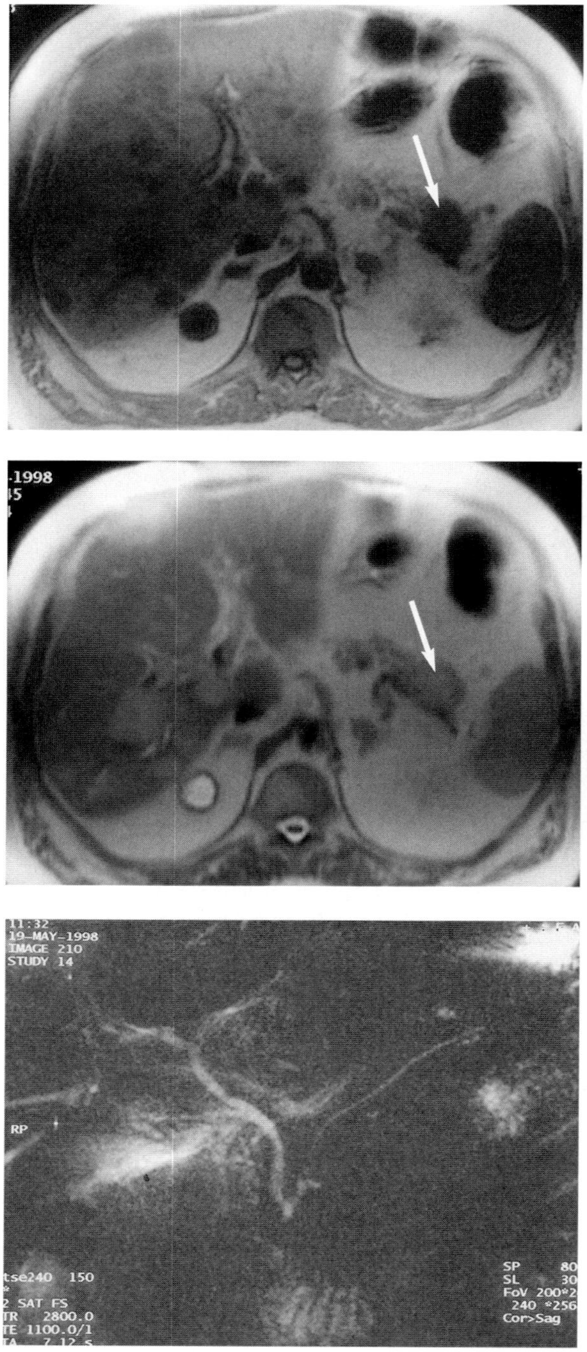

Fig. 8.42a–c. Adenocarcinoma. Ductal changes at magnetic resonance cholangiopancreatography. T1- (**a**) and T2- (**b**) weighted images show adenocarcinoma as markedly hypo- and slightly hyperintense, respectively (*arrows*). Also note presence of multiple liver metastases. **c** Cholangiographic image shows occlusion of the pancreatic duct in the pancreatic tail (*arrow*)

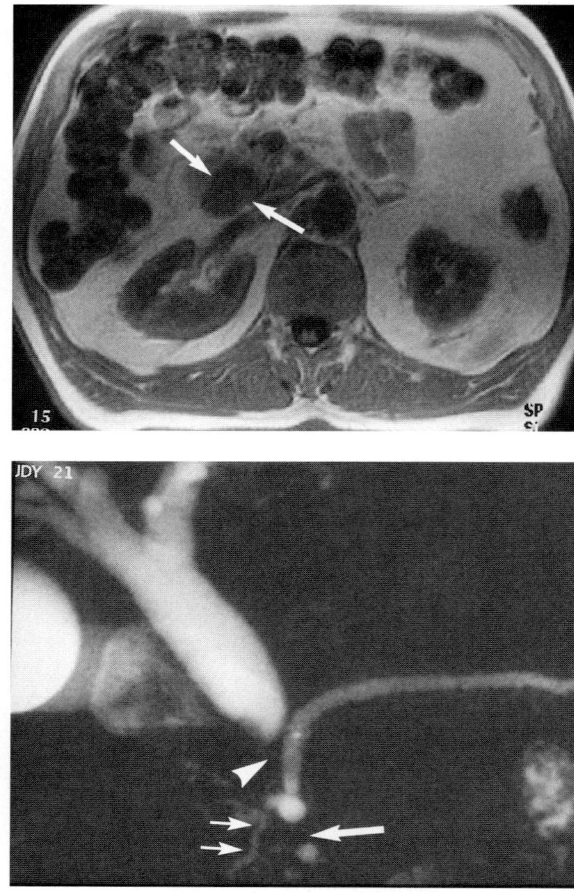

Fig. 8.43a,b. Adenocarcinoma. Ductal changes at magnetic resonance cholangiopancreatography. **a** T1-weighted image shows small hypointense tumor in the pancreatic head (*arrows*). **b** Cholangiographic image shows absence of the distal portion of the pancreatic duct and common bile duct (*arrow*), as well as severe narrowing of the common bile duct more proximally (*arrowhead*). Also note dilated side branch in the pancreatic head (*small arrows*) Note that in this patient, the obstruction of the pancreatic duct and bile duct was located at a different anatomical level, which is rather unusual

abnormalities are almost invariably present. The cholangiographic features in patients with ductal adenocarcinoma are well known from ERCP studies. Involvement of the main pancreatic duct may be seen as apparent occlusion (>50% of cases) or as a stenosis (Figs. 8.41, 8.42). Unlike in chronic pancreatitis, stenoses are usually rather long, solitary, and irregular with abrupt termination. Dilatation of the proximal main duct is also classic. In tumor of the pancreatic head, the double duct sign may be observed (Fig. 8.41). At the site of the tumor, side branches may be either invisible (normal or obliterated) or dilated (by obstruction), distorted, or displaced. An important sign is the absence of ductal abnormalities distal to the tumor (downstream). Furthermore, the portion of the main pancreatic duct that is dilated secondary to obstruction by tumor often has a more homogenous caliber; unlike in chronic pancreatitis, multiple short stenoses are usually not seen (this is not absolute, however, since chronic pancreatitis and pancreatic carcinoma may coexist). Similarly, dilated side branches usually have a somewhat more homogenous aspect without the typical morphologic features seen in chronic pancreatitis (clubbing, etc.).

Small lymph nodes are usually best seen on contrast-enhanced T1-weighted images obtained with fat suppression, and/or fat-suppressed T2-weighted images.

Liver metastases are usually well seen as hypointense nodules on T1-weighted non-contrast-enhanced snapshot turbo FLASH images. They are classically slightly hyperintense on T2-weighted images (Van Hoe et al. 1996). The conspicuity on these images depends on several factors including the technique used (spin echo, FSE, HASTE, etc.), sequence parameters (e.g., echo time), the size of the lesions, the presence of necrosis, the field strength, etc. Differentiating metastases from hemangiomas is usually easy when images with two different echo times are obtained (Bosmans et al. 1997). On contrast-enhanced images, liver metastases are hypointense. The peripheral wash-out sign is commonly observed on delayed scans.

8.4.3 Staging

The MRI criteria for defining non-resectability do not differ from those used in CT.

Peritoneal metastatic disease can be seen as peritoneal thickening in contrast-enhanced T1-weighted images obtained several minutes after injection of contrast medium (Low et al. 1997). Peritoneal metastases can also be suggested by the presence of ascites. By using heavily T2-weighted images, even small amounts of ascites are accurately detected (Bosmans et al. 1997).

8.4.4 Value

In a large multicenter study, Megibow et al. found no statistical differences between CT and MRI for evaluating vascular invasion of pancreatic carcinoma (Megibow et al. 1995). The results were rather disappointing for both techniques, with accuracies of 73% and 70% for CT and MRI, respectively. These poor results are obviously related to technical factors: The helical CT technique was not used and the MRI protocol was limited to cross-sectional imaging with spin echo techniques. More recently, Semelka et al. suggested that MRI could play a role in patients with pancreatic masses showing atypical features on spiral CT (Semelka et al. 1996).

While MRI has traditionally been used as a final diagnostic step in a limited number of patients, its role might change in the future. It has recently been shown that non-contrast-enhanced snapshot MRI competes favorably with contrast-enhanced helical CT in the detection of hepatic and extrahepatic upper abdominal disease (De Jaegere et al., in press). An important feature is the possibility to integrate different types of information: Besides morphologic information on the aspect of the tumors, MRI shows the signal intensity features of the tumors on T1-and T2-weighted images, the pattern of contrast uptake, and the secondary morphologic changes of the pancreatic duct. Moreover, vascular anatomy and disease can be assessed on contrast-enhanced MRA images. By integrating all these elements, it is usually possible to suggest or exclude primary pancreatic malignancy with a high degree of confidence.

In a recent study, ultrafast MRI (uMRI) yielded an accuracy of 89.1% (Trede et al. 1997). Even more importantly, MRI was equal or even superior to all other staging methods. Ichikawa et al. compared dynamic MRI with helical CT in the evaluation of tumor detection, local tumor extension, and vascular involvement. MRI tended to perform better than CT, although not all differences were statistically significant. The accuracy in detection of duodenal invasion, retroperitoneal extension, and portal venous system involvement with MRI was 88%, 90%, and 86%, respectively (Ichikawa et al. 1997). Interestingly, these authors relied entirely on state-of-the-art cross-sectional imaging: neither MRCP nor three-dimensional MRA was performed. In another recent study, a correct assessment of unresectability due to vascular involvement could be obtained in 22 of 23 patients (96%) (Catalano et al. 1998).

It remains unclear whether detection of small peritoneal metastases with MRI will be possible in the future. In a recent study, Low et al. used a dilute barium suspension combined with gadolinium-enhanced, fat-suppressed, T1-weighted MRI and reported good results in the detection of peritoneal implants (accuracy 86%) (Low et al. 1997). Interestingly, tumor detection was best on delayed contrast-enhanced images. It appears feasible, therefore, to perform dedicated sequences aimed at detecting peritoneal metastases as part of an "all-in-one" MR study. In any case, this approach deserves further research.

When state-of-the-art MRI equipment is used as a primary modality, it should be possible to avoid other diagnostic studies such as CT, catheter angiography, ERCP, EUS, and LUS in a large number of patients (Fig. 8.44) (Trede et al. 1997). It is clear that optimal results can only be obtained when high-end equipment is available (preferably 1.5 T with high-power gradients). Further studies are required to assess whether "all-in-one" pancreatic MRI will really prove to be a cost-effective primary diagnostic modality.

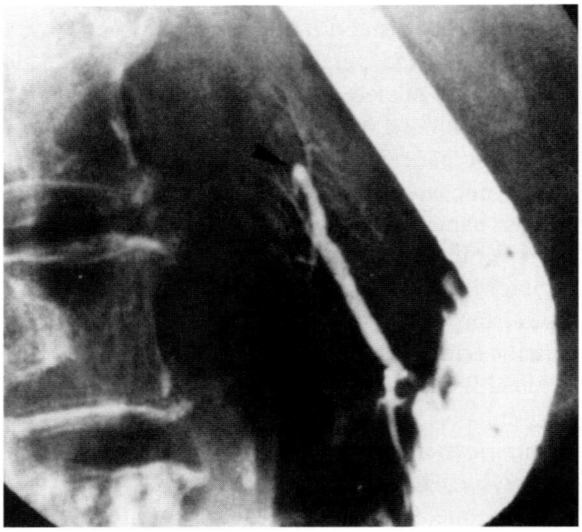

Fig. 8.45. Pancreatic adenocarcinoma. Endoscopic retrograde cholangiopancreatography (ERCP) features. ERCP shows obstruction of the pancreatic duct within the head of the pancreas

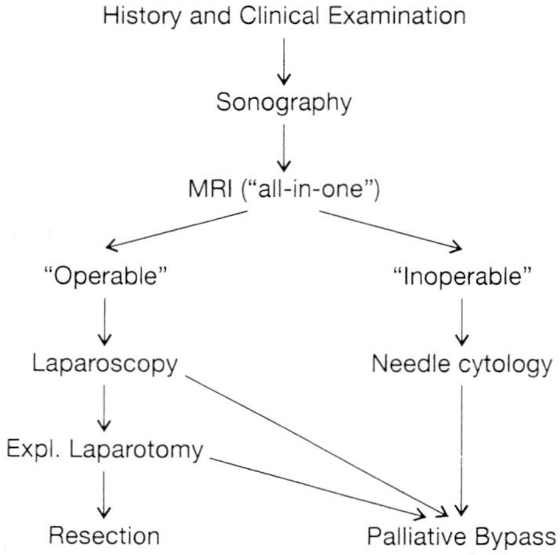

Fig. 8.44. Algorithm for the staging of pancreatic tumors. [Reprinted with permission from Gaa et al. (1997a)]

8.5 Endoscopic Retrograde Cholangiopancreatography

8.5.1 Findings

This technique is ideally suited for early detection of pancreatic adenocarcinoma because of the tumor's ductal origin. The two most common findings are main pancreatic duct stricture and complete main pancreatic duct obstruction (Fig. 8.45). The main pancreatic duct stricture tends to be relatively long in comparison to the typically short (<1 cm) stricture in chronic pancreatitis. The narrowing is more commonly irregular than regular. Importantly, aside from upstream dilatation, associated abnormalities of the main pancreatic duct are usually not seen. Extraductal extravasation of contrast medium may be associated with necrotic pancreatic carcinoma. The common bile duct may also be involved by pancreatic ductal carcinoma. An abrupt, irregular, distal stenosis favors malignant involvement. The double duct sign (narrowing or occlusion of adjacent segments of the pancreatic duct and common bile duct) is suggestive but not pathognomonic of ductal adenocarcinoma: it may also be seen in chronic pancreatitis. However, narrowing of the common bile duct in chronic pancreatitis is commonly more gradual than abrupt. Moreover, in chronic pancreatitis, the distal common bile duct is commonly displaced (pseudocysts) or attracted by a fibrotic mass. These morphologic features should be taken into account at image interpretation.

Ductal adenocarcinomas may also originate in side branches. In order to detect these tumors, adequate filling of side branches with contrast medium is mandatory.

8.5.2 Value

There is no doubt that ERCP is a very sensitive method for detecting pancreatic adenocarcinoma.

Unfortunately, the technique is much less specific. With the introduction of noninvasive diagnostic techniques such as US, CT, and MRI, the role of ERCP has changed. While ERCP is usually not the first diagnostic test performed, it now plays an important complementary role in a number of patients. The precise clinical indications to perform ERCP in patients with (suspected) pancreatic cancer may vary among institutions, reflecting local expertise and availability of other techniques. Although the decision to perform ERCP depends on several factors, indications may include: (1) palliative stent placement in patients with known unresectable pancreatic carcinoma invading the common bile duct; (2) obtaining tissue material in patients with atypical masses in the pancreatic head, particularly in the periampullary area; (3) suspicion of intraductal neoplasm; (4) difficult differential diagnosis between pancreatic cancer and chronic pancreatitis.

On the other hand, the systematic use of ERCP for preoperative placement of biliary stents to relieve jaundice and to get patients into better shape for the operation has to be condemned (Temudom et al. 1995). Indeed, stent placement may be harmful rather than beneficial in patients who are candidates for surgery, as has been demonstrated in several prospective randomized trials (Hatfield et al. 1982; McPherson et al. 1984; Pitt et al. 1985; Lai et al. 1994). Stent placement conveys the risk of preoperative cholangitis and probably increases the risk of postoperative septic complications (Helm and Stille 1984). Moreover, the stent often creates an inflammatory reaction around the bile duct, which can make surgical dissection more tedious (Gloor et al. 1997).

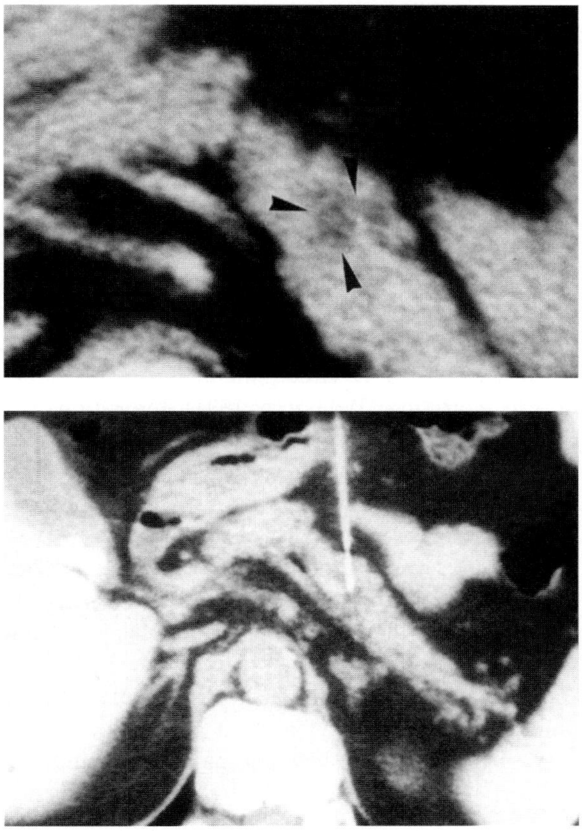

Fig. 8.46a,b. Computer tomography (CT)-guided needle puncture of a lesion in the pancreatic tail. **a** CT after IV iodinated contrast administration. A small area (*arrowheads*) with a lower degree of contrast enhancement relative to the normal pancreatic parenchyma is visible. **b** CT guidance allows correct placement of the needle tip in this area. Histopathologic study revealed ductal adenocarcinoma

8.6 Other Techniques

8.6.1 Percutaneous Transhepatic Cholangiography

Percutaneous transhepatic cholangiography (PTC) is most commonly used when endobiliary catheter placement is indicated in cases where ERCP is technically impossible. Diagnostic PTC has now been replaced by MRCP.

8.6.2 Radiologically-Guided Tissue Sampling

Fine needle aspiration may be performed under US, EUS, or CT guidance (Fig. 8.46). MR-guided tissue sampling is another alternative that will become available in the future. US-guided biopsies have the advantage of direct visualization of the needle as it progresses into the abdomen in the direction of the tumor. Direct correction of needle angulation can be made during the procedure. The limited acoustic window in transabdominal US may make percutaneous tissue sampling difficult or impossible in some patients. EUS-guided fine needle aspiration is commonly used to complement an EUS study. High positive predictive values have been reported with this technique. Negative fine-needle aspiration, however, does not rule out malignancy (Baron et al. 1997).

Depending on factors such as the size and location of the suspect lesion, CT-guided fine-needle aspiration or true cut biopsy (usually with an 18-gauge needle) may be performed. The complication rate of CT-guided fine needle aspiration for abdominal masses is less than 1% (Brandt et al. 1993; Edoute et al. 1991). While the true cut technique is somewhat more invasive, it offers better results and is safe in experienced hands (Levin and Bret 1991; Smith 1991). A point of concern is the increased prevalence of positive peritoneal cytologic washings in patients who have undergone prior percutaneous needle aspiration (Warshaw 1991). Indications for tissue sampling are therefore usually restricted to those cases where curative surgery is not considered and where alternative diagnoses (e.g., lymphoma, metastasis) have to be ruled out.

Brushings can be obtained by ERCP/PTC. The diagnostic yield in the diagnosis of pancreatic cancer is relatively low, except in periampullary tumors.

Overall, tissue sampling is required in only a minority of patients with suspected pancreatic carcinoma since helical CT and, in particular, "all-in-one" MRI commonly show pathognomonic findings (Gaa et al. 1997a,b; Van Hoe et al. 1998c).

8.6.3 Catheter Arteriography

Arteriographic findings in ductal adenocarcinomas include vessel narrowing by tumor (Fig. 8.47), encasement, and/or obstruction of the celiac, hepatic, splenic, gastroduodenal, or superior mesenteric artery, as well as of the pancreatic arteries (superior and inferior pancreaticoduodenal artery, dorsal pancreatic artery, or direct pancreatic branches from the splenic artery). Extrapancreatic tumor extension may cause displacement, narrowing, and/or occlusion of the large veins situated in the immediate proximity of the organ. The splenic and superior mesenteric veins are most commonly involved. Besides demonstrating vascular invasion, catheter angiography serves another important purpose: showing the arterial anatomy and detecting anatomic variants such as mesenteric origin of a right hepatic artery.

Currently, there is a tendency to replace catheter angiography by less invasive techniques. Several techniques (Doppler US, EUS, helical CT) have the ability to demonstrate vascular invasion (Gloor et al. 1997). It has recently been shown that thin-section helical CT provides the same information about vascular infiltration as angiography (Simon et al. 1997).

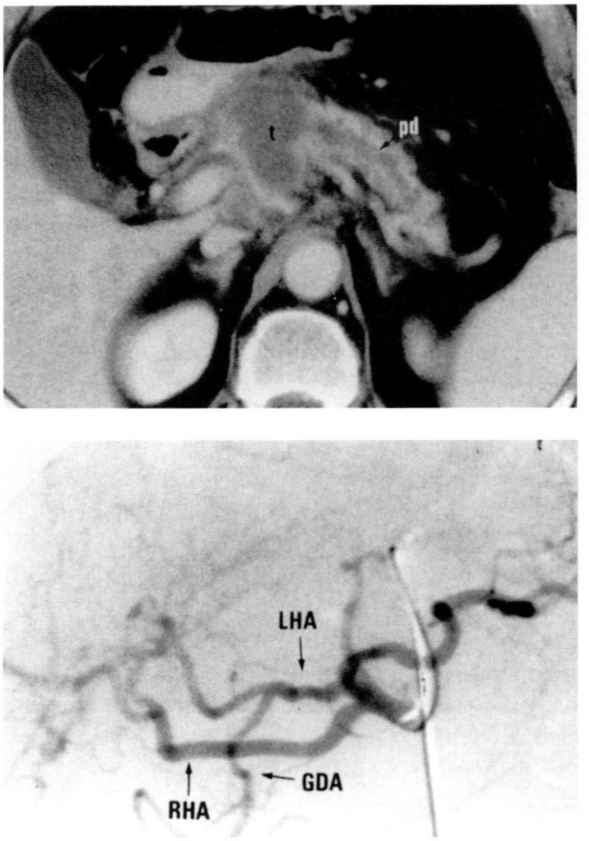

Fig. 47a,b. Unresectable adenocarcinoma of the pancreatic body. **a** Contrast-enhanced computed tomography image shows the tumor (*t*) as a hypodense mass. Note normal enhancement of parenchyma in the pancreatic tail and dilatation of the pancreatic duct (*pd*). **b** Arteriography shows narrowing and irregular outline of the left hepatic artery (*LHA*) and gastroduodenal artery (*GDA*) due to tumoral invasion. *RHA*, right hepatic artery

However, three-dimensional MRA will probably become the preferred technique because it uses no ionizing radiation and provides the surgeon with projective images showing all relevant anatomical features and resembling those obtained with conventional angiography.

8.7 Differential Diagnosis

8.7.1 Congenital Anomalies

In up to 35% of patients, the lateral margin of the head and neck of the pancreas may show a marked focal convexity, which could be mistaken for tumor

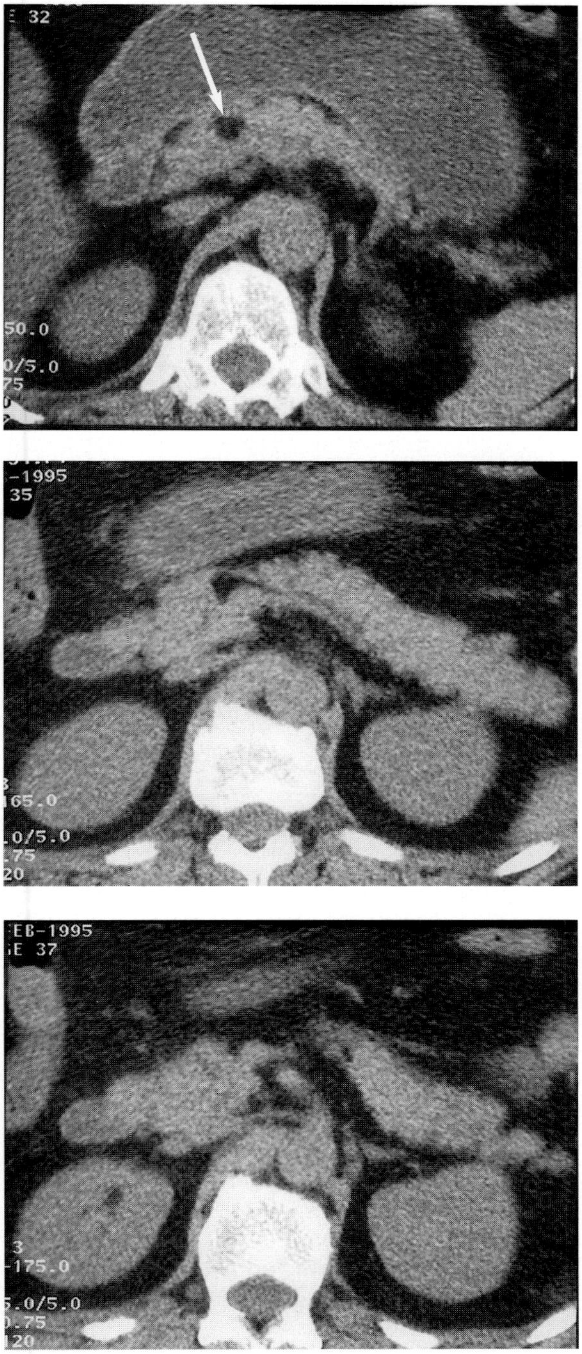

a b b

Fig. 8.48a–c. Focal lesion in the pancreatic neck: fat. **a** Non-contrast-enhanced image obtained at the level of the pancreatic neck shows focal lesion with negative density (*arrow*). **b,c** Images obtained at lower levels show that this "lesion" represents intrapancreatic extension of retroperitoneal fat

on CT or MR images (see Chap. 3) (Ross et al. 1996). Misdiagnosis can be avoided by assessing the enhancement pattern of the suspect "mass": unlike true neoplasms, these congenital lobules remain isodense to normal pancreatic parenchyma in all phases of perfusion.

Occasionally, intrapancreatic extension of fat mimics the appearance of a focal lesion on individual axial sections (Fig. 8.48).

8.7.2 Uneven Lipomatosis

In some patients with lipomatous pancreas, the uncinate process, which is derived from the ventral pancreatic bud, is spared from lipomatous infiltration. This non-lipomatous area may be seen as a hypoechoic area on US and may be mistaken for tumor (Marchal et al. 1989). On CT, the ventral part of the pancreatic head appears relatively hypodense relative to the uncinate process, both on non-contrast-enhanced and contrast-enhanced scans (Fig. 8.49). This appearance may be mistaken for tumor unless one is aware of this variant. The diagnosis is based on observation of a straight demarcation between the hypodense ventral part and the relatively hyperdense dorsal part of the pancreatic head (see Chap. 3). This transition line corresponds to the level of fusion between both embryonal portions of the organ. In MRI, the ventral and dorsal parts of the pancreatic head may also show different signal intensities. Again, this variant may be mistaken for tumor.

8.7.3 Focal Pancreatitis

8.7.3.1 Focal Acute Pancreatitis

This entity may mimic pancreatic cancer on all techniques. Features suggestive of focal pancreatitis are the presence of fluid adjacent to the pancreas, the absence of ductal dilatation and signs of parenchymal atrophy, and absence of ductal narrowing within the affected area. Besides imaging features, clinical data and laboratory values are important in distinguishing focal acute pancreatitis from tumor (Fig. 8.50).

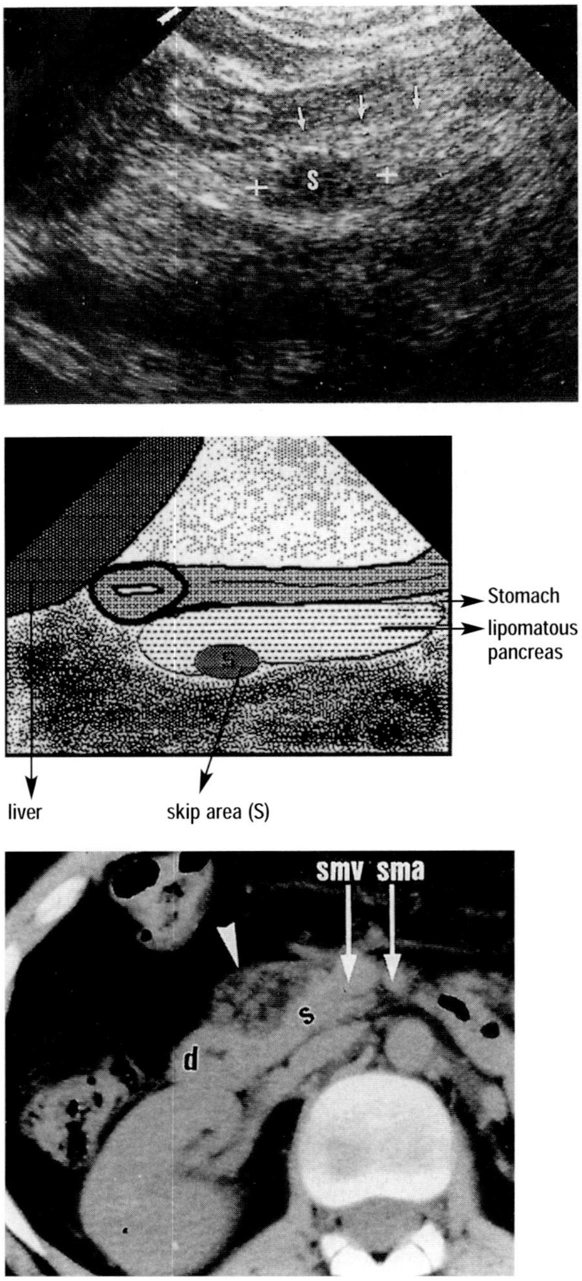

Fig. 8.49a–c. Uneven lipomatosis. **a** Ultrasonography; transverse section. Note the hyperechoic aspect of the pancreatic head and body (*arrows*). A zone of lower echogenicity is detected in the uncinate process, corresponding to the non-lipomatous skip area (*S*). **b** Schematic drawing of the same section. **c** Unenhanced computed tomography image. The lipomatous pancreas is demonstrated (*arrowhead*), with the exception of the uncinate process (*s*). *d*, Duodenum; *sma*, superior mesenteric artery; *smv*, superior mesenteric vein

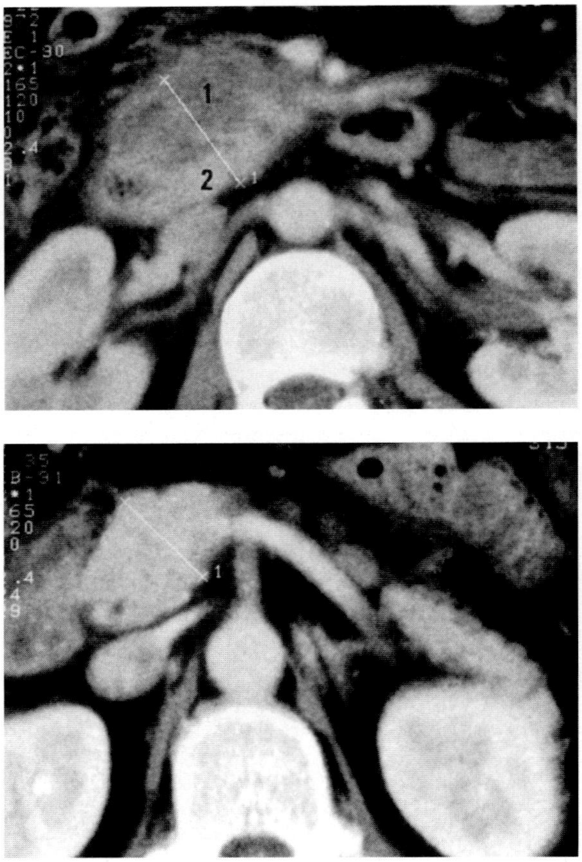

Fig. 8.50a,b. Focal acute pancreatitis simulating ductal adenocarcinoma. **a** Contrast-enhanced computed tomography (CT) image shows enlargement of the pancreatic head (diameter, 4.2 cm). The ventral portion of the head affected by acute edematous pancreatitis (*1*) is less enhancing (+42 HU) than the small remaining dorsal portion of normal pancreatic parenchyma (*2*), which is strongly enhancing (+101 HU). **b** Contrast-enhanced CT image obtained 3 months later. The head of the pancreas shows homogeneous enhancement (+110 HU). The diameter has decreased

8.7.3.2
Chronic Pancreatitis with Focal Inflammatory Mass

Enlargement of the pancreatic head is a common feature in chronic pancreatitis (Büchler et al. 1990). The following imaging findings can be helpful in the differential diagnosis with pancreatic carcinoma (Van Hoe et al. 1998c):

- Irregular and less pronounced dilatation of the pancreatic duct with a "beaded" aspect of the walls
- Presence of multiple small cavities within the mass representing dilated side branches of the pancreatic duct and/or small pseudocysts
- Intraductal or intraparenchymal calcifications

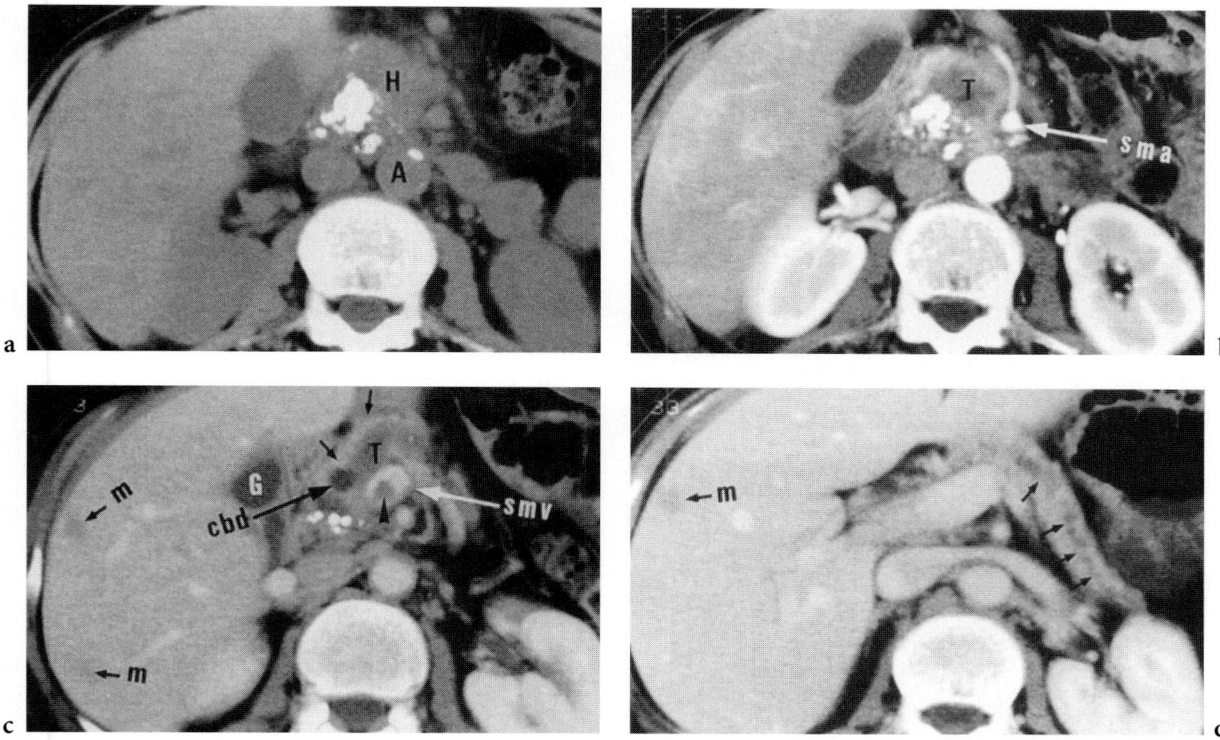

Fig. 8.51a–d. Chronic calcifying pancreatitis coexisting with ductal adenocarcinoma. **a** Unenhanced computed tomography (CT) image shows multiple calcifications in the pancreatic head (*H*), with loss of normal shape. Loss of fat plane with abdominal aorta (*A*). **b–d** Contrast-enhanced CT images. **b** Less enhancing area represents tumor (*T*), displacing a branch of the superior mesenteric artery (*sma*). **c** At a more cranial level, the weakly enhancing tumor (*T*) can be distinguished from the remnants of normal enhancing parenchyma (*arrows*). The common bile duct (*cbd*) is dilated, but the gallbladder (*G*) is not; this may be due to chronic cholecystitis. A non-enhancing area (*arrowhead*) within the superior mesenteric vein (*smv*) represents partial thrombosis or tumor invasion. *m*, Liver metastases. **d** At a still more cranial level, there is evident dilatation of the pancreatic duct (*arrows*), but with nonparallel serrated borders

- Less pronounced atrophy of the pancreatic parenchyma surrounding the dilated pancreatic duct
- Gradual – not abrupt – narrowing and obstruction of the dilated common bile duct.

One should be careful not to overlook tumors in patients with typical imaging features of chronic pancreatitis. Firstly, ductal adenocarcinoma may originate in a patient with pre-existing chronic pancreatitis (Fig. 8.51). The cumulative risk of pancreatic cancer complicating chronic pancreatitis has been estimated to be 1.8%–4% at 10 and 20 years follow-up (Lowenfels et al. 1993). Secondly, chronic (obstructive) pancreatitis may develop secondary to a ductal neoplasm.

8.7.4 Non-alcoholic Duct-Destructive Chronic Pancreatitis

Non-alcoholic duct-destructive chronic pancreatitis is an important new entity because it is a "cancer mimicker": cross-sectional studies typically show a mass lesion; cholangiographic studies usually show a relatively long stricture of the main pancreatic duct. Characteristic features on CT and MRI include the presence of a focal or more diffuse mass causing either regular or irregular narrowing of the main pancreatic duct, the absence of parenchymal atrophy and significant ductal dilatation proximal to the site of stenosis, and the absence of extrapancreatic spread (Van Hoe et al. 1998a) (Fig. 8.52).

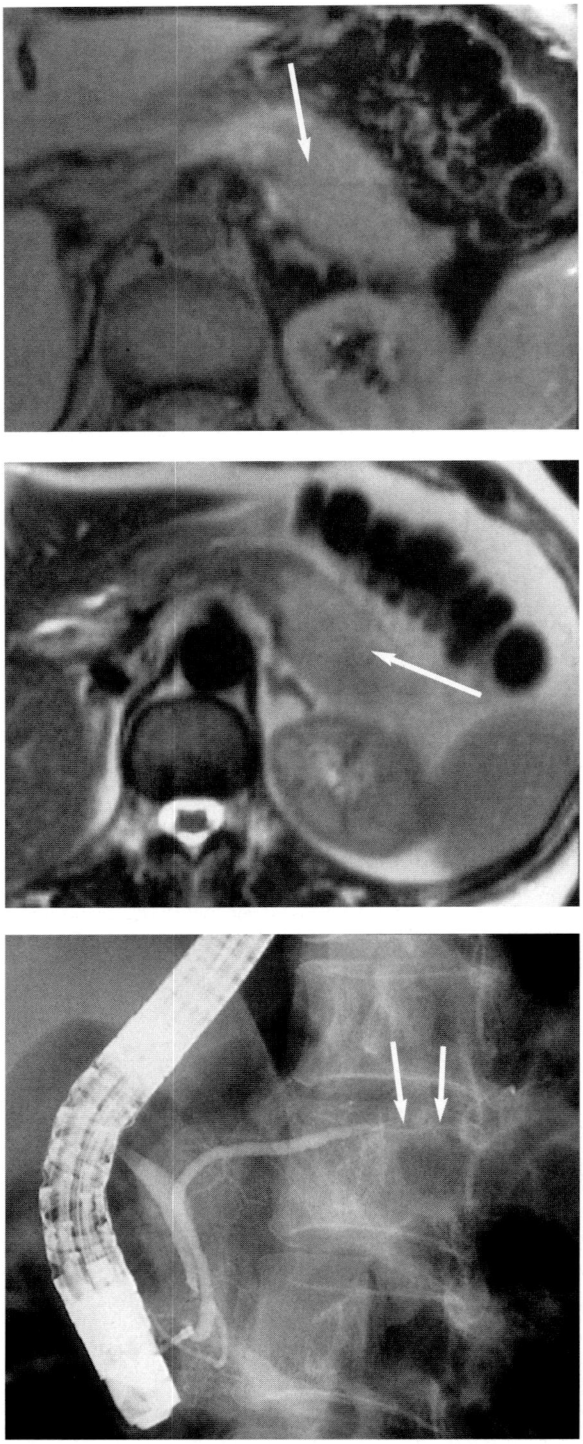

a b c

Fig. 8.52a–c. Non-alcoholic duct-destructive chronic pancreatitis. **a** Fat-suppressed T1-weighted image shows hypointense mass in the pancreatic tail (*arrowheads*). **b** T2-weighted image shows the mass as hyperintense (*arrowheads*). **c** Endoscopic retrograde cholangiopancreatography shows narrowing of the pancreatic duct in the pancreatic body/tail (*arrows*). Note that, despite its large size, the mass is relatively well-defined and limited to the confines of the pancreas

8.7.5 Cystic Neoplasms (see Chap. 9)

8.7.5.1 Serous Cystadenoma

These tumors are virtually always benign and show fairly typical imaging features: they consist of numerous small (<2 cm) cysts and a richly vascularized stroma. At contrast-enhanced helical CT or MRI scans obtained in the (late) arterial phase, part of the lesion may show significant enhancement (Itai and Ohtomo 1996).

8.7.5.2 Mucinous Cystic Neoplasms

These tumors may be either benign or malignant. They are seen as predominantly cystic lesions that may contain solid areas, internal septa, and/or small mural nodules. Unlike serous cystadenomas, the cyst walls lack a rich capillary network. The differential diagnosis with carcinoma is not always straightforward (Fig. 8.53).

8.7.6 Periampullary Tumors and Cholangiocarcinoma

8.7.6.1 Periampullary tumors

Periampullary tumors are those arising in the vicinity of the ampulla of Vater. Differentiating different

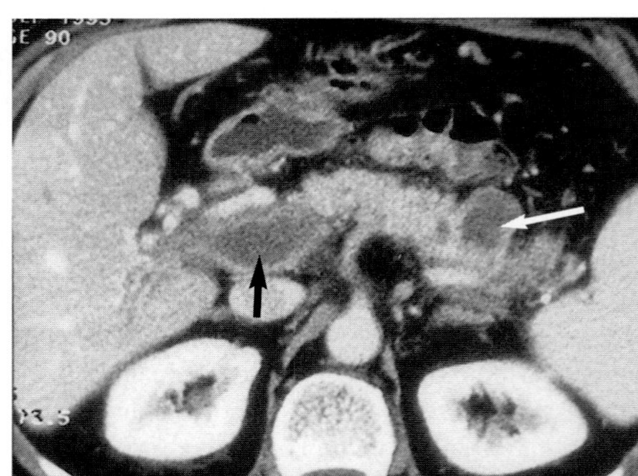

Fig. 8.53. Cystic pancreatic carcinoma. Computed tomography image shows predominantly cystic pancreatic carcinoma (*white arrow*), which was initially considered to represent a mucinous pancreatic neoplasm. Also note thrombosis of the portosplenic confluence (*arrow*)

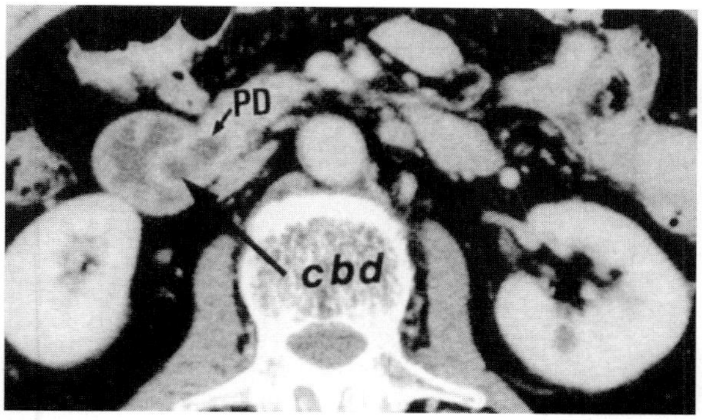

a

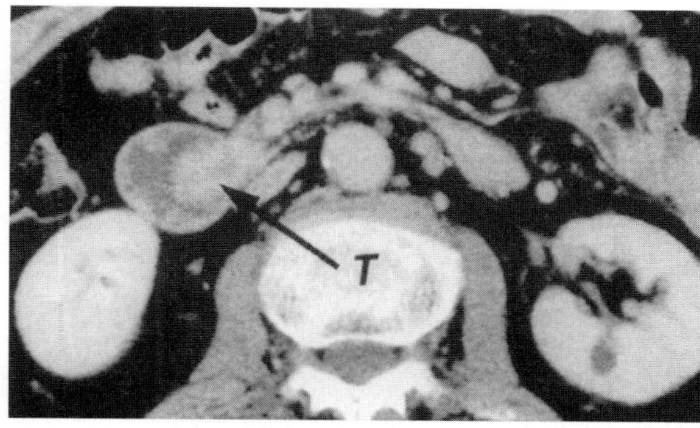

b

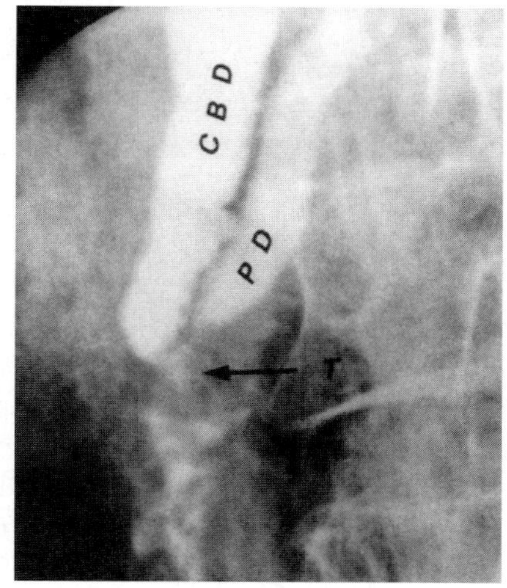

c

Fig. 8.54a–c. Small ampullary carcinoma causing bile duct and pancreatic duct dilatation. **a,b** Computed tomography (CT) of the ampullary region after IV iodinated contrast administration (incremental CT). A small mass (*T*) is protruding into the duodenal lumen. The duodenal loop is filled with pure tap water, which results in a good differentiation between the intraluminal tumor and the lumen itself. The double duct sign is demonstrated. *PD*, pancreatic duct; *cbd*, common bile duct. **c** Endoscopic retrograde cholangiopancreatography shows narrowing of the distal portion of the main bile duct and the pancreatic duct by the tumor. *CBD*, common bile duct; *PD*, pancreatic duct; *T*, tumor

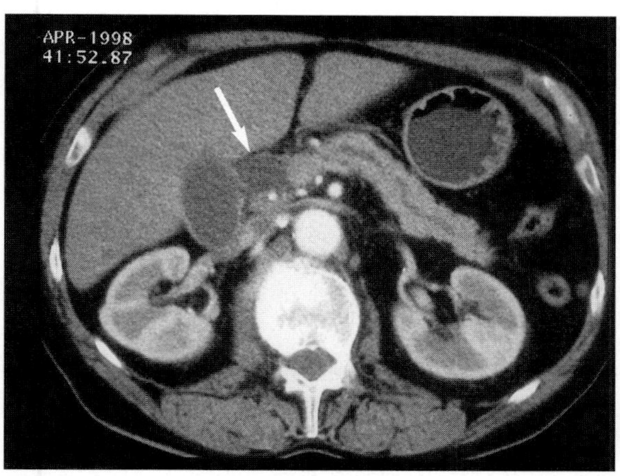

a

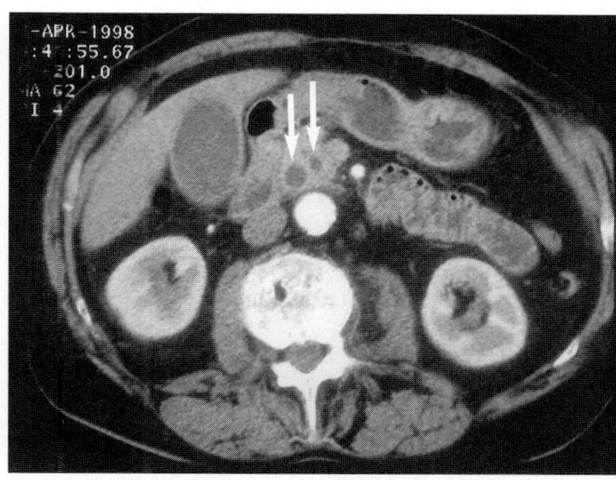

b

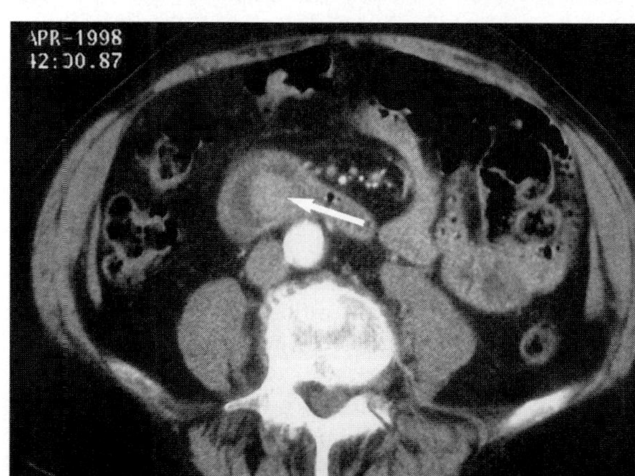

c

Fig. 8.55a–c. Ampullary carcinoma; the importance of oral contrast medium. **a,b** Images obtained at two different levels show dilatation of the common bile duct and pancreatic duct (*arrows*). **c** Image obtained at the level of the third portion of the duodenum shows a relatively large enhancing intraluminal mass representing a papilla enlarged by tumor (*arrow*) a 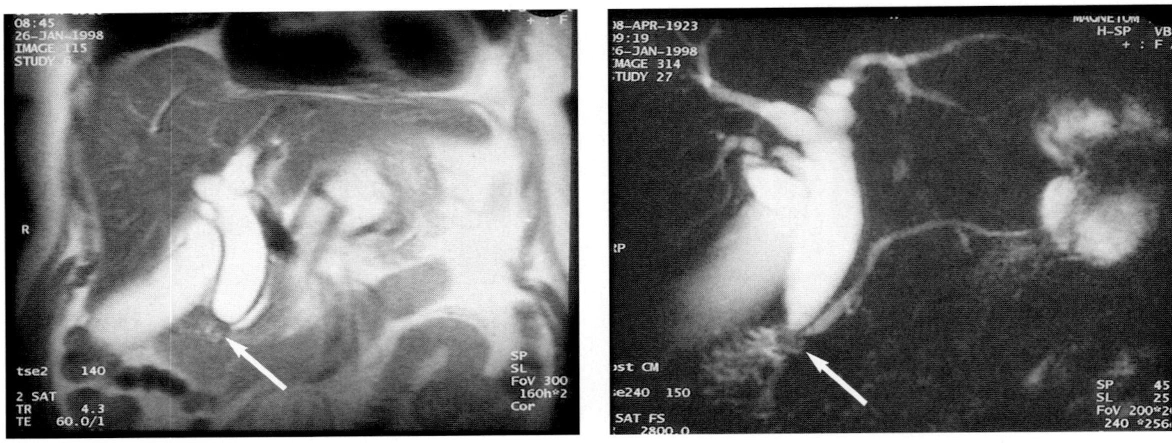 b

Fig. 8.56a,b. Ampullary carcinoma; magnetic resonance imaging (MRI). **a,b** Cross-sectional (**a**) and projective (**b**) T2-weighted MR images show dilated common bile duct and pancreatic duct with obstruction at the ampulla. The cause of the obstruction is a small ampullary carcinoma (*arrows*)

types of periampullary carcinoma (i.e., those originating from the duodenum, common bile duct, pancreatic duct, or ampulla) is usually difficult or impossible. One hallmark of the disease is dilatation of the common bile duct and pancreatic duct, including the supra-ampullary segments. The diagnosis of an ampullary tumor by imaging studies is particularly challenging because these tumors are usually small at the time of presentation (Fig. 8.54). Transabdominal US and dynamic CT perform rather poorly in the specific diagnosis of these tumors (Conlon et al. 1996). Adequate filling of the duodenum with tap water appears to facilitate tumor detection (Figs. 8.54, 8.55). EUS is better suited to diagnose small periampullary tumors. The value of MRI depends on the technique used. Classic cross-sectional MRI is less sensitive than EUS. By performing a dynamic MRCP study of the vaterian sphincter complex, periampullary abnormalities can be detected in an early stage (Van Hoe et al. 1998b). T2-weighted images obtained in the coronal plane are also useful (Fig. 8.56). An enlarged papilla is usually well seen if the duodenum is distended and filled with fluid. ERCP is commonly used as a final diagnostic step in these patients. If indicated, brushings can be obtained and a stent can be placed, either temporarily or as permanent palliative treatment.

Cholangiocarcinoma of the distal common bile duct may extend into the pancreatic duct and cause pancreatic duct dilatation. In such cases, the differ-

a 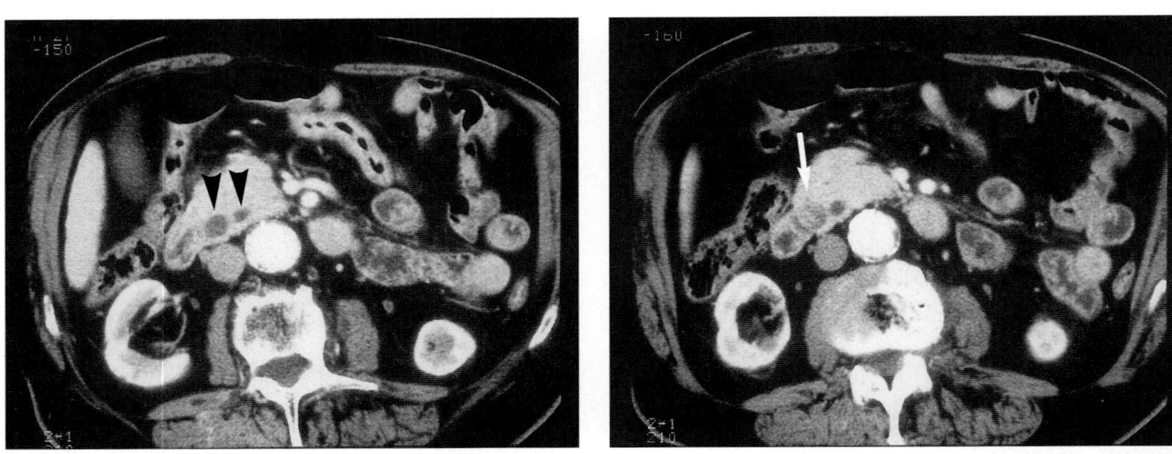 b

Fig. 8.57a,b. Cholangiocarcinoma. **a** Computed tomography (CT) image at the level of the pancreatic head shows dilatation of both the pancreatic and common bile ducts (*arrowheads*). **b** CT image obtained 10 mm more caudally shows soft-tissue mass centered in the lumen of the common bile duct: cholangiocarcinoma (*arrow*). There was secondary invasion of the pancreatic duct at the level of the papilla ential diagnosis with pancreatic carcinoma is impossible. More commonly, however, distal cholangiocarcinomas are detected in an earlier stage and seen as small neoplasms causing biliary duct obstruction without associated involvement of the pancreatic duct. With the use of helical CT, MRI, EUS, or ERCP, even relatively small cholangiocarcinomas can be detected as a soft-tissue mass within the common bile duct (Fig. 8.57).

8.7.7 Endocrine Tumors (see Chap. 10)

8.7.7.1 Functioning Endocrine Tumors

These tumors (85% of all endocrine pancreatic tumors) have quite characteristic imaging features: They are usually well vascularized and visible as hyperdense lesions on contrast-enhanced CT images. Small tumors may occasionally be seen only on images obtained in the arterial phase of perfusion (Van Hoe et al. 1995). On MRI, they are usually hypointense on T1-weighted images and hyperintense on T2-weighted images. Endocrine tumors may contain cystic or necrotic areas. Imaging is important for preoperative evaluation, not for diagnosis: The diagnosis is usually based on clinical signs and laboratory tests.

8.7.7.2 Non-functioning Endocrine Tumors

Unlike functioning endocrine tumors of the pancreas, non-functioning endocrine tumors are usually large and partially necrotic (Carlson et al. 1993). Thus, they may mimic the appearance of pancreatic adenocarcinoma. Differentiation may be possible in some cases because: (1) They usually show marked peripheral enhancement, and (2) they tend to cause displacement rather than obstruction of the main pancreatic duct.

8.7.8 Intraductal Mucinous Neoplasm

Mucin-producing tumors of intraductal origin are classified as follows (Itai and Ohtomo 1996):

A. "Peripheral type" (see Sect. 8.7.5.2)
B. "Branch type": mucin-secreting intraductal tumor usually located in uncinate process and causing localized dilatation of a side branch (Fig. 8.58)
C. "Duct ectatic type": mucin-secreting intraductal tumor characterized by diffuse dilatation of main pancreatic duct.

The mucin-secreting tumor is often too small to be visualized. One hallmark of the disease is marked focal or diffuse ductal dilatation. In branch-type tumors, a "polycystic" mass is seen in the uncinate process, actually representing focally dilated side branches filled with mucin. In tumors of the duct ectatic type, there is marked global dilatation of the main pancreatic duct without a demonstrable cause of obstruction. These tumors have malignant potential; therefore, early diagnosis is important.

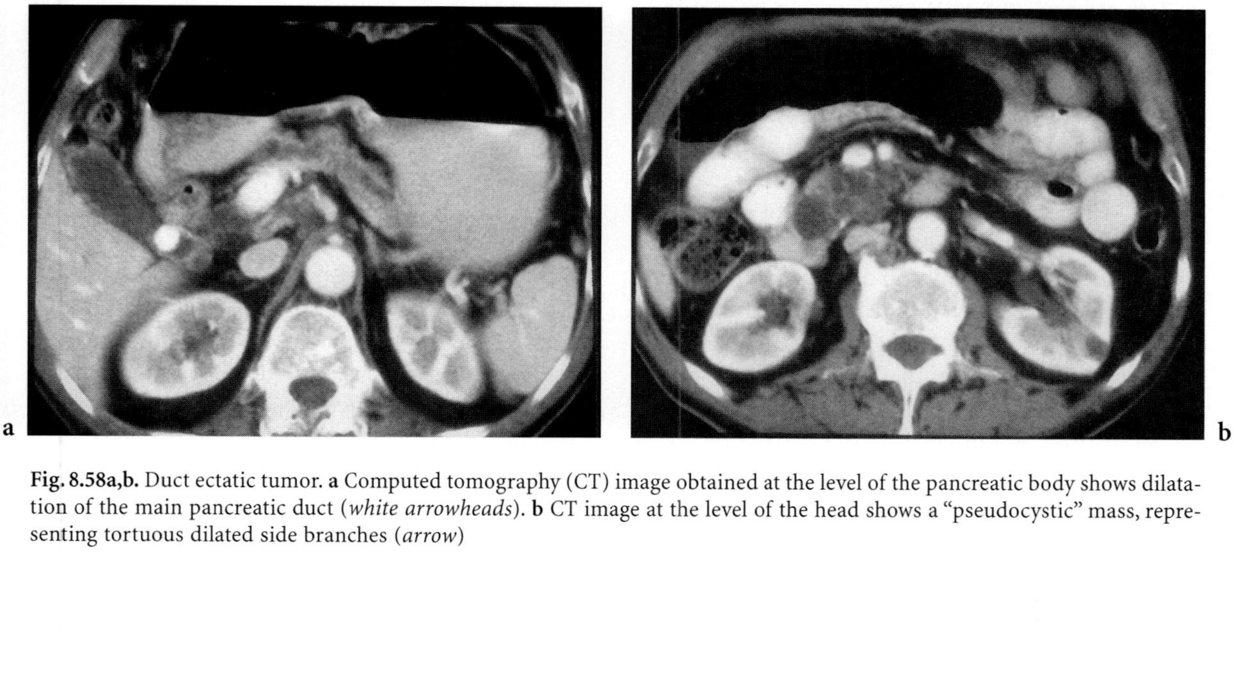

Fig. 8.58a,b. Duct ectatic tumor. **a** Computed tomography (CT) image obtained at the level of the pancreatic body shows dilatation of the main pancreatic duct (*white arrowheads*). **b** CT image at the level of the head shows a "pseudocystic" mass, representing tortuous dilated side branches (*arrow*)

8.7.9
Secondary Pancreatic Tumors (see Chap. 11)

8.7.9.1
Lymphoma

Differential features with ductal adenocarcinomas are the lower frequency of associated duct dilatation and the possible presence of retroperitoneal and upper abdominal adenopathies.

8.7.9.2
Metastases

Hypervascular pancreatic metastases (e.g., metastatic tumors from adenocarcinomas of the kidney) may mimic endocrine tumors. Most metastatic lesions, however, are hypovascular as compared with the normal pancreas. The diagnosis is based on: (a) clinical data, (b) absence of significant ductal dilatation, and (c) presence of multiple pancreatic lesions, usually associated with metastases in other organs.

8.8
Conclusions

Pancreatic carcinoma has a poor prognosis and is only curable by surgical resection. The task of imaging studies is twofold: (1) early tumor detection and (2) accurate selection of patients with resectable disease.

As illustrated in this chapter, a large number of diagnostic procedures are available to the clinician as he/she pursues the work-up of patients who are thought to have a pancreatic malignancy. As illustrated in Figs. 8.14 and 8.44, the approach chosen in different centers depends more on the local situation (personal interest and experience of clinicians, surgeons, and radiologists, availability of high-end technology, etc.) than on the results of large comparative studies. This is not surprising in view of rapid technical progress: Studies attempting to compare two state-of-the-art techniques may already be outdated by the time the material has reached the publication stage.

For preoperative staging, CT has classically been considered the best imaging technique (Freeny et al. 1988). This leading position of CT has been challenged in the last decade with the introduction of duplex abdominal sonography, EUS, and MRI. However, the recent introduction of thin-section dual-phase helical CT has dramatically improved the diagnostic accuracy of this noninvasive method, which, together with transabdominal US, is still used as the primary modality in many centers (Gloor et al. 1997).

Ultrafast interactive "all-in-one" MRI is another noninvasive technique that holds special promise by virtue of the fact that it provides the largest spectrum of information (cross-sectional T1- and T2-weighted imaging of the entire upper abdomen, cholangiopancreatography, arterial and venous angiography) and does not require the use of ionizing radiation (Trede et al. 1997). Because information on ductal anatomy, signal intensity, and contrast uptake pattern can be integrated, a specific diagnosis can be made in the majority of patients with pancreatic masses. However, because this technique is still evolving rapidly, its future role remains to be defined.

EUS has the disadvantage of being more invasive. On the other hand, it is, together with ERCP, the only non-surgical technique that allows tissue sampling without risk of peritoneal tumor spread. This technique will probably continue to play an important role in those patients where tissue sampling is warranted to differentiate benign from malignant disease, or to differentiate adenocarcinomas from other pancreatic tumors. On the other hand, the use of EUS as a primary technique is probably not justified since less invasive imaging methods are currently available (Dufour et al. 1997; Gloor et al. 1997).

Irrespective of the diagnostic strategy chosen, a combination of techniques will always be required in a number of patients. Moreover, since no single non-operative technique is 100% accurate, laparoscopy or surgical exploration will remain the decisive steps in tumor staging in a number of patients. LUS offers an exquisite detection of small hepatic metastases and may therefore be a valuable adjunct to laparoscopy. However, the value of laparoscopy and LUS remains to be determined. It has been suggested that most patients with micrometastases only detectable with laparoscopy or LUS present with clear signs of vascular involvement on helical CT (Gloor et al. 1997). Therefore, determination of the precise role of these techniques warrants further study.

Unfortunately, despite advances in pre- and peroperative staging of pancreatic carcinoma with all these new imaging techniques, patient survival remains essentially unchanged, mainly because of: (1) delayed presentation and (2) the absence of effective therapeutic options in patients with advanced disease (Vellet et al. 1992).

References

Angeli E, Venturini M, Vanzulli A et al (1997) Color Doppler imaging in the assessment of vascular involvement by pancreatic carcinoma. AJR 168:193–197

Aquino NM, Mortan R, Singh H (1989) Carcinoma of pancreas metastasizing to the tunica vaginalis testis. J Clin Ultrasound 17:287–290

Baert AL, Roex L, Marchal G, Hermans P, Dewilde D, Wilms G (1989) Computer-tomography of the stomach with water as an oral contrast agent: technique and preliminary results. J Comput Assist Tomogr 13:633–636

Baker ME, Cohan RH, Nadel SN, Leder RA, Dunnick NR (1990) Obliteration of the fat surrounding the celiac axis and superior mesenteric artery is not a specific CT finding of carcinoma of the pancreas. AJR 155:991–994

Baron PL, Abakken LE, Cole DJ et al (1997) Differentiation of benign from malignant pancreatic masses by endoscopic ultrasound. Ann Surg Oncol 4:639–643

Bemelman WA, de Wit LT, van Delden OM, Smits NJ, Obertop H, Rauws EAJ, Gouma DJ (1995) Diagnostic laparoscopy combined with laparoscopic ultrasonography in staging of cancer of the pancreatic head region. Br J Surg 82:820–824

Bluemke DA, Cameron JL, Hruban RH et al (1995) Potentially resectable pancreatic adenocarcinoma: helical CT assessment with surgical and pathologic correlation. Radiology 197:381–385

Bonaldi VM, Bret P, Atri M (1996) A comparison of two injection protocols using helical and dynamic acquisitions in CT examinations of the pancreas. AJR 167:49–55

Bonaldi VM, Bret PM, Atri M, Reinhold C (1998) Helical CT of the pancreas: a comparison of cine display and film-based viewing. AJR 170:373–376

Bosmans H, Van Hoe L, Gryspeerdt S, Kiefer B, Van Steenbergen W, Baert AL, Marchal G (1997) Technical note. Single-shot T2-weighted MR imaging of the upper abdomen: preliminary experience with the double echo HASTE technique. AJR 169:1291–1293

Brandt KR, Charboneau JW, Stephens DH, Welch TJ, Goellner JR (1993) CT- and US-guided biopsy of the pancreas. Radiology 187:99–104

Büchler M, Malfertheiner M, Friess H, Senn T, Beger HG (1990) Chronic pancreatitis with inflammatory mass in the head of the pancreas: a specific entity? In: Beger HG (ed) Chronic pancreatitis. Springer, Berlin Heidelberg New York, pp 41–46

Cahn M, Chang K, Nguyen P, Butler J (1996) Impact of endoscopic ultrasound with fine needle aspiration on the surgical management of pancreatic cancer. Am J Surg 172:470–472

Campbell JP, Wilson SR (1988) Pancreatic neoplasms: how useful is evaluation with US? Radiology 167:341–344

Carlson B, Johnson C, Stephens D et al (1993) MRI of pancreatic islet cell carcinoma. J Comput Assist Tomogr 17:735–740

Catalano C, Pavone P, Laghi A et al (1998) Pancreatic adenocarcinoma: combination of MR imaging, MR angiography and MR cholangiopancreatography for the diagnosis and assessment of resectability. Eur Radiol 8:428–434

Chen J, Baithun SI (1985) Morphologic study of 391 cases of exocrine pancreatic tumours with special reference to the classification of exocrine pancreatic carcinoma. J Pathol 146:17–29

Chezmar JL, Nelson RC, Small WC, Bernardino ME (1991) Magnetic resonance imaging of the pancreas with gadolinium-DTPA. Gastrointest radiol 16:139–142

Choi YH, Rubenstein WA, Ramirez De Arellano E, Intriere L, Kazam E (1997) CT and US of the pancreas. Clin Imaging 21: 414-440

Conlon KC, Dougherty E, Klimstra DS, Coit DG, Turnbull AD, Brennan MF (1996) The value of minimal access surgery in the staging of patients with potentially resectable peripancreatic malignancy. Ann Surg 223:134–140

Coombs RJ, Zeiss J, Howard JM, Thomford NR, Merrickx HW (1990) CT of the abdomen after the whipple procedure: value in depicting postoperative anatomy, surgical complications, and tumor recurrence. AJR 154:1011–1014

Cotton PB, Lees WR, Vallon AG, Cottone M, Grower JR, Chapman M (1980) Gray scale ultrasonosgraphy and endoscopic pancreaticography in pancreatic diagnosis. Radiology 134:453–459

Cuesta MA, Meijer S, Borgstein PJ, Sibinga Mulder I, Sikkenk AC (1993) Laparoscopic ultrasonography for hepatobiliary and pancreatic malignancy. Br J Surg 80:1571–1574

Crist DW, Sitzmann JV, Cameron LJ (1987) Informed hospital morbidity, mortality and survival after the Whipple procedure. Ann Surg 206:2284–2302

De Jaegere T, Van Hoe L, Van Steenbergen W et al Screening applications for MRI in the detection of upper abdominal disease: comparative study of non contrast-enhanced single-shot MR imaging and contrast-enhanced helical CT. Eur Radiol (in press)

DelMaschio A, Vanzulli A, Sironi S, Castrucci M, Mellone R, Staudacher C, Carlucci M, Zerbi A, Parolini D, Faravelli A, Cantaboni A, Garancini P, Di Carlo V (1991) Pancreatic cancer versus chronic pancreatitis: diagnosis with CA 19–9 assessment, US, CT, and CT-guided fine-needle biopsy. Radiology 178:95–99

Diehl SJ, Lehmann KJ, Sadick M, Lachmann R, Georgi M (1998) Pancreatic cancer: value of dual-phase helical CT in assessing resectability. Radiology 206:373–378

Dufour B, Zins M, Vilgrain V, Levy Ph, Bernades P, Menu Y (1997) Comparaison de la tomodensitométrie en mode hélicoidal et de l'échoendoscopie dans le diagnostic et le bilan des adénocarcinomes du pancréas. Gastroenterol Clin Biol 21:124–130

Earls JP, Rofsky NM, DeCorato DR, Krinsky GA, Weinreb JC (1997) Breath-hold single-dose gadolinium-enhanced three-dimensional MR aortography: usefulness of a timing examination and an MR power injector. Radiology 202:268–273

Edoute Y, Ben-Haim SA, Malberger E (1991) Value of direct fine needle aspirative cytology in diagnosis palpable abdominal masses. Am J Med 91:377–382

Engelhard K, Hollenbach HP (1997) High-resolution MRI of pancreatic masses with a new circularly polarized body phased-array coil. Eur Radiol 7:643–648

Faigel DO, Ginsberg GG, Bentz JS, Gupta PK, Smith DB, Kochman ML (1997) Endoscopic ultrasound-guided real-time fine-needle aspiration biopsy of the pancreas in cancer patients with pancreatic lesions. J Clin Oncol 15:1439–1443

Feng B, Song Q (1995) Does the common bile duct dilate after cholecystectomy? Sonographic evaluation in 234 patients. AJR 165:859–861

Frank K, Bliesze H, B^nhof JA, Beck K, Hammes P, Linhart P (1985) Laparoscopic sonography: a new approach to intraabdominal disease. J Clin Ultrasound 13:60–65
Freeny PC (1991) Radiology of the pancreas. Curr Opin Radiol 3:440–452
Freeny PC, Marks WM (1986) Hepatic perfusion abnormalities during CT angiography. Radiology 159:685–691
Freeny PC, Marks WM, Ryan JA (1988) Pancreatic ductal adenocarcinoma: diagnosis and staging with dynamic CT. Radiology 166:125–133
Freeny PC, Traverso LW, Ryan JA (1993) Diagnosis and staging of pancreatic adenocarcinoma with dynamic computed tomography. Am J Surg 165:600–606
Fuji M, Itoh K, Togashi K et al (1993) Spiral CT with a bolus of contrast material: efficacy in the detection of small pancreatic cancer. Radiology 189(p):230
Fukuda M, Mima S, Tanabe T, Hanui T, Suzuki Y, Hirata K, Terada S (1984) Endoscopic sonography of the liver – diagnostic application of the echolaparoscope to localize intrahepatic lesions. Scand J Gastroenterol 102:24–38
Fukuda M, Hirata K, Mima S (1992) Preliminary evaluation of sonolaparoscopy in the diagnosis of liver diseases. Endoscopy 24:701–708
Fukuya T, Honda H, Hayashi T et al (1995) Lymph-node metastases: efficacy of detection with helical CT in patients with gastric cancer. Radiology 197:705–711
Gaa J, Georgi M, Trede M (1997a) New concepts in MR imaging of pancreatic tumors. Imaging Decis MRI 1:2–7
Gaa J, Wendl K, Trede M, Georgi M (1997b) New concepts in MR imaging of pancreatic carcinoma: the all-in-one approach. In: Oudkerk M, Edelman R (eds) High-power gradient MR-imaging. Blackwell Science, Berlin, pp 425–430
Garber SJ, Lees WR (1992) The characterization of pancreatic and bile duct tumours by duplex Doppler. Clin Radiol 45:181–184
Gehl HB, Vorwerk D, Klose KC, Guenther RW (1991) Pancreatic enhancement after low-dose infusion of Mn-DPDP. Radiology 180:337–339
Gloor B, Todd KE, Reber HA (1997) Diagnostic workup of patients with suspected pancreatic carcinoma. Cancer 79:1780–1786
Gmeinwieser J, Feuerbach S, Hogenberger W et al (1995) Spiral CT in diagnosis of vascular involvement in pancreatic cancer. Hepatogastroenterology 42:418–22
Haase A (1990) Snapshot FLASH MRI- applications to T1,T2 and chemical shif imaging. Magn Reson Med 13:77–89
Haase A, Frahm J, Matthaei KD (1986) FLASH imaging: rapid NMR imaging using low flip angles. J Magn Reson 67:258–266
Hann LE, Conlon KC, Dougherty EC, Hilton S, Bach AM, Brennan MF (1997) Laparoscopic sonography of peripancreatic tumors: prelimionary experience. AJR 169:1257–1262
Hatfield AR, Tobias R, Terblanche J, Girdwood AH, Fataar S, Harries-Jones R et al (1982) Preoperative external biliary drainage in obstructive jaundice. Lancet 2:896–899
Heiken JP, Weyman PJ, Lee JK, Balfe DM, Picus D, Brunt EM, Flye ME (1989) Detection of focal hepatic masses: prospective evaluation with CT, delayed CT, CT during arterial portography, and MR imaging. Radiology 171:47–51
Heiken JP, Brink JA, Vannier MW (1993) Spiral (helical) CT. Radiology 189:647–656
Helm EB, Stille W (1984) Infective complications. In: Classen M, Geenen J, Kawai K (eds) Nonsurgical biliary drainage. Springer, Berlin Heidelberg New York, pp 111–119
Hennig J, Nauerth A, Friedburg H (1986) RARE imaging: a fast imaging method for clinical MR. Magn Reson Med 3:823–833
Hommeyer S, Freeny PC, Crabo LG (1995) Carcinoma of the head of the pancreas: evaluation of the pancreaticoduodenal veins with dynamic CT – potential for improved accuracy in staging. Radiology 196:233–238
Hyoty MK (1991) Computed tomography is important in assessing resectability of pancreatic carcinoma, even after ultrasonographic demonstration of the tumour. Ann Chir Gynaecol 80:259–262
Ichikawa T, Haradome H, Hachiya J (1997) Pancreatic ductal adenocarcinoma: preoperative assessment with helical CT versus dynamic MR imaging. Radiology 202:655–662
Itai Y, Ohtomo K (1996) Cystic tumors of the pancreas. Eur Radiol 6:844–850
John TG, Garden OJ (1993) Pancreatic cancer, part 1. Assessment of pancreatic cancer. In: Cuesta MA, Nagy AG (eds) Minimally invasive surgery in gastrointestinal cancer. Churchill Livingstone, London pp 95–111
John TG, Greig JD, Carter DC, Garden OJ (1995) Carcinoma of the pancreatic head and periampullary region. Tumor staging with laparoscopy and laparoscopic ultrasonography. Ann Surg 221:156–164
Kalender WA (1995) Technical foundations of spiral CT. JBR-BTR 78:68–74
Kalender WA, Seissler W, Klotz E et al (1990) Spiral volumetric CT with single-breathold technique, continuous transport and continuous scanner rotation. Radiology 176:181–183
Kalender WA, Polacin A, Sus C (1994) A comparison of conventional and spiral CT with regard to contrast and spatial resolution: an experimental study on the detection of spherical lesions. J Comput Assist Tomogr 18:167–176
Kettritz U, Warshauer D, Brown E, Schlund J, Eisenberg L, Semelka R (1996) Enhancement of the normal pancreas: comparison of manganese-DPDP and gadolinium chelate. Eur Radiol 6:14–18
Kiefer B, Grässner J, Hausman R (1994) Image acquisition in a second with half-Fourier acquisition single-shot turbo spin echo. JMRI (P) [Suppl]:86–87
Kim HS, Shin KH, Park CM et al (1996) Contrast enhancement of the pancreas and adjacent vessels during spiral CT: quantitative evaluation. Radiology 201(P):381
Klöppel G, Maillet B (1989) Classification and staging of pancreatic nonendocrine tumors. Radiol Clin North Am 27:105–119
Kobayashi G, Fujita N, Noda Y et al (1994) Evaluation of helical scanning in the diagnosis of pancreatic diseases. Nippon Shokakibyo Gakkai Zasshi 91:2083–2093
Korosec F, Frayne R, Grist T, Mistretta CA (1996) Time-resolved contrast-enhanced 3D MR angiography. Magn Reson Med 36:345–351
Kosuge T, Makuuchi M, Takayma T et al (1991) Thickening at the root of the superior mesenteric artery on sonography: evidence of vascular involvement in patients with cancer of the pancreas. AJR 156:69–72
Lai EC, Mok FP, Fan ST, Lo CM, Chu KM, Liu CL et al (1994) Preoperative endoscopic drainage for malignant obstructive jaundice. Br J Surg 81:1195–1198

Laing FC, Jeffrey RB Jr, Wing VW (1986) Biliary dilatation: defining the level and cause by real-time ultrasound. Radiology 160:39–42

Legmann P, Vignaux O, Dousset B et al (1998) Pancreatic tumors: comparison of dual-phase helical CT and endoscopic sonography. AJR 170:1315–1322

Lentschig MG, Reimer P, Rummeny E et al (1996) The role of spiral computed tomography and magnetic resonance imaging in the preoperative diagnostic of pancreatic carcinoma. Radiologe 36:406–412

Levin DP, Bret PM (1991) Percutaneous fine-needle aspiration biopsy of the pancreas resulting in death. Gastrointest Radiol 16:67–69

Lin JT (1988) Pancreatic carcinoma associated with chronic calcifying pancreatitis in Taiwan: a case report and review of literature. Pancreas 3:111–114

Loyer EM, David CL, Dubrow et al (1996) Vascular involvement in pancreatic adenocarcinoma: reassessment by thin-section CT. Abdom Imaging 21:202–206

Low RN, Barone RM, Lacey C, Sigeti J, Alzate G, Sebrechts C (1997) Peritoneal tumor: MR imaging with dilute oral barium and intravenous gadolinium-containing contrast agents compared with unenhanced MR imaging and CT. Radiology 204:513–520

Lowenfels AB, Maisonneuve P, Cavallini G et al (1993) Pancreatitis and the risk for cancer. N Engl J Med 328:1433–1437

Lu DS, Vedantham S, Krasny R et al (1996) Two-phase helical CT for pancreatic tumors: pancreatic versus hepatic phase enhancement of tumor, pancreas, and vascular structures. Radiology 199:697–701

Lu DS, Reber HA, Krasny RM, Kadell BM, Sayre J (1997) Local staging of pancreatic cancer: criteria for unresectability of major vessels as revealed by pancreatic-phase, thin-section helical CT. AJR 168:1439–1443

Marchal G, Baert A, Wilms G (1979) Intravenous pancreaticography in computed tomography. J Comput Assist Tomogr 3:727–732

Marchal G, Verbeken E, Van Steenbergen W, Baert AL (1989) Uneven lipomatosis: a pitfall in pancreatic sonography. Gastrointest Radiol 1989:233–237

Martin FM, Rossi RL, Dorrucci V et al (1990) Clinical and pathologic correlations in patients with periampullary tumors. Arch Surg 125:723–726

Matos C, Metens T, Devière J et al (1997) Pancreatic duct: morphologic and functional evaluation with dynamic MR pancreatography after secretin stimulation. Radiology 203:435–441

McPherson GAD, Benjamin IS, Hodgson HJF, Bowley NB, Allison DJ, Blumgart LH (1984) Preoperative percutaneous transhepatic biliary drainage: the results of a controlled trial. Br J Surg 71:371–375

Megibow AJ, Bosniak MA, Ambos MA (1981) Thickening of the coeliac axis and/or superior mesenteric artery: a sign of pancreatic carcinoma on computed tomography. Radiology 141:449–453

Megibow AJ, Zhou XH, Rotterdam H et al (1995) Pancreatic adenocarcinoma: CT versus MR imaging in the evaluation of resectability – report of the radiology diagnostic oncology group. Radiology 195:327–332

Minami M, Kawauchi N, Itai Y, Niki T, Sasaki Y (1992) Gastric tumors: radio-pathologic correlation and occurency of staging with dynamic CT. Radiology 185:173–178

Mitchell DG (1987) The superior mesenteric artery fat plane: is obliteration pathognomonic of pancreatic carcinoma? J Comput Assist Tomogr 11:247–253

Mitchell DG, Vinitski S, Saponaro S, Tasciyan T, Burk DL Jr, Rifkin MD (1991) Liver and pancreas: improved spin-echo T1 contrast by shorter echo time and fat suppression at 1.5 T. Radiology 178:67–71

Mori H, Miyake H, Aikawa H, Monzen Y, Maeda T, Suzuki K, Matsumoto S, Wakisaka M (1991) Dilated posterior superior pancreaticoduodenal vein: recognition with CT and clinical significance in patients with pancreaticobiliary carcinomas. Radiology 181:793–800

Müller MF, Meyenberger C, Bertschinger P et al (1994) Pancreatic tumors: evaluation with endoscopic US, CT, and MR imaging. Radiology 190:745–751

Muranaka T (1990) Morphologic changes in the body of the pancreas secondary to a mass in the pancreatic head. Analysis by CT. Acta Radiol 31:483–487

Murugiah M, Paterson-Brown S, Windsor JA, Miles A, Garden OJ (1993) Early experience of laparoscopic ultrasonography in the management of pancreatic carcinoma. Surg Endosc 7:177–181

Nelson RC, Chezmar JL, Sugarbaker PH, Bernardino ME (1989) Hepatic tumors: comparison of CT during arterial portography, delayed CT, and MR imaging for preoperative evaluation. Radiology 172:27–34

Niederau C, Grendell JH (1992) Diagnosis of pancreatic carcinoma. Imaging techniques and tumor markers. Pancreas 7:66–86

Nix GAJJ, Dubbelman C, Srivastava ED, Wilson JHP, Boender J, de Jongh FE (1991) Prognostic implications of the localization of carcinoma in the head of the pancreas. Am J Gastroenterol 86:1027–1032

Novick SL, Fishman EK (1998) Three-dimensional CT angiography of pancreatic carcinoma: role in staging extent of disease. AJR 170:139–143

Okita K, Kodama T, Oda M, Takemoto T (1984) Laparoscopic ultrasonography: diagnosis of liver and pancreatic cancer. Scand J Gastroenterol 94:91–100

Op den Orth JO (1987) Sonography of the pancreatic head aided by water and glucagon. Radiographics 7:85–100

Ormson MJ, Charboneau JW, Stephens DH (1987) Sonography in patients with a possible pancreatic mass shown on CT. AJR 148:551–555

Päivänsalo M et al (1988) US and CT in pancreatic malignancy. Acta Radiol 29:343–344

Paul MA, Sibinga Mulder L, Cuesta MA, Sikkenk AC, Lyesen GKS, Meijer S (1994) Impact of intraoperative ultrasonography on treatment strategy for colorectal cancer. Br J Surg 81:1660–1663

Pichler W, Frank W, Jantsch H et al (1989) Sonographic staging of pancreatic cancer. Report of 100 cases. Fortschr Röntgenstr 150:241–245

Pitt HA, Gomes AS, Lois JF, Mann LL, Deutsch LS, Longmire WP Jr (1985) Does preoperative percutaneous transhepatic biliary drainage reduce operative risk or increase hospital cost? Ann Surg 201:545–553

Prince MR, Yucel EK, Kaufman JA, Harrison DC, Geller SC (1993) Dynamic gadolinium-enhanced three-dimensional abdominal MR arteriography. J Magn Reson Imaging 3:877–881

Reimer P, Rummeny E (1998) Pancreatic receptors: contrast for MR imaging. Proceedings of the 9th annual meeting of the European Society of Gastrointestinal and Abdominal Radiology, Marbella, Spain, 24–28 May 1998, p 65

Rigauts H, Marchal G, Hupke R (1990) First experience with volume scanning. J Comput Assist Tomogr 14:675–682

Rigauts H, Marchal G, Baert AL (1992) Enhancement of the pancreas after single bolus injection combined with spiral scanning: a comparative study with conventional incremental scanning after biphasic contrast injection. Fortschr Rontgenstr 156:471–474

Robledo R, Prietro ML, Pérez M, Camunez F, Echenaguasia A (1988) Carcinoma of the hepaticopancreatic ampullary region: role of US. Radiology 160:39–42

Rohrman CA, Baron RL (1989) Biliary complications of pancreatitis. Radiol Clin North Am 27:93–104

Rösch T (1997) Endoscopic ultrasonography in pancreatic disease. In: Trede M, Carter DC (eds) Surgery of the pancreas, 2nd edn. Churchill Livingstone, London, pp 119–127

Rösch T (1998) Endoscopic ultrasonography. In: Howard J, Idezuki Y, Ihse I, Prinz R (eds) Surgical diseases of the pancreas. Williams and Wilkins, Baltimore, pp 185–192

Rösch T, Lorenz R, Braig C et al (1991) Endoscopic ultrasound in pancreatic tumor diagnosis. Gastrointest Endoscop 37:347–352

Ross B, Brooke Jeffrey R, Mindelzun R (1996) Normal variations in the lateral contour of the head and neck of the pancreas mimicking neoplasm: evaluation with dual-phase helical CT. AJR 166:799–801

Schulte SJ, Baron RL, Freeny PC, Patten RM, Horell HA, Maclin ML (1991) Root of the superior mesenteric artery in pancreatitis and pancreatic carcinoma: evaluation with CT. Radiology 180:659–662

Semelka RC, Marcos HB (1998) Nonendocrine tumors of the pancreas. In: Heuck A, Reiser M (eds) Magnetic resonance imaging of the abdomen. Springer, Berlin Heidelberg New York, pp 117–124

Semelka RC, Kroeker MA, Shoenut JP, Kroeker R, Yaffe CS, Micflikier AB (1993) Pancreatic disease: prospective comparison of CT, ERCP, and 1.5-T MR imaging with dynamic gadolinium enhancement and fat suppression. Radiology 181:785–791

Semelka RC, Kelekis NL, Molina PL et al (1996) Pancreatic masses with inconclusive findings on spiral CT: is there a role for MRI? JMRI 6:585–588

Simon C, Wunsch CS, Richter GM, Hoffmann V, Klar E, Kauffmann GW (1997) Will thin slice hydro CT replace angiography for staging of pancreatic carcinoma? Radiology 205(P):288

Smith EK (1991) Complications of percutaneous abdominal fine-needle biopsy: review. Radiology 178:253–255

Smits NJ, Reeders JWAJ (1995) Current applicability of duplex Doppler ultrasonography in pancreatic head and biliary malignancies. In: Tytgat GNJ, Reeders JWAJ (eds) Bailliere's clinical gastroenterology: diagnostic imaging of the gastrointestinal tract, part II. Bailliere Tindall, London, pp 153–172

Stephens DH (1996) Pancreatic adenocarcinoma. Abd Imaging 21:207–210

Temudom T, Sarr MG, Douglas MG, Farnell MB (1995) An argument against routine percutaneous biopsy, ERCP, or biliary stent placement in patients with clinically resectable periampullary masses: a surgical perspective. Pancreas 11:283–288

Tio TL, Tytgat GH, Cikot RJ et al (1990) Ampullopancreatic carcinoma: preoperative TNM classification with endosonography. Radiology 175:455–461

Trede M, Rumstadt B, Wendl K et al (1997) Ultrafast magnetic resonance imaging improves the detection and staging of pancreatic tumors. Ann Surg 226:393–407

Van Delden OM, Smits NJ, Bemelman WA, de Wit LT, Gouma DJ, Reeders JWAJ (1996) Comparison of laparoscopic ultrasound and transabdominal ultrasound in staging of cancer of the pancreatic head region. J Ultrasound Med 16:207–212

Van Delden OM (1997) Laparoscopic ultrasonography for abdominal tumor staging. Thesis, AZUA, Amsterdam, The Netherlands

Van Hoe L, Baert AL (1997) Pancreatic carcinoma: applications for helical computed tomography. Endoscopy 29:539–560

Van Hoe L, Gryspeerdt S, Marchal G et al (1995) Helical CT for the preoperative localization of islet cell tumors of the pancreas: value of arterial and parenchymal phase images. AJR 165:1437–1439

Van Hoe L, Bosmans H, Aerts P et al (1996) Focal liver lesions: evaluation of a half-Fourier RARE sequence. Radiology 201:817–823

Van Hoe L, Baert AL, Gryspeerdt S et al (1997) Dual-phase spiral CT of the liver: value of an early-phase acquisition in the differential diagnosis of focal lesions. AJR 168:1185–1192

Van Hoe L, Gryspeerdt S, Ectors N et al (1998a) Nonalcoholic duct-destructive chronic pancreatitis: imaging findings. AJR 170:643–647

Van Hoe L, Gryspeerdt S, Vanbeckevoort D et al (1998b) Normal Vaterian sphincter complex: evaluation of anatomy and contractility with dynamic single-shot MR cholangiopancreatography. AJR (to be published)

Van Hoe L, Vanbeckevoort D, Van Steenbergen W (1998c) Atlas of cross-sectional and projective magnetic resonance cholangio-pancreatography. Springer, Berlin Heidelberg New York

Van Hoe L, De Jaegere T, Bosmans H, Bogaert J, Oyen R, Marchal G Time-resolved MR angiography of the upper abdomen: initial clinical experience. Eur Radiol (submitted)

Vellet AD, Romano W, Bach DB, Passi RB, Taves DH, Munk PC (1992) Adenocarcinoma of the pancreatic ducts: comparative evaluation with CT and MRI imaging at 1.5 T. Radiology 183:87–95

Wang G, Brink JA, Vannier MW (1994) Theoretical FWTM values in spiral CT. Med Phys 21:753–754

Warshaw AL (1991) Implication of peritoneal cytology for staging of early pancreatic cancer. Am J Surg 161:26–29

Warshaw AL, Fernandez del Castillo C (1992) Pancreatic carcinoma. N Engl J Med 326:455–465

Warshaw AL, Gu ZY, Wittenberg J, Waltman AC (1990) Preoperative staging and assessment of resectability of pancreatic cancer. Arch Surg 125:230–233

Winter TC, Ager JD, Nghiem HV et al (1996) Upper gastrointestinal tract and abdomen: water as an orally administered contrast agent for helical CT. Radiology 201:365–370

Zeman RK, Cooper CC, Zeiberg AS et al (1997) TNM staging of pancreatic carcinoma using helical CT. AJR 169:459–464

9 Cystic Tumors of the Pancreas

V. VILGRAIN, D. MATHIEU, J.-M. BRUEL, J.-F. FLEJOU, A. RAHMOUNI, P. TAOUREL

CONTENTS

V. VILGRAIN, MD, Professor of Radiology, Hôpital Beaujon, Clichy, France
D. MATHIEU, MD, Professor of Radiology, Hôpital Henri Mondor, Université Paris 12, Val de Marne, France
J.-M. BRUEL, MD, Professor of Radiology, Hôpital Saint-Eloi, Montpellier, France
J.-F. FLEJOU, MD, Associate Professor, Department of Pathology, Hôpital Beaujon, Clichy, France
A. RAHMOUNI, MD, Assistant Professor, Hôpital Henri Mondor, Université Paris 12, Créteil, France
P. TAOUREL, MD, Assistant Professor, Department of Radiology, Hôpital Saint-Eloi, Montpellier, France

9.1 Introduction

Pancreatic carcinoma is the most frequent tumor of the pancreas. Cystic neoplasms of the pancreas are relatively rare, accounting for 1% of all pancreatic malignancies and 10%–15% of all pancreatic cysts (CUBILLA and FITZGERALD 1984). However, it is important to recognize these neoplasms because of their distinctive histomorphology and clinicopathologic features (KLÖPPEL 1984; KLÖPPEL and MAILLET 1989; CUBILLA and FITZGERALD 1975; YAMAGUCHI and MUNETOMO 1987; MATHIEU et al. 1989; FRIEDMAN and EDMONDS 1989; MOROHOSHI et al. 1983; WARSHAW et al. 1990; LACK 1989) and because the survival is better than in pancreatic carcinoma.

Most of cystic neoplasms are epithelial tumors of the exocrine gland. These lesions are developed from different cells including duct, acinar, and centroacinar cells. But in some cases, the origin of the tumor remains unclear and tumors with mixed endocrine and exocrine components may be observed. For this reason, electron microscopy or immunocytochemical studies now play a major role in assisting the diagnosis of these lesions.

9.2 Serous Cystadenomas

Serous cystadenoma, also called microcystic cystadenoma or glycogen-rich cystadenoma, is considered as a cystic tumor most frequently observed in middle-aged and elderly women (MATHIEU et al. 1989; WARSHAW et al. 1990; LACK 1989; ALBORES-SAAVEDRA et al. 1990; ALPERT et al. 1988; COMPAGNO and OERTEL 1978a; REMINE et al. 1987; BECKER et al. 1965; DIDOLKAR et al. 1975; TORRES-BARRERA et al. 1987; HODGKINSON et al. 1978a; RUBIN et al. 1991; SHORTEN et al. 1986; LO et al. 1977). The predominance of serous cystadenomas in women is demonstrated in all series, with a ratio of greater than 1.5:1, but is less significant than for mucinous cystic neoplasms (sex ratio 6:1). These lesions account for a small percentage of pancreatic neoplasms, but, despite its relatively uncommon occurrence, the microcystic adenoma is an important lesion to recognize radiologically. Unlike all of the other pancreatic neoplasms, which are considered frankly or potentially malignant, the serous cystadenoma is generally agreed to be benign (Albores-Saavedra et al. 1990; Alpert et al. 1988; Compagno and Oertel 1978a; Remine et al. 1987; Becker et al. 1965; Didolkar et al. 1975; Torres-Barrera et al. 1987; Hodgkinson et al. 1978a; Rubin et al. 1991; Shorten et al. 1986; Lo et al. 1977).

It can be found incidentally in 10%–30% of cases or, more commonly, may be revealed by abdominal pain or manifest as an abdominal mass (Mathieu et al. 1989; Lack 1989; Albores-Saavedra et al. 1990; Alpert et al. 1988; Compageno and Oertel 1978). The symptoms are nonspecific. Abdominal pressure or upper abdominal pain is the most frequent symptom described. Duration of abdominal discomfort ranges from a few days to several years. Other symptoms are rare and related to mechanical compression of adjacent structures: nausea or vomiting, obstructive jaundice in the case of cephalic location, and hematemesis secondary to segmental portal hypertension. Intestinal or peritoneal hemorrhage has rarely been described (Rubin et al. 1991). Asymptomatic cases account for the incidental findings during laparotomy or ultrasound examination performed for unrelated reasons. However, mild loss of weight is noticed in 40% of cases. Serous cystadenomas are slowly expanding tumors, and may produce quite large masses. Thus, 50% of the patients are found to have a round, firm palpable mass, discovered either by the patients themselves or at physical examination.

Multiple constitutional and pathologic abnormalities have been described in association with this tumor. Diabetes mellitus is seen in a large number of patients with serous cystadenoma. Compagno and Oertel (1978a) suggest that these abnormalities might be coincidental in elderly patients. Serous cystadenomas are found with increased frequency in patients with von Hippel-Lindau disease (Mathieu et al. 1989; Lack 1989; Albores-Saavedra et al. 1990).

Surgical excision remains the treatment of choice in most cases (Warshaw et al. 1990), but, in patients who are poor surgical candidates or in certain asymptomatic patients, follow-up examination alone seems to be an accepted form of treatment. Many of the previously reported microcystic adenomas were not resected, and none of those that were followed up (for many years in several cases) was found to have metastasized or invaded adjacent organs. In view of the morbidity and mortality associated with pancreatic surgery, it is important that the diagnosis of serous cystadenoma be made before surgery. However, an unusual case has be reported by George and coworkers (1989). They presented a primary tumor of the pancreas that was histologically indistinguishable from serous cystadenoma, but which behaved in a malignant fashion with metastases in the stomach and liver. They called this new entity serous cystadenocarcinoma. There is a wide variety of computed tomography (CT) and ultrasound features described in serous cystadenoma which can be attributed to the size of the cysts and to the amount of connective tissue between them (Lo et al. 1977; George et al. 1989; Friedman et al. 1983; Itai et al. 1982; Algard et al. 1986; Freeny et al. 1978; Buck and Hayes 1990; Wolson and Walls 1976; Caroll and Sample 1978; De Santos et al. 1978; Parienty et al. 1980; Kolmannskog et al. 1982; Wolfman et al. 1982; Zirinsky et al. 1984; Stovall 1986; Itai et al. 1988; Padovani et al. 1991; Fugazzola et al. 1991; Johnson et al. 1988). When this last component predominates, the diagnosis can be facilitated by the demonstration of predominant echogenic tumors at sonography and a hypervascular lesion with numerous small cysts and a calcified central scar on dynamic CT. Endosonography can be helpful in detecting the solid portion of the mass.

9.2.1 Pathologic Features

Macroscopically, serous cystadenomas are well-circumscribed, spherical to ovoid, multilocular cystic tumors (Lack 1989; Albores-Saavedra et al. 1990; Alpert et al. 1988). The edges are lobulated secondary to the bulging cysts. The junction with the adjacent pancreas is gross. Microscopically, a poorly defined fibrous capsule is seen only focally around the tumors. Cut sections of these tumors have a honeycombed or spongy appearance due to the presence of numerous cysts (Fig. 9.1). Some tumors are composed predominantly of cysts of 1–2 cm in diameter, whereas others consist predominantly of smaller cysts that are all less than 0.1 cm in diameter. Some tumors have a more varied mixture of cyst diameter. The fluid contained within the cyst is typically clear with no mucoid plugs. However, in resected speci-

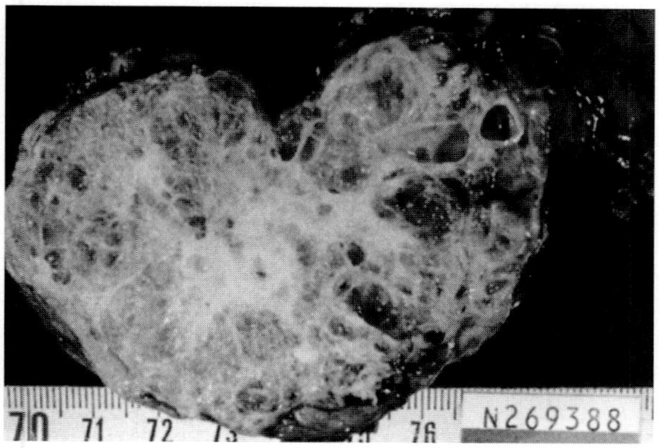

Fig. 9.1. Serous cystadenoma. Cross section of gross specimen shows numerous cysts separated by fibrous septa

mens, the cyst fluid frequently appears hemorrhagic; this may be partly attributed to fresh blood contaminating the fluid upon sectioning the fresh specimen. Nevertheless, the microscopic presence of abundant hemosiderin in the fibrous walls of most of the tumors indicates that spontaneous bleeding does occur in these tumors. Prominent fibrous bands are seen within the tumor, and the fibrosis may take the form of a central scar that may be calcified. These dystrophic calcifications are usually observed in tumors measuring 5 cm or more.

The histologic features are distinctive, with little variation from case to case. The cysts are lined by a single layer of flat or cuboidal epithelial cells and are separated by fibrous septa. Neither cytologic atypia nor mitotic figures are found (LACK 1989; ALBORES-SAAVEDRA et al. 1990; ALPERT et al. 1988; SHORTEN et al. 1986; LO et al. 1977). The presence of glycogen in the cells lining the cysts is a characteristic finding easily demonstrated by the presence of periodic acid–Schiff (PAS)-positive deposits that are digested by pretreatment with amylase. Intracellular mucins are not detected with special stains. The epithelium can be focally arranged in multiple papillary tufts without fibrovascular cores. Occasional true papillae are present, but no cytologic atypia are associated with these papillary formations. The stroma is highly vascular, creating a fine supporting network. In areas where the cysts are larger, the stroma appears collagenized. In these areas, the stroma often contains calcification, hemosiderin-laden macrophages, and cholesterol clefts. The pancreatic tissue immediately adjacent to the tumor is normal, or focally atrophic with or without mild chronic inflammation (ALBORES-SAAVEDRA et al. 1990; ALPERT et al. 1988).

The cell origin of serous cystadenoma has long been debated: centroacinar cell or ductal cell (LACK 1989; ALBORES-SAAVEDRA et al. 1990; ALPERT et al. 1988; COMPAGNO and OERTEL 1978a; SHORTEN et al. 1986; LO et al. 1977). However, the actual results of immunohistochemistry and ultrastructural findings seem to indicate that the centroacinar cell is the cell of origin of serous cystadenoma (ALPERT et al. 1988). Positive staining for tumor cells is found with epithelial membrane antigen and cytokeratins of low and broad molecular weights. Tumor cells are always negative for carcinoembryonic antigen (CEA). At the ultrastructural level, the tumor cells in serous cystadenoma most closely resemble centroacinar cells (ALPERT et al. 1988; SHORTEN et al. 1986; LO et al. 1977).

It is well established that serous cystadenoma is a strictly benign tumor. But the case of serous cystadenocarcinoma resembled histologically serous cystadenoma (GEORGE et al. 1989). This 11 cm tumor was observed in a 70-year-old man. Laparotomy revealed a large mass in the tail of the pancreas, involving the splenic hilum and the adjacent wall of the great curvature of the stomach, and liver metastases were present. On histologic examination, the findings of serous cystadenocarcinoma were associated with focal cytologic atypia, nuclear enlargement, and pleomorphism. Stains for mucin were negative, but abundant glycogen was demonstrated within the cells as PAS-positive, diastase-sensitive material. Histologically and clinically, the malignancy of this tumor was considered low grade. For these authors, this tumor could be the malignant counterpart of serous cystadenoma. However, no similar case with malignant behavior had been previously reported.

9.2.2 Imaging Procedures

Plain radiographs may show an upper abdominal soft tissue mass and sometimes the presence of calcifications within the tumor. FRIEDMAN and coworkers (1983) demonstrated calcifications more frequently in serous cystadenomas than in mucinous neoplasms (38% versus 16%, respectively). The calcification observed in serous cystadenomas is centrally located and either linear, arcuate, or globular (often described as "sunburst" calcification), and corresponds to the dystrophic calcification of the central scar. Gastrointestinal barium series occasionally demonstrate a widening of the duodenal loop or external displacement of the stomach or colon.

Sonographic appearance depends on the size of the microcysts (Mathieu et al. 1989; Friedman et al. 1983; Itai et al. 1982; Algard et al. 1986; Freeny et al. 1978; Buck et al. 1990; Wolson and Walls 1976; Wolfman et al. 1982; Johnson et al. 1988). When the tumor is only composed of cysts smaller than 2 mm in diameter, sonography shows a homogeneous, solid, well-encapsulated mass within the pancreas (Fig. 9.2). This mass is commonly hyperechoic relative to the adjacent pancreas. This structure is explained by the myriad of interfaces produced by the microscopic cysts (Fig. 9.3) (Mathieu et al. 1989; Johnson et al. 1988). The radiating septa and central scar are usually not visible. If the cysts are larger, they are depicted as anechoic structures of between 5 and 20 mm in diameter with regular, thin walls, often peripherally disposed. In the central area, calcification may be demonstrated as highly reflective echoes with acoustic shadowing.

On CT, the cystic spaces are visualized if they are not too small (Mathieu et al. 1989; Friedman et al. 1983; Itai et al. 1982; Algard et al. 1986; Buck and Hayes 1990; Caroll and Sample 1978; De Santos et al. 1978; Parienty et al. 1980; Kolmannskog et al. 1982; Wolfman et al. 1982; Zirinsky et al. 1984; Stovall 1986; Itai et al. 1988; Padovani et al. 1991; Fugazzola et al. 1991; Johnson et al. 1988). Before contrast, adenomas are hypodense (10–40 HU), encapsulated, and lobulated masses (Fig. 9.4). Bolus infusion and dynamic scan may show either diffuse homogeneous enhancement, or localized marked contrast enhancement of the solid portions of the tumor with stellate radiating bands of connective tissue and a linear peripheral ring. The septa are usually visible, and a honeycombed appearance is seen (Fig. 9.5). On post-contrast scans, the tumor may appear as a homogeneous or heterogeneous hypodense solid or polycystic mass. Foci of calcifications are better visualized in the central septa than on sonography. Cysts larger than 20 mm in diameter may exist at the periphery of the lesion (Fig. 9.6, 9.7).

In a review of 45 pathologically proven pancreatic cystic neoplasms, including 29 mucinous cystic tumors and 16 serous cystadenomas, Johnson et al. (1988) considered the number and size of the cysts present in the different lesions. When the diameter of the cysts was less than 2 cm and the number of cysts was greater than six, the application of these criteria for the diagnosis of adenoma led to a correct diagnosis on sonography in 78% and on CT in 93%.

On magnetic resonance imaging (MRI), serous cystadenomas show a lobulated external border, especially on spin echo images (Minami et al. 1989).

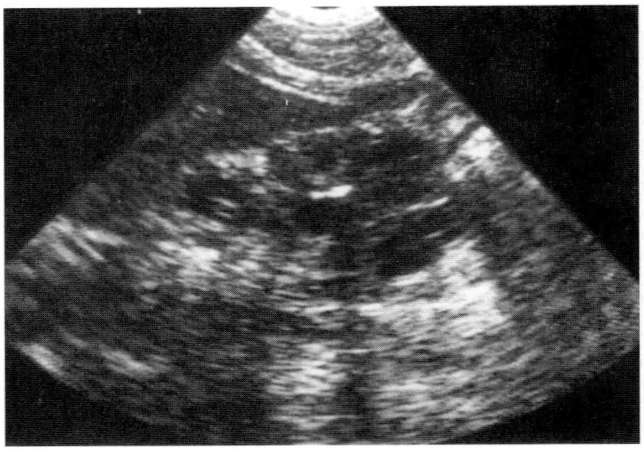

Fig. 9.2. Serous cystadenoma. Transverse sonogram demonstrating a hypoechoic mass of the head of the pancreas. Central calcifications with posterior shadowing are seen

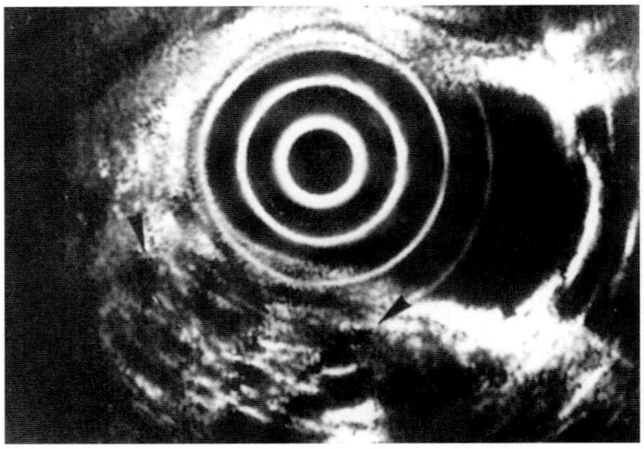

Fig. 9.3. Serous cystadenoma. Endosonography showing small cysts separated by echogenic septa

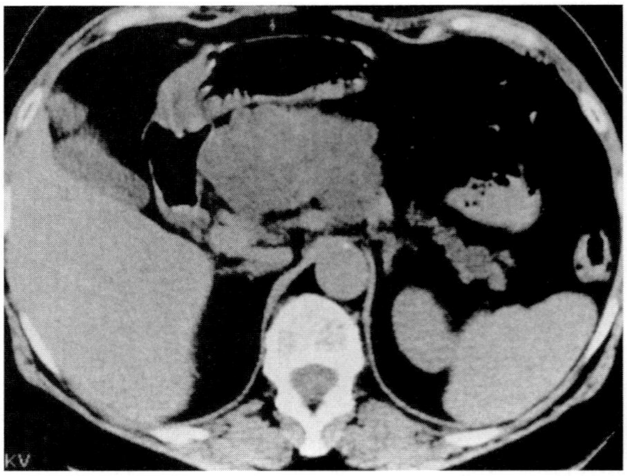

Fig. 9.4. Serous cystadenoma. Unenhanced computed tomography scan demonstrating the mass as hypodense and homogeneous

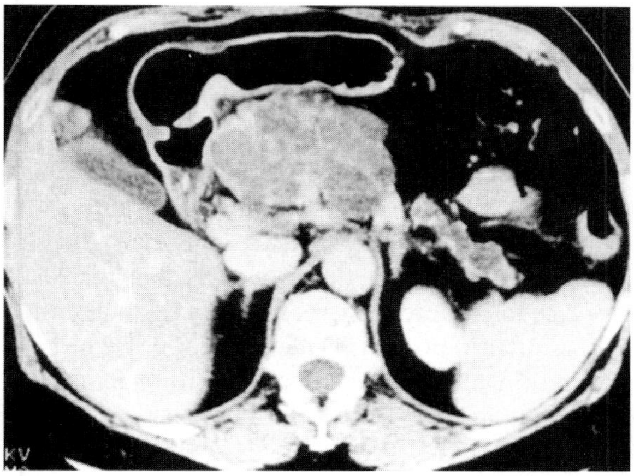

Fig. 9.5. Serous cystadenoma. Enhanced computed tomography scan (same patient as than Fig. 9.3) showing enhancement of the septa separating the cysts

a

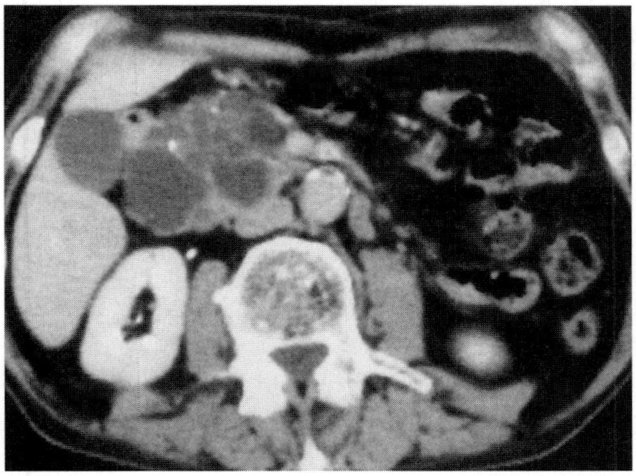

b

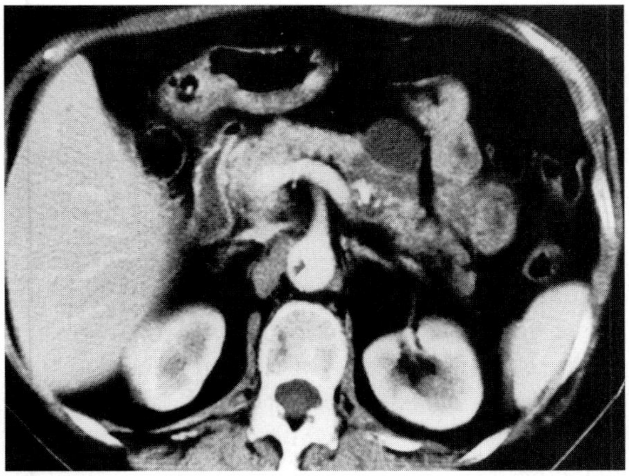

Fig. 9.6a,b. Serous cystadenoma. Computed tomography scans in two patients showing large cysts located at the periphery of the lesions

This new imaging modality shows that these tumors are composed of multiple compartments; their intensity is low on T1-weighted images and high on T2-weighted images. In a recent study, MRI was equal or slightly superior to CT in the diagnosis of this tumor, except in its limited ability to demonstrate calcifications of the tumor central scar and septa (MINAMI et al. 1989).

Selective angiography usually demonstrates the presence of a highly vascular tumor (MATHIEU et al. 1989; FRIEDMAN et al. 1983; FREENY et al. 1978). Enlarged pancreatic feeding arteries with celiac or mesenteric blood supply, tumor blush, some neovascularity, and large draining veins are visible. The tumor blush is homogeneous, but large cysts may produce lucent and avascular regions. The hypervascular nature of this cystic tumor is consistent with the extensive capillary network seen within the septa at microscopic examination. In the venous phase, the splenic or mesenteric veins may be displaced or obstructed.

Rarely, the serous cystadenomas have a morphologic variant differing from microcystic adenoma. It has a macrocystic appearance (LEWANDROWSKI et al. 1992). Five cases of macrocystic serous cystadenoma have been reported, two of which were of the unilocular type (LEWANDROWSKI et al. 1992). Imaging data of these cases were thought to represent either mucinous cystic neoplasms or pseudocysts. But microcystic and macrocystic serous tumors represent morphologic variants of the same pancreatic neoplasm.

Microcystic adenoma is a slow-growing tumor that exhibits benign behavior; however, it can become large enough to compress adjacent structures, thus leading to complications. Its potential for continued growth is illustrated in a few cases where resection was contraindicated. Thus, surgical excision remains the treatment of choice in most cases, but, in patients who are poor surgical candidates or in asymptomatic patients, follow-up examination alone seems to be an accepted form of treatment. Many of the previously reported microcystic adenomas were not resected, and none of those that were followed up (for many years in several cases) was found to have metastasized or invaded adjacent organs. In view of the morbidity and mortality associated with pancreatic surgery, conservative management seems advisable, particularly in elderly patients who are not likely to withstand rigorous surgery because of coexisting conditions, or in whom extirpation of a benign lesion seems unwarranted, particularly when in a cephalic location.

The diagnosis is usually made with a combination of sonography, endosonography, and CT, particularly when the solid components predominate upon the cystic areas. CT features of the central scar, especially when calcified, the enhancement of septations, and the sonographic findings of an echoic mass (due to the numerous interfaces produced by the microscopic cysts) are often diagnostic. When the lesion is composed of larger cysts, the distinction between serous cystadenoma and mucinous neoplasms is difficult; the management of these lesions depends upon the size and site of the tumor, as well as on the age of the patient. The role of percutaneous biopsies has not be clearly evaluated. Intraoperative biopsies can be an alternative for the exact histologic diagnosis and for the appropriate management of these tumors.

9.3 Mucinous Cystic Neoplasms

Mucinous cystic neoplasms of the pancreas are now regarded as either benign, but potentially malignant, or already malignant at the time of initial diagnosis (Mathieu et al. 1989; Warshaw et al. 1990; Albores-Saavedra et al. 1987, 1990; Compagno and Oertel 1978b; Leborgne et al. 1985; Hodgkinson et al. 1978b). Some tumors histologically do not display atypia and therefore could be considered benign. Other tumors show epithelial atypia, but malignant transformation cannot be proven. In these cases, tumors should be considered potentially malignant (borderline type). Finally, some tumors are obviously malignant at the time of diagnosis. Compagno and Oertel reported 41 mucinous cystic neoplasms: eight were considered histologically benign, 14 contained foci of atypical epithelium, and 19 contained foci of invasive adenocarcinoma (Campagno and Oertel 1978b).

Mucinous cystic neoplasms mainly occur in middle-aged women and usually cause epigastric pain and/or an abdominal mass. Signs and symptoms are nonspecific, and may be present for many years in some cases. They most likely result from pressure on contiguous structures by a slowly enlarging cystic mass. Very rarely, the initial symptoms are due to spread of the tumor into adjacent organs. A palpable mass, abdominal tenderness or pain, nausea, vomiting, diarrhea, bleeding, and weight loss are the most frequent complaints. These tumors are located within the tail or body of the pancreas in 70%–90% of cases, and in the head of the gland in 10%–30% of cases. Tumor size varies between 1 and 20 cm, and appears to correlate with the degree of malignancy: small tumors of less than 3 cm in diameter are histologically considered benign, whereas tumors with a diameter of 8 cm or more are considered malignant. Tumors involving the head of the pancreas may give rise to jaundice, whereas relatively small cystic masses often represent incidental radiologic or surgical findings. The lack of history of trauma or alcoholism can help to exclude the diagnosis of pseudocyst. However, in several patients, a clinical diagnosis of pseudocyst leads to various types of drainage procedures. These procedures are considered to be inappropriate for mucinous tumors. Systemic manifestations, probably due to excessive hormone production by the tumoral cells, have been occasionally described in the course of this tumor such as Zollinger-Ellison syndrome and watery diarrhea hypokalemia syndrome (Albores-Saavedra et al. 1987, 1990). Mucinous cystic neoplasms are slow-growing tumors that may be curable by a complete excision. Compagno and Oertel reported that 20 patients of the 27 who underwent total tumor removal survived without evidence of recurrence or metastasis after a mean follow-up of 6–7 years (range 3–10 years) (Compagno and Oertel 1978b). Similar results have been reported by Hodgkinson and coworkers; after complete excision, there was no recurrence of histologically benign tumors, and the 5-year survival rate of patients with malignant tumors was 68% (Hodgkinson et al. 1978b).

9.3.1 Pathologic Features

The gross appearance of mucinous cystic neoplasms varies. Most have a smooth external surface and are usually multilocular. The cysts are filled with thick mucoid material or hemorrhagic fluid. The inner surfaces of the cysts are smooth or trabeculated, but their walls may be thin and membranous, or thickened and composed of gray-white tissue (Fig. 9.8). The surface of the cysts may display large papillary projections within the cavities. Some neoplasms are unilocular, and others consist of a large cyst containing intramural gray-white, firm nodules. These mucinous cystic neoplasms have a dense, fibrous capsule that may have areas of dystrophic calcification or contain residual pancreatic tissue such as atrophic ducts or islets. Large connections between

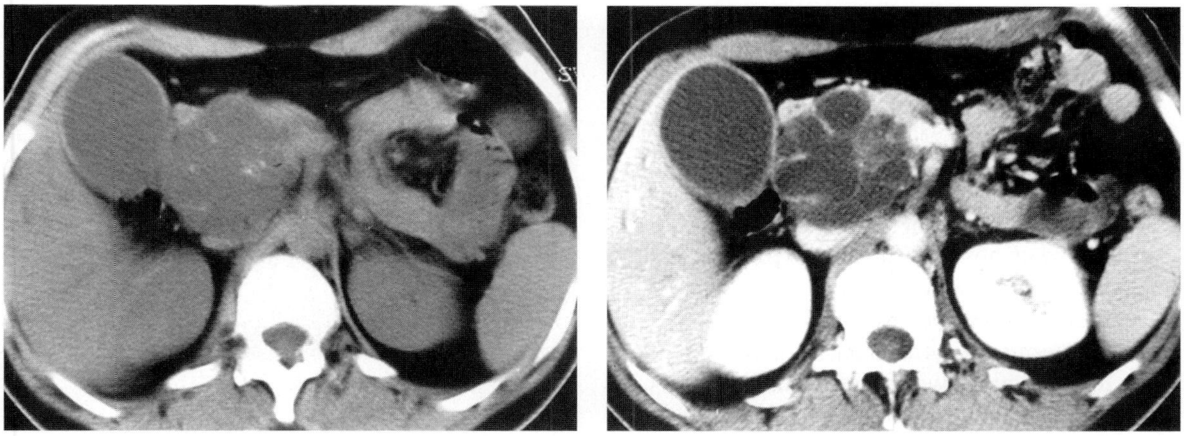

Fig. 9.7a,b. Macroscopic serous cystadenoma. Pre- (**a**) and post-contrast (**b**) computed tomography scans showing a multiloculated tumor containing large cysts

the tumor and the pancreatic duct may occur as fistulae. In the case of cephalic location, connection with the bile duct and/or the duodenum may be observed with massive excretion of mucin. In these rare circumstances, the distinction between intraductal mucin-hypersecreting tumors and mucinous neoplasms could be difficult and can be done only on the resected specimen.

Histologically, these tumors can be divided into three histologic variants: mucinous cystadenocarcinoma, the most common type, followed in frequency by mucinous cystic tumor, borderline type, and finally the rarest form of "benign" mucinous cystadenoma (LACK 1989; ALBORES-SAAVEDRA et al. 1987, 1990).

Typically, the cyst wall of all mucinous cyst tumors contains three distinct tissue layers: (a) an inner lining epithelium, (b) a middle zone of densely cellular primitive mesenchymal stroma resembling ovarian stroma, and (c) an outer layer of hyalinized connective tissue. However, in many cysts, these three layers are not clearly defined because the stroma is hypocellular or entirely fibrotic, or the hyalinized outer layer is absent.

In mucinous cystadenocarcinoma, the lining epithelium is quite variable, containing both benign-appearing, as well as malignant elements. The cysts are lined by a tall, mucin-producing columnar epithelium that shows intestinal differentiation as indicated by the presence of some goblet cells. The epithelial cells are positive for PAS and Alcian blue diastase-resistant. Occasional argentaffin and Paneth-like cells can be observed. The atypia of the cells lining the cysts varies considerably. Many tall columnar mucus-secreting cells and low cuboidal cells show little or no cytologic atypia, while others show nucleocytoplasmic abnormalities and pseudostratification with formation of papillary projections. Invasion of the stroma by neoplastic colonic-type glands is frequent, often inducing a desmoplastic reaction. Transitions between the different types of epithelial cells are seen in almost every tumor. Whether the benign-appearing epithelial cells behave as malignant cells remains an open question. The occasional presence of these benign-appearing cells in metastatic deposits suggests that they are truly malignant. Metastases in patients with adequately sampled mucinous cystadenomas and borderline tumors emphasize this point of view.

The borderline mucinous cystic tumors can have the same type of lining epithelial cells as cystadenocarcinomas, including their pseudostratification and cytologic atypia. However, the stromal infiltration lacks in borderline tumors. The primitive mesenchymal stroma often contains benign-appearing glands that should not be regarded as stromal infiltration. Some of these glands are pseudopyloric while others are colonic-like or appear to be lined by gastric-type superficial epithelium.

Mucinous cystadenomas differ from the borderline mucinous cystic tumors in that they lack epithelial pseudostratification and cytologic atypia. However, they share the characteristic mesenchymal stroma.

The epithelial cells of mucinous cystic tumors are positive for epithelial membrane antigen and low molecular weight keratin (MATHIEU et al. 1989; FRIEDMAN and EDMONDS 1989; LACK 1989; ALBORES-SAAVEDRA et al. 1990). CEA reactivity has been demonstrated in these tumors by immunohistochemical methods, although the intensity of the reaction varies from case to case and in different areas of the same tumor. Likewise, the cytoplasmic reaction appears to be more diffuse and stronger in cystadenocarcinomas than in cystadenomas. CEA positivity is also observed in the cystic fluid and in gland secretions. In a few cases, a high CEA concentration in cysts has been documented. This finding may be significant in the preoperative diagnosis of these lesions. However, the cellular localization of CEA by immunohistochemical studies does not allow distinctions between mucinous cystic tumors and the common ductal carcinomas, because most of the latter tumors are also CEA-positive. With immunohistochemical studies, different authors have demonstrated the tumor-associated antigen carbohydrate antigen 19–9 (CA 19–9) in the majority of pancreatic mucinous cystic neoplasms. A cytoplasmic reaction has been obtained in all types of mucinous tumors, although the reaction was stronger and more diffuse in cystadenocarcinomas than in cystadenomas. Recently, Albores-Saavedra et al. (1987) demonstrated that approximately 70% of mucinous cystic tumors of the pancreas express serotonin and, less frequently, a variety of peptide hormones such as somatostatin, pancreatic polypeptide, gastrin, and vasoactive intestinal peptide. The secretions of these peptide hormones probably explains some of the endocrine syndromes observed in association with these tumors, such as Zollinger-Ellison syndrome and the watery diarrhea hypokalemia syndrome. Although serotonin is the most common neuroendocrine marker in these mucinous tumors, carcinoid syndrome has never been reported in patients with these neoplasms.

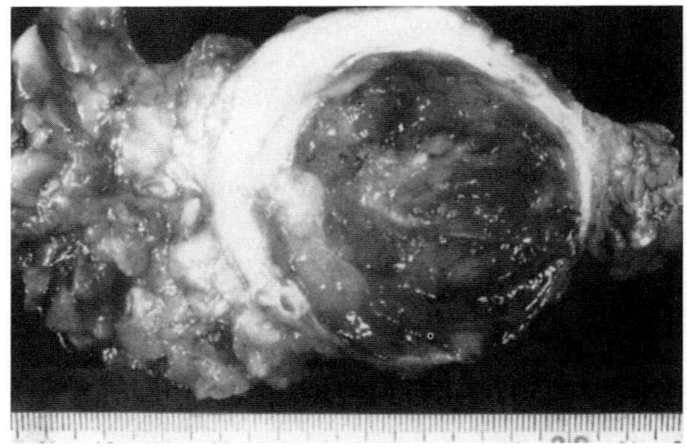

Fig. 9.8. Mucinous cystadenoma. Cross section of gross specimen showing a large cyst surrounded by a thick and irregular capsule

9.3.2 Imaging Procedures

Plain radiographs may, in 16% of cases, show the presence of calcifications, which are developed in the periphery of the tumor or in the wall of the cysts, arranged in amorphous clumps (Friedman et al. 1983). Since mucinous cystic neoplasms are quite large, gastrointestinal barium series can show extrinsic displacement. At sonography, mucinous cystic tumors are unilocular or more often multilocular cystic masses with strong posterior enhancement (Fig. 9.9) (Mathieu et al. 1989; Algard et al. 1986; Freeny et al. 1978; Wolson and Walls 1976; Caroll and Sample 1978; Padovani et al. 1991; Fugazzola et al. 1991; Johnson et al. 1988). The most important findings are the demonstration of internal septa separating the different cystic cavities and the possible visualization of nodular or papillary excrescences with irregular borders (Araki et al. 1982; Bastid et al. 1989). These internal septations and the irregularities of the cyst walls seem better demonstrated on sonography than on CT.

In a review of 45 pathologically proven pancreatic cystic neoplasms including 17 mucinous cystadenomas, 12 mucinous cystadenocarcinomas, and 16 microcystic adenomas, Johnson et al. (1988) considered the number and size of the cysts present in the different lesions. When the diameter of the cysts was greater than 2 cm and the number of cysts was six or fewer, mucinous tumors were correctly classified on sonography in 93% and on CT in 95%. CT demonstrates a round to oval, well-encapsulated lesion with a smooth external surface and a hypodense content (Figs. 9.10–9.11) (Mathieu et al. 1989;

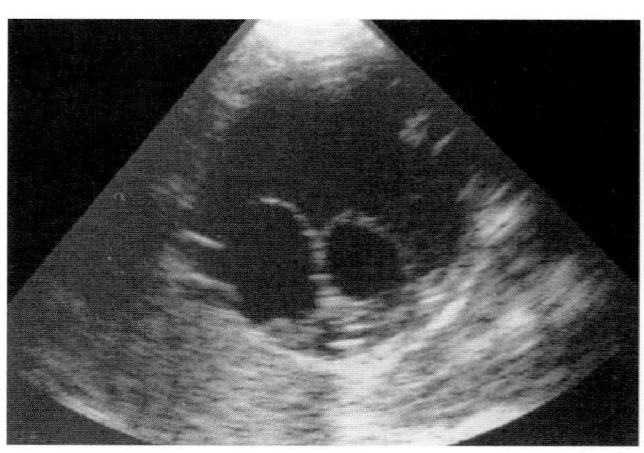

Fig. 9.9. Mucinous cystadenoma. Longitudinal sonogram of the left upper quadrant showing a large cystic lesion with septations

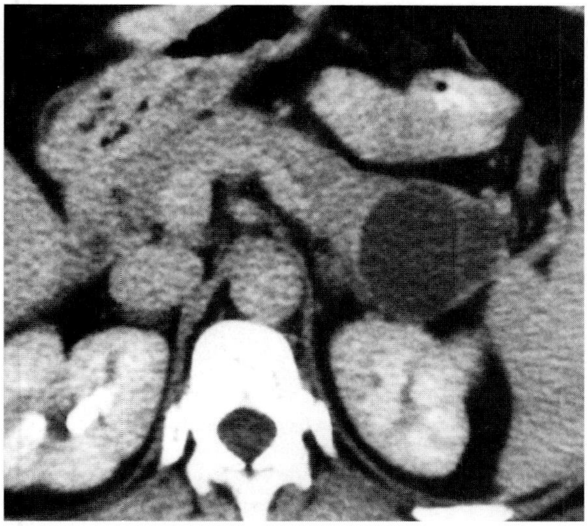

Fig. 9.10. Mucinous cystadenoma. Enhanced computed tomography scan. The lesion is hypodense and is surrounded by a thick vascularized capsule

ITAI et al. 1982; ALGARD et al. 1986; DE SANTOS et al. 1978; PARIENTY et al. 1980; KOLMANNSKOG et al. 1982; WOLFMAN et al. 1982; PADOVANI et al. 1991; FUGAZZOLA et al. 1991; JOHNSON et al. 1988; ARAKI et al. 1982). The mucinous tumors consist of one large cyst often associated with daughter cysts along its internal surface. Post-contrast CT demonstrates more clearly the enhancement of the cystic wall, the presence of thin, straight, or curvilinear septa, and is interesting for depicting a nodular thickening of the cystic wall (Fig. 9.11b). However, these septa and the eventual thickening of the cystic wall are well depicted on endosonography (Fig. 9.12). MRI seems to demonstrate clearly the septa and their thickness in all mucinous tumors, as well as the multilocularity of these lesions (MINAMI et al. 1989). Cystic compartments vary on T1- and/or T2-weighted images. The signal intensity is either low or high relative to the liver on T1-weighted images and slightly high relative to the adipose tissue on T2-weighted images. In the different reports, MRI is equal or slightly superior to CT in the diagnosis of these mucinous tumors, except in its limited ability to demonstrate calcifications of the tumor wall and septa. Based on a review of the literature and pathology reports, sonography, CT, angiography, and MRI are unable to differentiate mucinous cystadenoma from cystadenocarcinoma, except when invasion of adjacent organs or metastatic disease is present (Figs. 9.13–9.16). On angiography, mucinous cystadenomas are slightly hypervascular, and the majority demonstrate areas of lucency which correlate with the cystic component of the tumor mass. Arterial dilatation and neovascularity with faint blush are occasionally observed within the cyst wall or solid excrescences.

Only a few endoscopic retrograde pancreatography examinations have been reported in patients with mucinous cystic tumors (CROSS 1980). They may show displacement or encasement of the pancreatic duct or, more rarely, invasion of the duct with intraluminal defects or filling of the cystic cavity from the pancreatic duct.

Aspiration cytology of the pancreas is safe, accurate, and reliable, both intraoperatively and under imaging procedures (FOND et al. 1984). Most reports of pancreatic cytology have dealt with the distinction of classic ductal adenocarcinoma from benign or hyperplastic lesions. Some recent reports have emphasized the value of fine needle aspiration with appropriate stains in the diagnosis of mucinous cys-

a 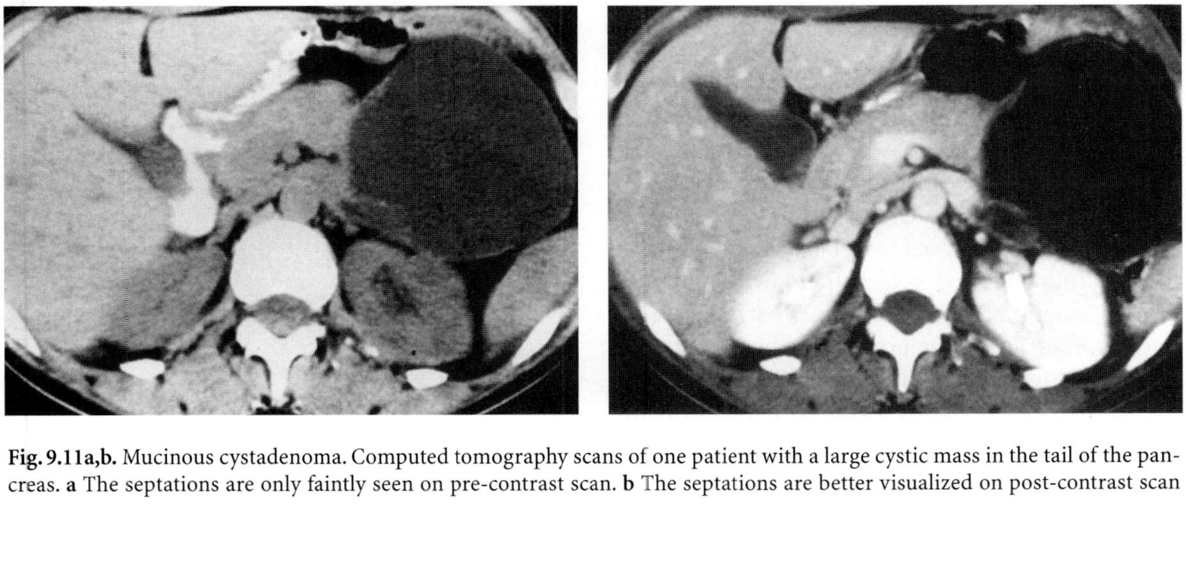 b

Fig. 9.11a,b. Mucinous cystadenoma. Computed tomography scans of one patient with a large cystic mass in the tail of the pancreas. **a** The septations are only faintly seen on pre-contrast scan. **b** The septations are better visualized on post-contrast scan

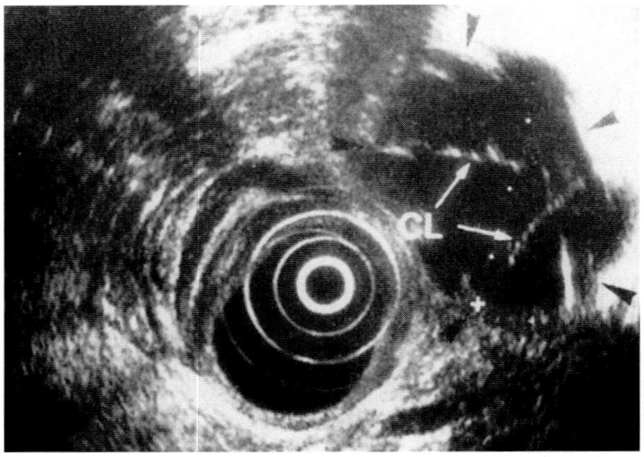

Fig. 9.12. Mucinous cystadenoma. Endosonography showing a large anechoic cyst containing internal septations

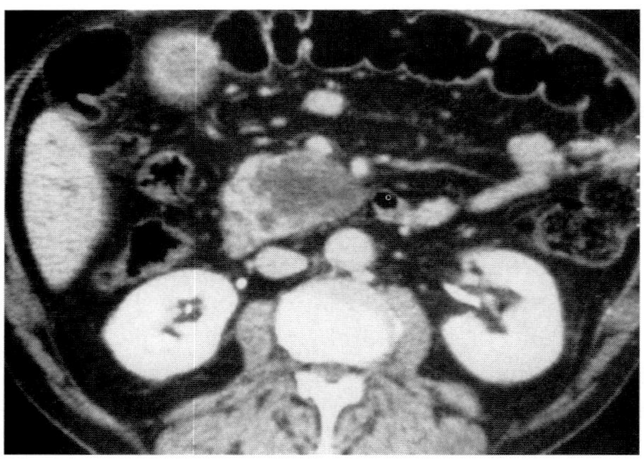

Fig. 9.13. Cystadenocarcinoma. Enhanced computed tomography scan showing an ill-defined and irregular lesion of the head of the pancreas

tadenocarcinoma (Emmert and Bewtra 1986; Vellet et al. 1988). The most important diagnostic criterion appears to be the presence of abundant mucin, appreciated both macroscopically, as the slides are spread, and microscopically, where it appears intracellularly and in the background (Emmert and Bewtra 1986; Vellet et al. 1988). Although it is enhanced by Giemsa staining, mucin can be recognized with Papanicolaou's stains, both by its color and consistency and by its parallel fibrillary structure. The necrotic background material in cavitating tumors of other types is more granular and flocculent in appearance. In two cases recently published, the cytologic presence of benign-appearing cell fragments in addition to malignant cells was described. The definitive diagnosis of adenocarcinoma rests, as always, on such nuclear signs as crowding, pleomorphism, and chromatin abnormalities.

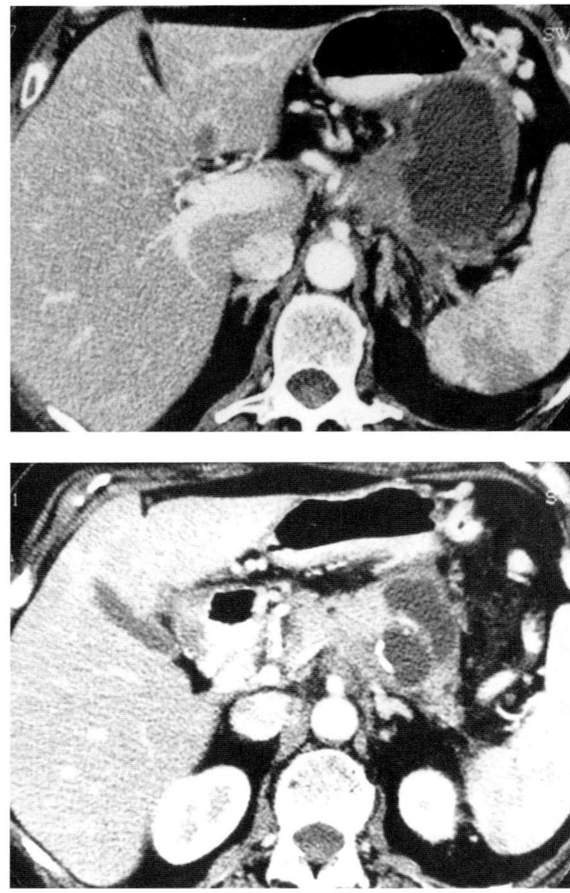

a

b

Fig. 9.14a,b. Cystadenocarcinoma (same patient). **a** Enhanced computed tomography (CT) scan showing an irregular hypodense lesion. **b** Enhanced CT scan obtained more caudally than (**a**). Note the encasement of the splenic and portal veins

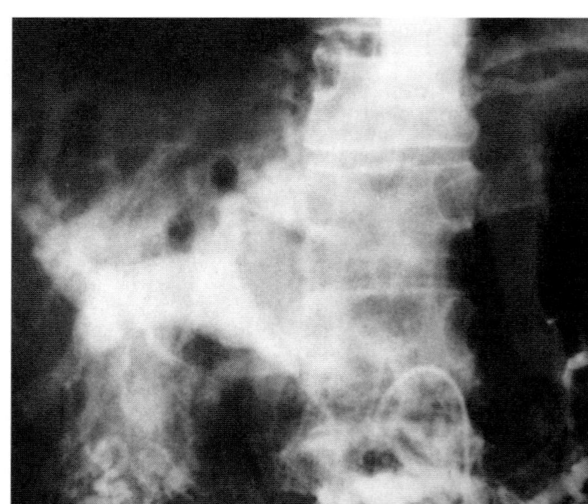

Fig. 9.15. Cystadenocarcinoma. Angiography demonstrating vascular invasion of the portal vein

However, the presence of regular cell aggregates with well-spaced nuclei in favor of benign mucinous cystadenoma does not exclude a malignant counterpart. As with histopathology, adequate sampling is essential. Different authors have also emphasized the value of the measurements of the CA 19–9 level in the aspirated cystic fluid of mucinous cystadenocarcinoma in comparison with benign lesions (NISHIDA et al. 1989).

9.4 Papillary Cystic Neoplasm

Recently, papillary cystic neoplasm (PCN) has been attracting attention as a new tumor (BALTHAZAR et al. 1984; BOOR and SWANSON 1979; CHOI et al. 1988; COMPAGNO et al. 1979; FARMAN et al. 1987; FRIEDMAN et al. 1985; MIETTINEN et al. 1987; SANFEY et al. 1983; SCHLOSNAGEL and CAMPBELL 1981; RUSTIN et al. 1986; MATSUNOU et al. 1990; MATSUNOU and KONISHI 1990; CAPPELLARI et al. 1990; STÖMMER et al. 1991; SCLAFANI et al. 1991; CUBILLA and FITZGERALD 1979; MOROHOSHI et al. 1983; LIEBER et al. 1987; BONDESON et al. 1984; LACK et al. 1983; BENJAMIN and WRIGHT 1980; WARREN 1985; MATSUDA et al. 1987; LEARMONTH et al. 1985; FOOTE et al. 1986; KATZ and EHYA 1990). From its gross and histologic features, PCN also has been described as papillary tumor, papillary epithelial neoplasm, solid and papillary neoplasm, papillary-cystic carcinoma, and papillary-cystic tumor. PCN is a rare tumor described essentially in young women (SCLAFANI et al. 1991; CUBILLA and FITZGERALD 1991; MOROHOSHI et al. 1983). Its incidence is extremely low: In a review of pathologic tissue from 747 patients with cancer of the pancreas seen between 1949 and 1972, only one case was found (CUBILLA and FITZGERALD 1979). Similarly, in a review from Hamburg based on histopathologic examination of 264 exocrine pancreatic tumors, only seven cases (2.7%) were found (MOROHOSHI et al. 1983). In a more recent series from 1984 to 1988, SCLAFANI et al. (1991) observed only two cases in 676 patients admitted for pancreatic malignancies. To study the natural history and malignant potential of this tumor, a review of the English literature was conducted by these authors on 58 well-documented cases reported between 1979 and 1991 (SCLAFANI et al. 1991). The age ranged from 11 to 47 years of age with 84% of patients younger than 35 years of age and 59% younger than 25 years of age. In a recent paper, MATSUNOU and KONISHI reported a case in an 8-year-old girl (MATSUNOU and KONISHI 1990). Only three men having this tumor were previously documented (MATSUNOU et al. 1990; SCAFANI et al. 1991).

The distribution in the pancreas included the head (38%), the body and/or tail (58%), and one tumor involved the entire pancreas (SANFEY et al. 1983). An abdominal mass was present in 65% of the cases and abdominal pain in 53%. In about 20% of PCNs, the lesion was an incidental finding at laparotomy or on radiographic studies (CUBILLA and FITZGERALD 1979). Hemoperitoneum was observed in only two cases (CUBILLA and FITZGERALD 1979). The average size of the tumor was 10 cm in diameter (range, 2.5–20 cm). Despite this large size, only two of 19 patients with tumors of the head of the pancreas, 20 cm and 5 cm, respectively, were jaundiced. The course of this tumor was usually indolent, with a favorable prognosis when total resection was performed.

Recurrence has only been documented in six cases. Liver metastases were reported in six cases. Five patients, aged between 18 and 42 years, underwent resection of metastases and were free of disease for between 15 months and 6 years (RUSTIN et al. 1986; CAPPELLARI et al. 1990; STÖMMER et al. 1991; WARREN 1985; MATSUDA et al. 1987). One 20-year-old woman with extensive bilobar metastases received tamoxifen because estrogen receptors were found in the tumors (SCLAFANI et al. 1991). This patient was asymptomatic 22 months later.

Operative and pathologic findings included invasion of the stomach, duodenum, or major blood vessels in nine of 58 patients (58%), and in six of nine patients the entire tumor was resected.

9.4.1 *Pathologic Features*

PCN is always surrounded by a fibrous capsule and shows extrapancreatic growth from the pancreas. The cross section is characterized by a mixture of solid and cystic portions, with frequent pseudocyst formations (Fig. 9.17). A lobulated, light brown tissue is mostly located at the periphery, whereas a zone of degeneration with hemorrhage and cystic spaces filled with necrotic debris is observed in the center of the tumor. These tumors are generally well-demarcated from the adjacent pancreatic tissue. Calcifications have been noticed occasionally in the periphery of this capsule.

Histologically, this hemorrhagic and necrotic lesion is surrounded by solid and pseudopapillary structures somewhat resembling an endocrine

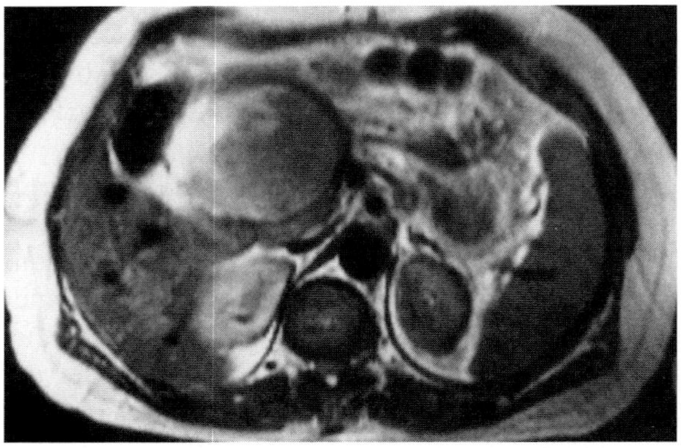

Fig. 9.16. Cystadenocarcinoma. Axial T1-weighted magnetic resonance image: the lesion is heterogeneous

tumor. The uniform cells containing round to ovoid nuclei have either a faint eosinophilic or a clear vacuolar cytoplasm. The cytoplasm of the clear cells occasionally contains tiny PAS-positive droplets. Larger, intercellular PAS-positive globules are also found. Mitoses are rare. The pseudopapillary structures have fibrovascular stalks, forming pseudoglandular patterns in some parts. In the margins of solid areas, aggregates of foamy cells, cholesterol granulomas, and fissure-like foci of hemorrhage are intermingled and show transition to the macroscopic cystic areas. These tumors are separated from the normal pancreas by a layer of connective tissue and may contain calcifications. The tumor cells occasionally show intracapsular invasion, but extracapsular growth within the pancreas is rarely observed. The prediction of metastasis or recurrence appears to be impossible from histologic evaluation of the primary tumor (Farman et al. 1987).

However, recently, Matsunou et al. (1990) observed four patients aged 39–51 years with tumors showing histologic features identical to PCN, but with clearly different growth patterns, suggesting a possible malignancy: lack of the capsule, infiltration into the pancreatic parenchyma, central fibrosis accompanied by dystrophic changes such as calcification and ossification, and presence of pleomorphic cells in some parts of the tumors. These tumors were designated as a solid, infiltrating variety of PCNs to differentiate them from common encapsulated PCNs.

Immunohistochemical studies have shown a constant positive staining for α_1-antitrypsin, characterized by a patchy distribution in the tumor tissue, but occasionally also for pancreatic enzymes such as amylase and lipase (Lack 1989; Miettinen et al. 1987; Matsunou et al. 1990; Matsunou and Konishi 1990; Stömmer et al. 1991; Lieber et al. 1987). These results indicate the undeniable presence of acinar components in PCN (Learmonth et al. 1985). α_1-Antitrypsin is considered to be an index of acinar cell differentiation, but its occurrence is not restricted to this tumor type. A positive reaction to α_1-antitrypsin has been reported in all acinar cell carcinomas and pancreatoblastomas, but also in other tumors. In PCN, a negative reaction was always demonstrated with antisera against CEA and CA 19-9. Occasionally, some of these tumors have revealed distinct positivity for the neuroendocrine cell marker neuron-specific enolase. In this last situation, PCN is indistinguishable pathologically from cystic nonfunctioning islet cell tumor.

In typical cases, electron microscopy reveals many „pale" cells (Lack 1989; Miettinen et al. 1987; Stömmer et al. 1991; Bondeson et al. 1984). Their cytoplasm displays abundant mitochondria, but is otherwise devoid of organelles. Ultrastructurally, well-developed Golgi apparatus and rough endoplasmic reticulum, and zymogen granules in the tumor cells of PCN show acinar cell differentiation. However, features of ductal cell differentiation have also been reported (Compagno et al. 1979). Moreover, the simultaneous presence of both duct cell differentiation and endocrine cells characteristics shown by neurosecretory granules has been noticed in some patients.

Due to the discrepancies of these results, various authors currently consider that PCN shows polymorphic differentiation and support the hypothesis of pancreatic primordial cell origin.

9.4.2
Imaging Procedures

There are several reports of the sonographic and CT findings in PCN (Mathieu et al. 1989; Friedman and Edmonds 1989; Balthazar et al. 1984; Farman et al. 1987; Friedman et al. 1985). All tumors demonstrate sharply defined, inhomogeneous, large pancreatic masses. The internal architecture of the lesion varies from solid to mixed solid and cystic to a thick-walled cyst, depending on the degree of hemorrhagic necrosis. Sonography depicts a well-demarcated echogenic mass with hypoechoic areas of varying number and size depending on the degree of hemorrhage and necrosis (Fig. 9.18a). CT shows a well-circumscribed muscle density mass containing low-density areas of variable size corresponding to hemorrhage and necrosis with an enhanced capsule (Fig. 9.18, 9.19). In cases of abundant hemorrhage, both modalities detect a thick-walled "cyst" with a

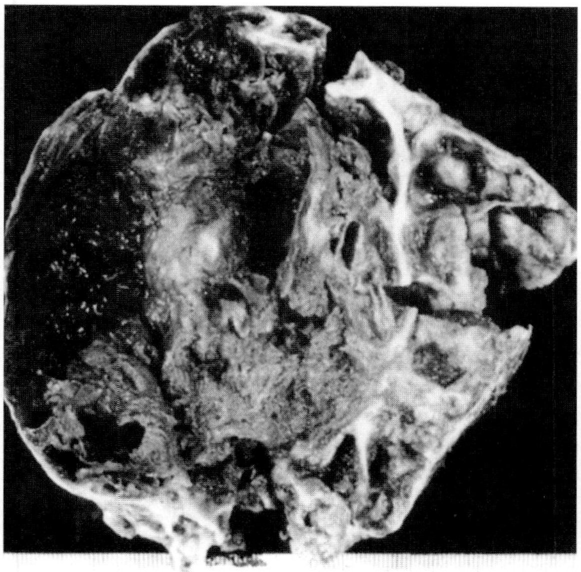

Fig. 9.17. Papillary cystic neoplasm. Cross section of gross specimen demonstrating a thick capsule and cystic components

ragged inner margin. The CT numbers in the "cysts" may be higher than water, correctly suggesting old blood and necrotic debris. Calcifications, either in the capsule or in the inner portion of the mass, have been noted in some reports. MRI may be helpful in demonstrating the presence of hemorrhage on T1-weighted images. Angiography generally shows a mildly vascular mass on celiac injection and a moderately vascular mass on supraselective injection.

As suggested by CHOI and coworkers (1988), PCN of the pancreas should be the primary diagnostic consideration when characteristic CT findings are detected in a young female patient. Guided percutaneous biopsy may be useful in selected cases (BONDESON et al. 1984; FOOTE et al. 1986; KATZ and EHYA 1990); however, most patients undergo surgery regardless of the results of needle biopsy.

9.5 Intraductal Pancreatic Tumors

These tumors have a relatively favorable prognosis and should be considered as low-grade malignancies (CUBILLA and FITZGERALD 1984; KLÖPPEL 1984; KLÖPPEL and MAILLET 1989; CUBILLA and FITZGERALD 1975; FRIEDMAN and EDMONDS 1989).

These pancreatic intraductal neoplasms are described in the literature under different terms (e.g., intraductal papilloma, adenoma, papillary adenoma, villous adenoma, adenomatosis, diffuse villous carcinoma, intraductal papillary adenocarcinoma, carcinoma in situ of the pancreas, and multiple primitive endoluminal tumors of the main pancreatic duct) (CONLEY et al. 1987; HALPHEN et al. 1988;

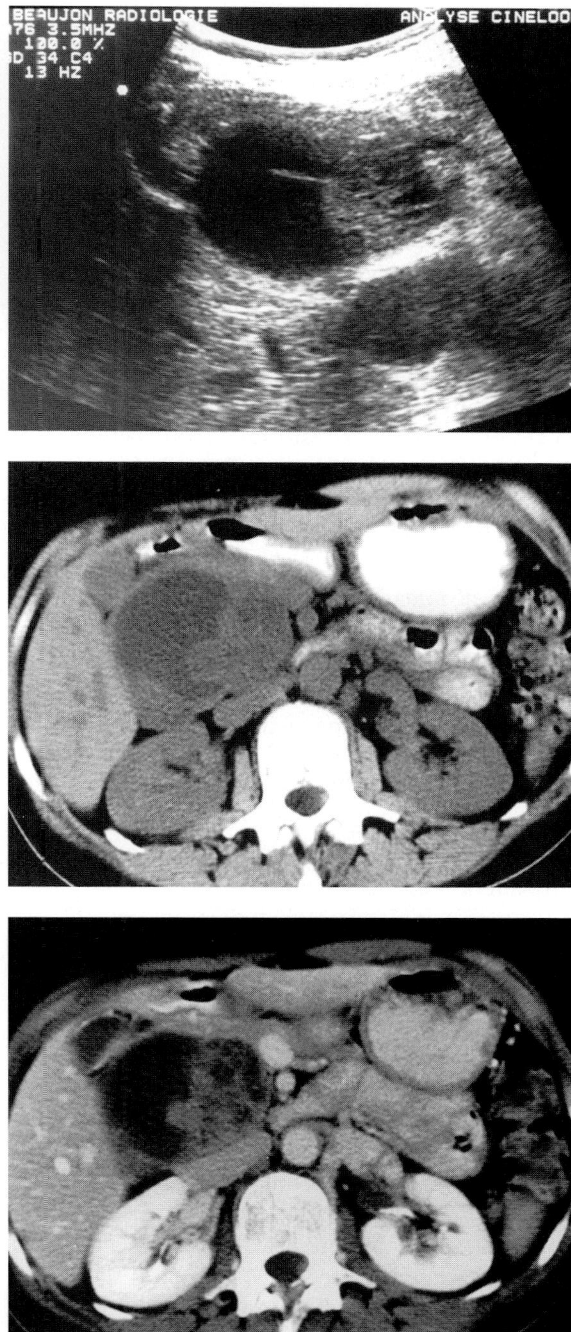

a b c

Fig. 9.18a–c. Papillary cystic neoplasm. **a** Transverse sonogram showing a solid and cystic mass of the head of the pancreas. **b,c** Computed tomography shows a heterogeneous lesion. No enhancement is noted within the cystic component

Caroli et al. 1975; Payan et al. 1990; Rogers et al. 1987; Warshaw et al. 1987; Ponsot et al. 1989; Place et al. 1985; Smith et al. 1986; Itai et al. 1987). Furthermore, intraductal mucin-hypersecreting tumors of the pancreatic ducts have recently received increasing attention (Morohoshi et al. 1989; Rickaert et al. 1991; Yamada et al. 1991). Therefore, it remains an open question whether these tumors can be considered as one entity or whether they belong to different categories. Another unsolved question is whether the group of pancreatic tumors recently described by Itai et al. as duct ectatic mucinous cystadenoma and cystadenocarcinoma, represents a separate entity or is merely a variant of these intraductal tumors (Itai et al. 1986; Agostini et al. 1989; Beaurain et al. 1991).

According to the different pathologic entities, we have separated this chapter into three different sections, i.e., intraductal papillary neoplasms, intraductal mucin-hypersecreting tumors of the pancreatic ducts, and duct ectatic mucinous cystadenoma and cystadenocarcinoma. Despite the actual confusing terminology observed in the pathologic literature, all these lesions can be considered histologically as papillary growths of ductal epithelium with various amounts of mucin production (Ponsot et al. 1989; Morohoshi et al. 1989; Rickaert et al. 1991; Yamada et al. 1991). Moreover, the radiologic appearances of all these lesions are quite similar: cystic dilatation and mucin production with or without visible tumoral lesion.

9.5.1 Intraductal Papillary Neoplasms

Some of these lesions are small nodules of hyperplastic ducts, rarely exceeding 1 mm in diameter. They may be termed ductal adenoma. However, they most likely represent reactive proliferations of ducts rather than true neoplasias, since they are most commonly observed in association with obstructive processes in the pancreas. These lesions are frequently found in association with pancreatic carcinomas obstructing the main pancreatic duct (Sommers et al. 1954; Klöppel et al. 1980). The aggregates of ducts are lined by a hypertrophic columnar epithelium sometimes forming papillary infoldings.

Papillary adenoma or papilloma of the pancreatic duct is an uncommon lesion (Conley et al. 1987; Halphen et al. 1988; Caroli et al. 1975; Payan et al. 1990; Rogers et al. 1987; Warshaw et al. 1987; Ponsot et al. 1989; Place et al. 1985; Morohoshi et al. 1989) which is developed in elderly patients (Klöppel 1984; Klöppel and Maillet 1989). The sex ratio is 1:1. Most patients have a long history of symptoms resembling those of chronic pancreatitis with pancreatic insufficiency. These pancreatitis-like episodes can be explained by temporary occlusions of the pancreatic ducts by viscous mucin plugs discharged by these tumors. The gross appearance of the pancreas is thickened and nodular, but no well-defined tumor is palpable. Cut sections demonstrate these tumors as soft intraductal masses within a dilated pancreatic duct, occurring predominantly in the head of the pancreas. In some cases, a multifocal tumor growth is observed with a diffuse spread over the pancreatic duct system (Halphen et al. 1988; Payan et al. 1990; Place et al. 1985).

The histologic structure of these tumors is characterized by a hyperplastic epithelium of the pancreatic ducts, with intraductal proliferation of tall, mucin-producing, columnar epithelium cells forming papillary, villous, and cribriform patterns (Ponsot et al. 1989; Morohoshi et al. 1989). Mitoses are rare. Foci of pronounced to severe cellular atypia are frequently observed (Halphen et al. 1988; Payan et al. 1990; Ponsot et al. 1989; Place et al. 1985). These findings are indistinguishable from lesions seen in the vicinity of well-differentiated invasive ductal carcinoma (Sommers et al. 1954; Klöppel et al. 1980). Then, the question remains open whether or not these carcinomatous areas in intraductal papillary neoplasms represent an early stage of invasive adenocarcinoma. The majority of tumor cells produce mucus staining positive with PAS and Alcian blue. The tumor cells are negative for CEA and CA 19–9, except in the areas marked by pronounced or severe atypia (Morohoshi et al. 1989).

9.5.2 Intraductal Mucin-Hypersecreting Tumors of the Pancreatic Ducts

In recent years, intraductal mucin-hypersecreting tumors of the pancreas have received increasing attention (Ponsot et al. 1989; Itai et al. 1987; Rickaert et al. 1991; Yamada et al. 1991). The various names given to these tumors, i.e., mucin-producing tumor, mucin-hypersecreting carcinoma, reflect their endoscopic, endosonographic, and radiologic findings.

An essential histologic characteristic of mucin-producing tumors is that a papillary growth of duct epithelium is present in the main pancreatic duct or in the small branch ducts of the gland. Mucus is produced mainly from this hyperplastic epithelium rather than from eventual cancerous epithelium. A large amount of mucin can then induce a passive dilatation of the main pancreatic duct and/or branch ducts. Subsequently, the major duodenal papilla was reported to have a specific appearance, that is, swollen with a wide open orifice and mucus excretion (RICKAERT et al. 1991). However, when the lesions are not developed in the main pancreatic duct close to the papilla, but in branch ducts, such tumors are not always accompanied by a specific appearance of the papilla or a remarkable dilatation of the main duct.

Grossly, the lesions present a large dilatation of the pancreatic ducts filled with sticky mucin. No distinctly elevated tumor is observed in these dilated ducts. These abnormalities can be confined to a localized or a distal pancreatic duct. The pancreatic tissue surrounding the cystic duct segments is usually sclerotic with fibrosis and atrophy on histology, but without tumoral involvement. There is no enlargement of the lymph nodes in the peripancreatic tissue. The histologic structure of these tumors is characterized by a hyperplastic epithelium of the pancreatic ducts, with intraductal proliferation of tall, mucin-producing, columnar epithelial cells forming papillary, villous, and cribriform patterns. These papillary projections contain a stromal stalk. Mitoses are rare. Foci of pronounced to severe cellular atypia are frequently observed. The majority of tumor cells produce mucus staining positive with PAS and Alcian blue. Immunocytochemically, the tumor cells can be positive for CEA and CA 19-9, particularly in the areas marked by pronounced or severe atypia (RICKAERT et al. 1991).

These intraductal mucin-producing tumors represent neoplasms with a low malignant potential. Absence of invasive tumor or metastasis, medical histories lasting for years, as well as the fact that the operated patients are alive up to many years after surgery without evidence of tumor recurrence clearly distinguishes these tumors from malignant lesions of the pancreas such as adenocarcinoma, mucinous cystadenoma, or cystadenocarcinoma (ITAI et al. 1987; RICKAERT et al. 1991). However, YAMADA et al. (1991) reported 12 malignant cases in a series of 22 mucin-producing tumors of the pancreas. In these malignant lesions, the tumors inside the ducts consisted of cancerous lesions over small areas with papillary or atypical hyperplasia. In some cases, a tumoral infiltration of the pancreatic parenchyma was observed invading the bile duct or duodenum. From histologic and histochemical studies, these authors consider that mucin-producing tumor and mucinous cystic neoplasm can be classified in the same conceptual category.

9.5.3 Duct Ectatic Mucinous Cystadenoma and Cystadenocarcinoma

Duct ectatic mucinous cystadenoma and cystadenocarcinoma can be classified hence into the group of intraductal mucin-hypersecreting neoplasms of the pancreas (ITAI et al. 1986; AGOSTINI et al. 1989; BEAURAIN et al. 1991). The first description of this disease was reported by ITAI and coworkers as a mass lesion that represents cystic dilatation of a side branch of the main pancreatic duct containing thick mucoid secretions (ITAI et al. 1986).

Macroscopically, the mass is covered by a thin rim of pancreatic parenchyma and consists of a conglomeration of communicating cysts, 1–2 cm in diameter, with thin fibrous capsules. Histologically, the findings consist of dilated ducts lined by papillary, hyperplastic epithelium with atypia. According to their clinical features and histologic appearances, they belong to the group of neoplasms that have been described as mucin-producing carcinomas, i.e., tumors with extreme, partly cystic dilatation of the duct system and mucin hypersecretion. There is no female predilection as observed in mucinous cystic neoplasms (BEAURAIN et al. 1991). Duct ectatic cystic lesions favor the uncinate process and head of the pancreas, whereas mucinous cystic neoplasms are usually in the tail. In the first description by ITAI et al., in all five cases, the lesions were located in the uncinate process (ITAI et al. 1986). However, AGOSTINI et al. (1989) reported a mucinous pancreatic duct ectasia in the body of the pancreas. Symptoms are nonspecific, and even the malignancies appear to be curable by pancreaticoduodenectomy if they are resectable at the time of diagnosis. In the 12 well-documented cases in the literature, occurring in seven females and five males (range, 30–76 years old, mean = 62 years), four presented foci of adenocarcinoma, three moderate to severe atypia, and five papillary and hyperplastic epithelium without atypia (BEAURAIN et al. 1991). The lesions were located in eight cases in the uncinate process, in three cases in the pancreatic head, and finally, in one case, diffusely in the body of the pancreas, this last case presenting a malignant transformation with signs of in situ carcinoma.

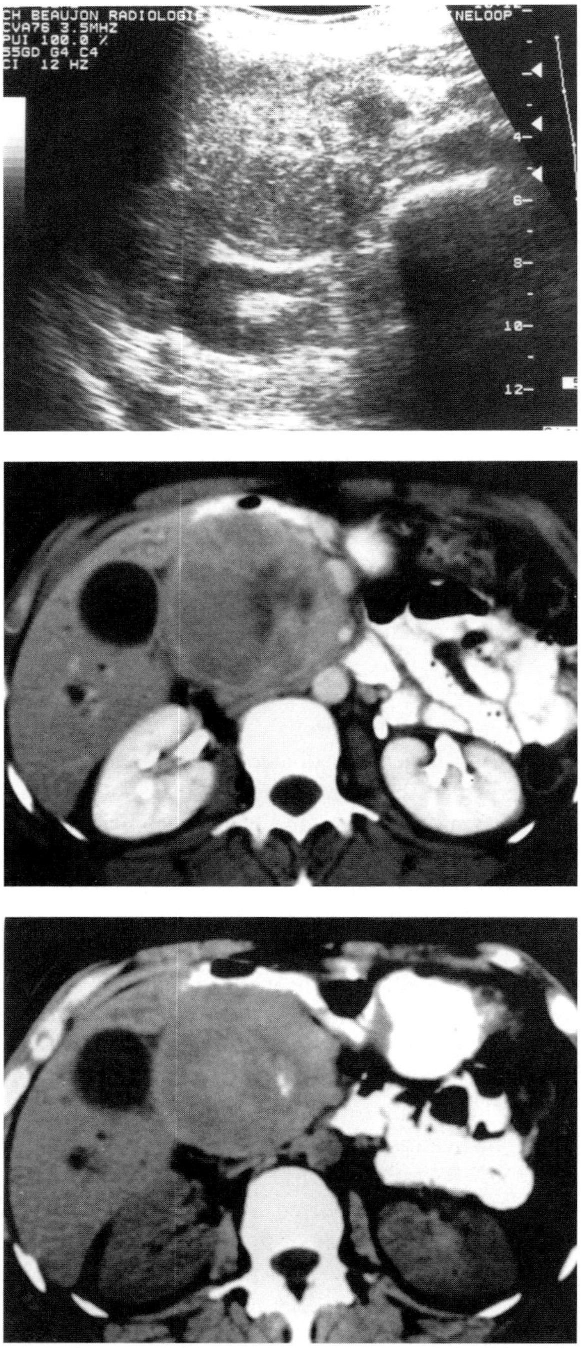

a

b

c

Fig. 9.19a–c. Papillary cystic neoplasm. **a** Transverse sonogram demonstrating a solid-appearance mass. **b,c** Pre- (**b**) and post-contrast (**c**) computed tomography scan in the same patient demonstrating a well-encapsulated heterogeneous lesion of the head of the pancreas with foci of hemorrhage

9.5.4 Imaging Procedures

The common features of papillary neoplasms are represented by the tumoral process itself and/or the consequences of mucoid plugs marked by cystic cavities and pancreatic duct dilatations. The lesions are located preferentially in the uncinate process as demonstrated by Itai et al. (1986). Sonography and CT show the small cystic lesions with round or lobulated margins. The tumor itself can be visualized at sonography or CT (Fig. 9.20). On CT scan, the tumor appears as a soft-density lesion. On post-contrast CT scan, there is an enhancement of the tumor nodule within the ducts. To our knowledge, only one case of mucinous ductal ectasia of the pancreas has be studied by MRI. MRI features demonstrate homogeneous signal intensities in each cyst. The separate cysts were clearly seen, especially on T2-weighted images. Dilatation of the main pancreatic duct was also depicted (Lee et al. 1992). Endosonography appears to be the method of choice for the evaluation of these lesions by demonstrating mucoid plugs, cystic dilatations, and tumor nodules. The exact location of these abnormalities can be determined precisely before surgery.

When the diagnosis remains uncertain, endoscopic retrograde pancreatography (ERP) is an excellent method for the diagnosis of this entity. Endoscopic observation can reveal an enlarged papilla with mucus flowing from a patulous orifice. ERP depicts the dilated main pancreatic duct or a localized and prominent cystic dilatation of a side branch of the main pancreatic duct, with grape-like clusters of pear-shaped pools of contrast material with amorphous or well-defined filling defects due to mucin or tumor mass(es) (Fig. 9.21). As suggested by Itai's group, when a cystic lesion is present in the uncinate process, ERP is mandatory to confirm or rule out a duct ectatic neoplasm (Itai et al. 1986). If ERP fails to confirm communication between the cyst and the duct, but demonstrates filling defects in the main pancreatic duct, percutaneous or operative pancreatography is recommended.

However, these cystic lesions can involve the whole parenchyma. In addition to the previous signs, all examinations demonstrate a diffusely dilated main pancreatic duct associated with dilatation of the side branch ducts filled as a result of mucin production (Fig. 9.22). The main limitation of imaging modalities is their inability to differentiate benign from malignant lesions. The sole method to affirm the benign or tumoral components of these lesions

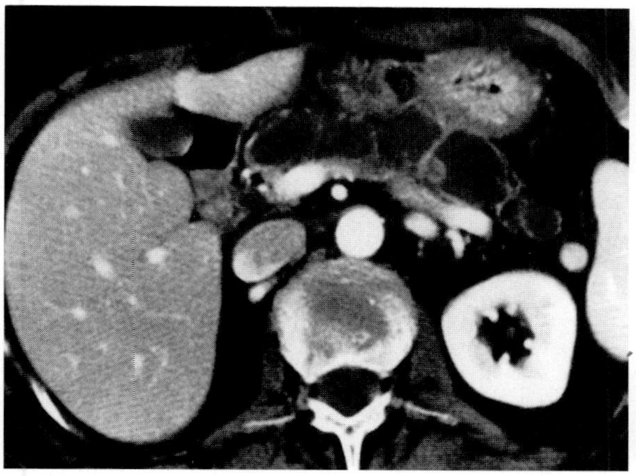

Fig. 9.20. Intraductal papillary-mucinous tumor. Enhanced computed tomography scan demonstrating marked dilatation of the main pancreatic duct with parenchymal atrophy. The nodules are intraductal malignant tumors

is represented by the entire histologic study of the resected specimen.

9.6 Other Cystic Neoplasms

Some other neoplasms have a cystic appearance.

9.6.1 Mucinous Carcinoma

This tumor is characterized by an extreme production of mucus (Cubilla and Fitzgerald 1975, 1984; Klöppel 1984; Klöppel and Maillet 1989). It is also termed colloid or gelatinous carcinoma. The location, sex distribution, and median age are similar to those of the common ductal adenocarcinoma. However, these lesions are usually large with a cystic appearance on cut sections due to the mucoid gelatinous material.

Histologically, there are large cystic spaces filled with mucin. These cystic areas are either lined by flattened mucin-producing cells or by simple connective tissue strands. In the mucus, there are frequently floating clusters of neoplastic cells. Pseudomyxoma peritonei from peritoneal metastases can occur during the evolution of the disease (Chefjec et al. 1986; Gustafson et al. 1984).

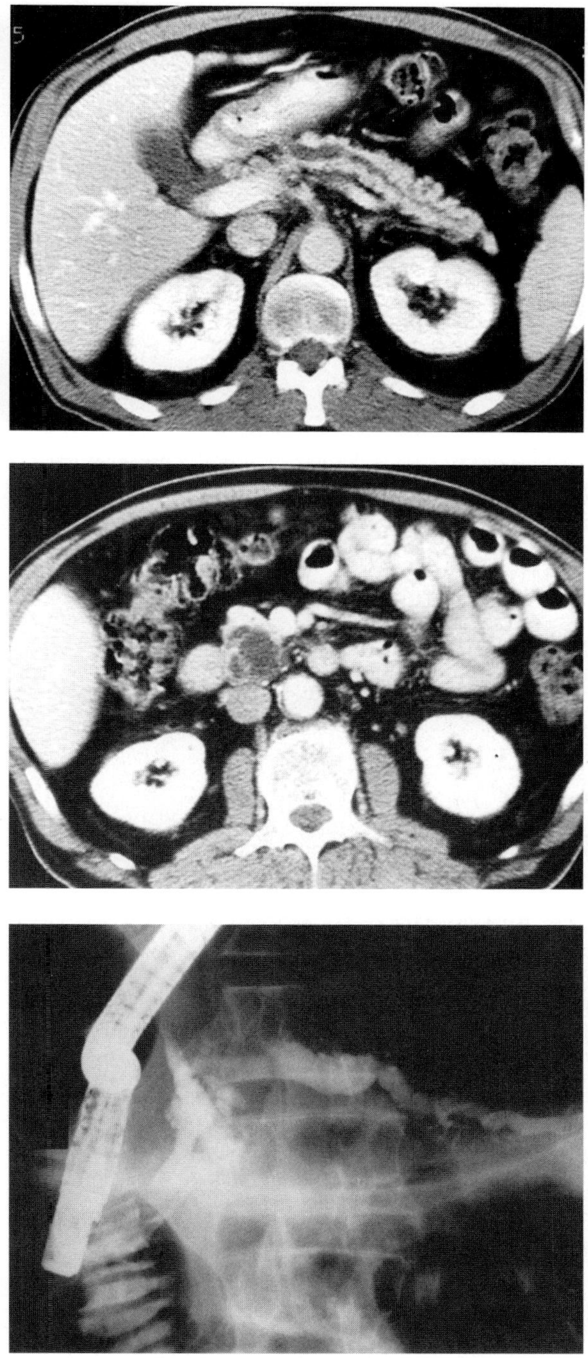

a b c

Fig. 9.21a–c. Intraductal papillary-mucinous tumor. **a,b** Post-contrast computed tomography showing moderate dilatation of the main pancreatic duct and dilatation of the branch duct of the head of the pancreas. **c** Endoscopic retrograde cholangiopancreatography demonstrating dilatation of the pancreatic ducts. Large filling defect in the main pancreatic duct due to mucoid secretion

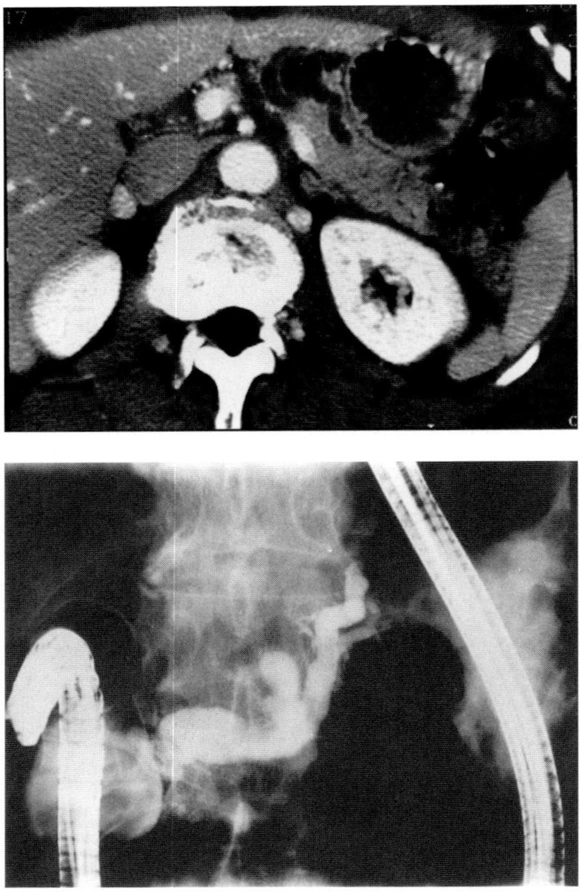

a

b

Fig. 9.22a–b. Intraductal papillary-mucinous tumor. **a** Enhanced computed tomography scan showing a moderately enlarged main pancreatic tumor and focal dilatation of branch ducts within the body of the pancreas. **b** Endoscopic retrograde cholangiopancreatography demonstrates the filling of dilated branch ducts

9.6.2 Sarcomas

This tumor is extremely unusual. Sarcomas of the mesenchymal supporting structures surrounding the pancreas can secondarily invade the pancreas itself (Neibling 1968). The specific histologic diagnosis and the determination of the exact site of origin is frequently difficult, even at the time of surgery or autopsy.

These rare tumors may be clinically silent and are often discovered only incidentally because of their large size, or may be symptomatic and produce findings that mimic carcinoma of the pancreas. When they are clinically silent, the patients are usually first examined late in the course of their disease. The tumors may be surgically resectable, but they are usually incurable. Following surgical resection, they may recur locally or with distant metastases, most frequently to the liver, lungs, lymph nodes, brain, skeleton, and peritoneum.

These tumors are usually huge with a well-defined mass and frequently have cystic components (Laverdiere et al. 1992).

9.6.3 Cystic Islet Cell Tumors

Islet cell tumors usually have a solid and hypervascular appearance. Cystic islet cell tumors are uncommon. However, some authors have reported an unusual case of cystic islet cell adenoma in which cyst aspiration was of value in confirming the diagnosis (Pogany et al. 1984). A recent case of low-density insulinoma was also described by Smith and Koenigsberg, presumably because it was less vascularized than was the surrounding normal pancreatic parenchyma (Smith and Koenigsberg 1990).

9.6.4 Pancreatic Metastases

The pancreas is a rare site of metastatic involvement. The majority of these patients also have metastases elsewhere in the body. The latter finding was confirmed in two recent series in the literature: Out of a total number of 16 patients with pancreatic metastases of various tumors, 14 patients had evidence of metastatic disease elsewhere in the body (Wernecke et al. 1986; Rumanick et al. 1984). Some tumors have a propensity to metastasize to the pancreas. These tumors are melanoma, carcinoma of the lung, ovary, breast, prostate, hepatocellular carcinoma, renal cell carcinoma, and a variety of sarcomas. These metastases may induce episodes of acute pancreatitis by pancreatic duct obstruction or may be discovered incidentally during routine evaluation or follow-up of the primary tumor. Pancreatitis can also occur owing to rapid lysis of pancreatic metastases during chemotherapy.

Pancreatic metastases may produce radiologic findings that are indistinguishable from those of primary pancreatic tumors. Some pancreatic metastases have a cystic appearance (Fig. 9.23). The primary tumor includes essentially carcinoma of the lung, ovary, and melanoma.

Percutaneous pancreatic biopsy may be helpful in the diagnosis.

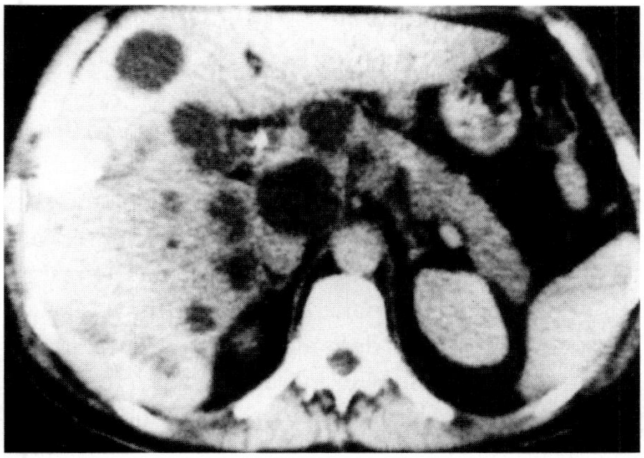

Fig. 9.23. Cystic pancreatic and hepatic metastases. Enhanced computed tomography scan demonstrating multiple cystic lesions. The primary tumor originates from the lung

9.6.5 Cystic Teratoma

This tumor is extremely rare, with only nine cases described in the literature (Assawamatiyanont and King 1977). The wall is well defined and inhomogeneous contents including hair, fat, and calcifications may be seen. Both US and CT scan demonstrate the cystic characteristics, as well as solid components and debris. CT and MRI may be helpful in demonstrating the presence of fat.

9.6.6 Pancreatic Lymphangioma

Lymphangioma of the pancreas has been rarely reported (Pandolfo et al. 1985). They are unilocular or multilocular and may contain serous or chylous fluid. They may be large and occasionally cause symptoms due to mass effect on adjacent structures. Calcifications occasionally occur in the dilated lymphatic spaces. The sonographic and CT characteristics of these lesions depends upon their vascularity and the presence of fat and fluid within the cystic spaces (Pandolfo et al. 1985; Salimi et al. 1991).

9.6.7 Cystic Schwannoma

Benign schwannomas are derived from the lining cells of the nerve sheath. Rarely, schwannomas can involve the abdomen. They often have a cystic appearance (Urban et al. 1992).

9.7 Other Cystic Lesions

9.7.1 True Cysts of the Pancreas

True cysts of the pancreas are derived from abnormal segmentation of the primitive ducts of the pancreas with resultant "sequestered" endoductal cells. These cells still have secretion of fluid, forming a cyst with a true epithelium lining the inner surface with no evidence of solid tissue component, internal septation, or tumor excrescences (Cubilla and Fitzgerald 1975, 1984; Klöppel 1984; Klöppel and Maillet 1989). This is an uncommon lesion and represents only 10%–15% of all pancreatic cysts. Most of these cysts are discovered in newborns. Their size varies from 1 to 13 cm. They may be uni- or multilocular. Congenital cysts are strictly avascular on angiogram. CT and ultrasonography findings include an anechoic mass with an attenuation coefficient of 0–20 HU, which demonstrates no contrast enhancement. These radiologic features allow the diagnosis of simple cyst (Mathieu et al. 1989).

9.7.2 Adult Polycystic Kidney Disease

Multiple true pancreatic cysts are seen in approximately 10% of patients with adult polycystic kidney disease (Cubilla and Fitzgerald 1975, 1984; Klöppel 1984; Klöppel and Maillet 1989). The cysts may be either diffuse or localized to one region of the pancreas. The number may vary from two to innumerable. Rarely, the pancreatic involvement may predominate over renal or hepatic involvement.

CT and sonographic findings are similar to those observed in single true cyst (Fig. 9.24) (Mathieu et al. 1989).

9.7.3 Von Hippel-Lindau Disease

Von Hippel-Lindau disease is an autosomally dominant disorder associated with neoplasms in many different organs. The major manifestations include retinal angiomatosis, hemangioblastoma of the central nervous system, renal cancer, and pheochromocytoma. Another frequent lesion observed in about 15% of patients is represented by the cystadenoma of the epididymis. Different cysts have also been described in this disease involving the pancreas and the kidney (NEUMANN et al. 1991). In some patients, serous cystadenomas have also been reported. Pancreatic islet-cell tumors, adenocarcinoma and hemangioblastoma have been occasionally observed in patients with this disease (NEUMANN et al. 1991).

The extent of the lesions varies from a few cysts to polycystic transformation of the enlarged organ (Fig. 9.25) (LEVINE et al. 1982). Several reports have mentioned pancreatic manifestations; however, few cases have been presented in detail. Most of these cystic pancreatic lesions were identified at autopsy, but a few were found intraoperatively. In general, cystic pancreatic lesions are asymptomatic or associated with only mild clinical symptoms (CHOYKE et al. 1990). Episodes of pancreatitis seem to be rare.

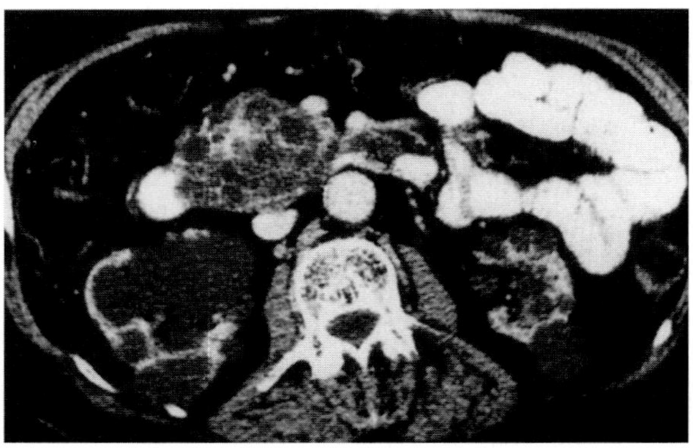

Fig. 9.24. Polycystic disease. Enhanced computed tomography scan demonstrating multiple pancreatic cysts associated with diffuse renal cysts

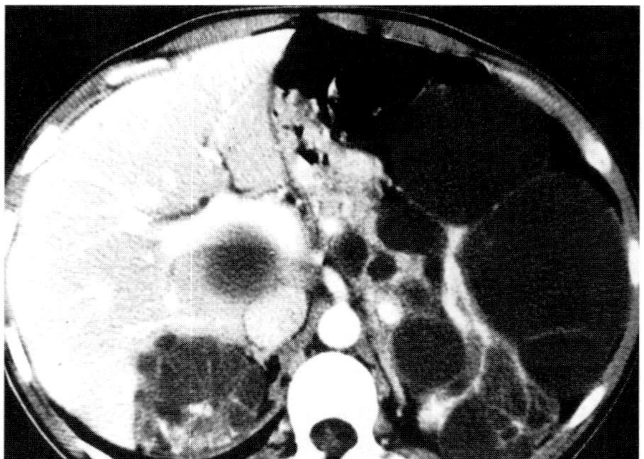

Fig. 9.25. Von Hippel-Lindau disease. Enhanced computed tomography scan showing multiple cysts within the pancreas, as well as complete replacement of the kidneys with cysts

9.7.4 Cystic Fibrosis

This disease is characterized by a progressive dilatation of the acini and pancreatic ducts, with secondary fibrosis leading to atrophy of the pancreatic parenchyma (HERNANZ-SCHULMAN et al. 1986). Fatty replacement and multiple true cysts that represent the remnants of the pancreatic ducts can be seen. These cysts can be demonstrated by both ultrasonography and CT. At sonography, the surrounding pancreatic parenchyma is hyperechoic due to fibrosis and fat replacement. On CT scan, the surrounding parenchyma is hypodense.

9.7.5 Primary Hydatid Disease of the Pancreas

Primary hydatid cyst of the pancreas is extremely rare; fewer than ten cases have been described in the literature (MISSAS et al. 1987). CT findings are nonspecific when the cysts appear well limited with a thin wall, but the diagnosis is suggested when curvilinear calcifications are present with a significant clinical history.

References

Agostini S, Choux R, Payan MJ, Sastre B, Sahel J, Clement JP (1989) Mucinous pancreatic duct ectasia in the body of the pancreas. Radiology 170:815–816

Albores-Saavedra J, Angeles-Angeles A, Nadji M et al (1987) Mucinous cystadenocarcinoma of the pancreas. Morphologic and immuno-cytochemical observations. Am J Surg Pathol 11:11–20

Albores-Saavedra J, Gould EW, Angeles-Angeles A, Henson DE (1990) Cystic tumors of the pancreas. Pathol Annu 26:19–50

Algard M, Ponsot P, Hautefeuille M et al (1986) Cystadénomes pancréatiques: intérêt diagnostique de l'échographie et de la tomodensitométrie. Gastroenterol Clin Biol 10:23–28

Alpert LC, Truong LD, Bossard MI et al (1988) Microcystic adenoma (serous cystadenoma) of the pancreas. A study of 14 cases with immunohistochemical and electron-microscopic correlation. Am J Surg Pathol 12:251–263

Araki T, Ohtomo K, Iai Y et al (1982) Demonstration of septa in cystic lesions. Comparative study by computed tomography and ultrasound. Clin Radiol 33:325–329

Assawamatiyanont S, King AD (1977) Dermoid cysts of the pancreas. Am J Surg 43:503–504

Balthazar EJ, Subramanyam BR, Lefleur RS et al (1984) Solid and papillary epithelial neoplasm of the pancreas. CT, sonographic and angiographic features. Radiology 150:39–40

Bastid C, Sahel J, Sastre B, Schurgers P, Sarles H (1989) Mucinous cystadenocarcinoma of the pancreas. Ultrasonographic findings in 5 cases. Acta Radiol 30:45–47

Beaurain P, Agostini S, Payan MJ et al (1991) Ectasies canalaires mucineuses du pancréas. Rev Im Med 3:639–644

Becker WF, Welch RA, Pratt HS (1965) Cystadenoma and cystadenocarcinoma of the pancreas. Ann Surg 161:845–860

Benjamin E, Wright DH (1980) Adenocarcinoma of the pancreas of childhood: a report of two cases. Histopathology 4:87–104

Bondeson L, Bondeson A-G, Genell S, Lindholm K, Thorstenson S (1984, Aspiration cytology of a rare solid and papillary epithelial neoplasm of the pancreas: light and electron microscopic study of a case. Acta Cytol 28:605–609

Boor PJ, Swanson MR (1979) Papillary cystic neoplasm of the pancreas. Am J Surg Pathol 3:69–75

Buck JL, Hayes WS (1990) From the archives of the AFIP. Microcystic adenoma of the pancreas. Radiographics 10:313–322

Cappellari JO, Geisinger KR, Albertson DA, Wolfman NT, Kute TE (1990) Malignant papillary cystic tumor of the pancreas. Cancer 66:193–198

Caroli J, Hadchouel P, Mercadier M, Lageron A (1975) Papillome bénin du canal de Wirsung: diagnostic par cathéterisme rétrograde. Med Chir Dig 4:163–166

Caroll B, Sample WF (1978) Pancreatic cystadenocarcinoma: CT body scan and gray scale ultrasound appearance. AJR 131:339–341

Chefjec G, Rieker WJ, Jablokow VR, Gould VE (1986) Pseudomyxoma peritonei associated with colloid carcinoma of the pancreas. Gastroenterology 90:202–205

Choi BI, Kim KW, Han MC et al (1988) solid and papillary epithelial neoplasms of the pancreas: CT fingings. Radiology 166:413–416

Choyke PL, Filling-Kaz MR, Shawker TH et al (1990) Von Hippel-Lindau disease: radiologic screening for visceral manifestations. Radiology 174:815–820

Compagno J, Oertel JE, Kremzar M (1979) Solid and papillary epithelial neoplasm of the pancreas, probably of small duct origin: a clinicopathologic study of 52 cases (ab). Lab Invest 40:248–249

Compagno J, Oertel JE (1978a) Microcystic adenomas of the pancreas (glycogen-rich cystadenomas). A clinico-pathologic study of 34 cases. Am J Clin Pathol 69:289–298

Compagno J, Oertel JE (1978b) Mucinous cystic neoplasms of the pancreas with overt and latent malignancy (cystadenocarcinoma and cystadenoma). Am J Clin Pathol 69:573–580

Conley CR, Scheithauer BW, Weiland LH, Van Heerden JA (1987) Diffuse intraductal papillary adenocarcinoma of the pancreas. Ann Surg 205:246–249

Cross MR (1980) Mucinous cystadenoma of the pancreas. Endoscopy as an aid to diagnosis. Gastroenterology 79:944–947

Cubilla AL, Fitzgerald PJ (1979) Cancer of the pancreas (nonendocrine): a suggested morphologic classification. Semin Oncol 6:285–297

Cubilla AL, Fitzgerald PJ (1984) Tumors of the exocrine pancreas. In: Atlas of tumor pathology, 2nd ser, fasc 19. Armed Forces Institute of Pathology, Washington DC

Cubilla AL, Fitzgerald PJ (1975) Morphological patterns of primary nonendocrine human pancreas carcinoma. Cancer Res 35:2234–2248

De Santos LA, Bernardino ME, Paulius DD, Martin RE (1978) Computed tomography of cystadenoma of the pancreas. J Comput Assist Tomogr 2:222–225

Didolkar MS, Malhotra Y, Holyoke ED et al (1975) Cystadenoma of the pancreas. Surg Gynecol Obstet 140:925–928

Emmert GM, Bewtra C (1986) Fine needle aspiration biopsy of mucinous cystic neoplasm: an unusual tumor. Diagn Cytopathol 2:69–71

Farman J, Chen CK, Schulze G et al (1987) Solid and papillary epithelial pancreatic neoplasm: an unusual tumor. Gastrointest Radiol 12:31–34

Ford A, Bret PM, Bretagnolle M et al (1984) Ultrasound and fine needle biopsy of cystic tumors of the pancreas. J Belg Radiol 67:277–284

Focte A, Simpson JS, Stewart RJ, St John-Wakefield J, Buchanan A, Gupta RK (1986) Diagnosis of the rare solid and papillary epithelial neoplasm of the pancreas by fine needle aspiration cytology. Light and electron microscopic study of a case. Acta Cytol 30:519–522

Freeny PC, Weinstein CJ, Taft DA et al (1978) Cystic neoplasms of the pancreas: new angiographic and ultrasonographic findings. AJR 131:795–802

Friedman AC, Edmonds PR (1989) Rare pancreatic malignancies. Radiol Clin North Am 27:177–190

Friedman AC, Lichtenstein JE, Dachman AH (1983) Cystic neoplasms of the pancreas. Radiological-Pathological correlation. Radiology 149:45–50

Friedman AC, Lichtenstein JE, Fishman EK et al (1985) Solid and papillary epithelial neoplasm of the pancreas. Radiology 154:333–337

Fugazzola C, Procacci C, Andreis IAB et al (1991) Cystic tumors of the pancreas: evaluation by ultrasonography and computed tomography. Gastrointest Radiol 16:53–61

George DH, Murphy F, Michalski R, Ulmer BG (1989) Serous cystadenocarcinoma of the pancreas: a new entity? Am J Surg Pathol 1:61–66

Gustafson KD, Karnaze GC, Hattery RR et al (1984) Pseudomyxoma peritonei associated with mucinous adenocarcinoma of the pancreas: CT findings and CT-guided biopsy. J Comput Assist Tomogr 8:335–338

Halphen M, Hoang C, Hautefeuille P et al (1988) Tumeurs intra-canalaires primitives multiples du canal de Wirsung. Démonstration d'une filiation entre tumeurs bénignes et malignes. Gastroenterol Clin Biol 12:163–168

Hernanz-Schulman M, Teele RL, Perez-Atayde A et al (1986) Pancreatic cystosis in cystic fibrosis. Radiology 158:629–631

Hodgkinson DJ, Remine WH, Weiland LH (1978a) Pancreatic cystadenoma. A clinicopathologic study of 45 cases. Arch Surg 113:512–519

Hodgkinson DJ, Remine WH, Weiland LH (1978b) A clinicopathologic study of 21 cases of pancreatic cystadenocarcinoma. Ann Surg 188:679–684

Itai Y, Moss AA, Ohtomo K (1982) Computed tomography of cystadenoma and cystadenocarcinoma of the pancreas. Radiology 145:419–425

Itai Y, Ohhashi K, Nagai H, Murakami Y, Kokubo T, Makita K, Ohtomo K (1986) "Ductectatic" mucinous cystadenoma and cystadenocarcinoma of the pancreas. Radiology 161:697–700

Itai Y, Kokubo T, Atomi Y, Kuroda A, Haraguchi Y, Terano A (1987) Mucin hypersecreting carcinoma of the pancreas. Radiology 165:51–55

Itai Y, Ohhashi K, Furui S, et al (1988) Microcystic adenoma of the pancreas: spectrum of computed tomographic findings. J Comput Assist Tomog 12:797–803

Johnson CD, Stephens DH, Charbonneau JW, Carpenter HA, Welch TJ (1988) Cystic pancreatic tumors: CT and sonographic assessment. AJR 151:1133–1138

Katz LBK, Ehya H (1990) Aspiration cytology of papillary cystic neoplasm of the pancreas. Am J Clin Pathol 94:328–333

Klöppel G (1984) Pathology, non-endocrine tumors. In: Klöppel G, Heitz PU (eds) Pancreatic pathology. Churchill Livingstone, New York, pp 9–113

Klöppel G, Maillet B (1989) Classification and staging of pancreatic nonendocrine tumors. Radiology Clin North Am 27:105–119

Klöppel G, Baummer G, Rückert K, Seifert G (1980) Intraductal proliferation in the pancreas and its relationship to human and experimental carcinogenesis. Virchows Arch [A] Pathol Anat Histol 387:221–233

Kolmannskog F, Schrumpf E, Valnes K (1982) Computed tomography and angiography in pancreatic apudomas and cystadenomas. Acta Radiol 23:365–372

Lack EE (1989) Primary tumors of the exocrine pancreas. Classification, overview, and recent contributions by immunohistochemistry and electron microscopy. Am J Surg Pathol 13:66–88

Lack EE, Levey R, Cassady JR, Wawter GF (1983) Tumors of the exocrine pancreas in children and adolescents: a clinical and pathologic study of eight cases. Am J Surg Pathol 7:319–327

Laverdiere JT, van Sonneberg E, Strum WB, Kuster GGR (1992) Pleomorphic pancreatic sarcoma mimicking pancreatic pseudocyst: CT appearance. AJR 158:87–89

Learmonth GM, Price SK, Visser AE, Emms M (1985) Papillary and cystic neoplasm of the pancreas – an acinar cell tumour? Histopathology 9:63–79

Leborgne J, Albisetti J, Heloury Y et al (1985) Les cystadénomes microkystiques et mucineux du pancréas. Réflexions à partir de 15 observations. Chirurgie 111:244–251

Lee MG, Auh YH, Cho KS, Chung YH, Han DJ, Yk ES (1992) Mucinous ductal ectasia of the pancreas: MRI. J Comput Assist Tomogr 16:495–496

Levine E, Collins DL, horton Wa, Schimke RN (1982) CT screening of the abdomen in von Hippel-Lindau disease. AJR 139:505–510

Lewandrowski K, Warshaw A, Compton C (1992) Macrokystic serous cystadenoma of the pancreas: a morphologic variant differing from microcystic adenoma. Hum Pathol 23:871–875

Lieber MR, Lack EE, Roberts JR Jr et al (1987) Solid papillary epithelial neoplasm of the pancreas: an ultrastructural and immunocytochemical study of six cases. Am J Surg Pathol 11:85–93

Lo JW, Fung CHK, Yonan TN, Martinez N (1977) Cystadenoma of the pancreas. An ultrastructural study. Cancer 39:2470–2474

Mathieu D, Guigui B, Valette PJ et al (1989) Pancreatic cystic neoplasms. Radiol Clin North Am 27:163–176

Matsunou H, Konishi F (1990) Papillary-cystic neoplasm of the pancreas. A clinicopathologic study concerning the tumor aging and malignancy of nine cases. Cancer 65:283–291

Matsuda Y, Imai Y, Kawata S et al (1987) Papillary cystic neoplasm of the pancreas with multiple hepatic metastases: a case report. Gastroenterol Jpn 22:379–384

Matsunou H, Konishi F, Yamamichi N, Takayanagi N, Mukai M (1990) Solid, infiltrating variety of papillary cystic neoplasm of the pancreas. Cancer 65:2747–2757

Miettinen M, Partanen S, Fraki O et al (1987) Papillary cystic tumor of the pancreas. An analysis of cellular differenciation by electron microscopy and immunohistochemistry. Am J Surg Pathol 11:855–865

Minami M, Itai Y, Ohtomo K, Yoshida H, Yoshikawa K, Iio M (1989) Cystic neoplasms of the pancreas: comparison of MR imaging with CT. Radiology 171:53–56

Missas S, Gouiamos A, Kourias E et al (1987) Primary hydatid disease of the pancreas. Gastrointest Radiol 12:37–38

Morohoshi T, Held G, Klöppel G (1983) Exocrine pancreatic tumors and their histological classification. Histopathology 7:645–661

Morohoshi T, Held G, Klöppel G (1983) Exocrine pancreatic tumours and there histological classification. A study based on 167 autopsy and 97 surgical cases. Histopathology 7:645–661

Morohoshi T, Kanda M, Asanuma K, Klöppel G (1989) Intraductal papillary neoplasms of the pancreas. A clinicopathologic study of six patients. Cancer 64:1329–1335

Neibling HA (1968) Primary sarcoma of the pancreas. Am Surg 34:690–693

Neumann HPH, Dinkel E, Brambs H et al (1991) Pancreatic lesions in the von Hippel-Lindau syndrome. Gastroenterology 101:465–471

Nishida K, Shiga K, Kato K et al (1989) Two cases of pancreatic cystadenocarcinoma with elevated CA 19–9 levels in the cystic fluid in comparison with two cases of pancreatic cystadenoma. Hepatogastroenterology 36:442–445

Padovani B, Neuveut P, Chanalet S et al (1991) Microcystic adenoma of the pancreas: report on four cases and review of the literature. Gastrointest Radiol 16:62–66

Pandolfo I, Scribano E, Gaeta M, Fiumara F, Longo M (1985) Cystic lymphangioma of the pancreas. CT demonstration. J Comput Assist Tomogr 9:209–210

Parienty RA, Ducellier R, Lubrano JM, Picard JD, Pradel J, Smolarski N (1980) Cystadenomas of the pancreas: diagnosis by computed tomography. J Comput Assist Tomog 4:364–367

Payan MJ, Xerri L, Moncada K et al (1990) Villous adenoma of the main pancreatic duct: a potentially malignant tumor? Am J Gastroenterol 85:459–463

Place S, Louvel A, Farhi JP, Chapuis S (1985) Adénocarcinome papillaire du canal de Wirsung. Gastroenterol Clin Biol 9:361–364

Pogany AC, Kerlan RK, Karam JH et al (1984) Cystic insulinoma. AJR 142:951–952

Ponsot P, Molas G, Vilgrain V, Gayet B, Fékété F, Paolaggi JA (1989, Adénomes, adénomatoses et adénocarcinomes pancréatiques intra-canalaires. Gastroenterol Clin Biol 13:663–670

Remine SG, Frey D, Rossi RL et al (1987) Cystic neoplasms of the pancreas. Arch Surg 122:443–446

Rickaert F, Cremer M, Deviere J et al (1991) Intraductal mucin-hypersecreting neoplasms of the pancreas. A clinicopathologic study of eight patients. Gastroenterology 101:512–519

Rogers PN, Seywright MM, Murray WR (1987) Diffuse villous adenoma of the pancreatic duct. Pancreas 23:727–730
Rubin GD, Jeffrey RB, Walter JF (1991) Pancreatic microcystic adenoma presenting with acute hemoperitoneum: CT diagnosis. AJR 156:749–750
Rumanick WM, Megibow AJ, Bosniak MA, Hilton S (1984) Metastatic disease to the pancreas: evaluation by computed tomography. J Comput Assist Tomogr 8:829–834
Rustin RB, Broughan TA, Hermann RE, Grundfest-Broniatowski F, Petras RE, Hart WR (1986) Papillary cystic epithelial neoplasms of the pancreas. A clinical study of four cases. Arch. Surg 121:1073–1076
Salimi Z, Fishbein M, Wolverson MK, Johnson FE (1991) Pancreatic lymphangioma: CT, MRI, and angiographic features. Gastrointest Radiol 16:248–250
Sanfey H, Mendelsohn G, Cameron JM (1983) Solid and papillary neoplasm of the pancreas. A potentially curable surgical lesion. Ann Surg 197:735–739
Schlosnagle DC, Campbell WG (1981) The papillary and solid neoplasm of the pancreas. Cancer 47:2603–2610
Sclafani LM, Reuter VE, Coit DG, Brennan MF (1991) The malignant nature of papillary and cystic neoplasm of the pancreas. Cancer 68:153–158
Shorten SD, Hart WR, Petras RA (1986) Microcystic adenomas (serous cystadenomas) of pancreas: a clinicopathologic investigation of eight cases with immunohistochemical and ultrastructural studies. Am J Surg Pathol 10:365–372
Smith RC, Kneale K, Goulston K (1986) In situ carcinoma of the pancreas. Aust NZ J Surg 56:369–373
Smith TR, Koenigsberg M (1990) Low-density insulinoma on dynamic CT. AJR 155:995–996
Sommers SC, Murphy SA, Warren S (1954) Pancreatic duct hyperplasia and cancer. Gastroentorology 27:629–640
Stömmer P, Kraus J, Stolt M, Giedl J (1991) Solid and cystic pancreatic tumors. Clinical, histochemical, and electron microscopic features in ten cases. Cancer 67:1635–1641
Stovall JM (1986) Microcystic adenoma: the specificity of computerized tomography in making the distinction. J Nat Med Assoc 78:1119–1121
Torres-Barrera G, Fernandez Del Castillo CA, Reyes E et al (1987) Microcystic adenoma of the pancreas. Dig Dis Sci 32:454–458
Urban BAZ, Fishman EK, Hruban RH, Cameron JL (1992) CT findings in cystic schwannoma of the pancreas. J Comput Assist Tomogr 16:492–493
Vellet D, Leiman G, Mair S et al (1988) Fine needle aspiration cytology of mucinous cystadenocarcinoma of the pancreas. Further observations. Acta Cytol 32:43–48
Warren RB (1985) Papillary cystic tumor of the pancreas. Arch Pathol Lab Med 109:706–707
Warshaw AL, Berry J, Gang DL (1987) Villous adenoma of the duct of Wirsung. Dig Dis Sci 32:1311–1313
Warshaw AL, Compton CC, Lewandrowski K, Da Cardenosa GH, Mueller PR (1990) Cystic tumors of the pancreas. New clinical, radiologic, and pathologic observations in 67 patients. Ann Surg 4:432–443
Wernecke K, Petters PE, Galanski M (1986) Pancreatic metastases: US evaluation. Radiology 160:399–402
Wolfman NT, Ramquist NA, Karstaedt N, Hopkins MBC (1982) Cystic neoplasms of the pancreas: CT and sonography. AJR 138:37–41
Wolson AH, Walls WJ (1976) Ultrasonic characteristics of cystadenoma of the pancreas. Radiology 119:203–205
Yamada M, Kozuka S, Yamao K, Nakazawa S, Naitoh Y, Tsukamoto Y (1991) Mucin-producing tumor of the pancreas. Cancer 68:159–168
Yamaguchi K, Munetomo E (1987) Cystic neoplasms of the pancreas. Gastroenterology 92:1934–1943
Zirinsky K, Abiri M, Baer JW (1984) Computed tomography demonstration of pancreatic microcystic adenoma. Am J Gastroenterol 79:139–142

10 Endocrine Tumors of the Pancreas

A. Roche, A.L. Baert, E. Thérasse, H. Rigauts, L. Van Hoe

CONTENTS

A. Roche, MD, Service de Radiodiagnostic, Unité de Radiologie Interventionnelle et Vasculaire, Institut Gustave Roussy, Rue Camille Desmoulins, F-94805 Villejuif Cédex, France
A.L. Baert, MD, Professor, Department of Radiology, University Hospital K.U.L., Herestraat 49, B-3000 Leuven, Belgium
E. Thérasse, MD, Service de Radiodiagnostic, Unité de Radiologie Interventionnelle et Vasculaire, Institut Gustave Roussy, Rue Camille Desmoulins, F-94805 Villejuif Cédex, France
H. Rigauts, MD, Resident, Department of Radiology, University Hospital K.U.L., Herestraat 49, B-3000 Leuven, Belgium
L. Van Hoe, MD, Assistant Professor, Department of Radiology, University Hospital K.U.L., Herestraat 49, B-3000 Leuven, Belgium

10.1 Classification and Clinical Aspects

A. Roche and E. Thérasse

10.1.1 Introduction

For almost 20 years, interest in endocrine tumors of the pancreas has been unflagging. In these tumors, the biologist has found a remarkable research model of the physiology of hormonal secretions. The clinician, armed with new methods of biologic diagnosis, has discovered that this pathology may be much more frequent than previously imagined (gastrinoma) and has acquired new therapeutic ammunition (somatostatin). To this model, the pathologist has added theories that go far beyond purely pancreatic and even digestive pathology. The radiologist, who has always encountered difficulties in exploring the pancreas, has forged new arms (intraoperative and endoscopic ultrasonography, functional methods of radioendocrinologic localization) specifically adapted to the detection problems presented by these tumors.

10.1.2 Terminology

The generic term "endocrine tumor of the pancreas" has superseded the previous concept of "tumor of the endocrine pancreas" (or insular tumor), which wrongly implied that the tumor could develop from the islets of Langerhans cells only. Indeed, tumors are also known to develop from pluripotent endocrine cells (nesidioblasts) located along the pancreatic canaliculi.

The terms "endocrine adenoma (or carcinoma) of the pancreas" and "nesidioblastoma" are still found in the literature and the term "nesidioblastoma" is often reserved – and wrongly so – for nonsecreting endocrine tumors of the pancreas.

Endocrine tumors of the pancreas that secrete a hormone normally produced by the pancreas (e.g., insulin or glucagon) are termed "orthoendocrine." Others secrete several hormones, either from the same lesion or in multiple intrapancreatic tumors. Still others may secrete hormones normally elaborated outside the pancreas (e.g., gastrin); these are called "paracrine."

This multiplicity of secretions can be explained if one admits that endocrine tumors of the pancreas develop from perfectly totipotent stem cells (nesidioblasts) prone to differentiation with varied secretory activities.

Digestive endocrine cells (among others) are termed "argentaffin" due to their ability to reduce silver salts they have absorbed. They share with other secretory cells, such as the pheochromocytes, the ability to extract and decarboxylate precursors of biogenic amines from the blood. This function is at the origin of the term denoting the system that groups these different cells: the APUD (amine precursor uptake decarboxylase) system. Tumors which develop from the cells of this vast system are generally called "apudomas."

Commonly encountered dysgenic or tumoral pathologic associations, accompanied by an abnormal secretion, are not fortuitous and may be understood thanks to theories such as Pearse's. These "polyadenomatoses," in reference to the neural crest which would give rise to the cells in question, are sometimes called "neurocristopathies." This concept is of obvious clinical interest, especially since there is a one-in-two familial incidence and a high degree of malignancy. Among the classifiable polyadenomatoses, "multiple endocrine neoplasias" (MEN) can affect the pancreas. For instance, Wermer's syndrome links prolactin-secreting hypophyseal adenoma, parathyroid adenoma, and endocrine tumor of the pancreas.

Clinically speaking, names for secretory tumors are conventionally derived from their symptomatic secretion: "insulinoma," "gastrinoma," "somatostatinoma," "vipoma," and so on. Insofar as these tumors are often multisecretory and comprised of pluripotent cells, a less restrictive denotation would be more appropriate; but for purposes of simplification, we will retain the sanctioned appellation.

10.1.3 Malignancy, Size, Localization

All endocrine tumors of the pancreas are potentially malignant (Martin et al. 1987), but it is not so much a question of cellular or even local tissular malignancy, in the usual sense of the term. Only by observing metastasis can one be certain of the tumor malignancy, especially since the development of malignant forms, even metastatic ones, may be extremely slow (>10 years). The various types of endocrine tumors of the pancreas do not all have the same potential of malignancy development (Table 10.1): insulinomas are nearly always benign, gastrinomas present malignancy criteria in about two-thirds of cases, and glucagonomas are almost invariably malignant from the outset. Metastases themselves present practically no histologic malignancy criteria. Their hormonal secretion may also differ from the primary lesion and, likewise, a tumoral response (sometimes complete) may often be noted under chemotherapy in hepatic metastases when, in the same patient, the primary lesion is totally unresponsive. It therefore could not be wrong to consider hepatic metastases and pancreatic tumor as the manifestations of notably different tumoral phenomena.

Tumor size at the time of diagnosis varies from one type of tumor to the next (Table 10. 1) and is a limiting factor for identification by morphologic examination. There is no direct correlation between the size of the lesion and the intensity of hypersecretion and of the resulting symptoms. The insulinoma measures less than 15 mm roughly two times out of three; gastrinomas are usually even smaller; the other types of tumors, however, are generally much larger at the time of diagnosis and, save for certain exceptions, their identification does not pose any problem. "Hidden" forms, in which microscopic lesions are discovered only after a meticulous examination of dozens of slices of the excised piece, are not uncommon, especially since pancreatic venous sampling makes the localization of tumors possible, regardless of their size. These differences are related to the presence or absence and to the greater or lesser effectiveness of compensatory mechanisms, triggered by abnormal hormonal hypersecretion. Thus, non-secretory tumors are generally very large when they become symptomatic. The same is true of glucagonoma, owing to the effectiveness of compensatory mechanisms of hypersecretion of glucagon. On the other hand, hypersecretion of gastrin is immediately symptomatic and gastrinoma may have clinical manifestations as early as the microscopic stage.

The possible multiplicity of intrapancreatic lesions must be taken into account (Table 10.1). Zollinger-Ellison syndrome is accompanied by mul-

Table 10.1. Main characteristics of pancreatic endocrine tumors

Pancreatic endocrine tumors	Relative Frequency	Secreted Hormone	Normal plasma level	Size (mm)	Frequency (%)				Frequency or no. of reported cases
					Ectopic	Multiples	Malignancy	MEN	
Insulinoma	56%	Insulin	3–21 mU/ml	<15 in 65%	2	22	16	8	0.3–1.3/year/million people (adults)
Gastrinoma	21%	Gastrin	<180 pg/ml	1 to 30	20 (duodenum)	50	60	25	1/year/million people (0.5% of ulcerous disease)
Nonsecreting tumor	15%			Large					
Glucagonoma	2.3%	Glucagon	<180 pg/ml	>30 in 80%	2	1	82	<5	150 cases
Vipoma	1.8%	VIP	<50 pg/ml	>30 in 78%	16 (neurologic)	20	60	10	<100 cases
Secreting carcinoid	<1%	5-HIAA, serotonin	<10 mg/day (urine), <150 ng/ml (blood)						Exceptional (0.05% of all carcinoid tumors)
Somatostatinoma	<1%	Somatostatin	<100 pg/ml						22 cases
PPoma	<1%	PP	<500 pg/ml						<10 cases
Somatocrinoma	<1%	(GRF) → GH	(Not dosable) → 0.5–10 mg/l						5 cases (0.08% in acromegaly)
Corticotrophinoma	<1%	ACTH 13–35 ng/ml							<20 cases
Paratyrinoma	<1%	PTH "like"	Not detectable						
Mixed tumors	1.5%								

VIP, vasoactive intestinal polypeptide; 5-HIAA, 5-hydroxyindoleacetic acid; PP, pancreatic polypeptide; GRF, growth hormone releasing factor; GH, growth hormone; ACTH, adrenocorticotropic hormone; PTH, parathyroid hormone tiple (or diffuse) tumors in one of every two cases. As a rule, insulinoma, vipoma, and glucagonoma are single tumors and very rarely develop as part of the MEN syndrome.

Localization of the tumor in any type of pancreatic gland can be cephalic, corporeal, or caudal, which definitely rules out blind surgical resection of hidden forms. Ectopic localization is possible but is of variable frequency, being exceptional for insulinoma and occurring in about 20% of cases of gastrinoma or vipoma.

10.1.4 Clinical Considerations, Diagnosis, and Treatment

10.1.4.1 Generalities

10.1.4.1.1 Epidemiology

Endocrine tumors of the pancreas are rare tumors. Insulinoma and gastrinoma (Zollinger-Ellison syndrome) are far more frequent (about one case per million inhabitants per year) than glucagonoma and vipoma (approximately 100–200 cases are described in the literature) (Table 10.1). One must bear in mind, however, that the identification and description of these tumors occurred relatively recently (insulinoma: 1902; gastrinoma: 1955; glucagonoma: 1966; somatostatinoma: 1977) and were linked to the development of hormonal assay possibilities. Zollinger-Ellison syndrome, at first considered extremely rare, now appears to be a fairly frequent lesion, with potentially 4000–6000 cases in France; this is far from the figure actually reported, implying that incomplete forms are largely unrecognized.

10.1.4.1.2 Diagnostic Principles

Clinical Diagnosis. When they are secretory, these tumors have the shared characteristic of manifesting themselves through common non-specific symptoms related to the abnormal hypersecretion - diarrhea, ulcers, neuropsychic disorders, diabetes, etc. - of which only the intensity or resistance to usual treatment is alarming, thus turning one's attention to an etiology that is just as rare. It is quite remarkable to be faced with a tumoral pathology in which the clinical manifestation is practically never the tumoral mass effect.

When the tumor is nonsecretory, the tumoral mass effect of the lesion is revealing and, as with all tumors of the pancreas, an extremely large lesion is often encountered from the outset. This is especially true for endocrine tumors of the pancreas, since even when very large or cephalic, these tumors have little or no biliary repercussions.

The slow clinical development of these tumors, even in certain malignant and metastatic forms, has already been pointed out.

Biological Diagnosis. Diagnosis of the secretory forms always hinges on the observation of a permanent and autonomous hormonal hypersecretion. Radiologic examination is useful only in localizing the tumors and should not be considered a diagnostic method. In other words, morphologic investigation can in no case precede a biologically established diagnosis. On the other hand, one must be aware that a hormonal hypersecretion in itself is not sufficient to confirm the diagnosis of endocrine tumor of the pancreas, just as the normality of secretions does not exclude it. Therefore , the radiologist must be advised of the main causes of increased serum levels of hormones other than pancreatic tumors (Table 10.2).

10.1.4.1.3 Principles of Treatment

Depending on the type of tumor, treatment will be more or less aggressive to control the abnormal secretion responsible for the symptoms and to control the tumoral mass effect for oncologic purposes. Thus, in insulinoma, control of hyperinsulinism is vital, while the oncologic problem is exceptionally of primary importance: simple enucleation or, when possible, medical treatment is therefore perfectly warranted. With Zollinger-Ellison syndrome, however, the oncologic problem is the major concern.

10.1.4.2 Principal Types of Tumors

10.1.4.2.1 Insulinoma

Clinical Manifestations. Clinical manifestations are very varied but, most importantly, neuropsychic. Since symptoms do not point directly to the disease, in 25% of patients it has already evolved for more than 5 years at the time of diagnosis. The appearance of signs during prolonged fasting or with exercise is the most distinctive feature.

Table 10.2. Other causes of increases in serum levels of gastrin, insulin, or glucagon

Gastrin	Insulin	Glucagon
Pyloric stenosis	Insulin administration and other causes of exogenous hypoglycemia	Chronic renal failure
2/3 Gastrectomy	Obesity	Hepatic failure, cirrhosis
Chronic renal failure	Reactive hypoglycemia (reactive to mild diabetes)	Portocaval shunt
Hepatic failure		Diabetes (failure in control, acidetosis)
Cirrhosis		Exogenous (diazoxide administration)
Portocaval shunt		Prolonged stress
Small bowel resection		Acute pancreatitis
Atrophic gastritis		
Truncal or supraselective vagotomy		

Diagnosis. The diagnosis is based mainly on the 48-h fasting test, with simultaneous assays of glycemia and insulinemia. A fall in blood glucose to below 0.5 g/l proves the organic nature of the hypoglycemia , while the unsuppressible character of the hyperinsulinemia proves its tumoral nature. A Turner ratio [glycemia (in mg/100 ml)/insulinemia (in mU/ml)] below 4 reveals this characteristic and is considered 100% positive at the 72nd hour of the test. The increase in circulating C peptide (which expresses the increase in proinsulin, the proportion of which rises in insulinoma) is also an excellent sign. Further, it allows differential diagnosis with factitious hypoglycemia due to surreptitious administration of insulin or sulfonamides, in which the insulin concentration is high.

Treatment. The treatment of choice is surgical, with simple enucleation if possible, which implies precise localization (Moreaux and Olivier 1987; Van Heerden et al. 1979; Xianju et al. 1980). Surgical mortality is low (6%). In rare cases of malignancy, systemic or locoregional hepatic chemotherapy (streptozotocin) may be administered. When surgical treatment is impossible, diazoxide, a hypoglycemic sulfonamide which blocks the secretion of insulin induced by glucose, can sometimes control the disease.

Most often, insulinoma is a benign ailment when it is diagnosed before a serious accident results in neurologic sequelae and when the tumor can be surgically removed after an accurate localization, in which the radiologist plays a leading role.

10.1.4.2.2 Gastrinoma (Zollinger-Ellison Syndrome; ZES)

Clinical Manifestations. The two key clinical signs are diarrhea and upper gastrointestinal ulcers. Ulcers, present in 85% of cases, are often multiple and may involve the gastrointestinal (GI) tract from the esophagus to the jejunum. ZES should be considered when these ulcers present one of the following distinctive characteristics: occurrence in a female or young person, positive familial antecedent, strong resistance to medical treatment , recurrent complications , association with diarrhea, vomiting not caused by a digestive stenosis, and proximity of the ulcer to Treitz's ligament, a rare but characteristic finding. Diarrhea, an essential element of the syndrome, is present in approximately 70% of cases and remains isolated or precedes the appearance of ulcers in 50% of cases.

Diagnosis. The diagnosis is based on confirmation of the gastric acid hypersecretion, which accounts for the radiologic characteristics of the disease: esophageal ulcerations and esophagitis , gastric ulcers developed on a hypersecreting stomach showing prominent rugal folds, and ulcerations and fold thickening of the duodenum and proximal jejunum. Biologic proof is supplied by the increase in basal acid output to above 15 mmol/h, with a basal acid concentration above 100 mmol/l. Hypergastrinemia is the second element of the biologic diagnosis, keeping in mind that there are numerous causes for high gastrin levels though these do not produce the very high levels associated with ZES. The sensitivity of the sign can be raised by injecting secretin, which normally lowers the gastrin levels, whereas these levels increase in ZES.

Treatment. Acid hypersecretion can be life-threatening and priority must be given to controlling it. Nowadays, total gastrectomies are rarely performed thanks to anti-H_2 drugs, which are almost always effective. Treating the tumoral mass is therefore an increasingly frequent concern, which has benefited from the possibilities of tumoral localization (Bonfils et al. 1981; Moreaux 1981). This oncologic approach to treatment is supported by the occurrence of apparently complete cures after certain exereses (Hautefeuille et al. 1979) and by the fact that hypergastrinemia could lead to the appearance of fundic carcinoid tumors (Mignon et al. 1987). Though the ideal treatment is surgical, exeresis is warranted only in cases of a simple procedure (tumor of the pancreatic tail or duodenal wall or very superficial tumor that can be enucleated). Surgical mortality in total pancreatectomies in patients with ZES is very high (around 35% in some reference series), and the probability of a complete exeresis is too low for one to suggest a cephalic pancreatoduodenectomy without reservation, even in cases where there is every indication that the lesions are restricted to the head. Conversely, from a very oncologic standpoint, total pancreatectomy could be proposed in some cases as a very aggressive attitude towards this illness, known to be malignant two-thirds of the time. In cases of malignancy, particularly with hepatic metastases, chemotherapy [intravenous (IV), intra-arterial (IA), or by chemoembolization] is generally suggested, using streptozotocin and/or 5 -fluorouracil (5-FU) and/or doxorubicin. Response rates vary between 40% and 60%, half of which are complete responses.

Prognosis. The poor prognosis of ZES is due to its frequent malignant development, despite an often slow progression (survival over 15 years is not exceptional with metastatic disease to the liver). The survival rate is 65% after 5 years and stabilizes at around 50% after 10 years. The best 5-year survivals are found in cases of ectopic tumors (69%) and with negative exploratory laparotomy (67%) (Mignon et al. 1987). The lowest survival rates are associated with metastatic disease to the liver (5-year survival of 27%) and with MEN (48%). In one out of four cases, the cause of death is a postoperative complication, and in one out of two cases it is the consequence of hepatic metastases.

10.1.4.2.3 Glucagonoma (Guillausseau et al. 1982; Stacpoole 1981)

Clinical Manifestations and Diagnosis. In 70% of the cases, the mucocutaneous syndrome leads to the diagnosis of the disease. It is a migratory necrolytic erythema affecting the friction zones and associated with mucosal manifestations (glossitis). Though its pathogenesis is unclear, a decrease in serum levels of glucagon often leads to the rapid and spectacular disappearance of the syndrome within a few days. Once the sickness is well established, this syndrome is absent in only one in ten patients. Other signs include: diabetes mellitus, anemia, diarrhea, and cachexia, which is sometimes associated with direct signs of pancreatic tumor. Diagnosis is based on the observation of a high serum level of glucagon, though there is also a fall in plasmatic amino acids.

Treatment. The ideal treatment is surgical. The usually slow tumoral progression sometimes justifies surgical debulking. Because of their slow growth, at the time of diagnosis these tumors have certainly been progressing for years and are almost invariably malignant. This is also a point in favor of early attempts at localization, the success of which would improve the effectiveness of surgical treatment, as in one of our cases. Systemic or locoregional chemotherapy (streptozotocin, 5-EU, Déticène) is suggested for malignant forms with metastasis. In one case, we managed to control tumoral development and the clinical syndrome by chemoembolization with doxorubicin. Somatostatin generally has a transient effectiveness in controlling the glucagon hypersecretion.

10.1.4.2.4 Vipoma (Pancreatic Cholera, Verner-Morrison Syndrome) (Rambaud and Jian 1987; Verner and Morrison 1974)

Clinical Manifestations. By definition, this condition is characterized by chronic diarrhea, a hydro-electrolytic, afecal, secretory diarrhea (persisting even during prolonged fasting) with daily discharge that can at times amount to 10 l. The other signs are mainly the consequences of dehydration which accompanies the major loss of water. Flush episodes occasionally occur, but gastro-intestinal hemorrhages are infrequent.

Diagnosis. The diagnosis is based on the demonstration of the secretory nature of the diarrhea, in the absence of gastric acid hypersecretion or other organic GI tract lesions. Under these conditions, the primary differential diagnoses are carcinoid tumors accompanied by hepatic metastases medullary thyroid carcinoma, and pheochromocytomas or ganglioneuro(blasto)mas. VIP elevation is sensitive and specific, but may be absent especially in hyperplasias.

Treatment. The treatment is based on the same principles as that of other slowly developing tumors. Only if the tumor is totally removed without hepatic metastases can one hope for a complete cure (i.e., in approximately 50% of the cases). Some cases of hyperplasia are cured after surgery, but surgical mortality is 30% with this disease.

10.1.4.2.5
Somatostatinoma (Ribet et al. 1987)

The symptomatology of this disease is nonspecific. It is the result of the inhibitory effect of somatostatin on the endocrine secretions of gastrin, insulin, cholecystokinin, and glucagon. It is this inhibitory effect which is turned to account to treat the other endocrine tumors of the pancreas with somatostatin analogs. The signs most often observed are deterioration in the general state of health, diabetes, and biliary lithiasis; other signs may include diarrhea with steatorrhea and gastric achlorhydria. The tumor often appears multisecretory, however, which enhances the symptomatology of unforeseen signs: hypersecretion of thyrocalcitonin, adrenocorticotropic hormone (ACTH), growth hormone releasing factor (GRF), gastrin, etc. In reported cases, the circulating somatostatin level rose to several thousand times the normal level. Localization of lesions is comparable to that of other large tumors and the principles of treatment are conventional: surgery if possible, chemotherapy otherwise.

10.2 Transabdominal Ultrasonography, Computed Tomography, and Magnetic Resonance Imaging

A.L. Baert, L. Van Hoe, H. Rigauts

10.2.1 Introduction

Patients with clinical symptoms suggesting an abnormal production of one or several hormones should initially be screened by radio-immunoassay and biochemical methods. The accuracy and specificity of these methods for the detection of elevated plasma or urine levels of the hormones is very high (Rossi et al.1989).

When clinical symptoms indicate a hormonally triggered disease and/or when abnormal levels of some hormones are established, radiologic investigation is indicated in order to localize the tumor, which is of essential help when surgical treatment is considered. Another important goal of imaging studies is the detection of metastatic disease (Thompson et al. 1994).

The radiologic detection of functioning endocrine tumors in the pancreas constitutes a major challenge, particularly in the case of suspected insulinoma or gastrinoma. This is mainly related to the size of these tumors: 70% of insulinomas are smaller than 1.5 cm, 38% of gastrinomas are smaller than 1 cm (Gunther et al. 1983; Krudy et al. 1984; Frucht et al. 1989). In patients with MEN-I syndrome, gastrinomas tend to be even smaller and multicentric. Failure of radiologic imaging techniques to demonstrate a focal lesion in patients with biochemical suspicion of an islet cell tumor of the pancreas may have two causes: the tumor may be too small to be detected or "diffuse neuro-endocrine cellular hyperplasia" or "microadenosis" may account for the clinical findings (Gunther et al. 1983).

10.2.2 Transabdominal Ultrasonography

10.2.2.1 Technique (see Chap. 8)

10.2.2.1.1
Findings

On ultrasonography, endocrine pancreatic tumors are usually hypoechoic when compared to surrounding normal glandular tissue (Fig. 10.1). A small hyperechoic capsule is sometimes detected in insulinomas (Gunther et al. 1983; Päivänsalo et al. 1989). The lesions are most commonly round or oval in shape and have a sharp interface with the surrounding normal pancreas. With the exception of the larger (mostly nonsecretory) islet cell tumors, the echo pattern is usually homogeneous. This is not absolute, however: even small lesions may contain cystic areas or calcifications. Invasion of peripancreatic fat and metastatic disease in the liver or lymph nodes is more frequently observed in nonsecretory endocrine tumors because these tumors are generally detected at a more advanced stage.

10.2.2.1.2
Value

Success rates of ultrasonography for the detection of insulinoma vary from 25% to 65% (Galiber et al. 1988; Gorman et al. 1986; Gunther et al. 1983). For

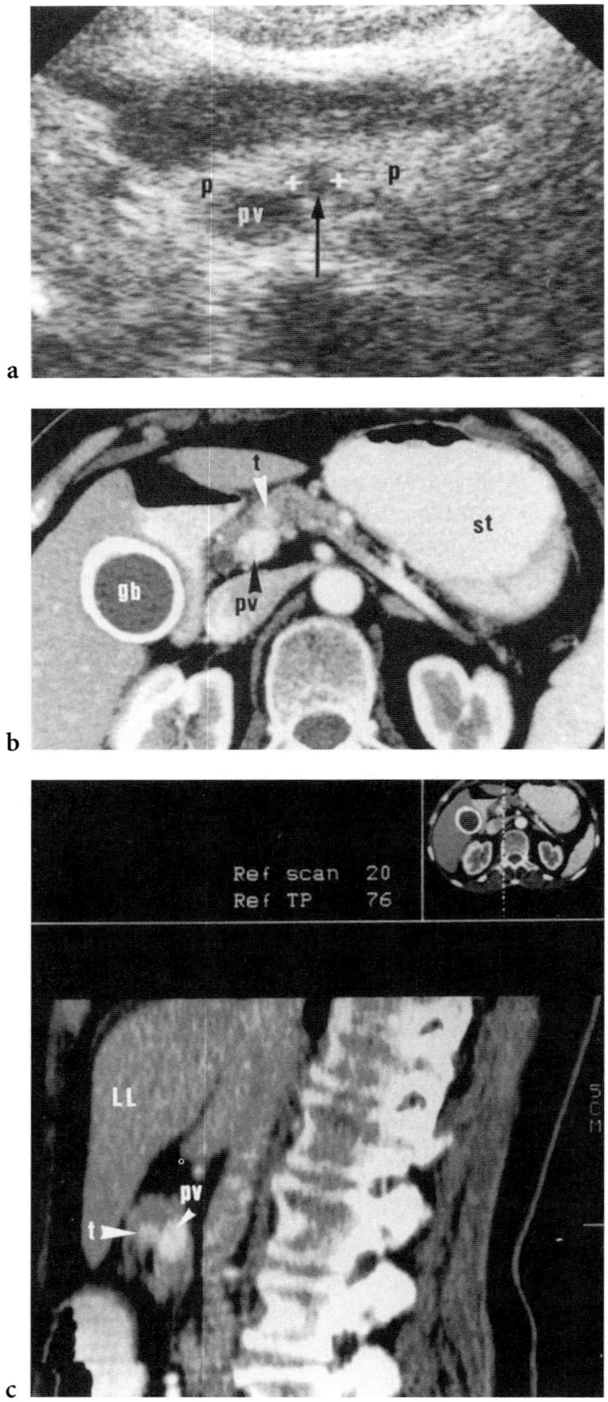

Fig. 10.1a–c. Small endocrine tumor (insulinoma). Typical ultrasonography (US) and computed tomography (CT) features. **a** US shows small (diameter 7–8 mm) hypoechoic lesion (arrow) in the dorsal portion of pancreatic neck. p, Pancreas; *pv*, portal vein. **b** Spiral CT following IV bolus injection of an iodinated contrast medium shows the insulinoma as a hypervascular lesion in the pancreatic neck (white arrowhead). *gb*, Gallbladder; *pv*, portal vein; *st*, stomach; *t*, tumor. **c** Sagittal reformatted image nicely displays the exact position of the lesion. *LL*, Left liver lobe; *pv*, portal vein; *t*, tumor

the detection of gastrinomas, the average success rate is only 20% (FRUCHT et al. 1989). The success rate depends on the expertise of the examiner, the body weight of the patient, and the technical quality of the apparatus used.

Although the diagnosis of functioning endocrine tumor is usually obvious if a focal pancreatic lesion is detected in a patient with a clinical diagnosis of functioning endocrine tumor, the morphologic features of these lesions are not really specific (FUGAZZOLA et al. 1990; PÄIVÄNSALO et al. 1989).

10.2.3 Computed Tomography

10.2.3.1 Technique

Accurate detection of endocrine pancreatic tumors requires helical (spiral) computed tomography (CT) technology (see Chap. 8). A non-enhanced scan of the pancreas is usually obtained to determine the appropriate coverage. Contrast material is injected in a cubital or antecubital vein with a mechanical power injector. A total of 100--150 ml iodinated contrast material (±350 Mg I/100 ml) is injected at a rate varying between 3 and 4 ml/s. If dual-phase helical CT is technically possible and if a sufficiently short rotation time can be used (0.75 s), two sets of images can be obtained within a very short time interval. Since functioning endocrine tumors tend to enhance before the onset of pancreatic enhancement, scanning in the late arterial phase seems appropriate (Fig. 10.2). The optimal scan delay time can be determined by the test bolus injection method (VAN HOE et al. 1995a). Alternatively, a predefined delay of approximately 15--25 s can be used, the exact timing depending on factors such as age and weight. Ideally, the liver should be included in this first scan (goal: detection of hypervascular liver metastases). A second helical scan includes the entire upper abdomen and is performed at 50–80 s, depending on the type of equipment and slice thickness chosen. While the first scan is best suited to the detection of small hypervascular tumors, the second scan better shows hypovascular or cystic lesions. Moreover, dual-phase CT enables one to take inter-individual variability in cardiac function into account: in patients with long circulation times, hypervascular lesions may be invisible on images obtained with the first acquisition. The following acquisition parameters are typi-

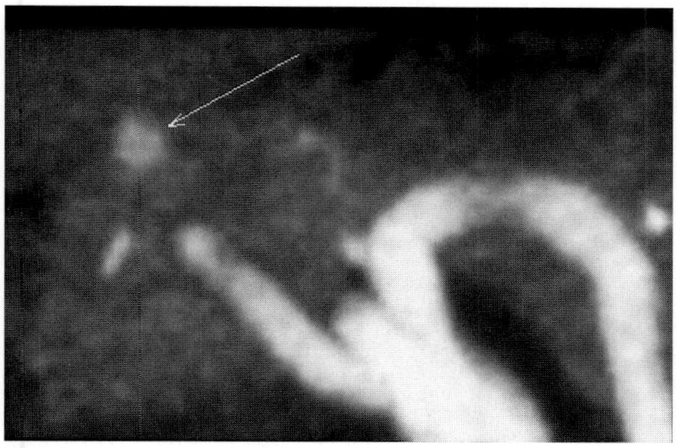

Fig. 10.2. Small endocrine tumor (4-mm gastrinoma). Detection with arterial-phase helical computed tomography (CT). Maximum intensity projection calculated from CT images obtained in the arterial phase shows hypervascular lesion in the pancreatic neck (arrow)

cally used: 3–5 mm collimation and a pitch of 1–1.5. Images are calculated at 2–4-mm increments.

Administration of a negative oral contrast (preferably 0.5--1 l tap water) and a spasmolytic agent is a crucial requirement to enable the detection of small tumors located in the wall of the duodenum.

Direct intra-arterial injection of iodinated contrast media has been advocated to obtain an adequate enhancement of islet cell tumors (AHLSTRÖM et al. 1990; KRUDY et al. 1984). This technique may increase the sensitivity of CT for the detection for small and/or less well perfused tumors (FINK et al. 1985; ROCHE et al. 1983).

10.2.3.2
Imaging Findings

In the pre-contrast series, functioning islet cell tumors are usually isodense and thus invisible. Insulinomas may contain small punctiform calcifications and their exact intrapancreatic location can therefore be suspected (Fig. 10.3). Cystic or partially necrotic endocrine tumors may contain low-density areas (Fig. 10.4).

Functioning endocrine tumors are typically seen as small, hyperdense masses on contrast-enhanced images (Fig. 10.1–10.8). It should be stressed that the contrast to surrounding pancreatic tissue may be low. This holds true particularly for images obtained in the parenchymal phase (phase of peak parenchymal enhancement) (Fig. 10.5). It is therefore necessary to pay particular attention to the presence of small, hyperdense lesions. Cine-display evaluation of images on the computer console is an essential part of the procedure. Occasionally, functioning endocrine tumors appear as partially cystic or necrotic lesions, or they may be relatively hypovascular (FINK et al. 1985; ROCHE et al. 1983). If water has been used as an oral contrast medium, endocrine tumors located in the duodenum (gastrinomas) can be detected as enhancing masses (WINTER et al. 1996) (Fig. 10.8). In general, liver metastases show the same features as the primary tumor; central necrosis may be somewhat more pronounced.

Non-functioning tumors are usually larger (4--15 cm). Large zones of intratumoral hemorrhage and necrosis are commonly detected (Fig. 10.9). Another typical feature is the presence of a strongly enhancing outer component.

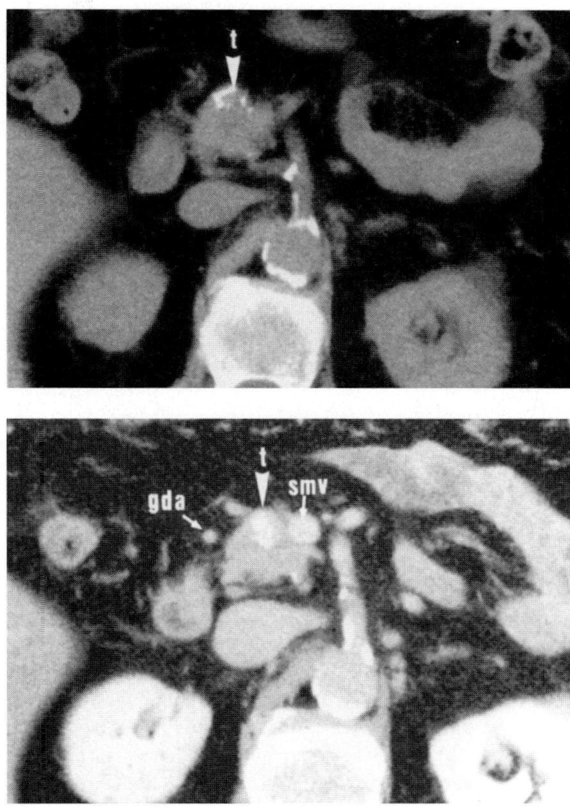

a

b

Fig. 10.3a,b. Calcified insulinoma. **a** Unenhanced computed tomography (CT) image shows calcifications *(arrowhead)* in the ventral portion of the pancreatic head. Note atheromatous calcifications in the abdominal aorta and in the superior mesenteric artery. **b** CT after IV injection of iodinated contrast medium. The calcification becomes invisible due to the marked enhancement of the small (diameter 6–7 mm) insulinoma. gda, Gastroduodenal artery; smv, superior mesenteric vein; t, tumor

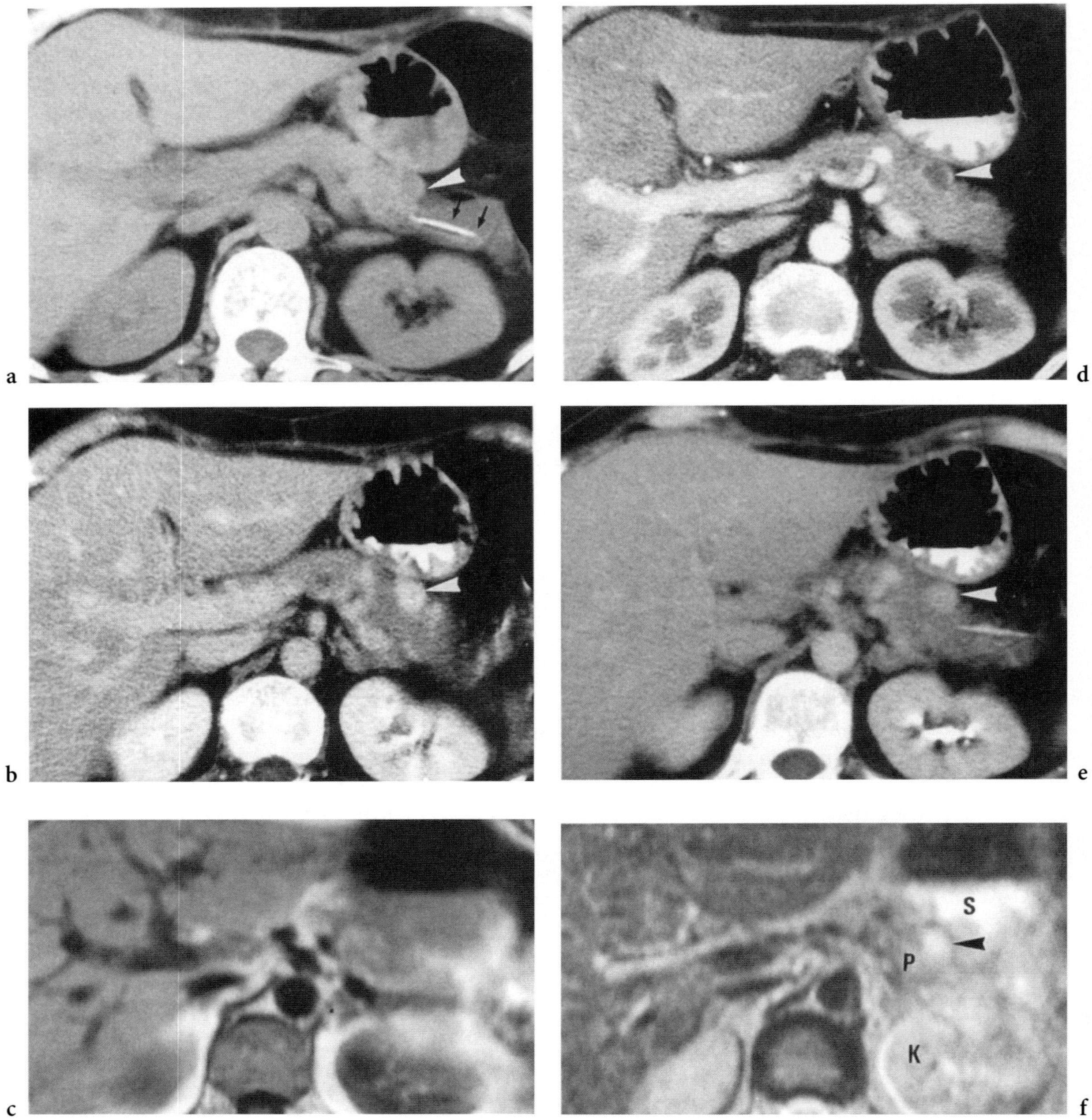

Fig. 10.4a–f. Partially necrotic gastrinoma. **a** Unenhanced computed tomography (CT) image shows small hypodense area (arrowhead) in the pancreatic tail. Slight bulging of the ventral border of the pancreatic tail. Intestinal tube *(arrows)* present. **b** Contrast-enhanced CT image obtained at 15 s shows typical ring-like peripheral contrast enhancement (arrowhead). **c** Contrast-enhanced CT image obtained at 100 s shows homogeneous enhancement of the lesion *(arrowhead)*. The increase in density of the central portion of the lesion may at least partially be explained by diffusion of contrast medium. **d** Contrast-enhanced CT image obtained at 5 min shows persisting enhancement of the lesion *(arrowhead)*. **e** T1-weighted spin echo magnetic resonance (MR) image fails to show the lesion. **f** T2-weighted spin echo MR image shows tumor as a moderately hyperintense lesion *(arrowhead)*. *P*, pancreatic parenchyma; *S*, stomach; *K*, left kidney

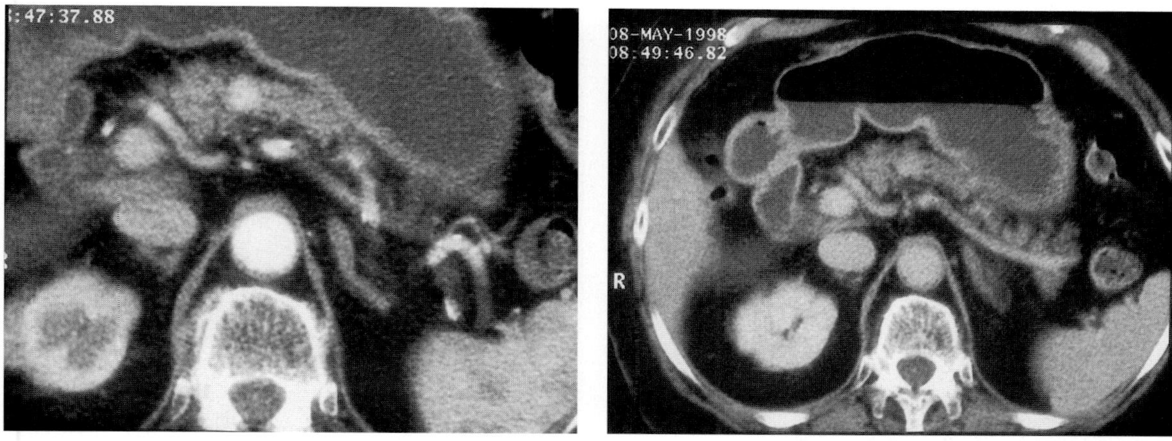

a b

Fig. 10.5a,b. Small functioning endocrine tumor (insulinoma). Typical features on dual-phase helical computed tomography (CT). a CT image obtained in the arterial phase shows a small hypervascular lesion in the pancreatic neck (arrow). b CT image obtained in the hepatic phase shows less contrast between the lesion and surrounding parenchyma

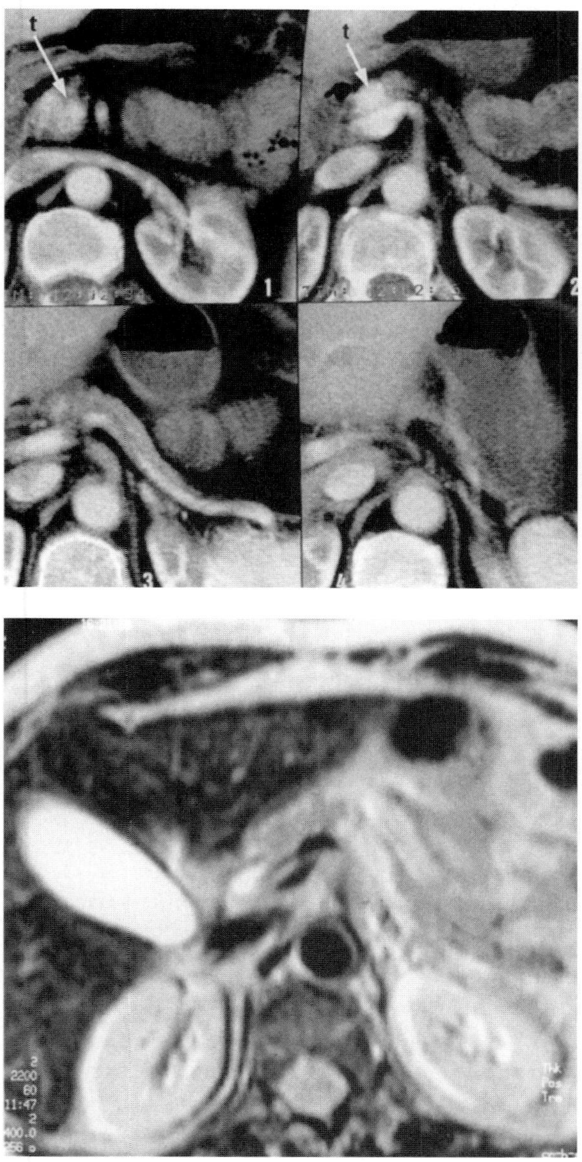

a

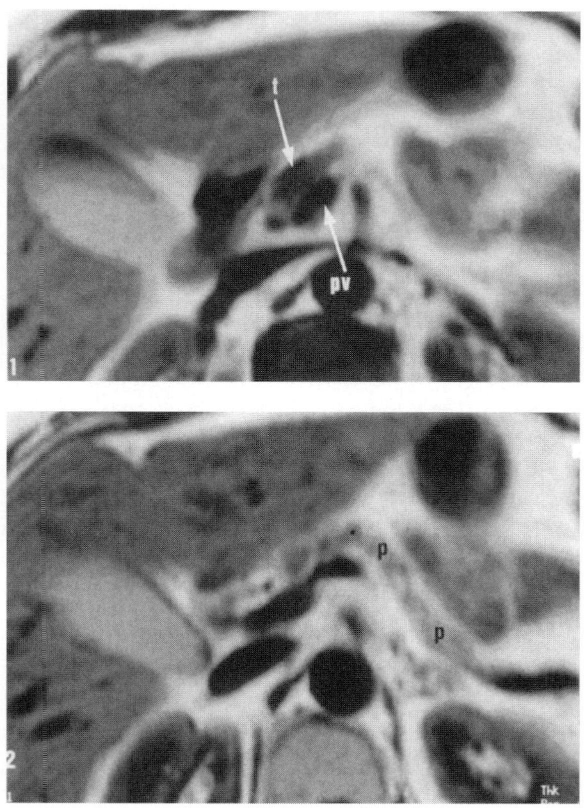

b c

d

Fig. 10.7a–d. Insulinoma. a Spiral computed tomography (*CT*) (1–4, four adjacent 5-mm slices). The tumor (*t*) is clearly seen as a small, strongly enhancing area in front of the portal vein on the most caudal slices (*1* and *2*). b,c T1-weighted spin echo magnetic resonance (MR) image shows the tumor as a hypointense lesion in the most caudal slice (**b**). *p*, pancreas; *pv*, portal vein; *t*, tumor. **d** T2-weighted spin echo MR image. The tumor is iso-intense with the pancreatic parenchyma and thus invisible

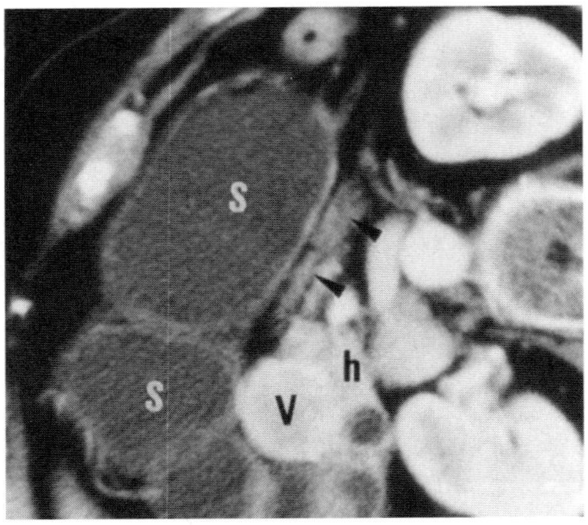

Fig. 10.6. Vipoma. Contrast-enhanced computed tomography (CT) image obtained with the patient in a right lateral decubitus position shows a strongly enhancing mass (*V*) in the pancreatic head (*h*). Atrophic pancreatic tail *(arrowheads)*. S, stomach

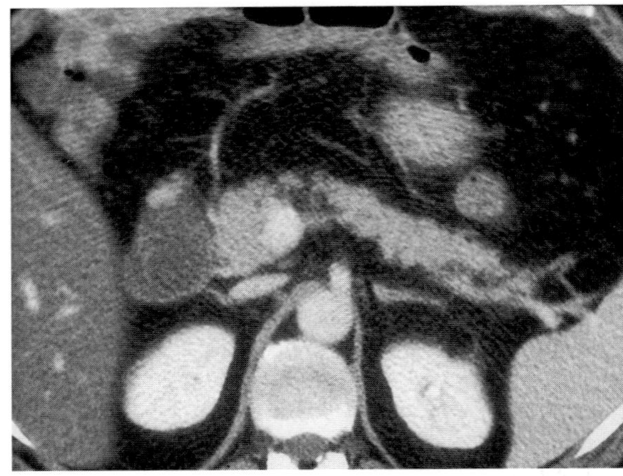

Fig. 10.8. Gastrinoma in the duodenal wall. Contrast-enhanced computed tomography image shows a hypervascular lesion in the ventral wall of the second part of the duodenum *(arrow)*: gastrinoma

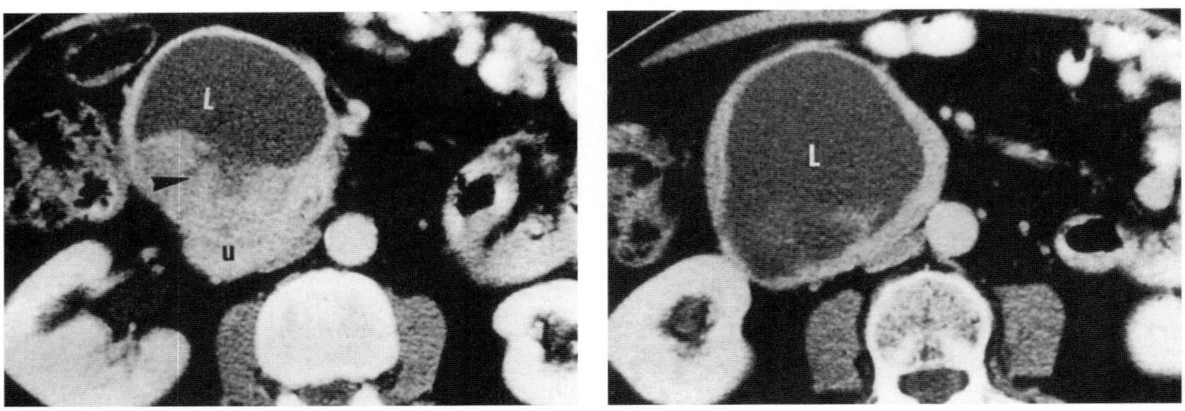

a b

Fig. 10.9a,b. Non-secreting "cystic" endocrine tumor. Contrast-enhanced computed tomography images show a thick-walled, fluid-containing mass originating from the uncinate process of the pancreas (u). The caudal and dorsal portion of the tumor contains a solid component (arrowhead). The ventral portion has a liquid (L) content

10.2.3.3
Value

Non-helical CT has given rather disappointing results for detecting endocrine tumors of the pancreas. Sensitivities reported vary between 50% and 80% (Krudy et al. 1984; Rossi et al. 1985). Initial experience with dual-phase helical CT has been promising (Van Hoe et al. 1995b). These results have been confirmed in recent studies (Chung et al. 1997; KING et al. 1998). In our experience, the overall sensitivity of helical CT is 80%--90%. It is clear that detection of very small tumors is beyond the scope of this technique. CT after direct intra-arterial injection of iodinated contrast media is probably more sensitive. However, because of its invasive character, it is not used in most centers.

10.2.4
Magnetic Resonance Imaging

10.2.4.1
Technique

The magnetic resonance imaging (MRI) technique used for the evaluation of endocrine tumors is essentially the same as that used for the evaluation of non-endocrine tumors (see Chap. 8). As in CT, administration of an oral contrast medium and a spasmolytic agent may be critical to detect lesions in the duodenal (or gastric) wall. Non-contrast-enhanced T1- and T2-weighted images and dynamic contrast-enhanced MR images are routinely obtained in order to optimize the detection of pancreatic tumors and hepatic metastases (SEMELKA et al. 1993). Dynamic gadolinium-enhanced imaging is usually performed using a multislice spoiled gradient echo sequence.

10.2.4.2 Imaging Findings

Most islet cell tumors are well visualized on T1-weighted MR images due to the high inherent contrast between hypointense tumors and hyperintense pancreas on T1-weighted images (particularly fat-suppressed images). The typical appearance of an endocrine pancreatic tumor on MR images is a hypointense aspect on T1-weighted images, a hyperintense aspect on T2-weighted images, and a hyperintense aspect on dynamic contrast-enhanced images (SEMELKA et al. 1993; KRAUS and ROS 1994; MITCHELL et al. 1992; PAVONE et al. 1993) (Fig. 10.10). However, the MRI appearance of the different types of endocrine tumors may be variable. Some tumors may, for instance, be isointense or even hypointense on T2-weighted images (VAN HOE et al. 1998) (see Fig. 10.7). Moreover, endocrine tumors may be invisible on contrast-enhanced images, because both the tumor and the surrounding tissue enhance significantly. Therefore, a combination of different types of images (T1-weighted, T2-weighted, and dynamic gadolinium-enhanced) is mandatory to detect as many lesions as possible. The same holds true for the detection and characterization of hepatic metastases: gastrinoma metastases usually

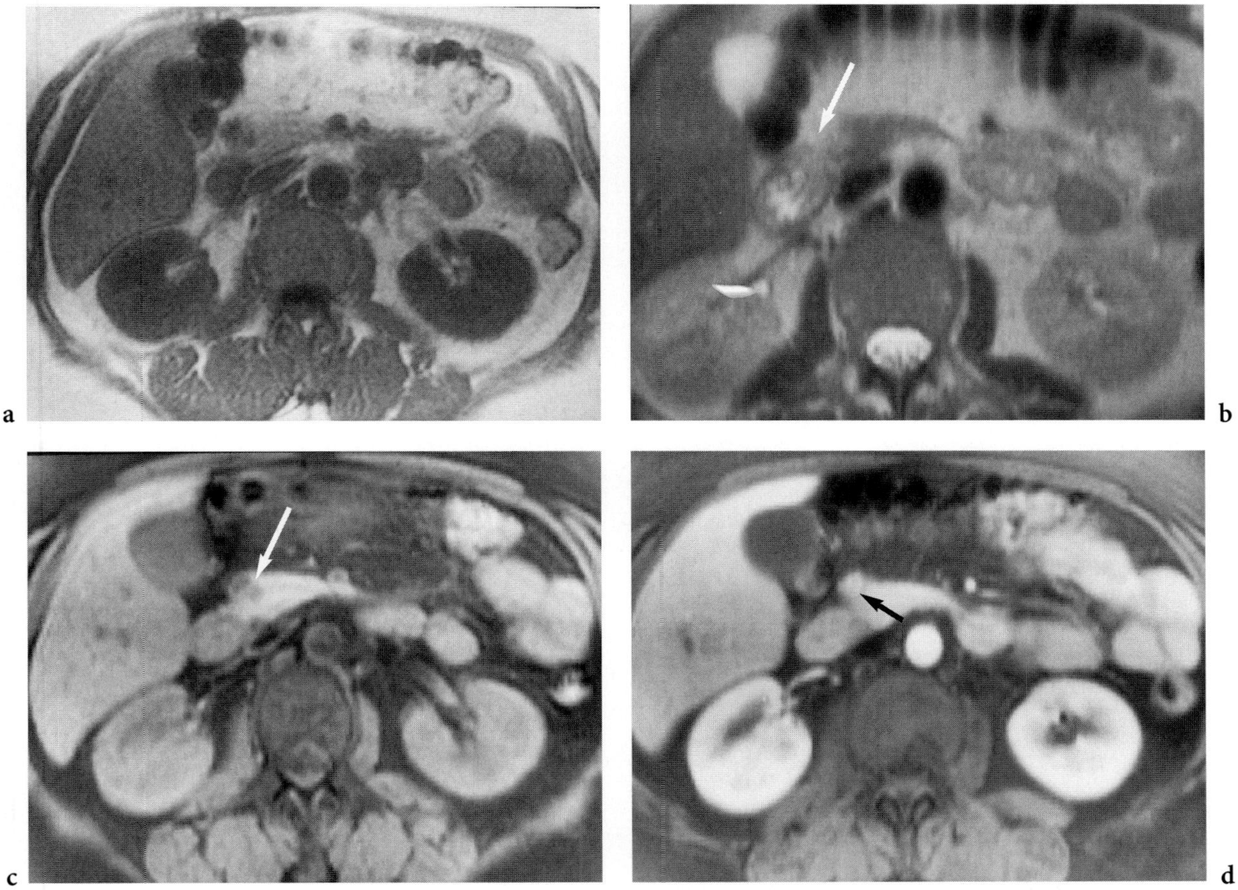

Fig. 10.10a–d. Small insulinoma. Magnetic resonance imaging features. **a** T1-weighted image shows small hypointense lesion in the pancreatic neck (arrow). **b** T2-weighted image shows the tumor as slightly hyperintense *(arrow)*. **c** Fat-suppressed T1-weighted image obtained before IV administration of contrast medium shows the tumor as hypointense *(arrow)*. **d** Fat-suppressed T1-weighted image obtained after IV administration of contrast medium shows the tumor as an enhancing mass *(arrow)*. Note that the tumor is now nearly ISO intense to normal pancreatic parenchyma

have very high signal intensity on T2-weighted images and may mimic hemangiomas. It has been demonstrated that the addition of delayed contrast-enhanced T1-weighted images is mandatory to differentiate metastases of gastrinomas from liver hemangiomas (Berger et al. 1996).

On dynamic contrast-enhanced images, endocrine tumors may appear as homogeneously enhancing masses or may show ring-like enhancement. The latter pattern of enhancement is most commonly seen in insulinomas (Semelka and Ascher 1993). Gastrinomas and insulinomas tend to be small. Occasionally, they contain cystic components. Functioning tumors other than insulinomas and gastrinomas are usually relatively large and heterogeneous. Non-functioning endocrine tumors are usually large and commonly contain large zones of intratumoral hemorrhage and/or necrosis.

10.2.4.3 Value

As in CT, the sensitivity of MRI largely depends on the technique used. In our experience, snapshot MRI has approximately the same sensitivity as dual-phase helical CT. Theoretically, MRI has the advantage of enabling lesion detection based on exploitation of more than one contrast mechanism: besides differences in contrast uptake patterns between endocrine tumors and normal parenchyma, differences in T1 and T2 relaxation rates are usually large enough to make these lesions visible. On the other hand, contrast-enhanced MR images may be somewhat less valuable than contrast-enhanced CT scans: since the normal pancreas has a high signal intensity on non-enhanced T1-weighted images (particularly on those obtained with fat suppression) and endocrine tumors tend to be hypointense on non-enhanced images, hypervascular lesions may become isointense after injection of contrast media.

Because MRI and CT exploit different contrast mechanisms, it is not surprising that applying both techniques may yield complementary results in individual patients.

10.2.5 Differential Diagnosis

Morphologic differentiation by radiological imaging methods of the different types of functioning endocrine pancreatic tumors is not possible. Only the diameter of some lesions may be indicative of their exact type.

Differentiation between primary and secondary (metastatic) hypervascular pancreatic tumors (renal cell carcinoma, thyroid carcinoma, malignant melanoma) may be equally difficult based on morphologic evaluation (Fig. 10.11); however, the clinical setting is usually quite different.

Cystic and hypovascular functioning endocrine tumors exist; however, they may be confused with other pancreatic neoplasms. Unlike in adenocarcinoma, obstructive dilatation of the pancreatic duct is rare in endocrine tumors.

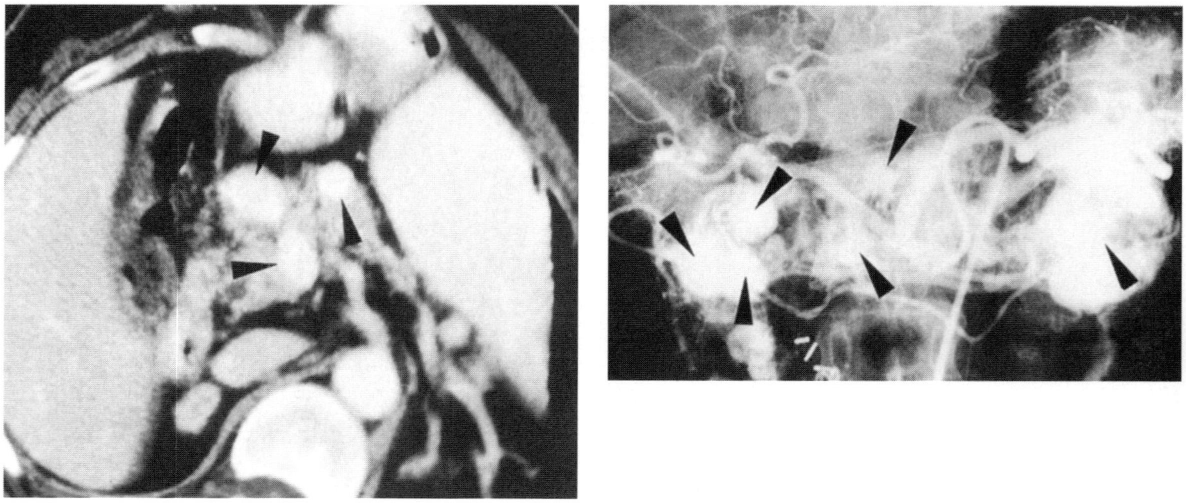

a b

Fig. 10.11a,b. Pancreatic metastases (renal adenocarcinoma). **a** Contrast-enhanced computed tomography image obtained with the patient in a right lateral decubitus position shows three strongly enhancing nodular structures (arrowheads) in the pancreatic head and body. **b** Arteriography confirms the presence of multiple hypervascular lesions of variable size

False positive findings are rare but may be the result of a misdiagnosis of a vascular anomaly such as an aneurysmal dilatation of the pancreaticoduodenal or splenic arteries or tortuosity of the splenic artery (Figs. 10.12, 10.13). These pitfalls are usually easily avoided by tracing the course on the artery on consecutive images. Arteriovenous malformations of the pancreas constitute another potential pitfall; the unsharp definition of the lesion may be a clue to a correct diagnosis (Fig. 10.14).

Finally, non-functioning endocrine tumors may be difficult to distinguish from cystic adenocarcinoma and mucinous cystic neoplasms.

a

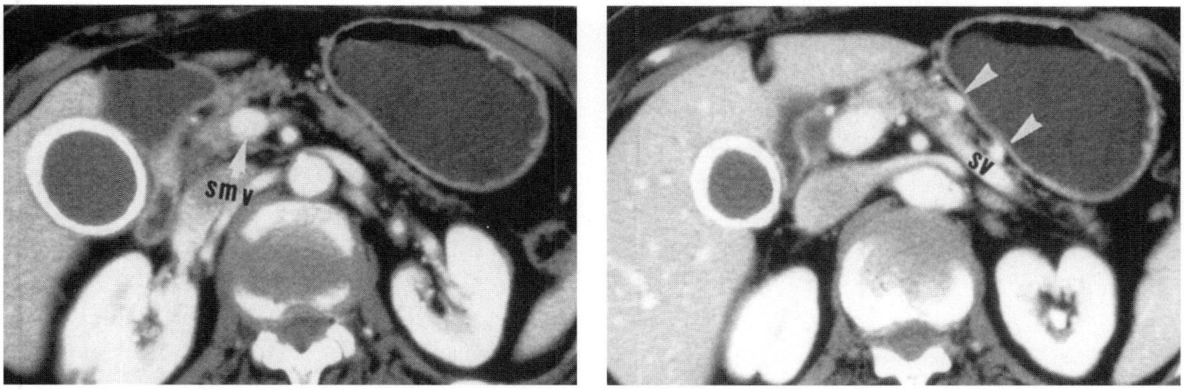

b

c

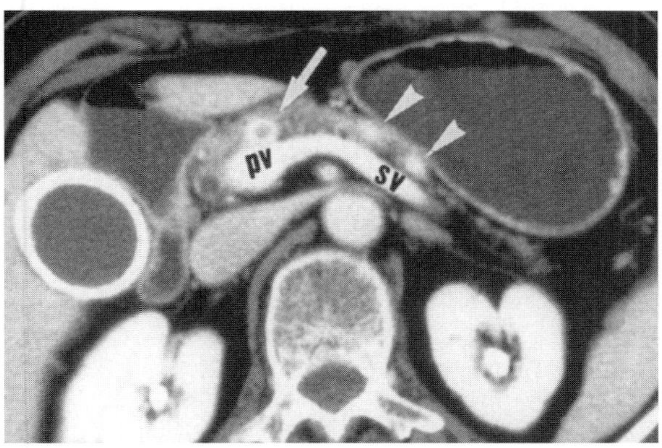

Fig. 10.12a–c. Nonsecreting endocrine tumor in the pancreatic neck; false image of endocrine tumor in the tail of the pancreas. **a–c** Computed tomography (*CT*) after IV iodinated contrast medium from caudally (**a**) to cranially (**c**). a Contrast-enhanced CT image shows atrophic pancreas. smv, Superior mesenteric vein. **b** Contrast-enhanced CT image obtained at a more cranial level reveals small (<10 mm) lesion with strong peripheral enhancement *(arrow)*, located close to the portal vein (pv). Two short segments *(arrowheads)* of tortuous splenic artery coursing ventrally and cranially to the pancreatic tail may erroneously suggest two additional pancreatic tumors. sv, Splenic vein. **c** On this more cranial section, the two round enhancing structures *(arrowheads)* are clearly situated outside the pancreatic tail

a

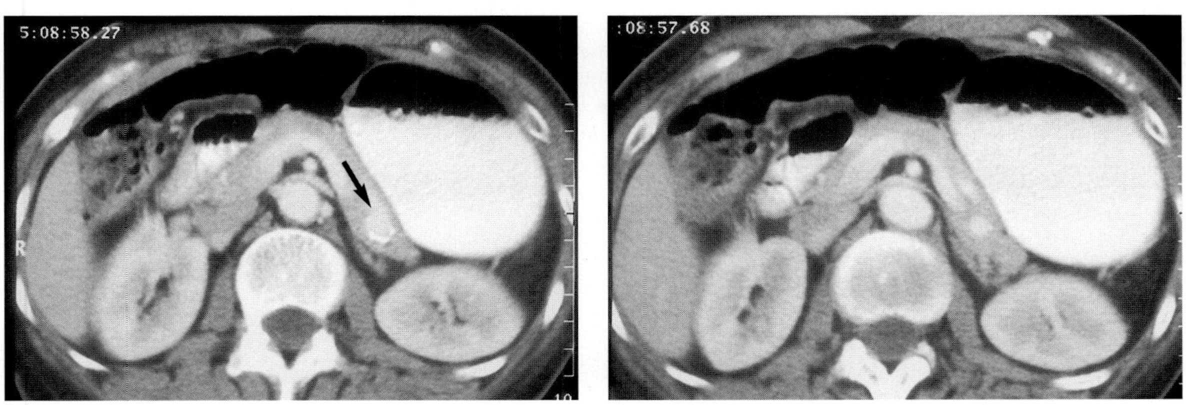

b

Fig. 10.13a,b. An aneurysm mimicking an endocrine tumor. **a** Contrast-enhanced computed tomography image obtained in the pancreatic phase shows a partially calcified hypervascular lesion in the pancreatic tail (arrow): endocrine tumor? **b** This contiguous image shows a normal splenic artery. The lesion shown in (**a**) represented a partially calcified aneurysm of the splenic artery

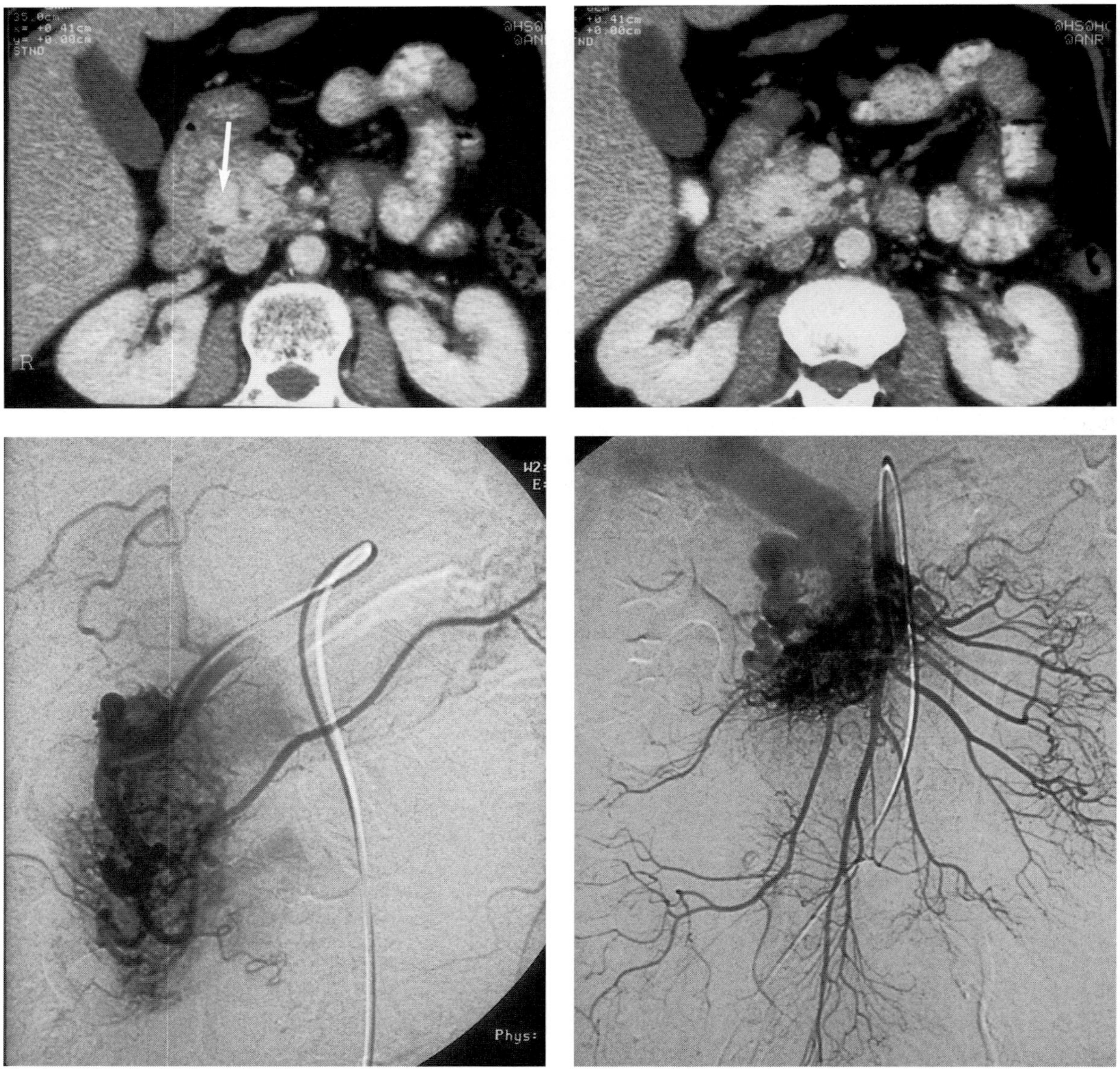

Fig. 10.14a–d. An arteriovenous malformation mimicking an endocrine tumor. **a** Contrast-enhanced image obtained at the level of the pancreatic head/neck shows a small hypervascular mass *(arrow)*: endocrine tumor? **b** Contrast-enhanced image obtained at a more caudal level shows a more diffuse hyperdense area surrounding the common bile duct and pancreatic duct: this appearance would be very unusual for a tumor. **c,d** Arteriographic images obtained after catheterization of the gastroduodenal (**c**) and superior mesenteric (**d**) arteries show the typical appearance of an arteriovenous malformation. Note enhancement of the portal vein in (**d**). (Courtesy of J. Callens, MD)

10.3 Endoscopic Ultrasonography

E. Thérasse and A. Roche

10.3.1 Introduction

Visualization of functioning pancreatic islet cell tumors is often difficult with most conventional imaging modalities, since patients are symptomatic at an early stage owing to the endocrine secretion while the tumor is still rather small. Though localization of vipomas and glucagonomas is less problematic [these tumors are usually larger (Gianello et al. 1988; Palazzo et al. 1992)J, CT, angiography, and transabdominal ultrasonography have a relatively high failure rate in the detection of insulinomas and gastrinomas (Galiber et al. 1988; Gianello et al. 1988; Glover et al. 1992; Grant et al. 1988; Palazzo et al. 1992; Rosch et al. 1992a). Intraoperative ultrasonography is highly accurate but prolongs the duration of the operation and requires diagnosis to be made confidently before surgery. Furthermore, since these tumors may not be palpable at surgery in up to 20% of cases (Norton et al. 1988; Rosch et al. 1992a), preoperative localization remains important and endoscopic ultrasonography is one of the best ways to achieve this goal.

10.3.2 Technique

Pharyngeal local anesthesia and intravenous sedation are given as for conventional endoscopy. The ultrasound probe, which is attached to the end of a side-viewing endoscope, is positioned down to the descending duodenal loop under fiberoptic guidance. To facilitate contact with the mucosa and to improve transmission of the ultrasound beam, the stomach is water filled and a balloon covering the transducer is inflated with water (Lightdale et al. 1991). The endoscope and attached transducer are then slowly withdrawn altogether while scanning through the duodenum pylorus, and stomach wall up to the esophageal hiatus (Glover et al. 1992). Rotation of the high-frequency (7.5–12 MHz) transducer provides real-time 360° axial images perpendicular to the long axis of the endoscope. Images of the pancreatic head are obtained from the duodenal loop and examination of the body and tail is done from the posterior wall of the gastric corpus and fundus (Rosch et al. 1991). The procedure may be repeated whenever necessary and the whole examination lasts 10–45 mm (Glover et al. 1992; Palazzo 1991; Rosch et al. 1992a).

10.3.3 Advantages

Endoscopic ultrasonography (EUS) allows scanning of the pancreas under ideal conditions for ultrasonographic imaging (Palazzo 1991): (a) high-frequency resolution, (b) very close proximity of the pancreas to the US probe, and (c) no bony or air interposition degrading the images.

The high-resolution imaging of EUS can distinguish structures as small as 2–3 mm in diameter (Rosch et al. 1992a), and lesions as small as 6 mm may be detected in most cases (Glover et al. 1992). EUS also provides good evaluation of bowel layers and this is important in cases of extrapancreatic gastrinomas, which are most often found in the duodenal wall (Glover et al. 1992). EUS is noninvasive and less time consuming than blood sampling or arteriography. Furthermore, EUS fine-needle (24G) aspiration biopsy has recently been described and this new technique may eventually reduce the false-positive rate of EUS (Vilman et al. 1992), especially in pancreatic head lesions.

10.3.4 Inconveniences

The depth of penetration of the ultrasound beam depends on the transducer frequency. Though very good resolution is obtained at 7.5–12 MHz imaging is limited to about 6–8 cm from the transducer (Glover et al. 1992; Kimmey et al. 1992) and large pancreatic lesions may not be adequately evaluated. In fact, this is rarely a problem since most islet cell tumors measure less than 2 cm (Galiber et al. 1988; Glover et al. 1992). EUS axial images are different from those usually provided by conventional ultrasonography and require experience to interpret. As with other imaging modalities, EUS may have blind areas and this is especially so in the region of the splenic hilum (Glover et al. 1992). The large diameter of ultrasonic endoscopes, their longer nonflexible tip, and their oblique viewing optic make duodenum entrance more difficult than with standard endoscopy, especially if scarring is present (Glover et al. 1992; Kimmey et al. 1992).

10.3.5 Features and Accuracy for Pancreatic Endocrine Tumors

The echo pattern of pancreatic endocrine tumors is variable but in most cases they appear as homogeneous hypoechoic lesions with clearly demarcated margins (Glover et al. 1992; Palazzo et al. 1992; Rosch et al. 1992a). However, heterogeneous, cystic, hyperechoic, or isoechoic patterns as well as calcifications have been reported, though much less frequently (Palazzo et al. 1992; Rosch et al. 1992a). Irregular margins, parapancreatic lymph nodes, and hepatic metastasis are suggestive of malignancy.

The diagnostic accuracy of EUS for pancreatic tumor detection has been reported to be high (Rosch et al. 1991, 1992b). In a large series of various pancreatic tumors with a predominance of carcinomas, Rosch et al. reported sensitivities of 99% , 90% , 77%, and 67% respectively for EUS, retrograde pancreatography (ERCP), CT, and transabdominal ultrasonography (Rosch et al. 1991). Though the mean tumor size was 4.5 cm, EUS sensitivity was 100% for the 27 lesions measuring less than 3 cm while the sensitivity of other techniques declined.

In most studies, EUS has proved far superior to transabdominal ultrasonography, CT, and angiography in detecting endocrine pancreatic tumors (Galiber et al. 1988; Gianello et al. 1955; Grant et al. 1988; Lightdale et al. 1991; Norton et al. 1956; Rosch et al. 1992a). In these studies, however, EUS was performed with knowledge of the results of other imaging modalities. Palazzo et al. (1992) reported overall diagnostic accuracy rates of 8.5%, 17%, and 87.5% respectively for transabdominal ultrasonography, CT, and EUS in the detection of endocrine pancreatic tumors.

In a large multicenter series of 39 islet cell tumors, EUS was able to localize 32 of the tumors (82% sensitivity) while 18 of 19 control patients were correctly rated as negative (95% specificity) (Rosch et al. 1992a). Moreover, all patients had negative results on transabdominal ultrasonography and CT, and mean tumor size was 1.4 cm. The accuracy of EUS is similar in all regions of the pancreas but detection is more difficult when the tumor is 1 cm or less in size, pedunculated, or isoechoic with the pancreatic parenchyma (Palazzo et al. 1992; Rosch et al. 1992a). Though parapancreatic lymph nodes may be misinter-preted as islet cell tumors, they usually are not palpable at surgery (Lightdale et al. 1991; Norton et al. 1955; Rosch et al. 1992a). EUS can accurately predict portal venous involvement, tumor size, and nodal involvement but is less reliable for the detection of arterial invasion (Rosch et al. 1992b). However, EUS is a locoregional imaging method and distant spread of malignancy has to be evaluated by other, conventional techniques.

10.3.6 Conclusion

Since pancreatic endocrine tumors are often small, conventional CT and transabdominal ultrasonography have a high failure rate for the detection of these lesions. EUS, on the other hand, has a very high accuracy rate even when these tumors measure less than 1 cm. Though no histologic diagnosis can be confirmed with EUS, visualization of a sharply marginated hypoechoic lesion is strongly suggestive of an endocrine tumor in the appropriate clinical setting.

10.4 Intraoperative Ultrasonography

E. Thérasse and A. Roche

10.4.1 Introduction

Preoperative localization of pancreatic islet cell tumors is not always possible and may be especially difficult for gastrinomas, with only 60%–74% of laparotomies finding the endocrine tumor in ZES (Cromack et al. 1957; Norton et al. 1986, 1988). Intraoperative failure to detect the endocrine tumor (by palpation) may lead the surgeon to perform a blind distal pancreatectomy, providing only a 36% success rate (Gianello et al. 1988). This could result in unnecessary morbidity and may also impede future surgical exploration because of post-inflammatory modifications. Therefore, whenever preoperative localization has failed, every effort should be made peroperatively to detect the occult pancreatic endocrine tumor, and intraoperative ultrasonography (IOUS) has been shown to be especially useful in this setting.

10.4.2 Technique

Before ultrasonographic examination, the lesser sac is surgically opened and the pancreas is dissected free so that the body and tail can be palpated and become easily accessible to ultra-sound scanning. After full operative exposure of the pancreas, the abdominal cavity is filled with warm saline to improve transmission of the ultrasound beam (Grant et al. 1988; Norton et al. 1988). Sterility is preserved by inserting the US probe into a long sterile plastic sleeve containing gel at the distal tip to provide additional acoustic coupling (Galiber et al. 1988; Norton et al. 1988). Repeated sagittal and longitudinal scanning is thoroughly performed with the transducer held 0.5–1 cm anterior to the pancreatic surface. Optimal scanning of the pancreatic head, uncinate process, and duodenum may be obtained after manual mobilization of these structures (Grant et al. 1988; Norton et al. 1988). Though earlier studies used 5- to 7.5-MHz probes, recent ones were performed with 10-MHz transducers (Galiber et al. 1988; Gianello et al. 1988; Norton et al. 1988).

10.4.3 Features and Accuracy for Pancreatic Endocrine Tumors

The appearance of most islet cell tumors on IOUS is similar to that described with preoperative US (Galiber et al. 1988; Norton et al. 1988). These lesions are typically hypoechoic in comparison with the pancreas and demonstrate discrete echoic borders. Isoechoic and hyperechoic lesions associated with a peripheral hypoechoic halo have also been reported, especially in young patients, who tend to present a less echoic surrounding pancreas (Gorman et al. 1986; Grant et al. 1988; Norton et al. 1988). Hyperechoic insulinomas may be accompanied by refractive shadows which may help their identification (Gorman et al. 1986). While tumoral size alone does not predict malignant potential (Norton et al. 1988), indistinct lesion margins with extension into adjacent pan-creas and obliteration of the pancreatic duct are findings suggestive of malignancy.

The sensitivity of IOUS is high, especially for the detection of insulinoma. Islet cell tumors as small as 3 mm have been detected (Gorman et al. 1986) and some series have reported up to 100% sensitivity when IOUS is used in association with intraoperative palpation (Galiber et al. 1988; Gianello et al. 1988; Norton et al. 1988). Studies including gastrinomas have generally yielded slightly less good results, mainly because of the relatively low detection rate of extrapancreatic tumors by IOUS (Cromack et al. 1987; Norton et al. 1988). Sensitivity also declines in cases of multiple small insulinomas (Gianello et al. 1988; Grant et al. 1988), which are almost always encountered in patients with clinically apparent MEN-1 syndrome. In fact, the low detection rate in these cases is not so problematic because enucleation of all the tiny tumors is not feasible and therefore subtotal panereateetomies are generally performed whatever the results of imaging modalities (Palazzo 1991 ; Palazzo et al. 1992).

In a study including 44 patients who underwent surgical exploration for suspected pancreatic endocrine tumor, either peroperative palpation or ultrasonography revealed a suspicious lesion in 39 patients, and 33 had one or more pathologically proven islet cell tumors (Norton et al. 1988). Excluding the five patients who showed no suspicious lesion using either method, intraoperative US sensitivity was 83% and 86% for gastrinomas and insulinomas respectively (Norton et al. 1988). Results were still better (93% overall) for intrapancreatic lesions because the detection rate of extrapancreatic tumors was only 53%. Unfortunately, IOUS showed 11 false-positive localizations which proved to be ectopic pancreas or lymph nodes in most cases. However, other authors have detected insulinomas of a mean diameter of 1.4 cm with 84% -90% sensitivity, without any false-positive results (Galiber et al. 1988; Gorman et al. 1986; Grant et al. 1988).

10.4.4 Advantages

Intraoperative ultrasonography may localize lesions that have not been detected by any imaging technique preoperatively (Galiber et al. 1988; Norton et al. 1988). IOUS imaging findings can suggest tumor malignancy and therefore prompt the surgeon to resect (instead of enucleate) the endocrine tumor (Norton et al. 1988). Since the majority of gastrinomas are malignant, this ability to assess malignancy may be more useful for these tumors than for insulinomas (Norton et al. 1988). IOUS also depicts the precise relationship of the islet cell tumor to the pancreatic and common bile ducts, helping the surgeon to determine the type of resection needed (Galiber et al. 1988; Gianello et al. 1988). Furthermore, IOUS is helpful in patients who have already undergone pancreatic surgical exploration, since the inflammatory reaction to the previous surgery often gives rise to a nodular-feeling pancreas, impeding localization by palpation (Grant et al. 1988).

10.4.5 Inconveniences

Intraoperative ultrasonography requires experience and adds time to the operation (Norton et al. 1988). Small tumors in the duodenum have a high likelihood of not being imaged (Norton et al. 1988), and IOUS may be more helpful in localizing insulinomas than gastrinomas, which are extrapancreatic in up to 50% of cases (Cromack et al. 1987; Norton et al. 1986, 1988). Because the transducer is difficult to position under the left costal margin, it may not be easy to accurately image the pancreatic tail, unless the spleen and tail of the pancreas are mobilized out of the retroperitoneum or unless a right-angle high-resolution transducer is used (Galiber et al. 1955; Norton et al. 1955). As with other imaging modalities, small impalpable false-positive images in the pancreatic head are problematic because the pancreatoduodenectomy necessary to remove a lesion in this area has a high (30%) morbidity and mortality (Cromack et al. 1957).

10.4.6 Conclusion

Intraoperative ultrasonography is particularly useful when preoperative localization of a pancreatic endocrine tumor has failed. However, even when preoperative localization is positive, bus is a useful adjunct to palpation and may affect surgical management either by demonstrat-mg further lesions that are not palpated or by suggesting malignancy not suspected by palpation alone. Furthermore, IOUS may ease the decision as to the optimal surgical approach by clearly depicting the vascular and pancreatic ductal anatomy.

10.5 Arteriography

A. Roche and E. Thérasse

10.5.1 Technique

Arteriographic investigation of the pancreas in search of endocrine tumors should opacify at least the celiac and superior mesenteric areas. The mesenteric injection should be sufficiently proximal as not to miss a proximally located dorsal pancreatic artery. These selective injections should precede any superselective catheterization maneuver, even if only with a guide wire. Superselective injections are then frequently necessary to clearly display the small lesions. In an effort to eliminate artifacts, it is always reassuring to analyze a pancreatic area from opacifications obtamed by the injection of two different pedicles. Study of the most distal portion of the tail of the pancreas, especially when the spleen is enlarged and superimposed, may necessitate oblique views or, even better, superselective injections. Subtraction images are indispensable. Digital sub-traction makes this possible, but even for the 1024 × 1024 matrices, loss of spatial definition often greatly impairs analysis of the very tiny vessels on which the diagnosis is usually based, and on the other hand, the higher contrast generates hyper-vascular false-positive images. For these reasons, we believe that conventional imaging with excel-lent photographic subtraction is still better, given the present state of digital subtraction angiography matrices.

The liver must always be carefully studied, in search of metastases which can be detected only by arteriography when they are tiny and hypervascularized.

The extrahepatic, peripancre atic portal system must also be perfectly analyzed, since invasion of these veins also indicates malignancy.

10.5.2 Signs

When the tumor is large, it is most often completely hypervascular with central hypodense zones. No doubt, these are not situations in which arteriography is most helpful; nevertheless, it has the advantage of differentiating quite clearly between a non-secreting endocrine tumor and a pancreatic adenocarcinoma that never has this appearance.

When the tumor is small, the most characteristic signs are the following:

1. Early opacification from peripheral vascularization (this is an adenoma) which forms a small, very localized mass effect. The pathologic nature of the arterial bowing can be easily asserted when it involves the intrapancreatic vessels since, normally, only the arterial branches that run along the pancreas from one surface of the organ to the other, form loops. This arterial bowing is a sign of primary importance since it is present even when the lesion is hypodense or isodense (Fig. 10.15).
2. During the capillary phase, the tumor stain is homogeneous, perfectly circumscribed, and more or less hypervascular, depending on its specific nature and on the arterial injection's degree of selectivity (Figs. 10.16, 10.17).
3. At later times, the hypervascularization often quickly vanishes and may have disappeared at the 15 th second.

Venous invasion by a malignant tumor is generally recognized by an abrupt occlusion and the development of a portoportal type of collateral circulation in the absence of an intra- or suprahepatic obstruction. Exceptionally, the tumor may present a macroscopic endovenous tumoral bud that follows the portal system in a hepatopetal fashion (Fig. 10.18) (Bok et al. 1984).

The tiny hepatic metastases are identical in character to the pancreatic tumor. The tumor stain may

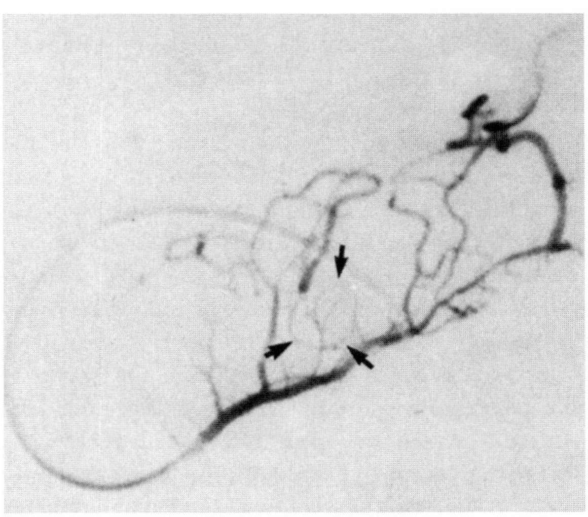

Fig. 10.15. Insulinoma of the body of the pancreas. No blush is visible, but small intraglandular corporeal arteries are abnormally displaced by the lesion *(arrows)*, permitting the diagnosis

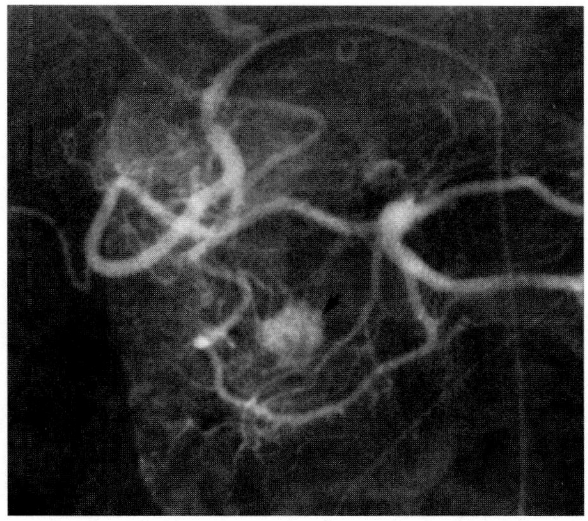

Fig. 10.16. Typical aspect of insulinoma: dense, early, homogeneous, and well-delimited staining of the adenoma (arrow). Note that tumoral branches exhibit a mass effect

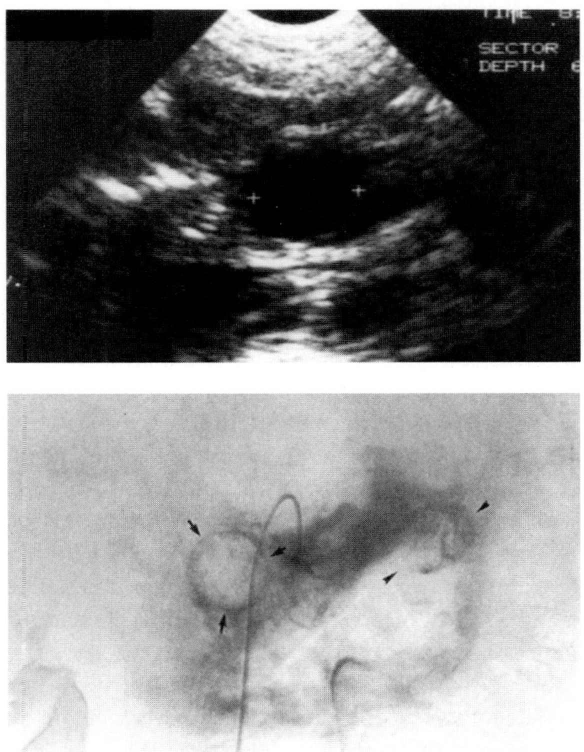

a

b

Fig. 10.17a,b. Exceptional case of cystic insulinoma. a Cystic mass developed into the right part of the pancreatic body and detected by ultrasonography. b Arteriography shows a round avascular mass presenting a very thin and regular hypervascular ring *(arrows)*. Also note a second, but typical, insulinoma of the tail *(arrowheads)*. At pathologic study, the cystic insulinoma presented only one layer of endocrine cells around the cyst, and cystic liquid contained a high level of insulin

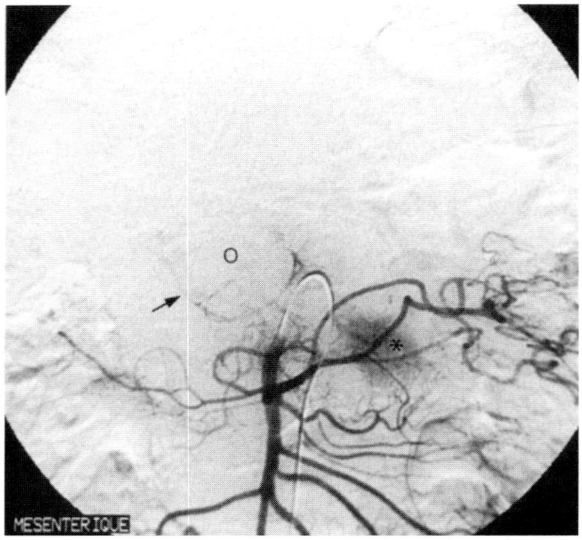

a

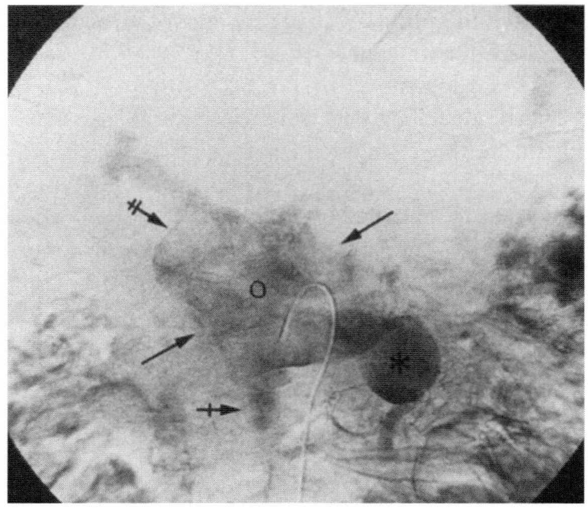

b

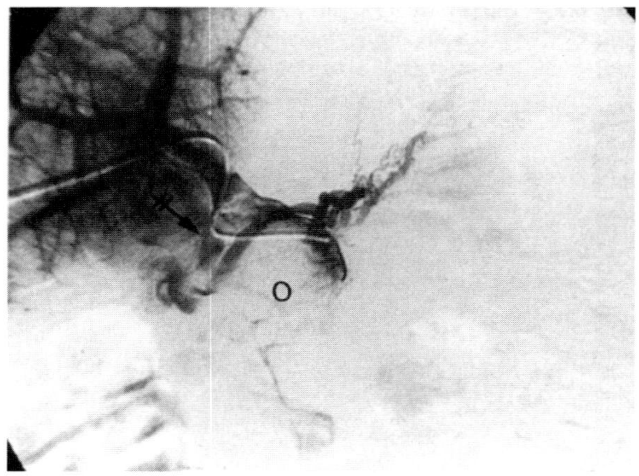

c

Fig. 10.18a–c. Malignant pancreatic endocrine tumor that secreted thyrocalcitonin. a,b Arteriography of the superior mesenteric artery. c Transhepatic portography. A tumoral cast (*black circle*) is seen growing into the lumen of the superior mesenteric (*crossed arrow*) and the portal veins (*double crossed arrow*), and deriving from the pancreatic tumor (*star*); the tumoral blush is highly typical of adenoma upon injection of the superior mesenteric artery (**a,b**) (early, dense, and well-limited blush). The tumoral endoluminal cast itself is mildly hypervascular (arrows). Transhepatic opacification of the portal vein (**c**) shows a tumoral lacuna (black circle) enlarging the vein and obviously coming from the pancreatic area

be relatively persistent and differentiation from a hemangioma is practically impossible if the lesion is very small. When the metastatic lesions are large, they often become heterogeneous, and at times are pseudocystic, even without treatment, as is frequent with hepatic metastases of endocrine origin.

Particularly in ZES, metastatic adenopathies often have the same features as the primary tumor. The adenom~ and one or more metastatic adenopathies may even coexist on the same image (Roche et al. 1982) (Fig. 10.19).

The main causes of false-positives are:

1. An accessory spleen: its hilar vascularization is a fundamental difference when compared to the adenoma. It remains hyperdense for a longer period, its dynamic being closer to the normal spleen.
2. Metastatic adenopathy: there is nothing to differentiate it from an adenoma and this is an insoluble problem in malignant tumors when the adenopathy is in close contact to the pancreas, particularly in ZES.
3. A duodenal ulcer (frequent in ZES), which may be hypervascular but shows no sign of a mass effect.
4. End-on vascularization of an anteroposteriorly oriented pancreatic tail.

False-negatives, other than lesions that are too small or insufficiently vascularized to be visualized, are most often the result of anatomic misinterpretations, which lead unknowingly to a mere partial opacification of the pancreas. In this regard, we must stress the importance of syste-matically opacifying at least the celiac trunk and the superior mesenteric artery, since certain tumors (such as some tumors of the pancreatic head) may be vascularized by the superior me-senteric artery only. We also stress the fact that a very high degree of catheterization selectivity in no way guarantees a better diagnosis if it precedes the selective injections. Because it causes spasms , superselective catheterization may on occasion have the opposite effect of masking the lesion.

a

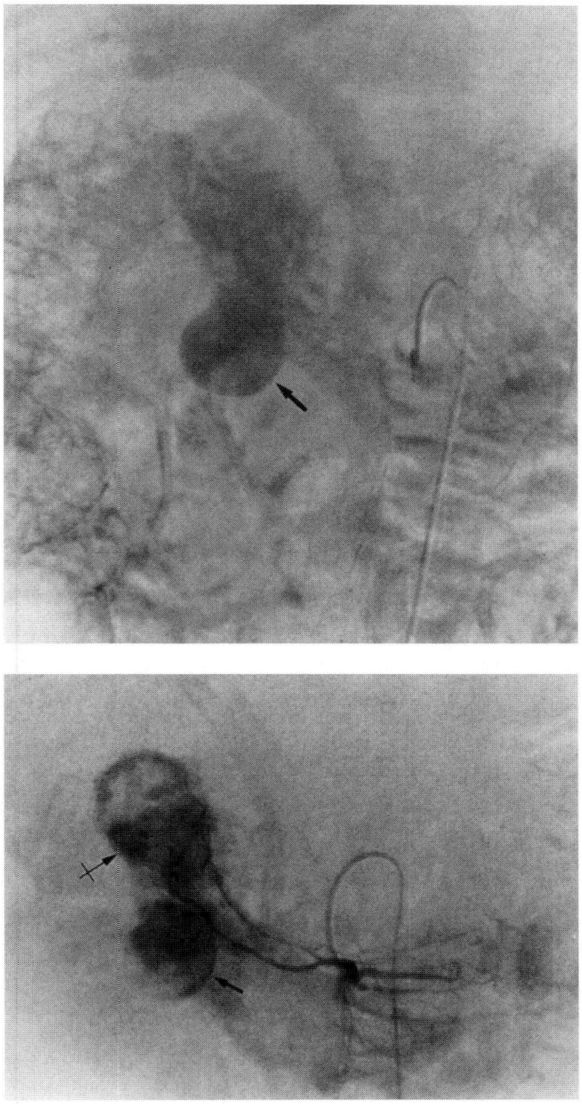

b

Fig. 10.19a,b. Metastatic adenomegaly mimicking gastrinoma in Zollinger-Ellison syndrome. **a** Opacification of the superior mesenteric artery shows typical signs of adenoma of the pancreatic head (*arrow*). **b** Selective opacification of the inferior duodenopancreatic artery shows the same lesion partially opacified (*arrow*) and another smaller blush (*crossed arrow*). At surgery, the larger lesion was a metastatic adenomegaly and the smaller one a gastrinoma

10.5.3 Results in the Different Types of Tumors

Detection of endocrine tumors of the pancreas is generally considered to be one of the great successes of diagnostic arteriography, with cer-tam small series reporting as high as 100 % sensitivity (Boijsen and Samuelsson 1970; Clouse et al. 1977; Collen et al. 1984; Fujii et al. 1974; Fulton et al. 1975; Hautefeuille et al. 1979; Huguet et al. 1978; Pistolesi et al. 1977). Though it is true that the signs can be particularly characteristic, in all series with more than 50 cases, arteriography's positivity is barely greater than 50 %.

In the large insulinoma series, arteriographic sensitivity remains between 50% and 55% (Galiber et al. 1988; Boissel and Proye 1985). It can drop below 30% when multiple lesions are involved (Galiber et al. 1988). Clearly artenography's performance is not as good as in the smaller series initially published, especially since 25% of diagnosed insulinomas are not hypervascular, or only slightly so (Roche et al. 1983).

In ZES the highest rate of positivity reported is 68% (Maton et al. 1987); however, the sensi-tivity usually reported for pancreatic tumors and for hepatic metastases is about 35% (Mignon et al. 1987). The false-positive rate for gastrinoma is high, from 8% to 35%. Like Mills et al. (1979), we have encountered a false-positive rate of about 30% (Roche et al. 1983), due essentially to confusion between gastrinoma and metastatic adenopathy (Fig. 10.19).

Because they are large and almost clearly malignant when diagnosed, rare or nonsecret-mg tumors pose no identification problems for arteriography.

10.6 Radioendocrinologic Localization Methods

A. Roche and E. Thérasse

10.6.1 Transhepatic Venous Sampling

10.6.1.1 Generalities

The techniques for entry and catheterization of the portal system were fine-tuned by the Swedish authors in the 1970s (Reichardt and Ingemansson 1980; Lunderquist et al. 1975; Ingemansson et al. 1975, 1976, 1977). These techniques allow for morphologic study of the pancreatic veins in cases of tumor or inflammatory disease and collection of pancreatic efferent venous blood samples to localize secreting tumors. This last application has benefited from the improved methods in radioimmunoassay, which now give very precise results on very small blood samples

10.6.1.2
Justification

Justification for the method stems from:

1. The small size of the most frequent endo-crine tumors of the pancreas (insulinoma, gastrinoma), which often eludes morphologic localization techniques
2. The possible presence of micropolyadenomatoses or hyperplasias which of necessity go undetected with morphologic examination

Pancre atic venous sampling circumvents these difficulties by localizing the tumor, not because of its space-occupying effect but through the abnormal secretions it produces and pours into its venous drainage system, the intensity of which is quite independent of tumoral size. Therefore, for each case study, this investiga-tion necessitates the most complete pancreatic venous mapping possible on which, point by point, will be reported the results of hormonal assays. An accurate knowledge of the anatomy of the pancreatic and peripancreatic veins is therefore indispensable in conducting and interpreting this examination.

10.6.1.3
Anatomy of the Pancreatic Veins

(Calas et al. 1956; Keller et al. 1980; Reichardt and Cameron 1980)

As always for venous systems, individual van-ations are frequent and dictate a personalized interpretation of each examination. An overall outline which is divided into three systems head, body and tail, and neck (or isthmus) – may, however, be described and serve as a reference (Fig. 10.20).

10.6.1.3.1
Veins of the Pancreatic Head

This system is composed of three superficial arcades (posterior, anterior, and inferior) and one intraglandular arcade. It has three principal efferent veins: the posterior superior, anterior inferior and posterior inferior pancreaticoduodenal veins.

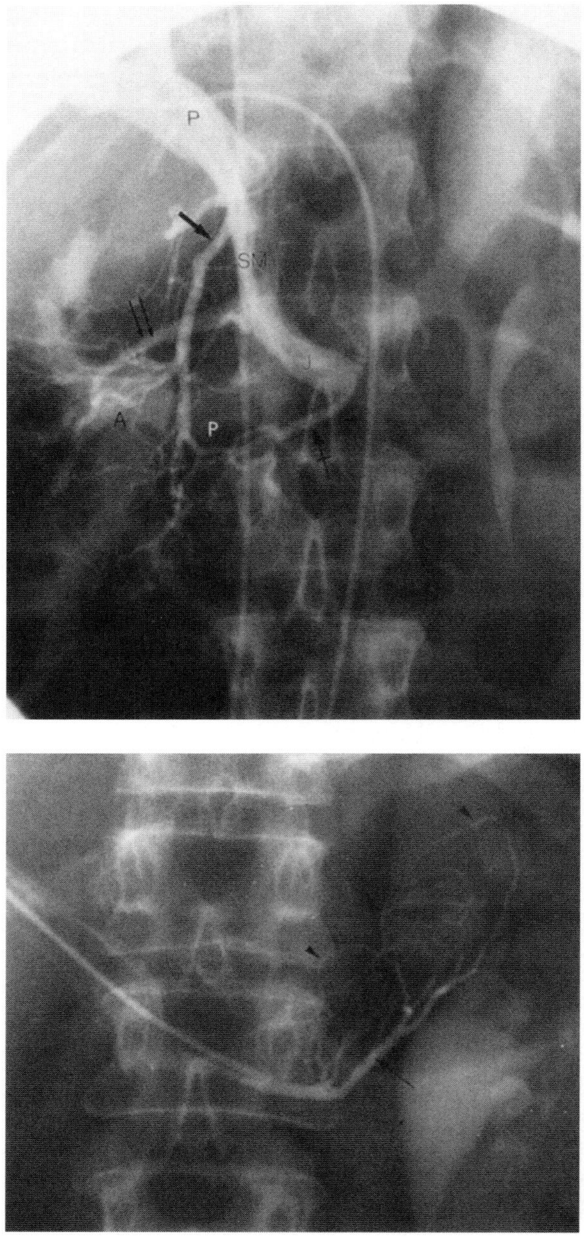

a

b

Fig. 10.20a,b. Radiologic anatomy of pancreatic veins. **a** Injection into the posterior superior duodenopancreatic vein (*arrow*) with opacification of the cephalic arcades – anterior (*A*), posterior (*P*), and inferior (*I*) – and of the anterior inferior (*double arrow*) and posterior inferior (*crossed arrow*) duodenopancreatic veins. *SM*, superior vein; *P*, portal vein; *J*, first jejunal vein. **b** Injection into the transverse pancreatic vein (*arrow*) with opacification of numerous dorsal pancreatic veins (*arrowheads*) draining into the splenic vein

Posterior Superior Pancreaticoduodenal Vein. In our experience, the posterior superior pancreati-coduodenal vein is the head's principal drainage pedicle in 940/o of cases. Usually it drains into the right posterior face of the inferior two-thirds of the main portal vein; much more rarely it drains into the angle it forms with the superior mesenteric vein and, exceptionally, into the superior mesenteric vein. Given the functional importance of this vein in the head's drainage, secreting cephalic tumors, regardless of their location, drain predominantly into this pedicle in more than three quarters of cases; its catheterization is therefore imperative.

Anterior Jnferior Pancreaticoduodenal Vein. The anterior inferior pancreaticoduodenal vein generally empties into the gastrocolic trunk. Remember that the latter is not constant and that its forming branches empty individually, or in-completely joined, into the superior mesenteric vein.

Posterior Jnferior Pancreaticoduodenal Vein. Most frequently, the posterior inferior pancreaticoduodenal vein empties into the first jejunal vein; sometimes its anastomosis slides into the second jejunal vein.

Posterior Cephalic Venous Arcade. The posterior cephalic venous arcade extends between the medial branch of the posterior superior vein and the superior branch of the posterior inferior vein. This arcade is located at the posterior surface of the gland and superior mesenteric vessels. It is generally easy to identify since it is clearly inside the other arcades of the head and, unlike them, is often straight or only slightly concave above and to the left. Compared with the anterior arcade, it receives few duodenal veins.

Inferior Cephalic Venous Arcade. The inferior cephalic venous arcade lies suspended between the medial branch of the anterior inferior vein and the inferior branch of the posterior inferior vein. It runs along the uncinate process and ascending duodenum from which it receives the respective branches and passes behind the superior mesenteric vessels. It is easy to identify, given its very inferior location running very closely along-side the duodenum and showing a very pro-nounced superior concavity.

Anterior Cephalic Venous Arcade. Lying between the lateral branch of the posterior superior vein and the lateral branch of the anterior inferior vein, the anterior cephalic venous arcade goes around the common bile duct on the outside. This cephalic arcade is the most difficult to identify clearly on venography because of the many super-imposed large duodenal pedicles it receives, as well as antral and pyloric veins which drain into the right gastroepiploic vein. Its general position is somewh~t vertical and slightly concave on the left. Throughout almost its entire course, it is generally the most lateral arcade.

Intrapancreatic Cephalic Veuous Arcade. The intrapancreatic cephalic venous arcade lies 5115-pended between the medial branch of the posterior superior vein and the medial branch of the anterior inferior vein. It descends between the common bile duct and the pancreatic duct and between the two pancreatic ducts. Seldom is it clearly identifiable on angiography. It then projects vertically between the anterior arcade (more laterally) and posterior arcade (more medially).

Anastomoses. Aside from their neck and corporeal venous anastomoses the cephalic veins are also anastomosed with the medial colic veins, the gastric veins, the biliary veins, and the intrahepatic portal system.

10.6.1.3.2 Veius of the Body aud Tail of the Pancreas

Two venous systems drain the body and tail of the pancreas: multiple and more or less vertical veins drain into the splenic vein, homologous to the pancreatic corporeal arteries, and there is also a horizontal venous axis, homologous to the transverse pancreatic artery.

Pancreatic Corporeal Veins. The corporeal veins are constant and empty into the splenic vein. The left gastric vein occasionally receives, at its ending, a large pancreatic vein which drains the right side of the body. The left gastroepiploic vein receives one or more small veins which drain the left extremity of the tail, homologous to the caudal pancreatic arteries. Depending on their relationship to the splenic and pancreatic veins, they can follow a descending or an ascending course. In the right part of the body, they most often follow an ascending, almost vertical course, since the splenic vein is generally above the pancreas. In the medial and left part of the body, their course usually slants towards the left and is close to horizontal.

Transverse Pancreatic Vein. The transverse pancreatic vein represents the longitudinal drainage axis of the body and tail. We found one or more well-defined transverse pancreatic veins in 56 cases in a series of 100 complete venographies. In three cases, there were two transverse veins of equal size. This vein empties into the inferior mesenteric vein half the time, but only, it would seem, when the latter drains markedly to the right, into the superior mesenteric vein or at the angle it forms with the splenic vein. In the other cases, it drains into the splenic vein's ending.

Anastomoses. The corporeal veins are extensively anastomosed to each other and to the transverse pancreatic vein. When the latter is not clearly individualized, the longitudinal anastomoses of the corporeal veins to each other are the equivalent. Both venous systems are anastomosed to the other isthmic and cephalic pancreatic veins. Like their homologous arteries, they are anastomosed to the middle colic veins, the veins of the left colic angle, and the gastric and epiploic veins, following a course similar to the arterial anastomoses.

10.6.1.3.3
Veins of the Neck ofthe Pancreas

The veins of the neck (or isthmus) of the pancreas form an anastomotic bridge between the cephalic and corporeal systems. Quite often, however, the drainage is well individualized, with two isthmic veins. On pancreatic venography, an isthmic vein is identified by its median position and by its anastomoses with the cephalic arcades and with the corporeal venous system.

Superior Jsthmic Vein. The superior isthmic vein empties into the splenic vein 5 ending, generally on its upper side. We have also seen it drain into the left gastric vein or the superior mesenteric vein.

Posterior Jsthmic Vein. The posterior isthmic vein empties into the inferior mesenteric vein, generally very close to its ending. Sometimes, it empties into the superior mesenteric vein just beneath the angle with the splenic vein into an accessory middle colic vein that drains into the superior mesenteric or even into the splenic vein.

10.6.1.4
Technique and Methodology
(Roche et al. 1982, 1983)

The technique of entry into the portal system has been well described in the literature (Doyon et al. 1979; Hoevels et al. 1978). For reasons of cornfort, the examination is usually conducted under general anesthesia, in which case it is important to ensure that the drugs used do not interfere with the metabolism of the hormones being assayed.

The venous sampling technique is subject to a few rules that limit the number of artifacts and errors in interpretation, as outlined in the following paragraphs.

Given the systematically laminar blood flow into the large trunks, it is vital that selective pancreatic samples be collected, to avoid very serious misinterpretation of assay results.

The small size of the veins used for blood sampling may sometimes necessitate a wedged catheterization which may artificially increase the hormone concentration in the blood sample, stopping the flow upstream. This risk may be avoided by comparing a simultaneous assay of another parameter, independent of the pathology being investigated.

The iodinated contrast media in the blood sample may interfere with the hormonal radioimmunoassay above a certain threshold (30% in the sample collected for gastrin). This can be avoided by collecting the blood samples either before any local injection or after careful aspiration of the contrast agent. As demonstrated for parathyroid adenomas (Doppman et al. 19~1b), contrast media may have a toxic effect on the endocrine tumor cells of the pancreas, leading to an inordinate release of hormones. However, this risk of inter-ference seems to be fairly low given the numerous anastomoses in pancreatic vascularization.

In our experience, the simultaneous use of stimulation tests does not help in localizing in-sulinomas and gastrinomas. In cases of insulinoma, however, it seems essential to keep the patient's glycemia low and stable, through close monitoring during examination. The aim is to preferentially lower physiologic secretion , since tumoral secretion is not very sensitive to the glucose stimulus. Hyperglycemic medications should be stopped at least 2 days before the examination. As for gastrinoma, anti-H_2 treatment is continued since it does not alter gastrin secretion, and its discontinuation could risk aggravating the disease.

Having taken these precautions, persistent errors in interpretation are linked to anatomy on the one hand, and to imperfect knowledge of normal secretory mapping on the other.

10.6.1.5
Indication

It should be kept in mind that transhepatic venous sampling is indicated strictly for localization purposes in patients whose diagnosis is otherwise formally established. In this regard, we must emphasize that while the pancreatic secretion of gastrin is in itself abnormal (even though it is practically impossible to differentiate between a duodenal and a cephalic pancreatic secretion) the same does not hold for insulin, whose physiologic secretion is also asymmetrical (being higher in the tail). In our experience, patients with insulin-secreting tumors always present high peripheral levels during the examination (systematically carried out at a low sugar level), in contrast to normal subjects. Conversely, some patients with insulinoma had an insulin level in the lesion's drainage vein that was lower in absolute terms than the levels sometimes encountered at the same location in normal subjects.

10.6.1.6
Overall Findings

According to the various reported series, the effectiveness of venous sampling for the purpose of localization ranges between 90% and 100% (ROCHE et al. 1982; BURCHARDT et al. 1979; DOPPMAN et al. 1981a; KALLIO and SUORANTA 1979; LARSSON et al. 1977; MILLAN et al. 1979; MITTY al. 1979; PASSARIELLO et al. 1975; PASSARO 1979; TURNER et al. 1978). One series involving only eight patients showed very poor results (DAGGETT et al. 1981) (62.5% false localizations). Our experience has led us to a different strategy, depending on the type of secreting tumor to be localized.

10.6.1.7
Localizing Value According to Tumor Type

10.6.1.7.1
INSULINOMA

The findings of different investigations in some important series are summarized in Table 10.3. The results of pancreatic venous sampling (PVS) (Tables 10.4-10.6) are excellent in insulinoma and we believe that PVS is currently indispensable for definitive preoperative localization of these endocrine tumors (HOULBERT et al. 1984) (Figs. 10.21-10.23). Indeed, this pathology is so rare, with almost no recurrences (FENICHEL et al. 1983), so benign after complete exeresis, and so serious after inappropriate pancreatic exeresis that it seems futile to discuss such and such an investiga-tive algorithm when all methods should be ex-hausted to ensure localization with certitude. In a series of 1067 cases collected by SEFANINI et al. (1974), the tumor was found in 76% of the cases with the first exploratory laparotomy procedure and in 11% of the cases with the second; 7% of tumors were never found. With knowledge of the preoperative radiologic examinations, the surgeon

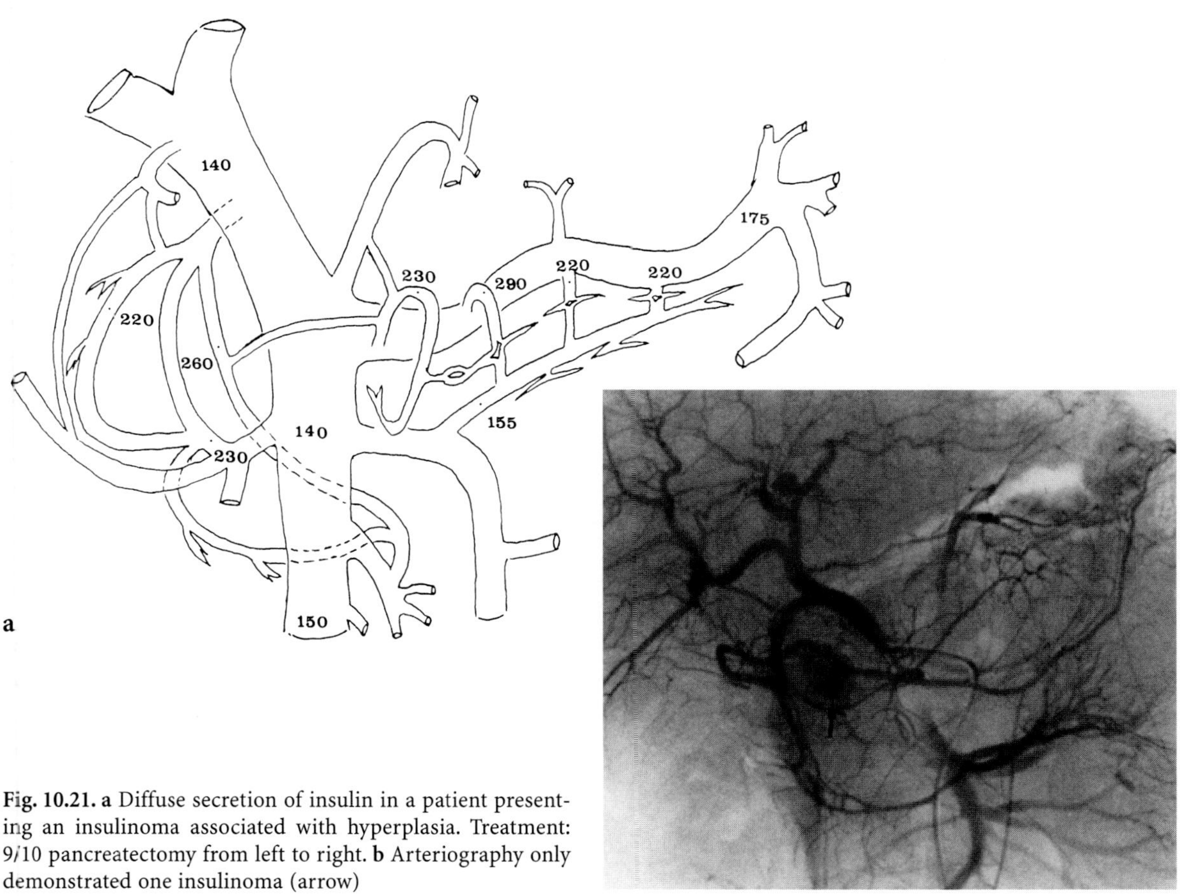

a

b

Fig. 10.21. a Diffuse secretion of insulin in a patient presenting an insulinoma associated with hyperplasia. Treatment: 9/10 pancreatectomy from left to right. b Arteriography only demonstrated one insulinoma (arrow)

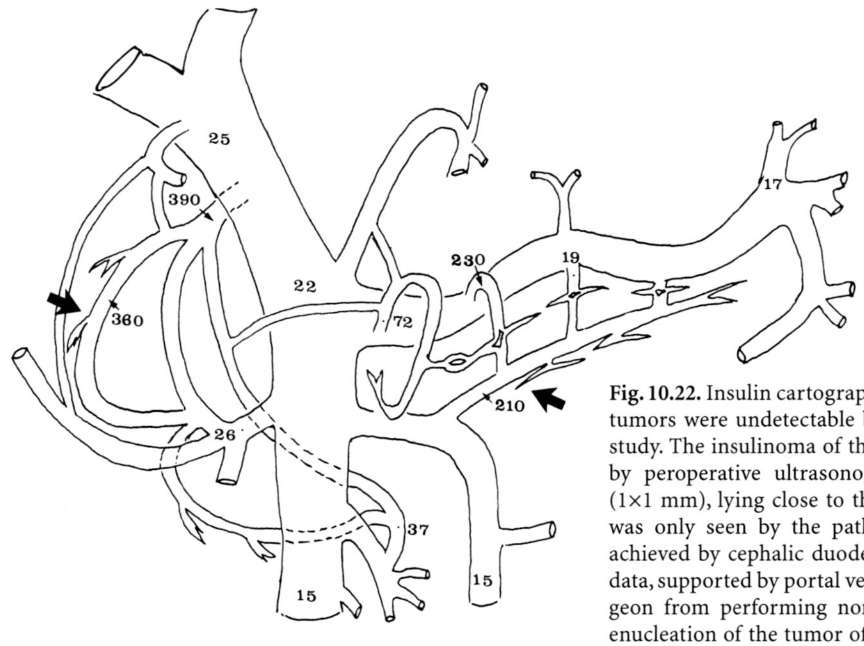

Fig. 10.22. Insulin cartography in a case of double tumor. Both tumors were undetectable by any preoperative morphologic study. The insulinoma of the body (10×10 mm) was detected by peroperative ultrasonography, but the cephalic tumor (1×1 mm), lying close to the second part of the duodenum, was only seen by the pathologist. Curative treatment was achieved by cephalic duodenopancreatectomy. (Preoperative data, supported by portal venous sampling, prevented the surgeon from performing noncurative left pancreatectomy or enucleation of the tumor of the pancreatic body)

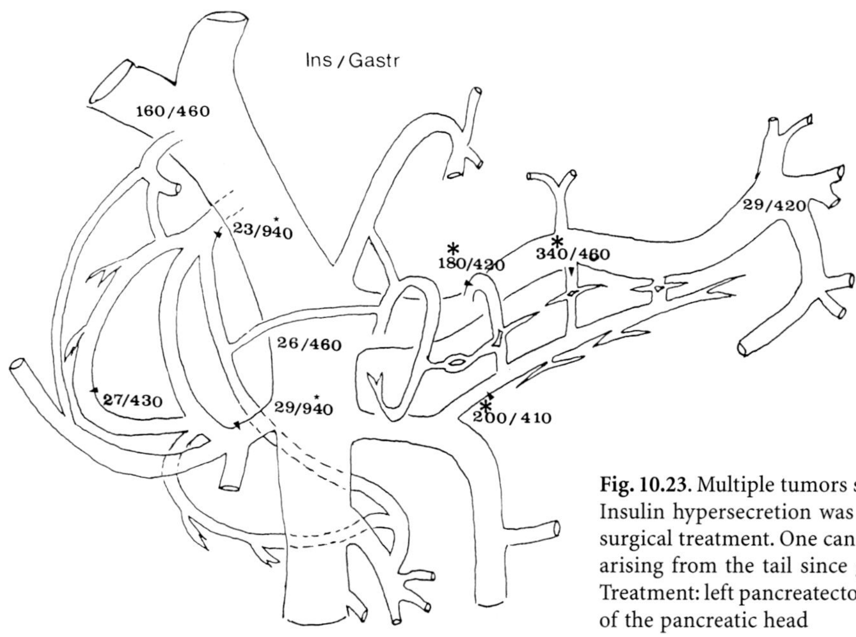

Fig. 10.23. Multiple tumors secreting either gastrin or insulin. Insulin hypersecretion was life-threatening and necessitated surgical treatment. One can ascertain that insulin secretion is arising from the tail since gastrin is secreted into the head. Treatment: left pancreatectomy and enucleation of the tumors of the pancreatic head

sees or palpates the lesion in 80%–90% of the cases. There remains at least one case in ten where he will have to resort to excision on the strength of radiologic examinations alone.

10.6.1.7.2 Zolliger-Ellison Syndrome

The results of radiologic examination and PVS are reported in Tables 10.7 and 10.8. In the experience of the Bichat Hospital (Mignon et al. 1987), when preoperative imaging was negative, surgical exploration found a macroscopic lesion in 77% of the cases, but three times out of four the tumor was ectopic (most often duodenal) (Fig. 10.24). The indication for PVS is very questionable in cases of ZES (Bonfils 1983). While preoperative localization of lesions is important for some (Vinik and Tompson 1986), others

Table 10.3. Sensitivity of morphologic explorations in localized insulinomas. The Mayo Clinic experience concerned 84 tumors in 52 patients (mean size: 14 mm), the AFC survey 240 tumors, and personal experience 88 tumors in 78 patients (mean size: 12 mm)

	US (%)	CT (%)	ART (%)	PVS (%)	POUS (%)	SP (%)	Positive POUS with negative SP (%)	Positive PVS with negative US, CT, ART, SP (%)
Mayo Clinic (Galiber et al. 1988)								
Single tumor	61	30	54		84		16	
Multiple tumors	15	8	29		36		8	
AFC survey (Boissel and Proye 1985)	23	31	53	71		92	0	
Personal series	28	23	55	98		82		16

US, preoperative ultrasonography; CT, computed tomography; ART, arteriography; PVS, pancreatic venous sampling; POUS, preoperative ultrasonography; SP, surgical palpation

Table 10.4. Location of insulinomas in 131 proven tumors (personal series)

Location of tumors	No. of tumors	%
Head	45	34
Neck	14	11
Body	38	29
Tail	34	26
Total	131	100

Table 10.5. Types of tumoral presentation in 110 operated patients with hyperinsulism

	Patients without MEN (%)	Patients with MEN (%)	Total of operated patients (%)
Single tumor	88	28	85
Multiple tumors	7	29	8
Hyperplasia	3	0	3
Hyperplasia + tumor(s)	2	43	4
Total	94%	6%	100

Table 10.6. Results of PVS in 136 patients suspected of having an insulinoma and explored by PVS (personal series)

Results of PVS	Operated					Not operated				
	No.	True localization	False localization	True negative	False negative	No.	Sulfonamide intoxication	Hyperplasia	Normal[c]	Lost to follow-up
Abnormal	103	102				14		7		7
Normal	4			1	3[b]	6	4		2	
Doubtful			1[a]			9			4	5
Total	107	102	1	1	3	29	4	7	6	12

[a] Lack of selectivity in sampling, negative surgical exploration, insulinoma of the pancreatic tail discovered 7 years later

[b] Lack of selectivity in sampling in one case; secretion of undedectable "insulin-like" hormone in two cases

[c] Patients were considered as normal, even if not operated on, when long follow-up (>5 years) showed no further clinical or biologic evidence of insulinoma

claim it does not change the surgical results (Cherner et al. 1986). Indeed, the tumors are multiple in the majority of the cases (McCarthy 1980) and more or less secreting in nature. Only tumors that are secreting sufficiently when samples are collected can be localized. In our experience, secretory localization is in the pancreatic head or in the duodenum in close to 90% of the cases. This means that, nine times out of ten, one would consider cephalic duodenopancreatectomy, since the tumor is too small and not found preoperatively in ca. 40% of Cases. However, authentic eases of complete cure after cephalic pancreatectomy guided by PVS findings have been reported (Hautefeuille et al. 1979). Nonetheless, this intervention seems all the more aggressive, know-mg that in more than 50% of the cases, the then nonsecreting corporeal localizations remain where they are (Deveney et al. 1978), and that in 25% of the cases ZES develops as part of an MEN-I syndrome.

10.6.1.7.3
Glucagonoma

Localization does not usually cause any problem, since the lesion is large when diagnosed. In rare cases where the diagnosis seems probable but the localizing morphologic examinations are negative or contradictory, one may resort to PVS. In six patients thus investigated (Table 10.9) we found evidence of and localized three glucagonomas. Two tumors measured less than 5 mm and one patient whom we hope to have cured completely presented no sign whatsoever of malignancy at the time of diagnosis. In all cases of known glucagonoma, the hormonal gradient in the pathologic area was more than ten times the peripheral value. One must nevertheless be cautious when interpreting these results, since regional or lymphatic secreting metastases are frequent and make the analysis of the hormonal mapping very delicate.

10.6.1.7.4
Vipoma and Other Rare Secreting Tumors

The remarks concerning glucagonoma also apply to vipoma. Venography does not seem to have played a contributing role. It remains, nonethe-less, the only examination that provides any hope of localization or even early diagnosis of these tumors before they reach a size where malignancy is the rule.

10.6.2 Localization Using the Intra-arterial Stimulation Test

10.6.2.1 The Principle

The principle underlying this method is to localize the area of the secreting lesion by identifying the arterial pedicle which, when infused with a product that stimulates tumoral secretion, sig-nificantly increases the hormonal output.

10.6.2.2 Technique

The stimulating agent is injected successively into the principal arteries vascularizing the potentially tumoral areas the splenic, gastroduodenal, and pancreatic arteries for the pancreas and the hepatic artery when liver metastases are suspected. Secretin, 20–30 units in 5 ml saline, is rapidly injected when looking for gastrinoma (Doppman et al. 1990; Imamura et al. 1989). The choice of stimulant is more controversial in cases of insulinoma. Calcium was selected since an IV injection stimulates tumoral secretin secretion (Brunt et al. 1986) without risk of severe hypoglycemia (Doppman et al. 1991). Dosages range from 0.01 (in the obese patient) to 0.025 mEq of Ca^{2+}/kg (recommended dosage for nonobese patients) as a rapid injection of calcium gluconate.

Venous sampling is simultaneously performed in the right and left hepatic veins, before and 30, 60, 90, and 120 s after the injection. Samples from these two hepatic veins are necessary (Doppman et al. 1990) since the splenic portal flow has a tendency to drain preferentially into the left liver, and the mesenteric flow into the right liver. Elevation in hormone levels has a localizing value only in the early samples since only these are affected by the first-pass effect, before systemic redistribution of the stimulant occurs.

10.6.2.3 Findings

Few teams have experience with the technique, but for those that do the results are encouraging.

In ZES, Imamura et al. (1989) reported 100% localization accuracy in 11 cases. They considered the test positive when the elevation in gastrin level was above 80 pg/ml (corresponding to a 120% elevation above the baseline level) after 40 s. Doppman et al. (1991) considered the test positive if the post-

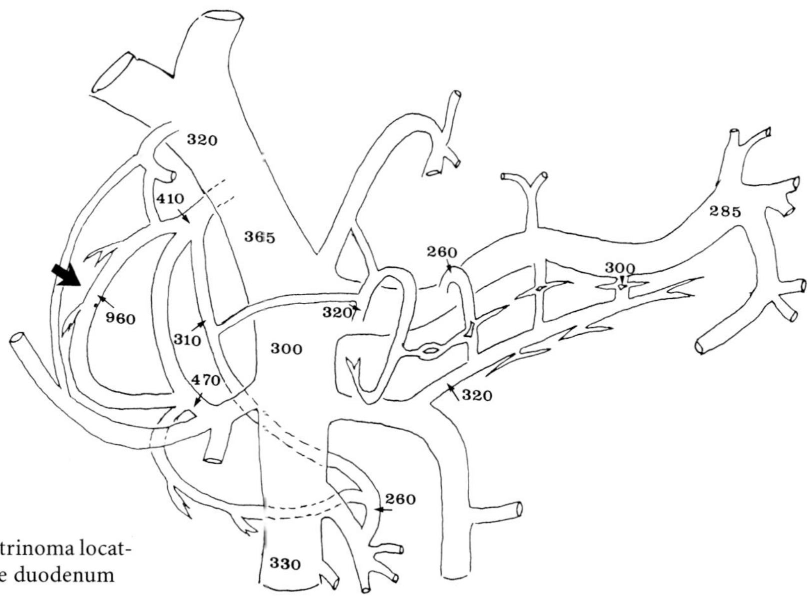

Fig. 10.24. Gastrin cartography in a gastrinoma located in the wall of the second part of the duodenum

Table 10.7. Results of morphologic explorations in ZES in the AFC survey (129 cases studied since 1965) and the Hôpital Bichat experience (69 patients explored from 1974 to 1985; laparotomy performed in all cases)

	US		CT		ART	
AFC survey [8]	VP (%)	FP (%)	VP (%)	FP (%)	VP (%)	FP (%)
	18	6	24	5	25	8
Hôpital Bichat experience [53]	Se (%)	SP (%)	Se (%)	Sp (%)	Se (%)	Sp (%)
Pancreatic tumors	28	93	35	83	35	84
Hepatic metastases	14	100	33	100	33	100

US, preoperative ultrasonography; CT, computed tomography; ART, arteriography; TP, true-positive; FP, false-positve; Se, sensitivity; Sp, specificity

Table 10.8. Comparative results of PVS and surgical exploration in ZES (53 operated patients; personal series)

	Type of lesions (% of patients			Location of lesions (% of patients)		
	Solitary lesion	Multiple lesion	Not identified	Head or duodenum	Body or tail	Head and/or duodenum + body and/or tail
PVS	92.5	7.5	–	86.5	5.6	7.6
Surgical findings	28.3	28.3	43.4	50.0	6.7	43.3

Table 10.9. Results of radiologic explorations in six cases investigated for suspected glucagonoma (personal series)

	US	CT	ART	PVS	Tumor size (mm)	Malignancy	Metastasis
#1	–	False +	–	True +	4	–	–
#2	False + –	–	–	True +	6	+	+ (lymph nodes)
#3	True +	–	True +	True +	25	+	+ (lymph nodes)
#4	–	–	–	–	Not operated on/proved to be normal (8 years' follow-up)		
#5	False +	–	–	–	Not operated on/proved to be normal (11 years' follow-up)		
#6	False +	–	–	–	Not operated on/proved to be normal (6 years' follow-up)		

US, preoperative ultrasonography; CT, computed tomography; ART arteriography; PVS, pancreatic venous sampling; –, negative; +, positive secretin/presecretin gradient was more than 50% after 30 s. The test enabled these authors to localize lesions in seven out of 13 cases investigated and, in one case, to differentiate between hemangioma and hepatic metastases. In this series, arteriography was positive in 38% of the cases, the IA test in 54%, and the PVS in 46%. Overall, the cojnbined score of arteriography and the IA test was 77% which given the mildly invasive nature of the exploratory method, is worthy of note.

In insulinoma the calcium IA test allowed accurate localization in the four cases studied (DOPPMAN et al. 1991), the chosen criteria being a doubling of the insulin level at 30 or 60 s. In the patient with multiple tumors associated with MEN-I syndrome, the tumors could be differen-tiated. The sensitivity ofthe method seems greater for cephalic localizations (Fig. 10.25–10.27). After con-firmation of these findings on more important series, it may well be fitting to add this technique to the arsenal of methods for localizing insulino-mas, especially since it is only mildly invasive.

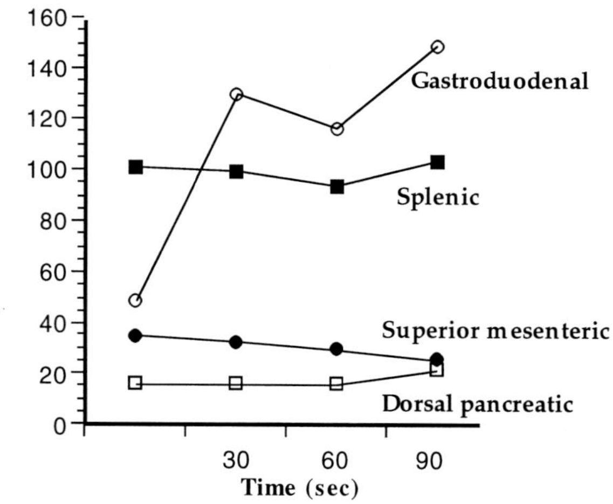

Fig. 10.25. Localization of an insulinoma in the pancreatic head by selective IA infusion of calcium. The gastroduodenal artery is clearly identified as the main feeding branch of the insulinoma. Dorsal pancreatic artery infusion induces very mild insulin secretion. There is no modification of insulin secretion after infusion of the splenic or superior mesenteric arteries

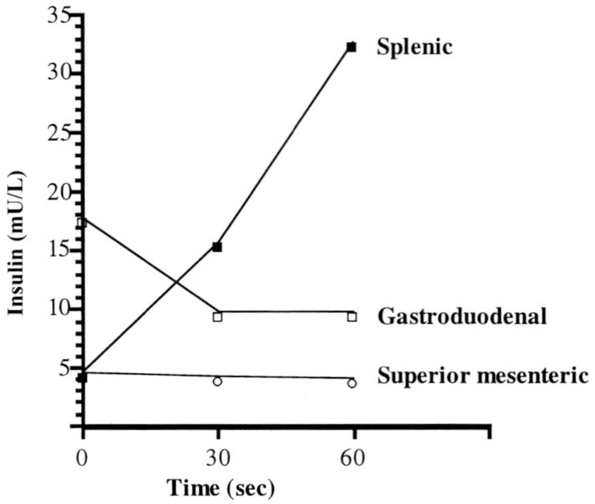

Fig. 10.26. Corporeal insulinoma feeded by the splenic artery

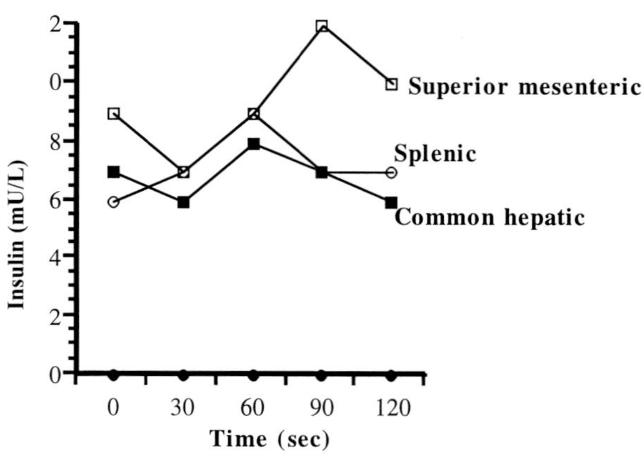

Fig. 10.27. Diffuse hyperplasia (surgical verified). IA calcium test failed to demonstrate any significant increase in insulin level after any selective arterial injection,

10.7 Diagnostic Algorithm

A.L. BAERT, L. VAN HOE, H. RIGAUTS

Controversy exists over the optimal diagnostic strategy in patients with clinical signs and laboratory findings suggestive of functioning endocrine tumors (KING et al. 1994). Many different techniques, including transabdominal and endoscopic sonography, CT, MRI, arteriography, transvenous sampling, and octreotide scanning have been proposed by different authors (KING et al. 1994; ROSCH et al. 1992a; ROSSI et al. 1989).

The following diagnostic algorithm could be proposed, taking into account the sensitivity and potential side effects of the different modalities.

If clinical data suggest the presence of a gastrinoma, thin-section helical CT or MRI can be used either as the first imaging modality or after transabdominal ultrasonography. The purpose is not only to localize the primary tumor, but also to detect (liver) metastases (present in 20%–30%). If metastatic disease is found, further imaging is not required. If a pancreatic (or duodenal) lesion is found, surgery may be the next step and peroperative ultrasonography may be used to confirm the diagnosis and to look for other lesions. If CT and/or MRI fail to show a suspect lesion, EUS is probably the best option. Selective angiography with secretin stimulation can be reserved for those cases with negative EUS results (Thompson et al. 1994).

In patients with suspected insulinoma, a different strategy is warranted: Since most insulinomas are benign and solitary, the single most important question is their exact location. Either transabdominal ultrasonography, EUS, MRI, or thin-section helical CT may be used as a first examination technique, and each may be used as a second technique in case of negative initial result. If these imaging modalities fail to reveal a focal lesion, selective angiography with calcium infusion and venous sampling should be performed in order to diagnose islet cell hyperplasia or nesidioblastosis, which accounts for 5%–10% of patients presenting with "insulinoma". While a more direct strategy consisting of exploration, palpation, and intraoperative ultrasonography has been proposed, this approach has two disadvantages: (1) the prolonged operation time and (2) the risk of removing the wrong part of the pancreas in patients with sonographically occult insulinoma and in those with hyperplasia/nesidioblastosis (THOMPSON et al. 1994).

Finally, octreotide scanning should be considered in patients presenting with persistent clinical symptoms after surgery.

References

Ahlström H, Magnusson A, Grama D, Eriksson B, Öberg K, Lörelius LE (1990) Preoperative localization of endocrine pancreatic tumors by intra-arterial dynamic CT. Acta Radiol 31(2):171--174

Berger JF, Laissy JP, Limot O, Henry-Feugeas MC, Cadiot G, Mignon M, Schouman-Claeys E (1996) Differentiation between multiple liver hemangiomas and liver metastases of gastrinomas: value of enhanced MRI. J Comput Assisted Tomogr 20:349--355

Boijsen E, Samuelsson L (1970) Angiographic diagnosis of tumors arising from the pancreatic islets. Acta Radiol (Diagn) 10:161--170

Boissel P, Proye C (1985) Les tumeurs endocrines du pancréas. Masson, Paris

Bok E, Cho KJ, Williams D, Brady T, Weiss CA, Forrest M (1984) Venous involvement in islet cell tumors of the pancreas. AJR 142:319--322

Bonfils S (1983) Les difficultés de la localisation topographique du gastrinome. Gastroenterol Clin Biol 7:639

Bonfils S, Landor J, Mignon M, Hervoir P (1981) Results of surgical management in 92 consecutive patients with Zollinger-Ellison syndrome. Ann Surg 194:692--697

Breathnach ES, Han SY, Rahatzad MT, Stanley RJ (1985) CT evaluation of glucagonomas. J Comput Assist Tomogr 9:25--29

Brunt L, Veldhuis J, Dilley W et al (1986) Stimulation of insulin secretion by a rapid intravenous calcium infusion in patients with b-cell neoplasms of the pancreas. J Clin Endrocrinol Metab 62:210--216

Burcharth F, Stage J, Stadil F, Jensen L, Fischermann K (1979) Localization of gastrinomas by transhepatic portal catheterization and gastrin assay. Gastroenterology 77:444--450

Calas F, Bouchet Y, Martin R, Couppie G (1956) Les veines du pancréas. 43° Réunion de l'Association des anatomistes, Lisbonne

Cherner J, Doppman J, Norton J et al (1986) Selective venous sampling for gastrin to localize gastrinomas: a prospective assessment. Ann Intern Med 105:841--847

Chung MJ, Choi BI, Han JK, Chung JW, Han MC, Bae SH (1997) Functioning islet cell tumors of the pancreas: localization with dynamic spiral CT. Acta Radiol 38:135--138

Clouse M, Costello P, Legg M, Soeldner S, Cady B (1977) Subselective angiography in localizing insulinomas of the pancreas. AJR 128:741--746

Cohen M, Doppman J, Krudy A et al (1984) Assessment of the ability of angiography to localize gastrinoma in patients with Zollinger-Ellison syndrome. Gastroenterology 86:1051

Cromack DT, Norton JA, Sigel B, Shawker TH, Doppman JL, Maton PN, Jensen RT (1987) The use of high-resolution intraoperative ultrasound to localize Gastrinomas: an initial report of a prospective study. World J Surg 11:648--653

Daggett P, Kurtz A, Morris D, Goodburn E, Lequesne L, Nabarro J et al (1981) Is pre-operative localisation of insulinomas necessary? Lancet 1:483--486

Deveney C, Deveney K, Way L (1978) The Zollinger-Ellison syndrome 23 years later. Ann Surg 188:384--391

Doppman J, Brennan M, Dunnick N, Kahn C, Gorden P (1981a) The role of pancreatic venous sampling in the localization of occult insulinomas. Radiology 138:557--562

Doppman J, Popovsky M, Girton M (1981b) The use of iodinated contrast agents to ablate organs: experimental study and histopathology. Radiology 138:333--340

Doppman J, Miller D, Chang R, Maton P, London J, Gardner J, Jensen R, Norton J (1990) Gastrinomas: localization by means of selective intraarterial injection of secretin. Radiology 174:25--29

Doppman J, Miller D, Chang R, Shawker T, Gorden P, Norton J (1991) Insulinoma: localization with selective intraarterial injection of calcium. Radiology 178:237--241

Doppman JL, Chang R, Fraker DL, Norton JA, Alexander HR, Miller DL, Collier E, Skarulis MC, Gorden P (1995) Localization of insulinomas to regions of the pancreas by intra-arterial stimulation with calcium. Ann Intern Med 123:269--273

Doyon D, Harry G, Roche A (1979) Techniques de la portographie. In: Ecoiffier J, Tessier JP, Roche A, Fischgold H (eds) Précis de techniques spécialisées en radiodiagnostic. Masson, Paris, pp 518--520

Eelkema EA, Stephens DH, Ward EM, Sheedy PF (1984) CT features of non-functioning islet cell carcinoma. AJR 143:943--948

Fenichel P, Rozo P, Hammou J, Harter M (1983) Double récidive d'un adénome bêtalangerhansien bénin. Nouv Presse Med 12:1018--1019

Fink IJ, Krudy AG, Shawker et al (1985) Demonstration of angiographically hypovascular insulinoma with intra arterial dynamic CT. AJR 144:555--557

Frucht H, Doppman JL, Norton JA, Miller DL, Dwyer AJ, Frank JA, Vinayek R, Maton PN, Jensen RT (1989) Gastrinomas: comparison of MR imaging with CT, angiography and US. Radiology 171:713--717

Fugazzola C, Procacci C, Andreis IAB et al (1990) The contribution of ultrasonography and computed tomography in the diagnosis of nonfunctioning islet cell tumors of the pancreas. Gastrointest Radiol 15:139--144

Fujii K, Yamagata S, Sasaki R, Ohneda A, Shoji T, Suzuki J (1974) Arteriography in insulinoma. AJR 120:634--647

Fulton R, Sheedy P, McIlrath D, Ferris D (1975) Pre-operative angiographic localization of insulin-producing tumors of the pancreas. AJR 123:367--377

Galiber AK, Reading CC, Charboneau JW, Sheedy PF, James EM, Gorman B, Grant CS, van Heerden JA, Telander RL (1988) Localisation of pancreatic insulinoma: comparison of pre- and intra-operative ultrasound with CT and angiography. Radiology 166:405--408

Gianello P, Gigot JF, Berthet F, Dardenne AN, Lambotte L, Rahier J, Otte JB, Kestens PJ (1988) Pre- and intra-operative localization of insulinomas: report of 22 observations. World J Surg 12:389--397

Gibril F, Doppman JL, Chang R, Weber HC, Termanini B, Jensen RT (1996) Metastatic gastrinomas: localization with selective arterial injection of secretin. Radiology 198(1):77--84

Glover JR, Shorvon PJ, Lees WR (1992) Endoscopic ultrasound for localisation of islet cell tumours. Gut 33:108--110

Gorman B, Charboneau JW, James EM, Reading CC, Galiber AK, Grant CS, van Heerden JA, Telander RL, Service FJ (1986) Benign pancreatic insulinoma: pre-operative and intra-operative sonographic localization. AJR 147:929--934

Grant CS, van Heerden J, Charboneau JW, James EM, Reading CC (1988) Insulinoma. The value of intra-operative ultrasonography. Arch Surg 123:843--848

Guillausseau P, Guillausseau C, Villet R, Kaloustian E, Valeur P, Hautefeuille P (1982) Les glucagonomes. Aspects cliniques, biologiques, anatomo-pathologiques et thérapeutiques. Revue générale de 130 cas. Gastroenterol Clin Biol 6:1029--1041

Gunther RW, Klose KJ, Ruckert K (1983) Islet cell tumours: detection os small lesions with CT and US. Radiology 148:485--489

Hautefeuille P, Valeur P, Gallian A, Roche A (1979) Surgical cure of malignant microscopic gastrinoma. Lancet 1:122

Hayashi T, Honda H, Yasumori K, Kawashima A, Kaneko K, Fukuya T, Tateshi Y, Ro T, Masuda K (1995) Selective intra-arterial injection of calcium for localization of insulinomas: proposed new criteria. Nippon Igaku Hoshasen Gakkai Zasshi 55(14):952--956

Hoevels J, Lunderquist A, Tylen U (1978) Percutaneous transhepatic portography. Acta Radiol (Diagn) 19:643--655

Houlbert D, Roche A, Dorf G, Gardies A, Roche D, Segrestaa J (1984) La localisation préopératoire des insulinomes est-elle nécessaire ? Ann Med Interne 13:16--20

Huguet J, Clement J, Jean P, Clerissi J, Burelle H (1978) Les tumeurs endocrines du pancréas. J Radiol Electrol 59:249--260

Imamura M, Takahashi K, Isobe Y, Hattori Y, Satomura K, Tobe T (1989) Curative resection of multiple gastrinomas aided by selective arterial injection test and intra-operative secretin test. Ann Surg 210:710--718

Imhof H, Frank P (1977) Pancreatic calcifications in malignant islet cell tumours. Radiology 122:333--338

Ingemansson S, Lunderquist A, Lundquist I, Lovdahl R, Tibblin S (1975) Portal and pancreatic vein catheterization with radio-immunologic determination of insulin. Surg Gynecol Obstet 141:705--711

Ingemansson S, Lunderquist A, Holst J (1976) Selective catheterization of the pancreatic veins for radio-immunoassay in glucagon-secreting carcinoma of the pancreas. Radiology 119:555--556

Ingemansson S, Kuhl C, Larsson L, Lunderquist A, Nobin A (1977) Islet cell hyperplasia localized by pancreatic vein catheterization and insulin radio-immuno-assay. Am J Surg 133:643--645

Kallio H, Suoranta H (1979) Localization of occult insulin secreting tumors of the pancreas. Ann Surg 189:49--52

Keller F, Niles N, Rosch J, Dotter C, Stenzel-Poore M (1980) Retrograde pancreatic venography: autopsy study. Radiology 135:285--293

Kimmey MB, Martin RW, Silverstein FE (1992) First clinical experience with ultrasound probes. Clinical application of linear ultrasound probes. Endoscopy 24 [Suppl 1]:364--369

King CMP, Reznek RH, Dacie JE, Wass JAH (1994) Imaging islet cell tumors. Clin Radiol 49:295--303

King AD, Ko GT, Yeung VT, Chow CC, Griffith J, Cockram CS (1998) Dual phase spiral CT in the detection of small insulinomas of the pancreas. Br J Radiol 112:20--23

Ko TC, Flisak M, Prinz RA (1992) Selective intra-arterial methylene blue injection: a novel method of localizing gastrinoma. Gastroenterology 102(3):1062--1064

Kraus BB, Ros PR (1994) Insulinoma: diagnosis with fat-suppressed MR imaging. AJR 162:69--70

Krudy AG, Doppman LJ, Jansen RT (1984) Localisation of islet-cell tumours by dynamic CT: comparison with plain CT, arteriography, sonography and venous sampling. AJR 143:585--591

Larsson L, Holst J, Kühl C, Lundquist G, Hirsch M, Ingemansson S, Lindkaer Jensen S, Rehfeld J (1977) Pancreatic somatostatinoma: clinical features and physiological implications. Lancet 1:666--668

Lightdale CJ, Botet JF, Woodruff JM, Brennan MF (1991) Localization of endocrine tumors of the pancreas with endoscopic ultrasonography. Cancer 68:1815--1820

Lunderquist A, Eriksson M, Ingemansson S, Larsson L, Reichardt W (1978) Selective pancreatic vein catheterization for hormone essay in endocrine tumors of the pancreas. Cardiovasc Radiol 1:117--124

Martin E, Bedossa P, Potet F (1987) Tumeurs et hyperplasies endocrines du pancréas. Caractères anatomopathologiques. In: Bonfils S, Mignon M (eds) Tumeurs endocrines du pancréas. Doin, Paris, pp 17--35

Maton P, Miller D, Doppman J et al (1987) Role of selective angiography in the management of patients with Zollinger-Ellison syndrome. Gastroenterology 92:913--918

McCarthy D (1980) The place of surgery in the Zollinger-Ellison syndrome. N Engl J Med 302:1344--1347

Mignon M, Rigaud D, Ruszniewski P, Vallot T, Rene E, Bonfils S (1987) Le syndrome de Zollinger-Ellison. Stratégie diagnostique et thérapeutique actuelle. In: Bonfils S, Mignon M (eds) Tumeurs endocrines du pancréas. Doin, Paris, pp 37--66

Millan V, Urosa C, Molitch M, Miller H, Jackson I (1979) Localization of occult insulinoma by superselective pancreatic venous sampling for insulin assay through percutaneous transhepatic catheterization. Diabetes 28:249--251

Mills S, Doppman J, Dunnick N, McCarthy D (1979) Evaluation of angiography in Zollinger-Ellison syndrome. Radiology 131:317--320

Mitchell D, Cruvella M, Eschelman D, Miettinen M, Vernick J (1992) MRI of pancreatic gastrinomas. J Comput Assist Tomogr 16:583--585

Mitty H, Efremidis S, Wertkin M, Dreiling D, Rayfield E (1979) Localization in insulinomas by radio-immuno-assay of blood obtained by the transportal route. J Clin Endocrinol Metab 48:1035--1037

Moreaux J (1981) Traitement chirurgical du syndrome de Zollinger-Ellison. Ses résultats chez 34 malades et son orientation actuelle. Chirurgie 107:557--565

Moreaux J, Olivier A (1987) Traitement chirurgical des tumeurs endocrines du pancréas. In: Bonfils S, Mignon M (eds) Tumeurs endocrines du pancréas. Doin, Paris, pp 201--215

Norton JA, Doppman JL, Collen MJ, Harmon JW, Maton PN, Gardener JD, Jensen RT (1986) Prospective study of gastrinoma localization and resection in patients with Zollinger-Ellison syndrome. Ann Surg 204:468--479

Norton JA, Cromack DT, Shawker TH, Doppman JL, Comi R, Gorden P, Maton PN, Gardner JD, Jensen RT (1988) Intraoperative ultrasonographic localization of islet cell tumors. Ann Surg 207:160--168

O'Shea D, Rohrer-Theurs AW, Lynn JA, Jackson JE, Bloom SR (1996) Localization of insulinomas by selective intraarterial calcium injection. J Clin Endocrinol Metab 81:1623--1627

Päivänsalo M, Mäkäräinen H, Siniluoto T, Stahlberg M, Jalovaara P (1989) Ultrasound compared with computed tomography and pancreatic arteriography in the detection of endocrine tumours of the pancreas. Eur J Radiol 9:173--178

Palazzo L (1991) Echo-endoscopie du tube digestif. Rev Prat (Paris) 41:225--231

Palazzo L, Roseau G, Salmeron M (1992) Endoscopic ultrasonography in the preoperative localization of pancreatic endocrine tumors. Endoscopy 24 [Suppl 1]:350--353

Passariello R, Rossi P, Simonetti G, Di Paolo A (1978) Cathétérisme portal transhépatique pour la localisation des tumeurs sécrétantes du pancréas. Ann Radiol 21:485--490

Passaro E (1979) Localization of pancreatic endocrine tumors by selective portal vein catheterization and radioimmuno-assay. Gastroenterology 77:806--807

Pavone P, Mitchell DG, Leonetti F, Di Girolamo M, Cardone G, Catalano C, Tamburrano G, Passariello R (1993) Pancreatic beta-cell tumors: MRI. J Comput Assisted Tomogr 17:403--407

Pereira PL, Roche AJ, Huppert PE, Maier G, Farnsworth CT, Duda SH, Damman F, Claussen CD (1998) Calcium arterial stimulation for insulinoma and hyperplasia: value of the intraarterial calcium test when morphological preoperative studies are negative. Radiology (to be published)

Pistolesi C, Frasson F, Fugazzola C et al (1977) Angiographic diagnosis of endocrine tumors of the pancreas. Radiol Clin 46:401--421

Rambaud JC, Jian R (1987) Choléra pancréatique (syndrome de Verner-Morrison). In: Bonfils S, Mignon M (eds) Tumeurs endocrines du pancréas. Doin, Paris, pp 101--114

Reichardt W, Cameron R (1980a) Anatomy of the pancreatic veins. A post mortem and clinical phlebographic investigation. Acta Radiol (Diagn) 21:33--41

Reichardt W, Ingemansson S (1980b) Selective vein catheterization for hormone assay in endocrine tumours of the pancreas: technique and results. Acta Radiol (Diagn) 21:177--187

Ribet A, Pradayrol L, Bommelaer G, Cloarec D (1987) Les somatostatinomes. In: Bonfils S, Mignon M (eds) Tumeurs endocrines du pancréas. Doin, Paris, pp 137--145

Roche A, Raisonnier A, Gillon-Savouret M (1982) Pancreatic venous sampling and arteriography in localizing insulinomas and gastrinomas: procedure and results in 55 cases. Radiology 145:621--627

Roche A, Capeau J, Halimi P (1983) Méthodes radiologiques de localisation des tumeurs endocrines du pancréas. Gastroenterol Clin Biol 7:49--58

Rosch T, Lorenz R, Braig C, Feuerbach S, Siewert JR, Schusdziarra V, Classen M (1991) Endoscopic ultrasound in pancreatic tumor diagnosis. Gastrointest Endosc 37:347--352

Rosch T, Lightdale CJ, Botet JF, Boyce GA, Sivak MV, Yasuda K, Heyder N, Palazzo L, Dancygier H, Schusdziarra V, Classen M (1992a) Localization of pancreatic endocrine tumors by endoscopic ultrasonography. N Engl J Med 326:1721--1726

Rosch T, Lorenz R, Braig C, Classen M (1992b) Endoscopic ultrasonography in diagnosis and staging of pancreatic and biliary tumors. Endoscopy 24 [Suppl 1]:304--308

Rossi P, Baert AL, Passariello R (1985) CT of functioning tumours of the pancreas. AJR 144:57--63

Rossi P, Allison DJ, Bezzi M, Kennedy A, Maccioni F, Wynick D, Maradei A, Bloom SR (1989) Endocrine tumors of the pancreas. Radiol Clin North Am 27:127--161

Semelka RC, Ascher SM (1993) MR imaging of the pancreas. Radiology 188:593--602

Semelka RC, Cumming MJ, Shoenut JP, Magro CM, Yaffe CS, Kroeker MA, Greenberg HM (1993) Islet cell tumors: comparison of dynamic contrast-enhanced CT and MRI with dynamic gadolinium enhancement and fat suppression. Radiology 186:799--802

Stacpoole P (1981) The glucagonoma syndrome: clinical features, diagnosis, and treatment. Endocr Rev 2:347--361

Stefanini P, Carboni M, Patrassi N (1974) Beta-islet tumors of the pancreas: results of a study on 1067 cases. Surgery 75:597--609

Sugimura H, Tamura S, Kodama T, Kakitsubata Y, Asada K, Watanabe K (1991) Metastatic pancreas cancer from the thyroid; clinical imaging mimicking non functioning islet cell tumor. Radiat Med 9:167--169

Thom AK, Norton JA, Doppman JL, Miller DL, Chang R, Jensen RT (1992) Prospective study of the use of intraarterial secretin injection and portal venous sampling to localize duodenal gastrinomas. Surgery 112(6):1002--1009

Thompson NW, Czako PF, Fritts LL et al (1994) Role of endoscopic ultrasonography in the localization of insulinomas and gastrinomas. Surgery 116:1131--1138

Tjon A Tham RTO, Falke THM, Jansen JBMJ, Lamers CBHW (1989a) CT and MR imaging of advanced Zollinger-Ellison Syndrome. J Comput Assist Tomogr 13:821--828

Tjon A Tham RTO, Jansen JBMJ, Falke THM, Roelfsema F, Griffioen G, van den Sluys Veer A, Lamers CBHW (1989b) MR, CT, and ultrasound findings of metastatic vipoma in pancreas. J Comput Assist Tomogr 13:142--144

Turner R, Morris P, Lee E, Harris E (1978) Localisation of insulinomas. Lancet 1:515--518

van Heerden J, Edis A, Service F (1979) The surgical aspects of insulinomas. Ann Surg 189:677--682

Van Hoe L, Marchal G, Baert AL et al (1995a) Determination of scan delay time in spiral CT angiography: utility of a test bolus injection. J Comput Assist Tomogr 19:216--220

Van Hoe L, Gryspeerdt S, Marchal G, Baert AL, Mertens L (1995b) Helical CT for the preoperative localization of islet cell tumors of the pancreas: value of arterial and parenchymal phase images AJR 165:1437--1439

Van Hoe L, Gryspeerdt S, Baert AL (1998) Endocrine tumors of the pancreas. In: Heuck A, Reiser M (eds) Abdominal and pelvic MRI. Springer, Berlin Heidelberg New York, pp 109--116

Verner J, Morrison A et al (1974) Endocrine pancreatic islet disease with diarrhea. Report of a case due to diffuse hyperplasia of nonbeta islet tissue with a review of 54 additional cases. Arch Intern Med 133:492--500

Vilman P, Jacobsen GK, Henriksen FW, Hancke S (1992) Endoscopic ultrasonography with guided fine needle aspiration biopsy in pancreatic disease. Gastrointest Endosc 38:172--173

Vinik A, Thompson N (1986) Controversies in the management of Zollinger-Ellison syndrome. Ann Intern Med 105:956--959

Wilms G, Baert AL, Dardenne AN, Mathurin P, Staels P, Bouillon R, Lerut J, Lerut T (1990) Percutaneous transhepatic venous sampling of the pancreas in localizing insulinomas. J Belg Radiol 73:453--457

Winter TC, Freeny PC, Nghiem HV (1996) Extrapancreatic gastrinoma localization: value of arterial-phase helical CT with water as an oral contrast agent. AJR 166:51--52

Xianju Z, Yu Z, Weiran W, Tonghua L (1980) Insulinoma diagnostic and therapeutic experiences in 60 cases. Clin Med J 93:149--158

11 Rare and Secondary Tumors of the Pancreas

P. Legmann, O. Vignaux, B. Dousset, and J. Grellet

CONTENTS

11.1 Introduction

The use of ultrasonography (US), helical computed tomography (CT), and magnetic resonance imaging (MRI) with fast sequences and contrast medium administration has improved the visualization of pancreatic tumors (Semelka et al. 1991; Kelekis and Semelka 1997). Indications for the use of endoscopic ultrasonography are now better defined and this technique provides detailed images of the pancreatic and peripancreatic area, and is most useful as a preoperative procedure to improve detection and staging of tumors (Botet and Lightdale 1992; Rösch et al. 1991; Klöppel and Maillet 1989). Although staging of pancreatic neoplasms has improved, and high accuracy for the detection and staging of tumors has been achieved, patient outcome remains uniformly poor (Baytor and Berg 1973). It seems that the main role of imaging is to prove inoperability of patients with tumors to prevent needless postoperative morbidity and mortality. Helical CT has decreased the role of other diagnostic tests like endoscopic retrograde cholangiopancreatography (ERCP) and angiography (Freeny and Lawson 1982; Friedman and Edmonds 1989). The origin of the tumoral cells are also more specifically defined by means of ultrastructural and immunohistochemical investigations, and it is now possible to describe imaging signs characteristic of most of the different histologic types of pancreatic tumor, including some rare ones (Cubilla and Fitzgerald 1979; Morohoshi et al. 1983, 1987). Percutaneous fine-needle biopsy under US or CT guidance enables preoperative diagnosis in numerous cases. Use of fine-needle biopsy can avoid useless laparotomy and reduce hospitalization (Freeny 1988).

P. Legmann, MD, Hôpital Cochin, Service de Radiologie, Assistance Publique, Hôpitaux de Paris, 27 rue du Faubourg Saint-Jacques, F-75679 Paris Cédex 14, France

O. Vignaux, MD, Hôpital Cochin, Service de Radiologie, Assistance Publique, Hôpitaux de Paris, 27 rue du Faubourg Saint-Jacques, F-75679 Paris Cédex 14, France

B. Dousset, MD, Hôpital Cochin, Service de Chirurgie Digestive, Assistance Publique, Hôpitaux de Paris, 27 rue du Faubourg Saint-Jacques, F-75679 Paris Cédex 14, France

J. Grellet, MD, Groupe Hospitalier Pitié – La Salpétrière, Service Central de Radiologie, Assistance Publique, Hôpitaux de Paris, 47–83 Boulevard de l'Hôpital, F-75651 Paris Cédex 13, France

11.2 Histogenesis of Tumors of the Exocrine Pancreas

Most (>95%) pancreatic tumors are of epithelial origin deriving from the ductal cell. A few originate from the acinar cell or have a mixed origin. The histogenesis of certain tumors (solid-cystic tumor, anaplastic tumor) remains uncertain. In addition to these tumors of epithelial origin, we give due consideration in this chapter to metastases, nonepithelial tumors, and malignant lymphomas. Cystic tumors and endocrine tumors are described in Chap. 9 (Cubilla and Fitzgerald 1984; Klöppel and Maillet 1989; Morohoshi et al. 1987).

11.3 Rare Pancreatic Tumors of Ductal Cell Origin

Ductal adenocarcinoma is by far the most frequent tumor. Rare ductal neoplasms include mucinous carcinoma, adenosquamous carcinoma, pleomorphic giant cell carcinoma, and giant cell carcinoma osteoclast-type.

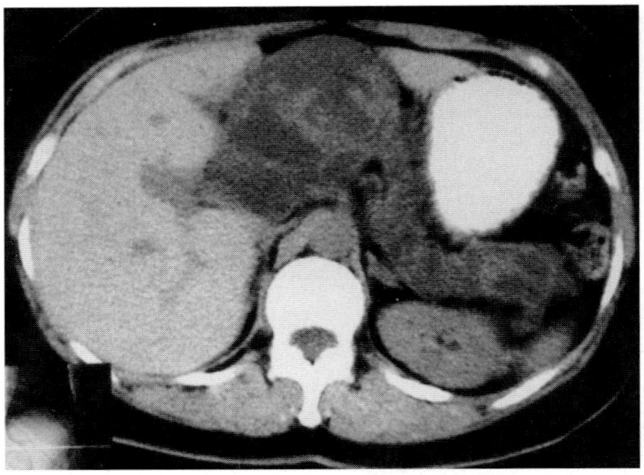

a

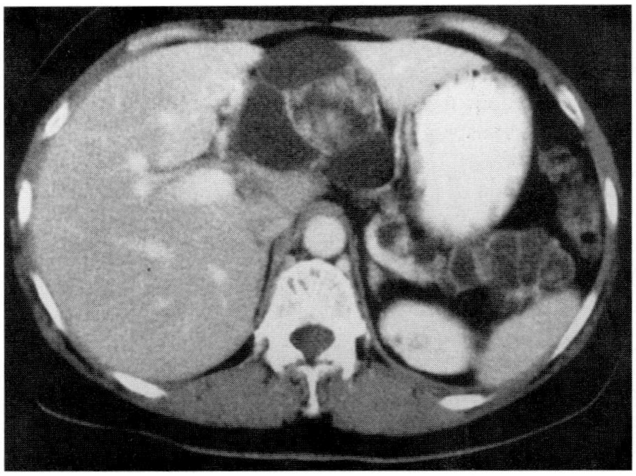

b

Fig. 11.1a,b. Patient with mucinous adenocarcinoma. Computed tomography before (**a**) and after (**b**) intravenous injection of iodinated contrast showing large cystic areas bordered by polypoid nodules enhanced after injection

11.3.1 Mucinous Carcinoma (Adenocarcinoma)

The clinical presentation is very similar to that of ductal adenocarcinoma. A unique feature of this tumor is that its density may be lower than that of ductal carcinoma; it may also be cystic (Cubilla and Fitzgerald 1984; Mathieu et al. 1989).

Mucinous carcinomas tend to be larger with broad cystic spaces filled with squamous substances bordered by malignant cells. Pseudocystic areas filled with mucin substances appear anechoic or hypoechoic on US, and hypodense on CT. Following chemotherapy, calcifications may appear within the tumor or its metastases. Cytodiagnosis is possible by means of fine-needle aspiration biopsy, but false-negatives are frequent owing to the relative rarity of malignant cells. The excessive mucin production may cause biliary obstruction and renal tubular obstruction in these patients. Pseudomyxoma peritonei can occur (Hertzana et al. 1989).

Mucinous adenocarcinomas are larger and softer than duct cell adenocarcinoma. The mucin-hypersecreting carcinomas limited to the duct consist of flat or polypoid tumors confined to the main pancreatic duct and its side branches. These tumors have been reported to spread along the duct and frequently invade the parenchyma or extend outside the gland. The pancreatic ducts are dilated and filled with mucin produced by the tumor. Sonography of mucinous adenocarcinoma limited to the duct reveals a diffusely dilated main pancreatic duct filled with mucin of varying degrees of echogenicity. Contrast-enhanced CT may depict enhancing tumor nodules within the ducts. Otherwise, the mucin-filled ducts have a homogeneous or slightly inhomogeneous low attenuation. The parenchyma is generally atrophic (Fig. 11.1a,b).

Contrast-enhanced MRI may reveal large hypointense cystic areas on T1-weighted spin echo sequences. Polypoid nodules are enhanced after injection of gadolinium (Fig. 11.2a,b).

Endoscopic US, is remarkable for its ability to strikingly depict dilated main pancreatic ducts filled

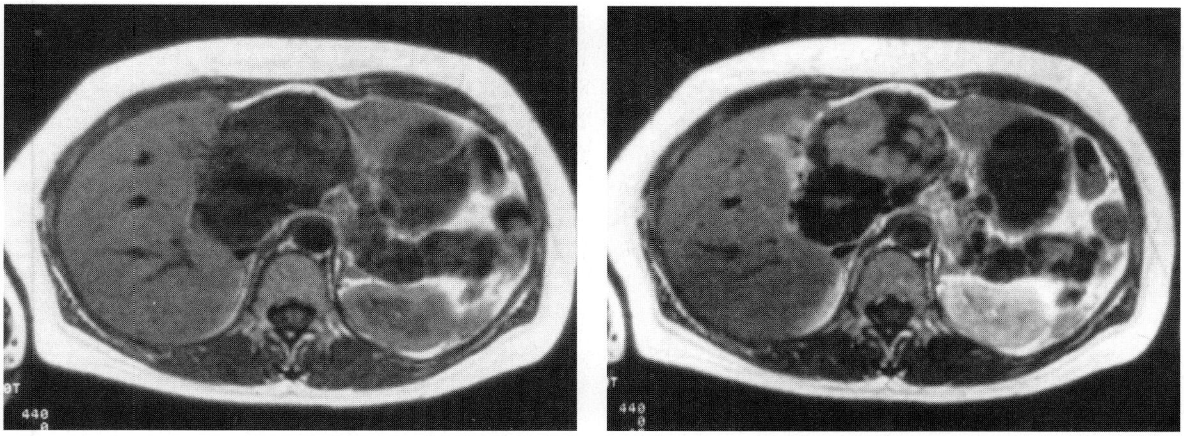

a b

Fig. 11.2a,b. Patient with mucinous adenocarcinoma. T1-weighted spin-echo sequence before (**a**) and after (**b**) injection of gadolinium showing large cystic areas with polypoid nodules enhanced after injection

with amorphous or well-defined filling defects due to mucinous tumor masses. Endoscopic observation typically reveals an enlarged papilla with mucus flowing from a patulous orifice (Botet and Lightdale 1992; Rösch et al. 1991). The diagnostic key with this particular entity is the correlation of clinical factors with the imaging appearance. The mean survival is 11 months.

11.3.2 Adenosquamous Carcinoma

Squamous or adenosquamous carcinoma is a rare variant with some specific differential pathologic and radiographic findings, but the outcome and prognosis are not much different from ordinary adenocarcinoma. In several large series, squamous or adenosquamous carcinoma occurred in less than 0.5% of all cases of carcinoma (Cihak et al. 1972). The two components of the carcinoma (adenoid cells and epidermal cells) are variably distributed throughout the tumor. The epidermal component presents a tendency to necrosis. This carcinoma is seen to occur predominantly in males. Radiologically, the tumor appears solid or partially necrotic, the necrosis sometimes being widespread. The appearance is somewhat characteristic because the density of the tumor appears to be low, resulting from necrosis within the mass. Survival is 0% at 1 year (Wilczynski et al. 1984; Friedman and Edmonds 1989).

11.3.3 Pleomorphic Giant Cell Carcinoma

Histologically, pleomorphic giant cell carcinoma presents the same characteristics as sarcoma, with a mixture of anaplastic mononucleated cells, pleomorphic multinucleated cells, and fusiform cells. These large and markedly necrotic tumors (Wolfman et al. 1985; Guillan 1985) are widely metastatic at the time of their detection. Radiologic signs include large tumors with necrotic and hemorrhagic cavities, widespread peripancreatic adenopathies, direct extension to the surrounding organs, and metastatic dissemination with hematogenous spread and ascites. This unusual neoplasm has an age distribution and sex ratio similar to duct cell adenocarcinoma. Location is about evenly distributed between the head, body, and tail of the gland. Small areas of mucin-producing adenocarcinoma can be found. Sonography and CT will depict this neoplasm as a cystic mass with thick margins when hemorrhagic necrosis predominates (Laverdière et al. 1992). CT numbers of the cystic component are compatible with old blood. Otherwise pleomorphic carcinomas are solid or mixed, and well-demarcated at enhanced CT. Lymphadenopathy is striking and hematogenous metastases are frequently present. Significant direct extension to the surrounding organs with metastatic dissemination to the liver, lungs, and peritoneal cavity, is a suggestive finding. Fine-needle aspiration biopsy can be performed to exclude lymphoma, which could be treated efficiently (Pinto et al. 1986). It may be quite difficult to obtain an adequate tissue sample for cytologic and biochemical study. Prognosis is poor, with a mean survival of 2 months.

11.3.4 Giant Cell Carcinoma, Osteoclast-Type

Osteoclast-type giant cell tumors of the pancreas (OGTP) were reported in 1968 for the first time (Baniel et al. 1987). Most authors have presumed an epithelial origin from acinar tissue, but recent evidence supports a mesenchymal origin. OGTP is histologically indistinguishable from giant cell tumor of bone (Rosai 1968). The reported age range is large. There is no significant sex predilection or particular site of origin within the gland. The diagnosis of OGTP can be strongly suggested by the results of fine-needle aspiration cytology combined with clinical and imaging data. OGTP are large neoplasms with well-defined or locally invasive margins, with often large multifocal regions of hemorrhagic necrosis. The giant cells resemble benign osteoclasts and may contain up to 100 nuclei, but do not exhibit mitotic figures. OGTP are well vascularized by cavernous or sinusoidal blood spaces. Zymogen granules found in OGTP are cited as evidence for their origin from acinar cells. CT and sonography reveal large, partially or multifocally necrotic masses of pancreatic origin. Giant cell carcinoma of the osteoclast type appears as a tumor with cystic cavities. Liver metastases and extensive local invasion are less likely to be seen. Although the prognosis is poor, about 25% of reported cases have experienced long-term survival after surgery. Prognosis is better than with ductal cell adenocarcinoma or pleomorphic giant cell carcinoma.

11.4 Tumors of the Exocrine Pancreas with an Acinar Cell Origin

11.4.1 Acinar Cell Carcinoma

Acinar cell tumors arise from acinar elements of the pancreas. Acinar cell carcinomas are often voluminous: They are of soft consistency and present areas of necrosis. Microscopically, their acinar aspect suggests an endocrine tumor, but the existence of zymogen granules indicates their exocrine origin. Ultrastructurally, the tumor cells are polyhedral, arranged in distinct acini and connected by desmosomes that contain multiple electron-dense cytoplasmic secretary granules. These tumors develop at a late age in both sexes. They are rare and have been reported to comprise 1%–13% of non-endocrine pancreatic malignancies. An association with subcutaneous and intraosseous fat necrosis identical to the syndrome more commonly occurring in the context of pancreatitis is occasionally present. The patients present metastatic fat necrosis due to systemic release of lipase by functioning tumors cells. About two thirds of reported cases of metastatic fat necrosis due to pancreatic neoplasms have been in documented acinar cell carcinomas (Cantrell et al. 1981). These patients present with skin or bone and joint lesions frequently associated with fever, leukocytosis and eosinophilia. Serum lipase elevation in the presence of a normal serum amylase is characteristic. The presentation comprises subcutaneous fat necrosis composed of nodules resembling those of erythema nodosum, but with widespread distribution, and polyarthralgia associated with articular swelling that affects the distal articulations of the extremities, commencing at the elbows and knees. These radiologic lesions are situated in the neighborhood of the subcutaneous nidi of fat necrosis. Skeletal radiographs reveal lytic bone lesions, accompanied by distal skin lesions. Periosteal reaction may be present, but is not common. Patients with acinar cell carcinoma and metastatic fat necrosis usually have liver metastasis at presentation. In the cases reported, CT showed the well circumscribed mass with some central necrosis. The unique aspect of these cases is the presence of a permeative lytic process which may involve the phalanges of the hands and feet. The prognosis of this disease is poor, the mean survival being 7 months, with patients living 2–11 months (Radin et al. 1986).

11.4.2 Pancreatoblastoma

Pancreatoblastoma is a rare epithelial tumor with a protracted malignant course, occurring in children. Pancreatoblastoma in childhood is a rare pancreatic tumor of acinar cell origin, comprising 0.5% of epithelial tumors of the pancreas, and progresses with a slow, sluggishly malignant course. Characteristics of pancreatoblastoma include nests of squamoid cells and a pattern of epithelial cells. The correct diagnosis is best made on histopathologic findings seen on light microscopy, electron microscopy, and histochemistry. US-guided fine-needle biopsy can be helpful (Baniel et al. 1987). Characterization of this tumor with electron microscopy is very important; the presence of zymogen-like granules helps in making the diagnosis of pancreatoblastoma (Bucchino et al. 1984). Detection of pancreatoblastoma in adults has been reported (Palosaari et al. 1986). The neoplasm is often misdiagnosed as neuroblastoma or hepatoblastoma. It tends to be large (7–12 cm), soft, and rounded, with central necrosis, and to occur in the head or tail of the pancreas. Excision of the primary mass without metastases leads to a good prognosis. But if metastases are present at the time of diagnosis, the prognosis is very poor. The most frequent site of metastases has been described as the liver. Metastases may be present very early. A metastatic lesion in the liver can be falsely identified as hepatoblastoma or fibrolamellar hepatocellular carcinoma.

Initial signs and symptoms may include a palpable mass, anorexia, and vomiting.

11.4.2.1 Imaging

US findings show a well-demarcated, septated, heterogeneous mass with multiple cystic portions and multiple spotty calcifications, or a well-demarcated solid mass with slightly lower echogenicity than liver. Sometimes, it appears as a mixed echogenic mass (Lumkin et al. 1993).

CT depicts the tumor as an inhomogeneous solid mass inseparable from the pancreas. CT findings include a well-encapsulated, enhancing, huge pancreatic mass with areas of calcification or hemorrhage and necrosis. A multiloculated appearance by enhancing septa has been demonstrated in reported cases.

Some tumors may show well-defined margins. All tumors are predominantly solid, containing areas of focal or multifocal lower attenuation that suggest cystic, hemorrhagic, or necrotic portions. After administration of contrast material, CT shows a mass with a multiloculated appearance and enhancement of internal septa. Density of tumors is lower than that of adjacent liver (Herman et al. 1994; Capelle 1986).

MRI shows a hypointense tumor on T1-weighted sequences and a highly hyperintense mass on T2-weighted sequences (Lumkin et al. 1993; Stephenson et al. 1990).

The short-term prognosis of pancreatoblastoma is more favorable than that of other malignant tumors of the pancreas.

11.5 Tumors of the Exocrine Pancreas of Uncertain Origin

11.5.1 Solid and Papillary Epithelial Neoplasm (Solid-Cystic Tumor, Papillary Cystic Tumor)

Solid and papillary epithelial neoplasm (SPEN) is an uncommon, low-grade malignant tumor found in young women. Although SPEN can appear at any age, even in childhood, they typically occur in adolescent or young adult females, and display a black racial predilection (Amar et al. 1991). Only 5% of cases occur in males. SPEN or solid-cystic tumors are often discovered incidentally after abdominal trauma or during gynecologic surgery. They may also be discovered in the presence of increasing abdominal discomfort or in the context of polyarthralgia and/or eosinophilia due to intravascular release of lipase.

Macroscopically, SPEN present as large masses (mean diameter of 10 cm), with no preferential localization within the pancreas and with the characteristic of being easily resected (Kissane 1994).

Grossly, a SPEN is a large, well-encapsulated mass, that usually demonstrates variable degrees of internal hemorrhage and cystic degeneration. Areas of hemorrhagic degeneration vary from solid friable areas to frankly cystic cavities. This tumor may appear as solid, cystic, or mixed solid and cystic. Initially, the solid tumor is constituted of monomorphic cells of rather small size, arranged in „rosettes“ around the vascular axes. Later, the cellular regions farthest from the vessels are excavated by pseudocysts. The noninvaded cellular capsules around the vessels are constituted of pseudopapillae protruding into the cystic area. Extensive hemorrhage changes the composition of the cystic areas. Characterization of the pathologic process of hemorrhagic degeneration can demonstrate the presence of blood products. Fluid debris levels may be present in solid or cystic areas. Calcifications are rare: They can be peripheral or capsular, or situated in the center of the tumoral mass and seem to be a more common feature with peripheral location (Procacci et al. 1995).

US shows a well-defined echogenic mass containing cystic areas of variable echogenicity: hyperechoic, anechoic, or hypoechoic, without dorsal reinforcement. Hyperechoic areas correspond to areas that are solid and hemorrhagic, or cystic and hemorrhagic. The most frequent signs observed on US show a well-defined echogenic mass containing cystic areas of variable echogenicity (Balthazar et al. 1984).

On CT, the well-defined tumoral mass contains cystic areas of a density higher than that of water. After administration of contrast medium, enhancement of the solid components is evident; but the degree of enhancement of the solid portion of the tumor remains inferior to that of normal pancreas. Hyperattenuating areas correspond to solid hemorrhagic regions. Areas of intermediate attenuation are solid hemorrhagic areas or cystic hemorrhagic areas (Fig. 11.3a,b). In cases of extreme hemorrhage or abundant necrosis, US and CT show a cystic cavity with thick walls and irregular internal borders. The density of the cystic content varies according to its composition (old blood, necrotic material). Metastases may develop in lymph nodes and liver (Choi et al. 1988; Savci et al. 1996).

T1-weighted images demonstrate areas of high signal intensity distributed diffusely, peripherally, or centrally. On T2-weighted images, these areas are depicted as areas of high signal intensity or of mixed low and high signal intensity. Areas of high signal intensity on T1-weighted MR images correspond to areas of hemorrhagic necrosis or hemorrhagic debris that are solid or cystic. High signal intensity on T2-weighted images are seen in solid hemorrhagic areas or cystic areas. A discontinuous low-signal-intensity rim can be seen on T2-weighted images. Peripheral enhancement can be noted.

Fluid-debris levels can be present as a direct sign of hemorrhagic cystic degeneration. With MRI, this effect may be seen in solid or cystic areas of hemorrhagic degeneration. This feature can help to characterize this tumor (Ohtomo et al. 1992).

Fine-needle aspiration biopsy is possible. However, it entails a risk of hemorrhage and cytologic features alone can be inadequate to confirm the diagnosis.

The prognosis of these tumors is good: They are not very invasive, they display low-grade malignancy, and are slow growing. Local recurrence is rare and occurs only when resection is incomplete. This tumor is a low-grade malignancy that is apparently curable with surgical excision.

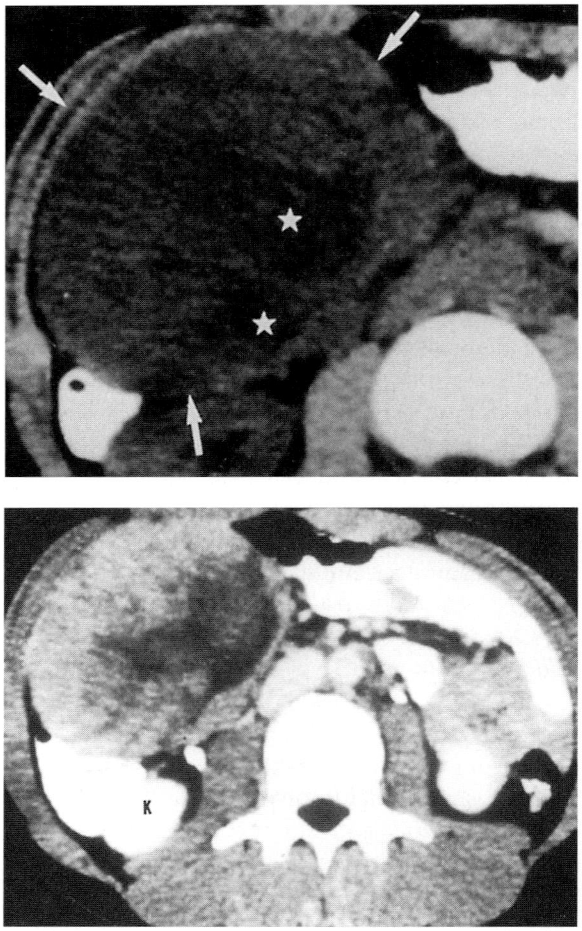

a

b

Fig. 11.3a,b. Pancreatic solid cystic tumor in a 68-year-old female. A large mass was present in the epigastrium and right hypogastrium. **a** Computed tomography (CT) before intravenous injection of iodinated contrast reveals a large mass (6_5 cm) of the pancreatic head (*arrow*), with heterogeneous density. Relatively hypodense „cystic" areas (*asterisks*) with an attenuation value of 45 HU are visible. **b** Following CT after intravenous injection of iodinated contrast, the heterogeneous aspect of the tumor is better visible due to the enhancement of the peripheral solid portion of the lesion. Note the absence of septations. *K*, kidney

11.5.2 Other Tumors of the Pancreas of Uncertain Origin

The radiologic appearance of some rare tumors of the pancreas have not been described. The tumors belonging to this group include anaplastic carcinoma with little pleomorphism and predominantly small cells, pure small cell carcinoma, ciliated cell carcinoma, oncocytic carcinoma, and clear cell carcinoma.

11.6 Mixed Tumors

The pancreas can be the site of several nonepithelial neoplasms that can also occur in other organs. The recent literature contains isolated reports of such exceptional tumors and tumor-like conditions, e.g., pleomorphic pancreatic sarcoma, intrapancreatic lipoma, liposarcoma, pancreatic sarcoidosis, and hemangioma (MANGIN et al. 1985; SAGALOW et al. 1988) (Fig. 11.4).

Pancreatic lymphangioma exhibits the pattern of sunburst calcification similar to the appearance described as specific for serous cystadenoma or phleboliths visible on standard radiographs. On CT, the density of the lobulated mass is usually equivalent to that of water, due to the lipid content of the lymphatic fluid. After intravenous injection of iodinated contrast medium, heterogeneous enhancement occurs. The MRI signal of lymphangioma is slightly hypointense in comparison with the liver on T1-weighted spin-echo sequences, and strongly hyperintense on T2-weighted spin-echo sequences. Needle biopsy will reveal chylous liquid (HANELIN and SCHIMMEL 1977; SALIMI et al. 1991).

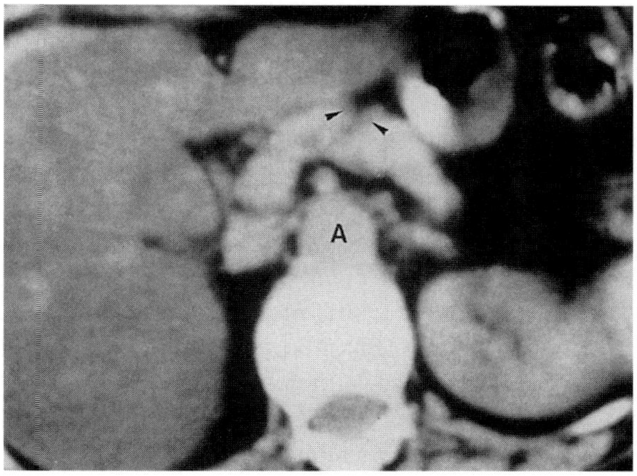

Fig. 11.4. Liposarcoma of the pancreas in a 64-year-old female with general symptoms. A hypoechoic lesion was detected on ultrasonography (not shown). Computed tomography (CT) after intravenous injection of iodinated contrast shows a small mass (diameter, 1 cm; *arrowheads*) enhancing less than the adjacent normal pancreas. CT-guided needle biopsy revealed a liposarcoma composed of round and fusiform cells with a low degree of differentiation. *A*, aorta

11.7 Intrapancreatic Lipoma

Lipomas are common benign mesenchymal neoplasms. In the digestive tract, lipomas are frequently seen in the colon; however, they are uncommon in the pancreas. Usually, there are no specific clinical findings. Sonographic findings show hypoechoic areas with well-defined margins. CT study confirms the presence of the mass and analyzes attenuation values, showing homogeneously distributed tissue of fat density with no central or peripheral contrast enhancement. This finding enables the diagnosis of proven lipoma. Values ranging from 80–120 HU indicate a lesion composed of fat. Other tissues, both benign and malignant, may have negative attenuating values. Malignant neoplasms containing fat such as liposarcomas are characterized by higher densitometric values, greater size, areas of solid or fluid densities, and by blurred outlines (BANKS et al. 1975). Nevertheless, a well-defined liposarcoma may mimic a benign lesion at radiologic examination because of the homogeneity of fat tissue density and the sharply defined margins of the liposarcoma. Helical scanning, with multiple reconstruction, allows CT to be a reliable noninvasive tool to enable diagnosis of intrapancreatic lipoma.

11.8 Pancreatic Plasmocytoma

Pancreatic plasmocytoma is very rare. It is usually associated with multiple myeloma or with a focal bone lesion. US and CT show a focal mass, isodense with the normal gland, and slightly hypodense after administration of contrast medium. Pancreatic plasmocytoma can show an attenuation value similar to that of the pancreatic parenchyma both before and after intravenous injection of contrast medium (FUKUYA et al. 1989).

In the case of multiple myoma, the presence of a focal pancreatic mass should lead to the diagnosis. Percutaneous biopsy allows diagnosis of the tumor. Usual treatment is irradiation (MITCHELL and HILL 1985; OLSON et al. 1993).

11.9 Pancreatic Schwannoma

Pancreatic schwannomas are derived from Schwann cells, the lining cells of the nerve sheath (BURD et al. 1992; DAS GUPTA et al. 1969). Rarely, intrapancreatic schwannomas have been described. Masses can occupy the body and tail of the pancreas and mimic a pancreatic pseudocyst (EGGERMONT et al. 1987).

Other appearances of pancreatic schwannoma include a large necrotic mass with biliary obstruction. Tumors with pronounced degenerative changes include cyst formation, calcification, or hemorrhage. Many lesions can present as a cystic pancreatic mass. Microscopic evaluation can reveal intrapancreatic schwannoma with cystic degeneration including a laminar aspect of the cyst with dense fibrous layers of connective tissue and numerous hemosiderin-laden macrophages (Ferrozzi et al. 1997).

CT findings of schwannoma include areas of low CT attenuation with soft tissue density. The low density lesions are homogeneous and result from a combination of factors including high lipid content and cystic degeneration (Moller et al. 1982).

11.10 Pancreatic Hemangioma

Pancreatic hemangioma is a rare benign lesion. It is a tumor of connective tissue origin. This tumor can be asymptomatic. Ultrasound shows a heterogeneous lesion with hypoechoic or anechoic areas. CT reveals a hypodense lesion before administration of contrast medium, and peripheral enhancement after injection. Diagnosis can be suggested by these findings. Other benign diseases can include Castleman disease, pancreatic fibromas, and sarcoidosis (Mangin et al. 1985; Chaulin et al. 1994; Mathieu et al. 1989) (Figs. 11.5, 11.6).

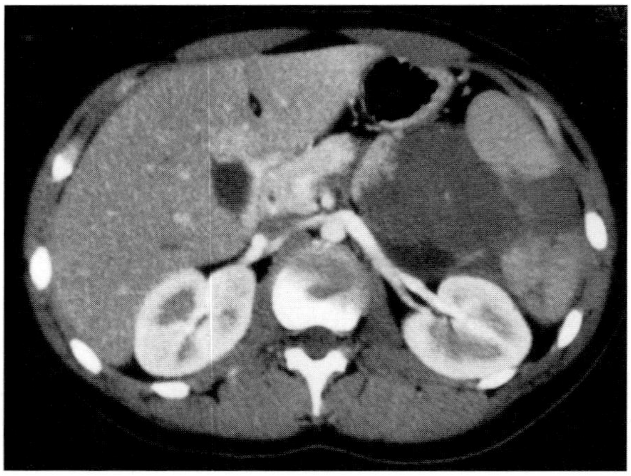

Fig. 11.5. Malignant histiocytic fibroma in a 16-year-old girl. Computed tomography after intravenous injection of iodinated contrast reveals a large mass of the pancreatic tail with hypodense density and heterogeneous aspect of the spleen owing to encasement of splenic vessels

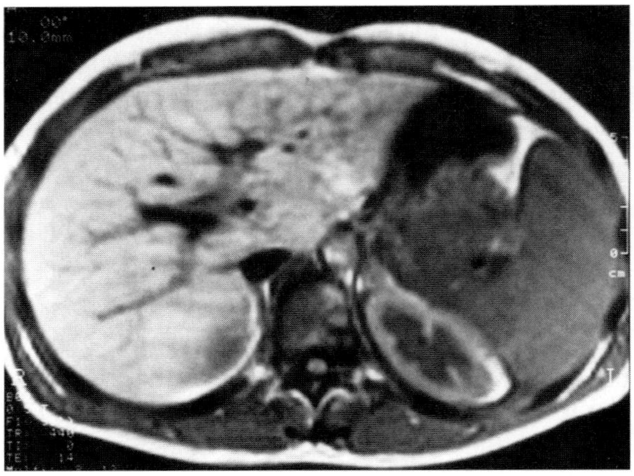

Fig. 11.6. Same patient as in Fig. 11.5. Magnetic resonance imaging of malignant histiocytic fibroma: gradient-recalled echo T1-weighted sequence without gadolinium, showing large hypointense lesion

11.11 Pancreatic Lymphoma

Pancreatic lymphoma is rare, comprising less than 0.2% of pancreatic malignancies and less than 1% of non-Hodgkin's lymphomas (NHL)(Ackerman et al. 1976; Borrowdale and Strong 1994).

Pancreatic involvement by malignant lymphoma is reported in autopsy series and could occur in one third of all patients with malignant lymphomas. Two histologic types are mainly reported, „diffuse histiocytic" and „diffuse mixed histiocytic". Histopathologic analysis can reveal low- or high-grade lymphoma. Pancreatic involvement is estimated to occur in 82% of cases of Burkitt's lymphoma (Banks et al. 1975; Burgener and Hamlin 1981).

NHL is frequently seen in patients who are immunocompromised owing to chemotherapy for malignant affections, organ transplantation, or acquired immunodeficiency syndrome (AIDS). These NHLs are very aggressive. Their predilection for extranodular sites is evidenced by the high frequency of hepatic localizations (Cappel et al. 1989).

Fine-needle aspiration biopsy is of limited value in identifying the histologic subtype of lymphoma and surgery may still be needed for a definite diagnosis. It is mandatory to make efforts to establish the diagnosis of lymphoma because it is potentially curable even at an advanced stage.

The pancreas may be involved by widespread NHL or may be the primary or predominant site of involvement. Pancreatic lymphoma is a somewhat ambiguous term. Indeed, it may be very difficult to distinguish between an intrinsic pancreatic abnormality and pancreatic invasion from adjacent lymphadenopathy. Pancreatic invasion from surrounding tissue with retroperitoneal and mesenteric lymphadenopathy comprises between 30% and 80% of all cases. Primary involvement of the pancreas is rare and has been reported in only a few cases. Lymphoma predominantly involving the pancreas at presentation causes a diagnostic challenge because it mimics carcinoma of the pancreas in its clinical and radiological appearance. However, differentiation is important because pancreatic lymphoma may respond favorably to chemotherapy. There is no age or sexual predominance. The mean age of presentation is 50 years. Signs and symptoms include epigastric pain, jaundice, and fatigue. Serum pancreatic enzyme levels may be elevated and cholestasis may be present (Costello et al. 1984; Ehrlich et al. 1968; Fischer and Kabakow 1987).

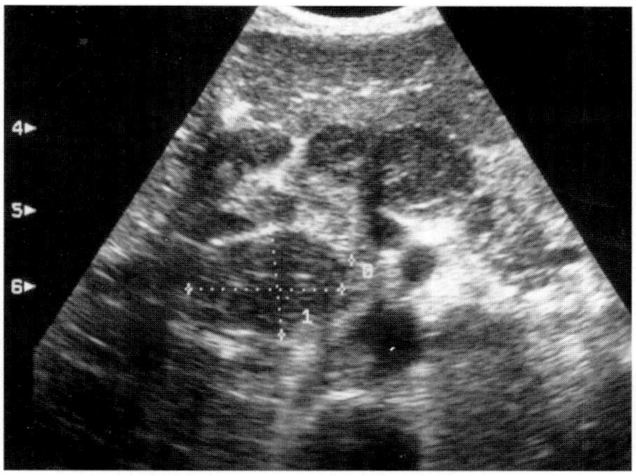

Fig. 11.7. Patient with primary lymphoma of the pancreas. Ultrasound shows multiple hypoechoic masses with enlargement of the pancreas

11.11.1 Imaging

11.11.1.1 Ultrasound

US may reveal a focal hypoechoic mass as a round lesion with well-defined contours. Sometimes, it appears as an infiltrating lesion, grossly reproducing the shape of the pancreas and presenting poorly-defined contours. The tumors are usually not calcified.

The mean diameter of the pancreatic mass is usually larger than carcinoma of the pancreas. Lymph nodes, when present, involve the retroperitoneal region below the level of the renal veins, and this sign is considered to strongly suggest the diagnosis of pancreatic lymphoma. When lymphoma involves the head of the pancreas, biliary ductal dilatation is usually present; however, unlike in carcinoma, pancreatic ductal dilatation is uncommon in lymphoma (Sthamler et al. 1988; Wittenberg et al. 1982) (Fig. 11.7).

11.11.1.2 Computerized Tomography

Numerous CT findings suggestive of pancreatic lymphoma have been described, including large homogeneous masses infiltrating surrounding tissue, with or without retroperitoneal and mesenteric lymphadenopathy (Prayer et al. 1992). Recently, two patterns of pancreatic lymphoma have been described: a large infiltrating lesion with poorly-defined contours, and rounded, well-delineated masses. At dynamic CT, the tumor appears heterogeneous. Stranding of retroperitoneal fat and thickening of anterior pararenal fascia can be encountered (Teefey et al. 1986). This may be related to tumorous infiltration, but also to tumor-induced pancreatitis suggested by high serum pancreatic enzyme levels. Pancreatitis may be associated with pancreatic tumors. Diffuse swelling of the pancreas simulating acute pancreatitis at CT, has been reported in lymphomas and carcinomas (Francis and Glazer 1982; Levine 1981). Pancreatitis associated with tumor lysis may also occur following institution of a chemotherapeutic regimen. Lymphadenopathy may or may not be present with pancreatic lymphoma. The presence of enlarged retroperitoneal lymph nodes below the level of the renal veins is considered suggestive of the diagnosis (Zeman et al. 1985) (Fig. 11.8).

Changes involving the fat around the celiac trunk and the superior mesenteric artery can also be a sign in pancreatic lymphoma, although less frequently than in the case of ductal adenocarcinoma. Signs of venous occlusion or stenosis can be present. Venous involvement may be a frequent finding in pancreatic lymphoma. The majority of patients with lymphoma primarily involving the pancreas at clinical and radiologic presentation may have widespread disease. Lesions at other sites may help to suggest the diagnosis of lymphoma. Lymphoma can best be con-

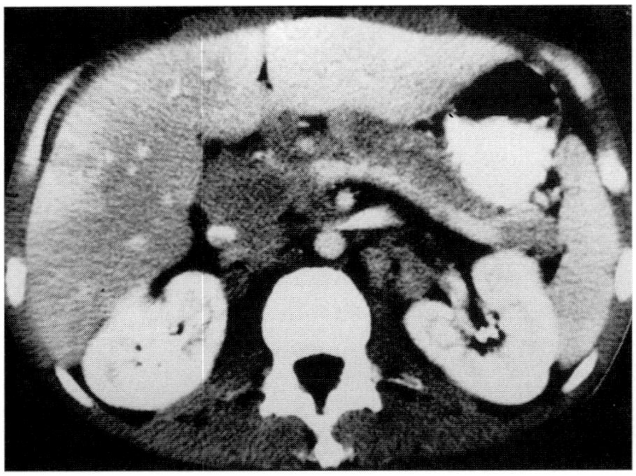

Fig. 11.8. Same patient as in Fig. 11.7. Primary lymphoma of the pancreas. Computed tomography after intravenous injection of contrast medium shows hypodense mass with enlargement of the head and body of the gland with retroperitoneal nodes along the left renal vein

sidered to primarily involve the pancreas on findings at biopsy and/or from imaging features such as dilatation of the pancreatic duct or presence of a „beak sign“ at the interface between tumor and pancreas. However, some patients may have lymph node involvement, limited to the area of the pancreas without intrinsic pancreatic disease. From a clinical point of view, this distinction is not important because the diagnostic challenge and the treatment of both entities are the same. Small tumor volume, well-defined contours, tumor heterogeneity, pancreatic duct dilatation, and venous invasion are not arguments against the diagnosis of pancreatic lymphoma. Distinction between pancreatic lymphoma and pancreatic carcinoma cannot be reliably made by CT criteria, although the presence of enlarged retroperitoneal lymph nodes or peripancreatic lymphadenopathy should suggest the diagnosis of primary pancreatic lymphoma. However, the diagnosis of pancreatic lymphoma must ultimately be made with biopsy. Differentiation of pancreatic lymphoma from ductal tumors of the pancreas is essential because of the differences in clinical management, treatment, and prognosis. The prognosis of pancreatic lymphoma compared to pancreatic adenocarcinoma appears to be favorable in most cases. Chemotherapy may be effective in patients with pancreatic lymphoma to provide palliation, increase patient survival, and produce an occasional cure. The role of surgery for the diagnosis and treatment of patients with primary pancreatic lymphoma is debated (Mansour et al. 1989; Webb et al. 1989). The necessity and method of obtaining an accurate preoperative histopathologic diagnosis remain controversial.

Pancreatic lymphoma may be distinguished from pancreatic adenocarcinoma by several factors, including patient age, presence of a palpable epigastric mass, tumor size, duration of clinical symptoms, enlarged retroperitoneal lymph nodes, and lesions at other sites. A high index of suspicion is important in establishing an accurate diagnosis, which depends on biopsy and histologic examination. Excellent response and remission rates can be expected with completed chemotherapeutic protocols. Average survival for patients with primary pancreatic lymphoma may be years longer than expected with ductal tumors of the pancreas. Pancreatic lymphoma should be considered in the differential diagnosis of most patients with undiagnosed pancreatic tumors. Prompt and accurate diagnosis, combined with the proper treatment, may be rewarding and result in long-term survival for many patients with primary pancreatic lymphoma.

11.12 Pancreatic Sarcoma

Sarcoma of the pancreas is an extremely unusual lesion accounting for fewer than 1% of pancreatic tumors (Alguacil-Garcia and Weiland 1977; Chevrel 1968; Neibling 1968). Histologic differential diagnosis of sarcoma include leiomyosarcoma, fibrosarcoma, carcinosarcoma, rhabdomyosarcoma, liposarcoma, hemangio-endothelioma, malignant neurilemoma, malignant hemangiopericytoma, and malignant fibrous histiocytoma (Gogquin and Salembier 1971; Marini and Vidiri 1993; Rus 1993). One case of pleomorphic pancreatic sarcoma has been reported (Laverdière et al. 1992). US and CT findings in pancreatic sarcoma include a huge, well-defined mass that may occupy much of the abdominal cavity. In some cases, a low-density center in the tumor has been described, with a peripheral, circumferential, thick, spiculated capsule enhanced after intravenous administration of contrast medium (Fig. 11.9). Pseudocystic masses have also been described with wall thickness and spiculation in a case of cystic pleomorphic sarcoma of the pancreas, mimicking pancreatic pseudocyst (Laverdière et al. 1992). CT permits visualization of tumor nodularity, calcification, and vascularity, thereby aiding in the differentiation of other cystic pancreatic masses. Treatment remains one of surgical resection, but may be difficult because of peri-

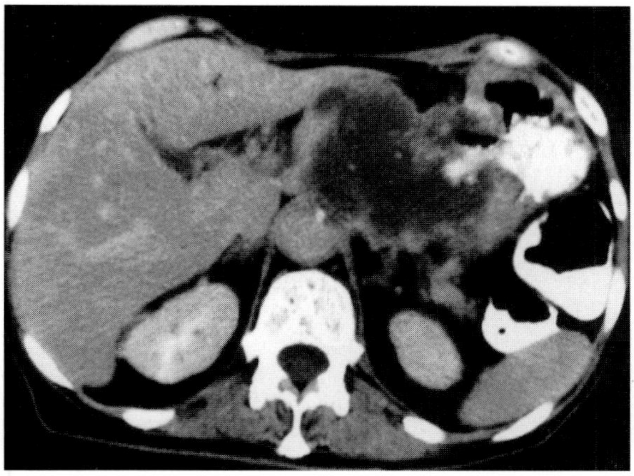

Fig. 11.9. Patient with sarcoma of the pancreas. Computed tomography (CT) after intravenous injection of iodinated contrast shows large cystic and necrotic mass with enlargement of the body and tail of the pancreas. Cytologic diagnosis was made after fine-needle biopsy. CT shows large extension of the tumor towards the celiac trunk and mesenteric vessels

pancreatic extension. Prognosis is limited, with an only 13% survival rate at 5 years.

11.13 Intrapancreatic Metastases

The frequency of intrapancreatic metastases is underestimated and varies considerably in the literature: from 11% of patients with neoplasms in an autopsy series to 4.5% of patients with pancreatic tumors in clinical series. These lesions may appear a long time after the primary neoplasm. Clinically, the pancreas is infrequently involved by metastatic disease and such involvement is usually from direct extension from a contiguous organ. Only 3% of patients with advanced remote primary malignancy are reported to have metastasis to the pancreas. The incidence is higher in patients with melanoma (37.5%), breast carcinoma (19%), and bronchogenic carcinoma (8.4 %). Other malignancies reported to metastasize to the pancreas include ovarian, prostatic, gastric, hepatocellular, colonic, esophageal, biliary, renal, and cervical carcinomas, and various sarcomas (Hamilton et al. 1982; Mulligan et al. 1997; Opocher et al. 1982; Whittington et al. 1982).

Metastasis to the peripancreatic nodes is not uncommon, and secondary invasion of the pancreas from tumor in these nodes is difficult to differentiate from direct metastasis to the pancreas. US and dynamic CT examination of the pancreas help to increase detection of metastasis (Biset et al. 1991). Percutaneous guided biopsy serves for planning therapy as it differentiates metastases from primary ductal adenocarcinoma. If the primary tumor is responsive to chemotherapy or hormonal manipulation, the pancreatic metastasis has a better prognosis than primary ductal adenocarcinoma (Derias and Chong 1993). Pancreatic metastasis are usually not symptomatic. When symptoms are present, they are often nonspecific and include jaundice, gastrointestinal hemorrhage, or acute pancreatitis. Practically, metastases of all neoplasms may spread to the pancreas, but the most frequent primary tumors are those with hematogenous dissemination. Primary tumors are more often melanoma, lung cancers, breast cancers, and renal cell carcinoma. The high incidence of renal cancers seems to be related to their latency, to the occurrence of hematogenous solitary metastasis, and to the high survival rate after surgery (Carini et al. 1988; Portal et al. 1992). Melanoma as a primary tumor may also be related to patient survival with chemotherapy (Johansson et al. 1970) (Figs. 11.10, 11.11a,b). US is the first method to be used. Pancreatic metastases are usually small, between 1.5 and 2 cm. In most cases, metastases are hypoechoic and well defined. Anechoic lesions can be related to several primary tumors such as melanoma, ovarian carcinoma, or sarcoma.

CT examination reveals intense enhancement in the arterial phase, in the case of metastatic renal cancer. This feature may also be observed in breast cancer. Solitary lesions of the head of the pancreas are particularly difficult to differentiate from adenocar-

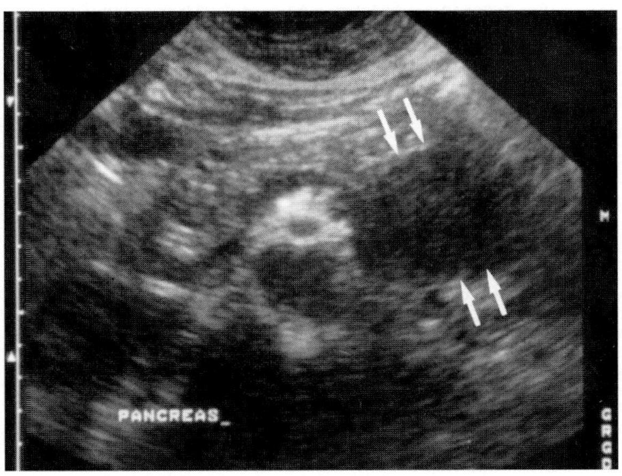

Fig. 11.10. Patient with pancreatic metastases from a melanoma. Ultrasound of the body and tail of the pancreas showing hypoechoic mass metastatic from a melanoma (*arrows*)

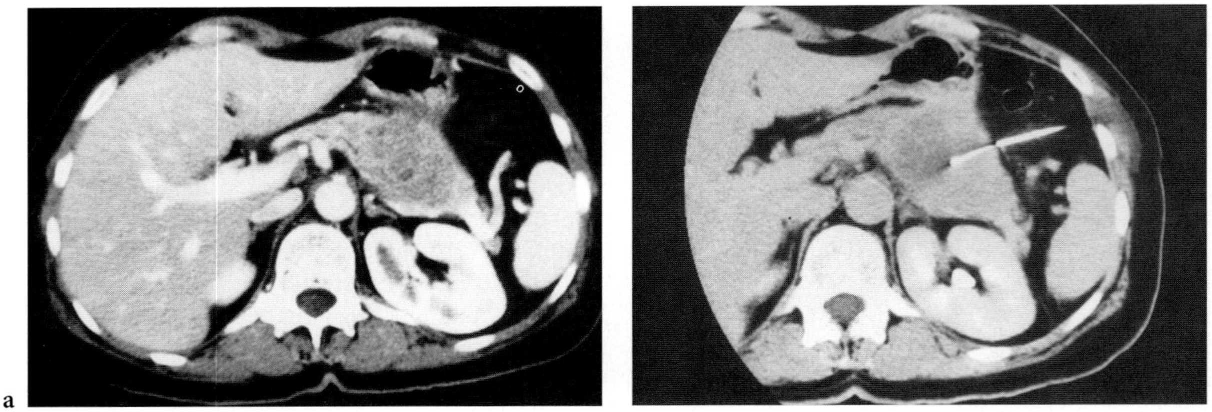

Fig. 11.11a,b. Patient with pancreatic metastases from a melanoma. **a** Computed tomography (CT) after injection of iodinated contrast showing a large mass of the body and tail of the pancreas with encasement of splenic vessels. **b** CT-guided biopsy of the pancreatic mass

cinoma. Duct dilatation may be observed, but less often than with carcinoma of the pancreas. Dynamic CT shows dissemination of the lesion to two or more parts of the pancreas, nonobliteration of the retropancreatic fat, and absence of dilatation of the biliary tree in the case of a voluminous tumor of the pancreatic head. Only positive results of percutaneous punctures must be considered. Difficulties in interpretation concern metastasis from a primary glandular cancer which has the same appearance as carcinoma of the pancreas. Laparotomy should be avoided. Chemotherapy may be guided by cytologic and histologic samples and improves prognosis according to the chemosensitivity of the primary neoplasm. Surgery is indicated for tumors with slow evolution, for gastro-intestinal hemorrhage requiring hemostasis, and for metastases of renal or breast cancer, particularly if the lesion occurs late and appears solitary (STANKARD and KARL 1992). The evolution of metastases of melanoma or lung cancer is usually rapid, but survival after chemotherapy is significantly better than in adenocarcinoma of the pancreas. Survival may be long, as in one case of renal metastases with 5 years' survival after surgery (STRIJK 1989).

When pancreatic metastasis is isolated, it should be detected at a stage at which effective treatment is still possible. The lesion can be small, with a diameter of between 0.5 cm and 2 cm.

11.13.1 Imaging

OnUS, metastases appear as hypoechoic nodules (WERNECKE et al. 1986). Multiple localizations of such nodules help to establish the metastatic origin of the images. Most frequently, pancreatic metastatic lesions are visible as a single pancreatic mass or as multiple nodular masses disseminated throughout the organ. The performance of CT has improved with helical CT, and this may result in higher sensitivity of CT in the detection of small metastatic intrapancreatic tumors.

On CT, small metastases may appear hypodense before and hyperdense after intravenous injection of iodinated contrast medium, and it is rather difficult to detect them as long as there is no modification of the pancreatic contour (MURANAKA et al. 1989; RUMANCIK et al. 1984).

Metastatic disease from primary adenocarcinoma of the right side of the colon has been reported. Clinical and CT findings in cases of pancreatic metastases from carcinoma of the colon cannot be distinguished from those of a primary ductal adenocarcinoma. CT findings show CT density of between 20 and 30 HU, consistent with areas of tumor necrosis or mucin production. This feature of hypodensity (scirrhous area or fibrosis of tumor) has a prevalence similar to that observed in primary ductal adenocarcinoma. Some masses can be isodense with the pancreas, and extend up along the hepatoduodenal ligament, with infiltration around the head and body of the pancreas. The most likely mode of spread in most of these cases is the lymphatic system. Progression of nodal metastases from carcinoma of the cecum, ascending colon, and transverse colon is likely to involve pancreatic parenchyma, and the tumor is likely to become inseparable from the pancreas.

Pancreatic metastasis from renal cancer has been reported to be hypervascular on angiography, this finding being considered characteristic of these lesions. On US, their appearance is nonspecific and can be hypoechoic and hyperechoic (Fig. 11.12). CT findings include heterogeneous as well as homogeneous enhancement, with hypo-, iso-, or hyperdense lesions. Even cystic masses have been reported on non-contrast CT (Ferrozzi et al. 1997). An intense early enhancement is very uncommon in pancreatic ductal adenocarcinomas. Distinction between renal cancer pancreatic metastasis and islet cell tumors is more problematic. Intense ring enhancement is typical for both of these tumors. Clinical history should permit distinction and a hypervascular pancreatic tumor in a patient with a history of renal cancer should be considered a metastasis from renal cancer until proven otherwise (McNichols et al. 1981; Rypens et al. 1992; Strijk 1989) (Fig. 11.13).

The possible clinical importance of MRI for establishing the diagnosis of pancreatic metastasis from renal cancer may include early detection, early guidance to surgical management, and avoidance of biopsy which might result in substantial hemorrhage (Py et al. 1984).

MRI of pancreatic metastases from renal cancer are mostly hypointense with normal pancreas on T1-weighted images, and hyperintense on T2-weighted images (Kelekis et al. 1996). Following contrast agent administration, lesions become hyperintense (comparable with renal cortex on immediate post-gadolinium, T1-weighted images). Intense enhancement on early post-gadolinium images is a finding consistent with the reported appearance on angiography.

A high-intensity signal on T2-weighted images, intense early enhancement in a homogeneous fashion in small tumors, and rim enhancement in large tumors can be considered as distinctive MRI findings for diagnosis of pancreatic metastasis from renal cell carcinoma.

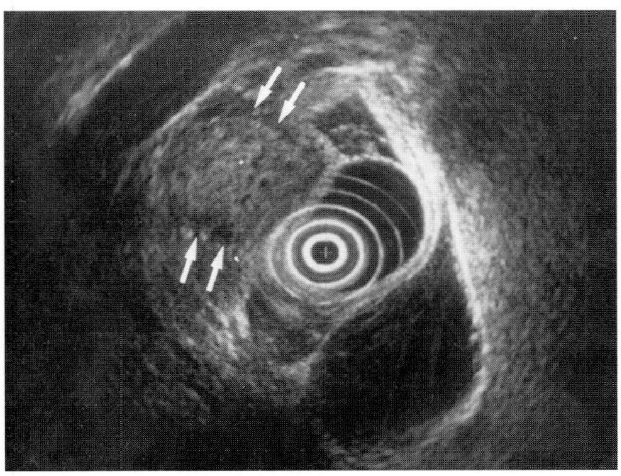

Fig. 11.12. Pancreatic metastasis from renal carcinoma. Endoscopic ultrasound shows a mixed hypoechoic and hyperechoic mass of the head of the pancreas (*arrows*)

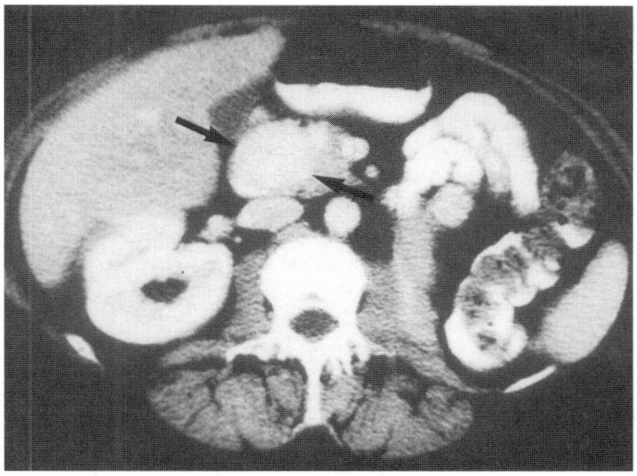

Fig. 11.13. Same patient as Fig. 11.10. Patient with pancreatic metastasis from renal carcinoma. Computed tomography shows a hypervascular mass of the head of the gland (*arrows*)

11.14 Conclusion

Knowledge of the morphologic aspects of rare neoplasms of the pancreas permits diagnosis on the basis of imaging data. Nevertheless, the diagnosis of rare tumors of the pancreas can be difficult by imaging. The tumor may be characterized by a „solid" aspect (e.g., common ductal adenocarcinoma), a mixed aspect (solid components and liquid necrosis or fluid-filled cysts), or by a predominantly cystic aspect.

The diagnosis of pancreatic metastasis and lymphoma can be assisted by US, helical CT, or MRI, as well as specific tumors such as lipomas, hemangiomas, or lymphangiomas.

Finally, diagnosis can be made by CT- or US-guided percutaneous biopsy. In addition to imaging findings, fine-needle aspiration biopsy often yields results decisive for the diagnosis. Great diagnostic precision is required given the extremely varied pathology and the fact that some conditions require specific therapy. In some tumors (such as mucinous cystic tumor and solid-cystic tumor), surgical excision is required, and in others, survival will depend on chemotherapy or antibiotic therapy. Finally, in elderly patients presenting with a benign lesion, no treatment would be advisable, according to imaging findings and biopsy results.

References

Ackerman AB, Aust JC, Bredenberg CE, Hanson VA, Rogers LS (1976) Problems in differentiating between pancreatic lymphoma and anaplastic carcinoma and their management. Ann Surg 184:705–708

Alguacil-Garcia A, Weiland LH (1977) The histologic spectrum, prognosis and histogenesis of the sarcomatoid carcinoma of the pancreas. Cancer 39:1181–1189

Amar A, Jougon J, Laban P, Jouanelle A, Marry JP, Edouard A (1991) Trois cas de tumeur solides et papillaires du pancreas chez la femme de la race noire. Semin Hop Paris 67:1001–1005

Balthazar E, Subramanyam B, Lefleur R, Barone C (1984) Solid and papillary epithelial neoplasm of the pancreas: radiographic, CT, sonographic, and angiographic features. Radiology 150:39–40

Baniel J, Konichezky M, Wolloch Y (1987) Osteoclast-type giant cell tumor of the pancreas: case report. Acta Chir Scand 153:67–69

Banks PM, Arseneau JC, Granlick MR, Canellos GP, De Vita VT, Bernard CW (1975) American Burkitt's lymphoma. A clinicopathologic study of 30 cases. Pathologic correlations. Am J Med 58:322–329

Baytor SM, Berg JW (1973) Cross classification and survival characteristics of 5,000 cases of cancer of the pancreas. J Surg Oncol 5:335–358

Biset JM, Laurent F, De Verbizier G, Houang B, Constantes G, Drouillard J (1991) Ultrasound and computed tomography findings in pancreatic metastasis. Eur J Radiol 12:41–44

Borrowdale R, Strong RW (1994) Primary lymphoma of the pancreas. Aust N Z J Surg 64:444–446

Botet JF, Lightdale C (1992) Endoscopic ultrasonography of the upper gastrointestinal tract. Radiol Clin North Am 30:1067–1083

Buchino JJ, Castello FM, Nagaraj MS (1984) Pancreatoblastoma. A histochemical and ultrastructural analysis. Cancer 53:963–969

Burd DA, Tyagi G, Bader DA (1992) Benign schwannoma of the pancreas. AJR 159:675

Burgener FA, Hamlin DG (1981) Histiocystic lymphoma of the abdomen: Radiographic spectrum. AJR 137:337–342

Cantrell BB, Cubilla AL, Erlandson RA, Fortner J, Fitzgerald PJ (1981) Acinar cell cystadenocarcinoma of human pancreas. Cancer 47:410–416

Capelle J (1986) Pancreatoblastome. Aspects échographiques et tomodensitométriques. A propopos d'un cas clinique. J Radiol 67:345–347

Cappel MS, Yao F, Cho KC, Axiotis CA (1989) Lymphoma predominantly involving the pancreas. Dig Dis Sci 34:942–947

Carini M, Selli C, Barbanti G, Bianchi S, Muraro G (1988) Pancreatic late recurrence of bilateral renal cell carcinoma after conservative surgery. Eur Urol 14:258–260

Chaulin B, Pontais C, Laurent F, De Mascarel A, Drouillard J (1994) Pancreatic castleman disease: CT findings. Abdom Imaging 19:160–161

Chevrel BB (1968) Sarcome du pancréas. Ann Chir 22:3–4, 199–203

Choi B, Kim Y, Kim C, Kim K, Han M (1988) Solid and papillary epithelial neoplasms of the pancreas: CT findings. Radiology 166:413–416

Cihak RW, Kawashima T, Steer A (1972) Adenoacanthoma (adenosquamous carcinoma) of the pancreas. Cancer 19:1133–1140

Costello P, Duszlak EJ Jr, Kane RA et al (1984) Peripancreatic lymph node enlargement in Hodgkin's disease, non-Hodgkin's lymphoma, and pancreatic carcinoma. CT 8:1–11

Cubilla AL, Fitzgerald PJ (1979) Classification of pancreatic cancer (nonendocrine). Mayo Clin Proc 54:449–458

Cubilla AL, Fitzgerald PJ (1984) Tumors of the exocrine pancreas. In: Hartmann WH (ed) Atlas of tumor pathology, fasc 19, ser 2. Armed Forces Institute of Pathology, Washington DC, pp 1–288

Das Gupta TK, Brasfield RD, Srong EW, Hajdu SI (1969) Benign solitary schwannomas (neurilemomas). Cancer 24:355–366

Derias NW, Chong WH (1993) Fine needle aspiration diagnosis of a late solitary pancreatic metastasis of renal adenocarcinoma. Cytopathology 4:369–372

Eggermont A, Vuzevski V, Huisman M, De Jong K, Jeekel J (1987) Solitary malignant schwannoma of the pancreas: report of a case and ultrastructural examination. J Surg Oncol 36:21–25

Ehrlich AN, Stalder G, Geller N, Sherlock P (1968) Gastrointestinal manifestations of malignant lymphoma. Gastroenterology 54:1115–1121

Ferrozzi F, Bova D, Campodonico F et al (1997) Pancreatic metastases: CT assessment. Eur Radiol 7(2):241

Fischer MG, Kabakow B (1987) Lymphoma of the pancreas. Mt Sinai J Med 50:492

Francis IR, Glazer GM (1982) Burkitt's lymphoma of the pancreas presenting as acute pancreatitis. J Comput Assist Tomogr 6:395–397

Freeny PC (1988) Radiology of the pancreas: two decades of progress in imaging and intervention. AJR 50:975–981

Freeny PC, Lawson RL (1982) Radiology of the pancreas. Springer, Berlin Heidelberg New York, p 514

Friedman AC, Edmonds PR (1989) Rare pancreatic malignancies. Radiol Clin North Am 27:177–190

Fukuya T, Yoshimitsu K, Kitagawa S et al (1989) Plasmacytoma of the pancreatic head. Gastrointest Radiol 14:226–228

Gogquin B, Salembier Y (1971) Les sarcomes fuso-dellaires du pancréas, à propos de deux observations. J Chir 102:217–226

Guillan RA (1985) Pleiomorphic adenocarcinoma of the pancreas. An analysis of five cases. Cancer 56:918–928

Hamilton I, Reis LD, Rashid SA, Clayden AD, Benson EA, Axon AT (1982) Association between carcinoma of the pancreas and carcinoma of the breast. Clin Oncol 8:89–90

Hanelin LG, Schimmel DH (1977) Lymphangioma of the pancreas exhibiting an unusual pattern of calcification. Radiology 122:636

Herman TE, Siegel MJ, Dehner LP (1994) CT of pancreatoblastoma derived from the dorsal pancreatic anlage. J Comput Assist Tomogr 18:648–650

Hertzana Y, Bar-Ziv J, Freund U (1989) Computed tomography of unusual calcified pancreatic tumors. J Comput Assist Tomogr 13:75–76

Johansson H, Krause V, Oldling L (1970) Pancreatic metastases from a malignant melanoma. Scand J Gastroenterol 5:573–575

Kelekis NL, Semelka RC (1997) MRI of pancreatic tumors. Eur Radiol 7(6):875

Kelekis NL, Semelka RC, Siegelman ES (1996) MRI of pancreatic metastases from renal cancer. J Comput Assist Tomogr 20:249

Kissane JM (1994) Pancreatoblastoma and solid anc cystic papillary tumor: two tumors related to pancreatic ontogeny. Semin Diagn Pathol 11:152–164
Klöppel G, Maillet B (1989) Classification and staging of pancreatic non-endocrine tumors. Radiol Clin North Am 27:105–119
Laverdière JT, Van Sonneberg E, Strum WB, Kuster GGR (1992) Pleomorphic pancreatic sarcoma mimicking pancreatic pseudocyst: CT appearance. AJR 158:87–89
Levine E (1981) Carcinoma of the pancreas presenting as acute pancreatitis: CT diagnosis. Gastrointest Radiol 6:29–33
Lumkin B, Anderson MW, Ablin DS, McGahan JP (1993) CT, MRI, and color Doppler ultrasound correlation of pancreatoblastoma: a case report. Pediatr Radiol 23:61–62
Mangin P, Perret M, Ronjon A (1985) Hémangiome du pancréas. J Radiol 66:381–384
Mansour GM, Cucchiaro G, Niotis MT, Fetter BF, Moore J et al (1989) Surgical management of pancreatic lymphoma. Arch Surg 124:1287–1289
Marini M, Vidiri A (1993) Case of malignant fibrous histiocytoma of the pancreas: computed tomography (CT) and ultrasound (US) appearance. Eur Radiol 3(1):86
Mathieu D, Guigui D, Valette PJ et al (1989) Pancreatic cystic neoplasms. Radiol Clin North Am 27:163–176
Mc Nichols DW, Segura JW, Deweerd JH (1981) Renal cell carcinoma: long term survival and late recurrence. J Urol 126:17–23
Mitchell DG, Hill MC (1985) Obstructive jaundice due to malignant myeloma of the pancreatic head, CT evaluation. J Comput Assist Tomogr 66:381–384
Moller Pedersen V, Hede A, Graem N (1982) A solitary malignant schwannoma mimicking a pancreatic pseudocyst. A case report. Acta Chir Scand 148:697–698
Morohoshi T, Held G, Klöppel G (1983) Exocrine pancreatic tumors and their histological classification: a study based on 167 autopsy and 97 surgical cases. Histopatology 7:645–661
Morohoshi T, Kanda M, Horie A et al (1987) Immunocytochemical markers of uncommon pancreatic tumors. Acinar cell carcinoma, pancreatoblastoma, and solid cystic (papillary-cystic) tumor. Cancer 59:739
Mulligan ME, Fellow DW, Mullen SE (1997) Pancreatic metastasis from Ewing's sarcoma. Clin Imag 21:23
Muranaka T, Teshima K, Honda H, Nanjo T, Hanada K, Oshuimi Y (1989) Computed tomography and histologic appearance of pancreatic metastases from distant sources. Acta Radiol 30:615–619
Neibling HA (1968) Primary sarcoma of the pancreas. Am Surg 34:690–693
Ohtomo K, Furui S, Onoue M (1992) Solid and papillary epithelial neoplasms of the pancreas: MR imaging and pahtologic correlation. Radiology 184:567–570
Olson MC, Kalbhen CL, Posniak HV (1993) Pancreatic plasmacytomas in a patient with multiple myeloma: CT and ultrasound findings. Abdom Imaging 18:323–324
Opocher E, Galleoti F, Spina GP, Battaglia G, Hernandez C (1982) Diagnosis of secondary tumors of the pancreas. Analysis of 13 cases. Minerva Med 73:577–581
Pinto MM, Monteiro NL, Tizol DM (1986) Fine needle aspiration of pleomorphic giant-cell carcinoma of the pancreas: case report with ultrastructural observations. Acta Cytol 30:430–434
Palosaari D, Clayton F, Seaman J (1986) Pancreatoblastoma in an adult. Arch Pathol Lab Med 110:650–652
Portal I, Barthet M, Alemy M, Payan MJ, Sastre B, Sahel J (1992) Recurrent pancreatic metastases from a hypernephroma. Press Med 38:1822
Prayer L, Schurawitzki H, Mallek R, Mostbeck G (1992) CT in pancreatic involvement of non-Hodgkin lymphoma. Acta Radiol 33:123–127
Procacci C, Graziani R, Bicego E et al (1995) Papillary cystic neoplasm of the pancreas: radiological findings. Abdom Imag 20:554
Py JM, Arnaud JP, Cinqualbre J, Adolff M, Bollack C (1984) Les métastases pancréatiques des néphro-épithéliomes. A propos de 2 observations. Acta Chir Belg 84:117–121
Radin DR, Colletti PM, Forrester DM et al (1986) Pancreatic acinar cell carcinoma with subcutaneous and intraosseous fat necrosis. Radiology 158:67–68
Rosai J (1968) Carcinoma of the pancreas simulating giant cell tumor of bone. Cancer 22:333–344
Rösch T, Lorenz R, Braig C et al (1991) Endoscopic ultrasound in pancreatic diagnosis. Gastrointest Endosco 37:347–352
Rumancik WM, Megibow AJ, Bosniak MA, Hilton S (1984) Metastatic disease to the pancreas: evaluation by computed tomography. J Comput Assist Tomogr 8:829–834
Rus PD (1993) Leiomyosarcoma of the pancreatic bed dectected on CT scans. AJR 161:210
Rypens F, Van Gansbeke D, Lambilliote JP, Van Regemorter G, Verhest A, Struyven J (1992) Pancreatic metastasis from renal cell carcinoma. Br J Radiol 65:547–548
Sagalow BR, Miller CL, Wechster RJ (1988) Pancreatic sarcoidosis mimicking pancreatic cancer. JCU 16:131
Salimi Z, Fishbein M, Wolverson MK, Johnson FE (1991) Pancreatic lymphangioma: CT, MRI, and angiographic features. Gastrointest Radiol 16:248–250
Savci G, Kilicturgay S, Sivri Z, Parlak M, Tuncel E (1996) Solid and papillary epithelial neoplasm of the pancreas: CT and MR findings. Eur Radiol 6:68–88
Semelka RC, Kroeker MA, Shoenut JP, Kroeker R, Yaffe CS, Micflikier AB (1991) Pancreatic disease: prospective comparison of CT, ERCP, and 1,5-T MR imaging with dynamic gadolinium enhancement and fat suppression. Radiology 181:785–791
Stankard CE, Karl RC (1992) The treatment of isolated pancreatic metastases from renal cell carcinoma: a surgical review. Am J Gastroenterol 87:1658–1660
Stephenson CA, Kletzel M, Seibert JJ, Glasier CM (1990) Pancreaticoblastoma: MR appearance. J Comput Assist Tomogr 14:492–493
Sthamler B, Bickel A, Manor E, Shahar MB, Kuten A, Suprun H (1988) Primary lymphoma of the head of the pancreas. J Surg Oncol 38:48–51
Strijk SP (1989) Pancreatic metastases of renal cell carcinoma: report of two cases. Gastrointest Radiol 14:123–126
Teefey SA, Stephens DH, Sheedy PF (1986) CT appearance of primary pancreatic lymphoma. Gastrointest Radiol 11:41–43
Webb TH, Lillemoe KD, Pitt HA, Jones RJ, Cameron JL (1989) Pancreatic lymphoma. Is surgery mandatory for diagnosis or treatment? Ann Surg 209:25–30
Wernecke K, Peters PE, Galanski M (1986) Pancreatic metastases: US evaluation. Radiology 160:399–402
Whittington R, Moyland DJ, Dobelbower RR, Kramer S (1982) Pancreatic tumors in patients with previous malignancy. Clin Radiol 33:297–299

Wilczynski SP, Valente PT, Atkinson BF (1984) Cytodiagnosis of adenosquamous carcinoma of the pancreas. Use of fine-needle aspiration. Acta Cytol 18:733–736

Wittenberg J, Simeone JF, Ferruci JT Jr, Mueller PR, Van Sonnenberg E, Neff CC (1982) Non-focal enlargment in pancreatic carcinoma. Radiology 144:131–135

Wolfman NT, Karstaedt N, Kawamoto EM (1985) Pleomorphic carcinoma of the pancreas: computed tomographic, sonographic and pathologic findings. Radiology 154:329–332

Zeman RK, Schiebler M, Clark LR et al (1985) The clinical and imaging spectrum of pancreaticoduodenal lymph node enlargement. AJR 144:1223–1227

12 Pancreatic Trauma

C. DOUWS, N. GRENIER, and J. C. BRICHAUX

CONTENTS

12.1 Introduction

Traumatic injuries of the pancreas are rare and difficult to diagnose. The retroperitoneal location of the pancreas explains the attenuated symptomatology early after the trauma, and there is no specific biologic paraclinical test. Therefore, these lesions are often not detected until complications arise.

Although computed tomography (CT) has transformed the management of blunt trauma of the abdomen, notably as far as detection of injuries of solid organs are concerned, the imaging of pancreatic lesions remains difficult. The diagnosis of these injuries is nevertheless fundamental since they are associated with a high mortality.

12.2 Epidemiology

Pancreatic injuries are present in 2% (Dodds et al. 1990; NORTHRUP and SIMMONS 1972) to 7% (NILSSON et al. 1956; PATEL and BAUX 1955) of cases of closed abdominal trauma, far behind injuries to the liver at 47% , the spleen at 44%, and the kidneys at 34% (TAYLOR et al. 1959). These injuries are rarely isolated (PATEL and BAUX 1955), and 60% of the injuries are duodenopancreatic. In 90% of the cases, an associated lesion is found in another abdominal organ (DODDS et al. 1990).

Mortality ranges from 16% (JONES 1955) to 20% (JEFFREY et al. 1953; JEFFREY 1990; CALEN et al. 1957), an approximately equal number of deaths being caused by (a) hemorrhage and hypovolemic shock (BROOKE JEFFREY 1990) and (b) serious infection with septic shock, this being a function of the level of the lesion and of the associated injuries. Morbidity is also high. Complications arise in 33% (LEPPÄNIEMI et al. 1955) of cases when injury of the ducts of the pancreas is not detected early.

12.3 Anatomic Injuries and Mechanisms

The pancreas is a deep, retroperitoneal, solid organ located behind the lesser sac. It surrounds the vertebral body of L1. At the time of violent shock, it is crushed on the "chopping block" of the vertebrae. In order of frequency, injuries involve the body, the head, and the tail of the pancreas (BROOKE JEFFREY 1990).

Three types of impact can be distinguished (NORTHRUP and SIMMONS 1972):

1. When the impact is to the right of the vertebral column, the lesion will involve the head of the pancreas; hepatic and especially duodenal injuries are therefore often associated findings.
2. If the impact is median, the body is injured, with clean-cut, complete fractures and transections.
3. If the impact is to the left, the tail of the pancreas is contused due to a pulling mechanism (PATEL and BAUX 1955) involving traction on the splenic vessels. Left renal, left colic, and splenic injuries are therefore often observed.

C. Douws, MD, N Grenier, MD, J. C Brichaux, MD, Service de Radiologie Groupe Hôspitalier Pellegrin, Place Amέle-Raba-Léon, F-33076 Bordeaux Cédex, France

Hypotonia of the abdominal wall at the time of the shock explains the high frequency of these injuries in children and in alcoholic patients (PATEL and BAUX 1955). They follow falls onto bicycle or motorcycle handles or from substantial heights (CALEN et al. 1987). In adults, crushing against car steering wheels (BASS et al. 1988) is the most frequent cause.

Contusions of the pancreas can be complicated by early pancreatitis following the attrition of the parenchyma. The latter occurs in the hours following the injury, which explains why a pancreatic lesion may be overlooked if the explorations are performed too early. The anatomic lesions are therefore classified according to the damage to the parenchyma and pancreatic ducts. There are several classifications, but the most noteworthy take into account the risk of hemorrhage, of tissular attrition, and of acute pancreatitis, thereby guiding the therapeutic approach. However, only rupture of the pancreatic duct requires surgery.

Grade 1 is a simple contusion of the parenchyma or a small hematoma, without capsular rupture.

Grade 2 corresponds to small fractures and hematomas without any injury of the pancreatic duct.

Grade 3 is a clean-cut section of the pancreas over more than 50% of its thickness with rupture of the pancreatic duct.

Grade 4 corresponds to crushing of the entire pancreatic gland (JEFFREY 1990).

Complications are a function of the severity of the injury and the rapidity of the management. Fistulas, pseudocysts, and abscesses are the most frequent (NORTHRUP and SIMMONS 1972). Fistulas are not always considered a complication since they avoid the formation of pseudocysts thanks to the free flow of pancreatic secretions. Contusions of the pancreatic tail cause fewer fistulas than those of the head. Pseudocysts occur in 10% of the cases. The current treatment by percutaneous drainage (BASS et al. 1988; JAFFE et al. 1989) makes it possible to avoid the occurrence of secondary infection, spontaneous perforation, massive hemorrhage, obstruction of the biliary ducts, and acute intestinal occlusion. These pseudocyst complications are aggravated by high mortality.

Pseudoaneurysms of pancreaticoduodenal arteries, secondary hemorrhages, persistent or recurrent pancreatitis, insufficiency of the exocrine function or diabetes, or a residual stenosis of the pancreatic duct appear more rarely.

12.4 Clinical and Laboratory Findings

At the time of the initial clinical evaluation, upon arrival in an emergency trauma center, the symptoms in favor of a pancreatic lesion are very often absent (two-thirds of the cases) because they become evident quite late. Due to the retroperitoneal location of the pancreas, there are few irritative phenomena of the peritoneum within the hours following the accident (thus explaining this time lag).

When interrogation of the patient is possible, the patient may report initial and brief post-traumatic epigastric pain that has entirely sub-sided. A supramesocolic impact may be visible on the skin. Traditionally, the pain is deep and posterior with epigastric guarding. Pain may be absent for several days, even in the case of complete transection with avulsion of the pancreatic duct. In fact, there is no correlation between clinical findings and the severity of the lesions.

Not only are the symptoms discrete, but the clinical signs are often absent. If palpation causes epigastric or supramesocolic pain, this should arouse suspicion of a pancreatic lesion. Contracture is mild or absent.

In isolated forms, the clinical manifestations may only appear with late complications, such as pseudocysts, which may occur weeks, months, or even years later. This delay may be due to inhibition of the pancreatic secretions or to the impossibility of activating the pancreatic enzymes (NORTHRUP and SIMMONS 1972).

The laboratory analyses are not characteristic either. The increase in serum and urine amylase levels can be delayed (CALEN et al. 1987; NILSSON et al. 1986; NORTHRUP and SIMMONS 1972; PATEL and BAUX 1985; MEREDITH and TRUNKEY 1985). Furthermore, this finding is not specific, also being encountered in injury of the digestive tract, the salivary glands, or other intra-abdominal organs. However, a progressive increase in amylase over more than 6 days should arouse suspicion of a pancreatic complication. In the absence of fistulas, the persistence of a high level of amylase first suggests a pseudocyst. The presence of amylase upon peritoneal lavage is indicative of pancreatic injury, but its absence does not exclude it (NORTHRUP and SIMMONS 1972; MEREDITH and TRUNKEY 1988). Hyperleukocytosis is not very valuable.

In view of the above, the history and mechanism of the impact quite often constitute the only criteria for suspecting the diagnosis and the only indications for imaging studies.

12.5 Radiologic Findings

The currently preferred approach to the imaging of closed abdominal injuries is combined use of CT and ultrasonography. The detection of renal, splenic, and hepatic injuries has been markedly improved by such an approach, but this is not true to the same extent for injuries to the pancreas and hollow viscera.

12.5.1 Plain Films

Plain films of the abdomen are not worthwhile for the diagnosis of isolated injury of the pancreas. However, extraperitoneal gas, suggesting a rupture of the duodenum, constitutes a reason to search for an associated pancreatic lesion.

12.5.2 Ultrasonography

Ultrasonography is better suited for the follow-up of an already proven lesion than for immediate diagnosis since intestinal gaseous distention usually prevents visualization of the pancreas in the initial hours following trauma (DODDS et al. 1990). Nevertheless, when the pancreas is visible, any fractures can be shown (Fig. 12.1); furthermore, acute pancreatitis, and the complications resulting from it, does not pose any major diagnostic problems (i.e., hematomas, peripancreatic fluid collections, pseudocysts, and abscesses can all be identified).

12.5.3 Computed Tomography

Computed tomography (CT) seems to offer most advantages in the exploration of the pancreas following blunt abdominal trauma. Indeed, CT is often the only technique to permit the diagnosis; as such, it is extremely important and must be rigorously applied.

Upper digestive tract opacification with diluted water-soluble contrast medium must be performed: filling of the duodenum with contrast medium facilitates study of the head of the pancreas, while the nonopacified duodenum may suggest an increase in the volume of the head. Presence of fluid in the duodenal lumen can simulate a peripancreatic fluid collection.

The intravenous injection of iodinated contrast medium is fundamental for showing the thin fractures which do not enhance after injection in relation to the pancreatic parenchyma.

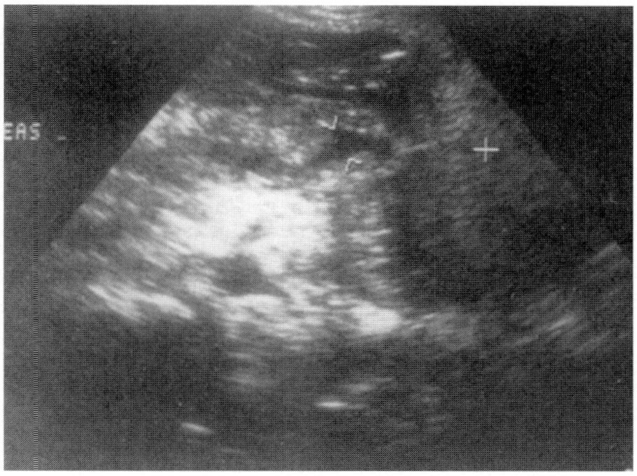

Fig. 12.1. Transverse sonogam showing a hypoechoic fracture of the body of the pancreas *(arrows)*

In spite of all these precautions, the quality of CT examinations is often impaired by the patient's agitation or an incapacity for adequate apnea. Sedation can therefore be useful. However, streak artifacts related to the water-air interfaces of the digestive tract are difficult to avoid.

Currently, helical CT provides excellent images, even in patients with multiple trauma and severe pain. Breath-holding is no longer necessary. The speed with which the sections are obtained makes it possible to acquire isolated arterial-phase and tissue-phase images, and to repeat the examination using thin sections to more precisely evaluate small organs like the pancreas. The detection of limited pancreatic fractures is facilitated by this. An initial acquisition of 7-mm sections may be followed by the use of helical CT centered on the pancreas to obtain 5-mm or 3-mm slices. The only artifacts still present are those due to the air-water interfaces of the digestive tract.

If the results are inconclusive, a repeat CT examination should be performed a few hours later. It should be read by radiologists with adequate training, if indeed one can acquire expertise in this type of trauma, which is, as mentioned above, extremely rare (JEFFREY 1990).

The indications for CT can be evident when the injury of the pancreas is combined with other abdominal injury, notably when hemoperitoneum is detected on ultrasonography. However, when the injury of the pancreas is isolated, the history and the mechanism of the impact at the epigastric level are sufficient grounds for requesting a CT study.

The fractures are generally very thin (Fig. 12.2), often at the limit of the spatial resolution of CT. The pancreatic parenchyma itself does not show any changes in density even in the presence of a complete fracture (Jeffrey 1990). Sometimes the two edges of the fracture separate and the lesion is therefore obvious after intravenous contrast enhancement (Fig. 12.3). It appears hypodense as compared with the normal parenchyma, even if the fracture space is filled by a hematoma. These fractures can assume several aspects: rectangular, irregular, or in waves.

When there is damage to great vessels, notably the splenic artery and the splenic vein, substantial peripancratic hematoma will result, often being located at the level of the mesenteric root. Some injuries, even large ones, may not bleed and as a result hematomas are frequently absent.

Rupture of the pancreatic duct is not directly visible. There is a leak of hypodense pancreatic liquid which is hypodense when pure but is often mixed with a hematoma, which prevents its identification.

The contusions cause a partial or total increase in the volume of the gland, which appears hypodense and heterogeneous after injection of the contrast medium (Fig. 12.4). Associated duodenal contusions can also be identified (Fig. 12.5). Intramural hematomas are seen as collections adjoining the head of the pancreas. Pneumoretroperitoneum in the right anterior pararenal space leads to suspicion of a duodenal rupture, all the more so when there is a leak of the water-soluble contrast medium on the opposite side.

In its early stage, pancreatitis following trauma has a CT appearance which can be identical to that of pancreatitis due to other causes (Fig. 12.6). Infiltration of the peripancreatic fat can be observed, with thickening of Gerota's fascia or infiltrations of the anterior pararenal space [even when it occurs in isolation, this is considered a very important sign by many authors (Jeffrey al. 1983; Jeffrey 1990; Calen et al. 1987; Dodds et al. 1990)], a local or diffuse increase in the volume of the pancreas, and a heterogeneous aspect of the parenchyma. These lesions are often delayed, and sufficient time must be allowed if discernible modifications are to be observed at the time of the CT examination. According to Jeffrey et al. (1983), there appears to be a high number of false-negatives (Peitzman et al. 1986) when the CT scan is performed too early, for instance less than 12 h after the trauma. False-positive findings are due to artifacts (Dodds et al. 1990)

Lane et al. (1994) have reported a new sign which seems to have good sensitivity. In their retrospective

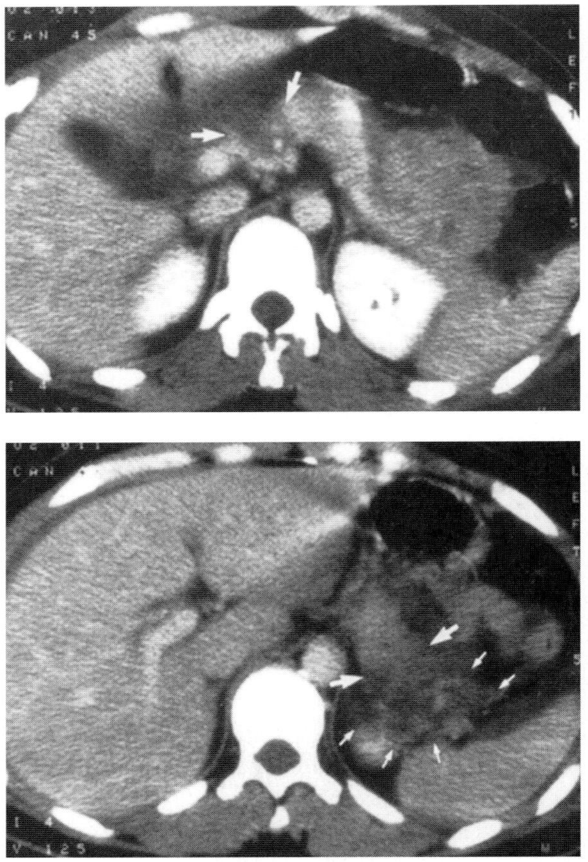

Fig. 12.3a,b. Contrast-enhanced CT. **a** The pancreatic parenchyma appears abruptly sectioned at the junction between the body and the head *(arrows)*. **b** At an upper level, the tail is enlarged *(thick arrows)* with irregular margins and a peripancreatic fluid collection *(thin arrows)*

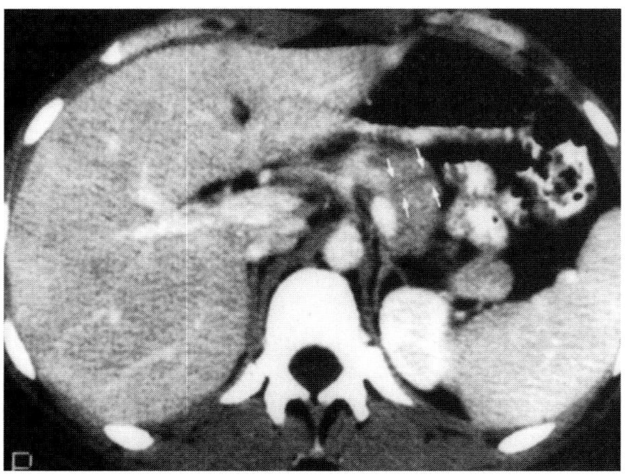

Fig. 12.2. Contrast-enhanced CT scan demonstrating anterior laceration of the body of the pancreas *(thin arrows)*

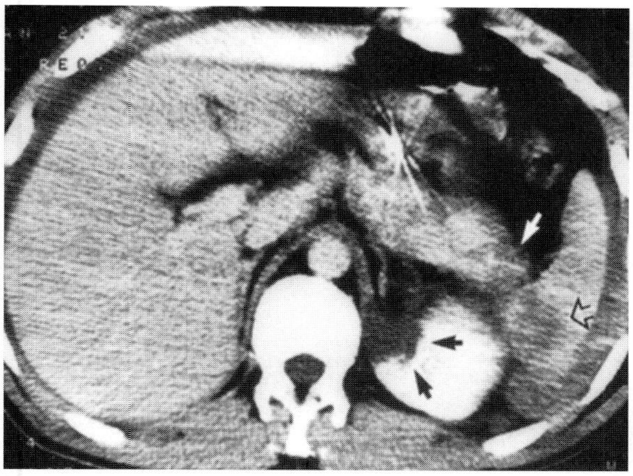

Fig. 12.4. Contrast-enhanced CT scan shows a heterogeneous tail of the pancreas *(white arrow)* with a thin peripancreatic fluid collection. A splenic *(open arrow)* and a left renal *(black arrow)* contusion are also present

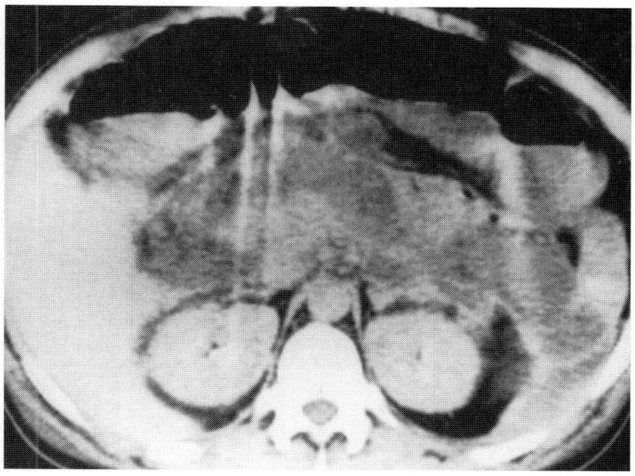

Fig. 12.6. Pancreatitis occurring 2 days after trauma

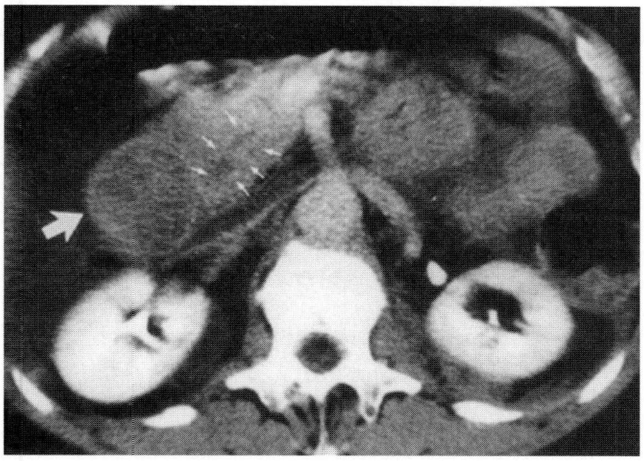

a

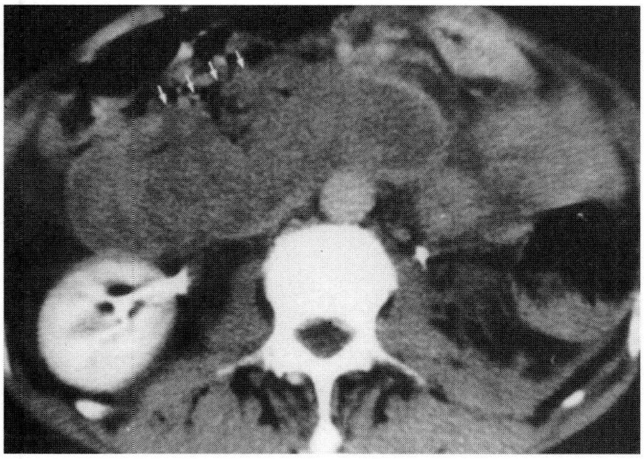

b

Fig. 12.5a,b. Laceration of the pancreas with rupture of the duodenum. **a** This contrast-enhanced CT scan demonstrates enlargement of the pancreatic head with a parenchymal fissure *(thin arrows)*. The lumen of the duodenum is dilated by blood *(thick arrow)*. **b** This scan at a lower level shows the third part of the duodenum with an enlarged lumen and distruption of its anterior wall *(arrows)*

analysis, 90% of patients with pancreatic trauma had fluid separating the splenic vein from the pancreas adjacent to the site of injury. Because blunt pancreatic trauma is very rare, this sign would be difficult to evaluate prospectively. Nevertheless, radiologists should look for it along with the other signs described above.

Imaging characteristics of complications of post-traumatic pancreatitis are not substantially different from those seen in acute pancreatitis of other etiology (Peitzman et al. 1986). Pseudocysts are often located in the anterior pararenal space (Figs. 12.7, 12.8) and very rarely in the transverse mesocolon. They are generally encapsulated, causing a mass effect.

Abscesses take on variable patterns. Gas bubbles are sometimes seen. They are difficult to differentiate from normal intestinal air except when they are located in the center of the pancreatic parenchyma.

As far as pseudoaneurysms are concerned, CT shows a hypodense mass before the injection of contrast; the mass enhances strongly, similar to the great vessels, during the bolus. Angiography confirms the diagnosis and permits endovascular treatment.

Once again, it should be emphasized that these diagnoses are extremely difficult and require substantial expertise. Due to the rarity of this type of trauma, the sensitivity of CT in the detection of traumatic injuries of the pancreas has never really been evaluated (Jeffrey et al. 1983; Jeffrey 1990; Dodds et al. 1990). The interpretation of these examinations must be meticulous: thickening of the anterior pararenal fascia or vague infiltration of the peripan-

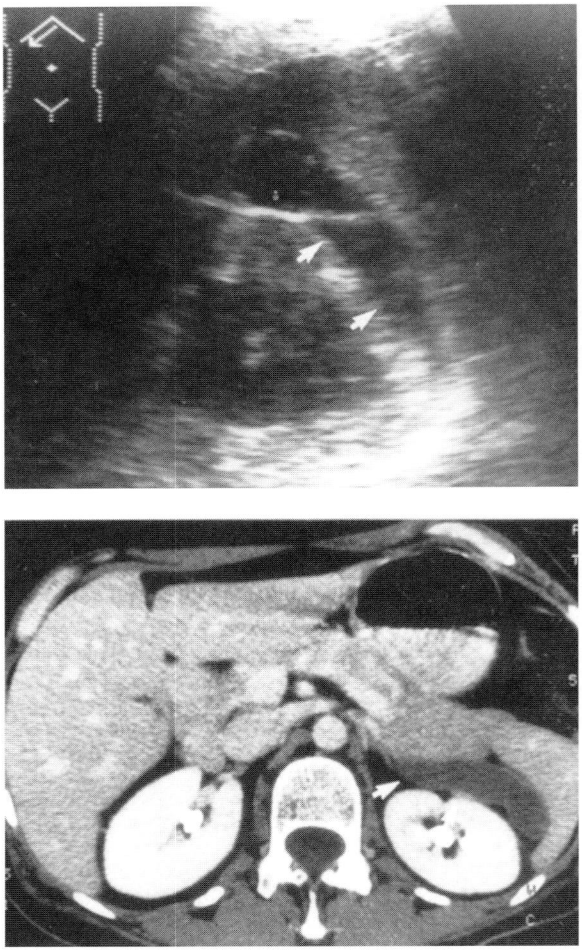

a

b

Fig. 12.7.a,b. Post-traumatic pancreatic pseudocyst. **a** This transverse sonogram shows a hypoechoic collection *(arrows)* at the posterior aspect of the tail of the pancreas. **b** Contrast-enhanced CT demonstrates the same collection *(arrow)* within the anterior pararenal space

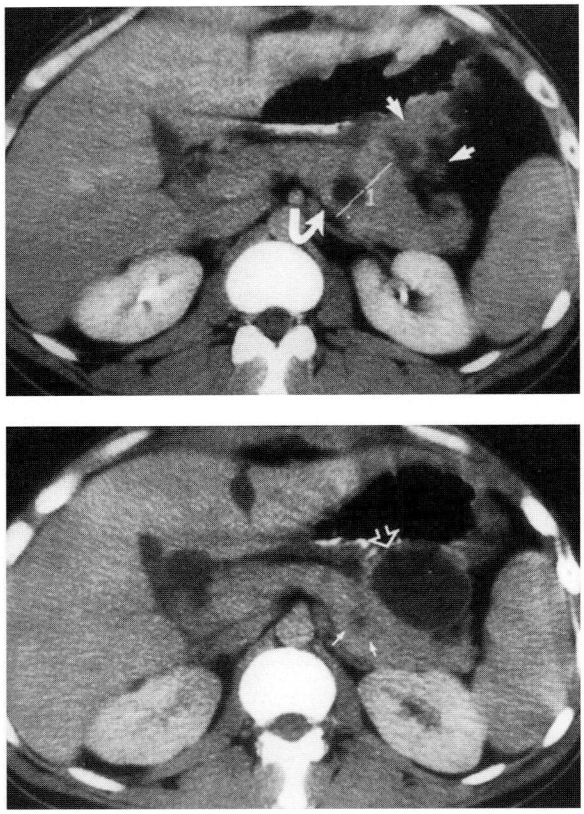

a

b

Fig. 12.8. Contrast-enhanced CT. a Two days after the trauma, CT shows an intrapancreatic hematoma at the surface of the tail (curved arrow) and a hematoma within the laser sac (arrows). b Two weeks later, the intrapancreatic collection has decreased (white arrows), but a pseudocyst has appeared anteriorly (open arrow)

creatic fat, although nonspecific, should lead to the performance of a further CT study within the next 24 h.

12.5.4
Endoscopic Retrograde Cholangiopancreatography

Retrograde catheterization of the biliary and pancreatic ducts remains worthwhile. It enables the detection of injury of the pancreatic duct requiring a surgical suture . Faced with suspicion of pancreatic trauma some authors still perform retrograde catheterization of the papilla with opacification to check the integrity of the ducts (Richieri et al. 1980). When the clinical picture is highly evocative, but the CT examination is negative or doubtful, ERCP is worthwhile. If there is no pancreatic duct injury, conservative treatment is sufficient.

References

Bass J, DiLorenzo M, Desjardins JG, et al. (1988) Blunt pancreatic injuries in children: the role of percutaneous external drainage in the treatment of pancreatic pseudocysts. J Pediatr Surg 23:721–724

Calen S, Moreno P, Nicolau H, Winnock S, Janvier G, Videau J (1987) Traumatismes duodéno-pancréatiques: Considération diagnostiwues et thérapeutiques à propos de 25 cas. J Chir 124:263–271

Dodds WJ, Taylor AJ, Erickson SJ, Lawson TL (1990) Traumatic fracture of the pancreas: CT characteristics. J Comput Assist Tomogr 14:3745–378

Jaffe RB, Arata JA, Matlak ME (1989) Percutaneous drainage of traumatic pancreatic pseudocysts in children. AJR 152:591–595

Jeffrey RB Jr (1990) Pancreas, retroperitoneal duodenum, colon, and vascular trauma. In: McCort JJ (ed) Trauma radiology. Churchill Livingstone, New York, pp 215–230

Jeffrey RB Jr, Federlem P, Crass RA (1983) Computed tomography of pancreatic trauma. Radiology 147:491–494

Jones RC (1985) Management of pancreatic trauma. Am J Surg 150:698–704Leppäniemi A, Haapiainen R, Kiviluoto T, Lempinen M (1988) Pancreatic trauma: acute and late manifestations. Br J Surg 75:165–167

Lane MJ, Mindelzun RE, Sandhu JS, McCormick VD, Jeffrey RB (1994) CT diagnosis of blunt abdominal trauma. AJR 163:833–835

Meredith JW, Trunkey DD (1988) CT scanning in acute abdominal injuries. Surg Clin North Am 68:155–264

Nilsson E, Norrby S, Skullman S, Sjödahl R (1986) Pancreatic trauma in a defined population. Acta Chir Scand 152:647–651

Northrup WF, Simmons RL (1972) Pancreatic trauma: a review. Surgery 71:27–43

Patel JC, Baux D (1985) Les contusions duodénopancréatiques. Rev Prat 35:34–42

Peitzman AB, Makaroun MS, Slasky BS, Ritter P (1986) Prospective study of computed tomography in initial management of blunt abdominal trauma. J Trauma 26:585–592

Richieri JP, Gioan JA, Martin M, Pin G, Allio P, Jean E (1980) Pancréatographie endoscopique: sa place dans l'exploration des traumatismes du pancréas. Nouv Press Med 9:387

Taylor GA, Guion CJ, Potter BM, Eichelberger MR (1989) CT of blunt abdominal trauma in children. AJR 153:555–559

13 Pancreatic Transplantation

N. Grenier, H. Trillaud, C. Douws

CONTENTS

13.1 Introduction

Treatment of diabetes mellitus has improved in recent years thanks to progress in insulin therapy. However, this illness remains extremely severe. Approximately 50% of subjects who have had diabetes for more than 20 years have complications or secondary signs of the disease (nephropathy, neuropathy, retinopathy, enteropathy, and arteriopathy) (West et al. 1980).

The aim of treatment is at present to obtain a stable glycemia with intermittent administration of exogenous human insulin. The Diabetes Control and Complications Trial Research Group (1993) reported that intense insulin therapy has a beneficial effect on the occurrence and progression of secondary complications. However, this therapy does not avoid the onset of complications and leaves the patient exposed to accidents related to hypo- or hyperglycemia.

The goal of transplantation therapy is to restore endogenous secretion of insulin by implanting a whole pancreas from a donor. Better patient selection, improvements in surgical techniques, preservation of grafts with University of Wisconsin solution, and improved immunosuppression have increased survival rates. Most pancreas transplants are simultaneous pancreas-kidney transplants, which give higher pancreas graft survival rates. The results of simultaneous pancreas-kidney transplantation in patients with insulin-dependent diabetes mellitus and end-stage renal disease have improved significantly over the last decade. The 1-year patient, pancreas, and kidney survival rates reported by the International Pancreas Transplant Registry (1995) were 91%, 74%, and 84%, respectively. The 1-year graft survival rate in isolated pancreas transplantation was 52%.

This technique of transplantation allows patients to recover normal and stable glucose and glycosylated hemoglobin levels (Robertson 1992), improves quality of life (Hathaway et al. 1994), and could stop the evolution of certain complications (Kennedy et al. 1990; Gaber et al. 1995) and reverse that of others such as diabetic nephropathy (Abouna et al. 1983).

13.2 Indications

Initially, pancreas transplantation was proposed only to patients with severe involvement complicated by micro-angiopathy and renal insufficiency justifying a concomitant renal transplantation. Now, in some centers (Sutherland et al. 1987), even patients who have proliferative retinopathy and progressive kidney involvement without renal insufficiency are considered as good candidates.

N. Grenier, MD, Professor of Radiology, Service de Radiologie, Groupe Hôspitalier Pellegrin, Place Amélie-Raba-Léon, F-33076 Bordeaux Cédex, France
H. Trillaud, MD, Fellow in Radiology, Service de Radiologie, Groupe Hôspitalier Pellegrin, Place Amélie-Raba-Léon, F-33076 Bordeaux Cédex, France
C. Douws, MD, Radiologist, Service de Radiologie, Groupe Hôspitalier Pellegrin, Place Amélie-Raba-Léon, F-33076 Bordeaux Cédex, France

Another particular indication is severe glycemic instability despite intensive glucose monitoring and insulin therapy, with the risk of life-threatening hypo- and hyperglycemic episodes (Dunn and Sutherland 1991).

13.3 Surgical Techniques

Two main techniques were initially used by the various surgical teams, either transplantation of a segmented pancreas (body and tail) or transplantation of the whole gland with a duodenal segment. Segmental transplantation (Fig. 13.1), with either pancreatic duct occlusion by neoprene, polymer injection, or drainage into a Roux-en-Y jejunal loop, has at present been abandoned because of the high number of complications (severe pancreatitis and collections). Although more complicated, total pancreatic transplantation is now the most widely used technique (Fig. 13.2). The gland is retrieved in totality with a duodenal segment and the graft is positioned within the peritoneal cavity. The celiac trunk and the superior mesenteric arteries are implanted with a common aortic patch (Fig. 13.3) on the common iliac artery. If the liver is also retrieved from the same donor, the celiac trunk is no longer available for the pancreatic graft. Therefore, the splenic artery is anastomosed to the superior mesenteric artery or a Y arterial iliac graft is interposed. The venous blood is drained into the portal vein via the splenic and superior mesenteric veins. The portal vein is then implanted on the common iliac vein. Portal drainage of the pancreatic venous flow via an anastomosis on the superior mesenteric vein of the receiver offers no advantages.

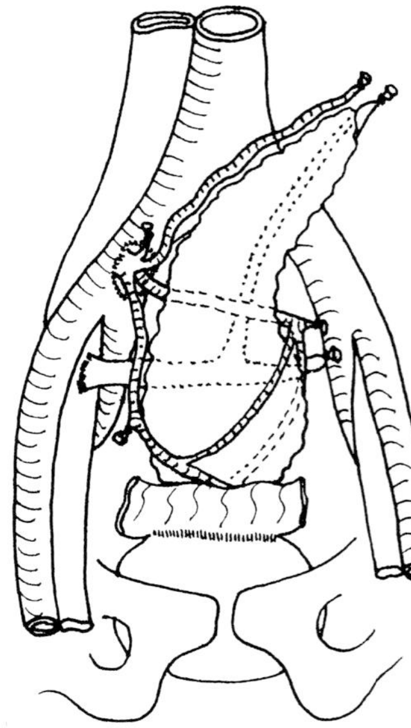

Fig. 13.2. Total pancreas transplantation with bladder drainage. Duodenocystectomy is performed with a complete duodenal segment. [Modified from Dunn and Sutherland (1991)]

Exocrine secretions are now more commonly drained into the bladder than into the bowels. Although bladder drainage lessens the risk of leaks and collections and permits monitoring of amylase in the urine, this technique leads to more urological complications (Hickey et al. 1997).

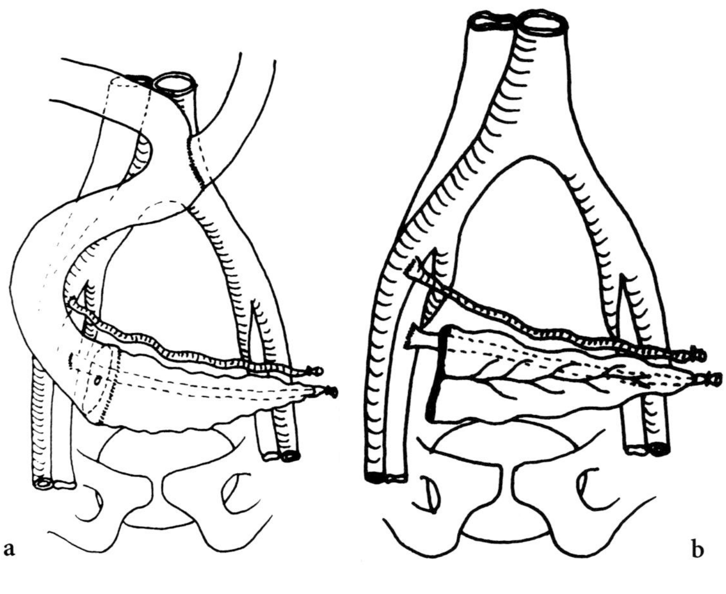

13.1a,b. Segmental pancreas transplantation. **a** Exocrine secretions are drained in a Roux-en-Y bowel loop. **b** Exocrine secretions are suppressed by pancreatic duct occlusion (neoprene). [Modified from Dunn and Sutherland (1991)]

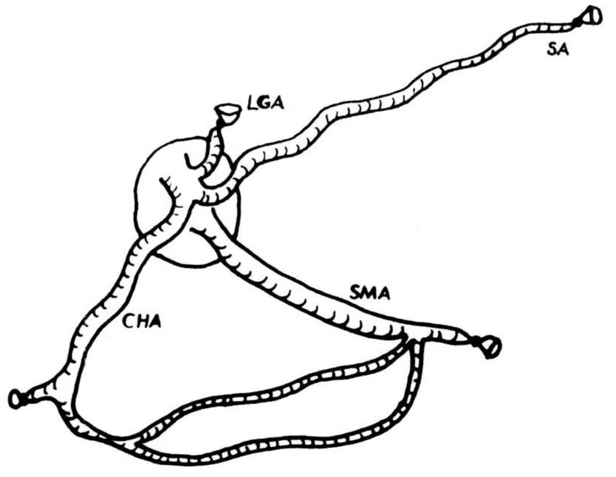

Fig. 13.3. Pancreatic allograft arteries. Usually, the celiac trunk and the superior mesenteric arteries are retrieved on the same aortic patch. The left gastric and hepatic arteries are ligated.

13.4 Radiologic Imaging Methods

13.4.1 Technique and Normal Findings

Because of its size and location in the abdominal cavity, imaging of a grafted pancreas is more difficult than that of liver or kidney transplants.

Radionuclide studies are considered very useful in many centers (KUNI et al. 1989). Technetium-99m diethylenetriamine penta-acetic acid studies are most commonly used and allow the evaluation of both pancreatic perfusion and renal function. For pancreatic perfusion, the normal delay between the arterial and parenchymal peak is 4 s or less. Bladder scintigraphy is also performed to detect urinary leaks (ECKHOFF et al. 1994).

Ultrasonography is the first-line examination when pancreatic function is impaired (LOW et al. 1990). However, sonography can be difficult in total pancreatic transplantation because the graft is often obscured by bowel loops and because the limits of the gland are sometimes hard to determine precisely. A filled bladder helps in visualizing the lower portion of the graft. A normal pancreatic parenchyma shows intermediate homogeneous echogenicity (Fig. 13.4) and the pancreatic duct, when visualized, does not exceed 2–3 mm in diameter. Color Doppler may help in identifying the gland by showing the arterial and venous pedicles and the intrapancreatic vessels (Fig. 13.5a,b) (YANG et al. 1990). It is important to show the anastomoses and assess the permeability of the splenic artery and vein. As the blood flow in these vessels is slow, low pulse repetition frequency settings are required. On spectral waveforms, the arterial flow generally demonstrates low resistance with a resistive index lower than 0.7 (PATEL et al. 1989) (Fig. 13.5c).

Abdominal computed tomography (CT) is also very useful for the follow-up of pancreatic transplants (LOW et al. 1990; MOULTON et al. 1989). Opacification of the bowel loops and colon is mandatory to correctly identify the graft. Intravenous infusion of iodine contrast agent should be performed only when necessary and if renal function is not impaired. When an anastomotic leak is suspected, a concomitant retrograde opacification of the bladder should be performed. Use of a 3% dilution of contrast is recommended for this (LONGLEY et al. 1990; BISCHOF et al. 1995). The pancreatic graft is usually located in the right iliac fossa, extending cephalad along the right colon. Normal grafts display homogeneous density and well-defined contours (Figs. 13.6, 13.7). Presence of gas is possible around the graft in the immediate postoperative period. After intravenous injection of contrast, the normal pancreatic parenchyma shows a homogeneous enhancement allowing better delineation of collections. Segmental grafts, usually implanted in the pelvis, are easier to identify (Fig. 13.6). When the pancreatic duct has been occluded with neoprene, its density is spontaneously high.

Magnetic resonance imaging (MRI) has been proposed by several authors to evaluate pancreatic allografts (KELCZ et al. 1991; VALHEY et al. 1988; YUH et

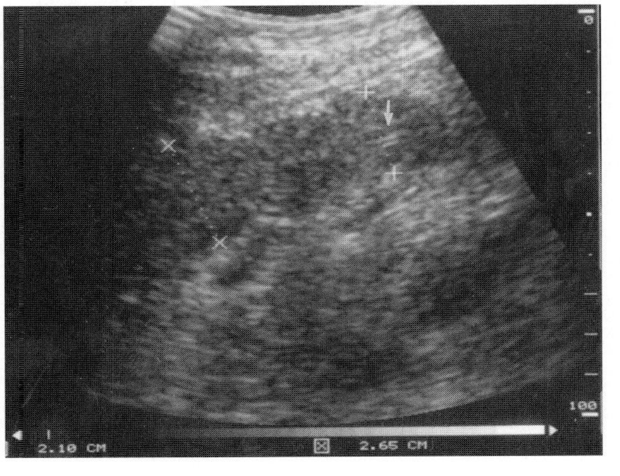

Fig. 13.4. Ultrasound of a normally functioning graft. The echo texture of the pancreatic parenchyma is homogeneous and of medium intensity. The pancreatic duct is visible (*arrow*) and of normal size

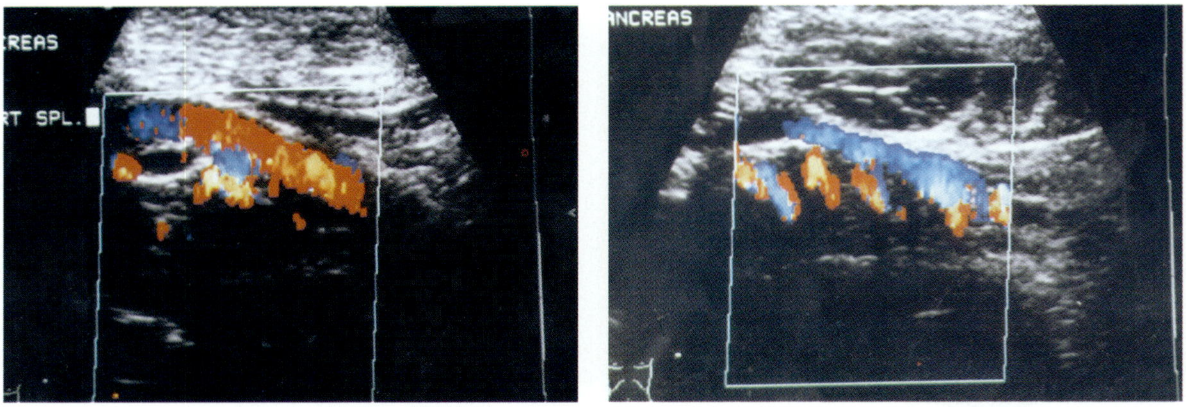

a b

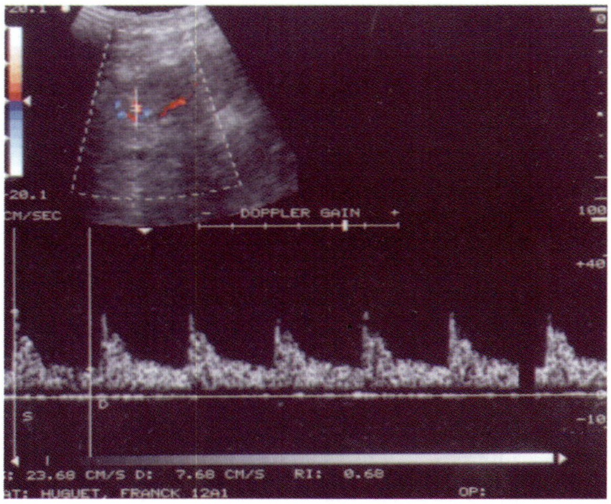

c

Fig. 13.5a–c. Color Doppler flow imaging. Normal splenic artery (a) and normal splenic vein (b) with intrapancreatic vessels on a segmental pancreatic transplant. c The arterial spectral waveform shows low resistance

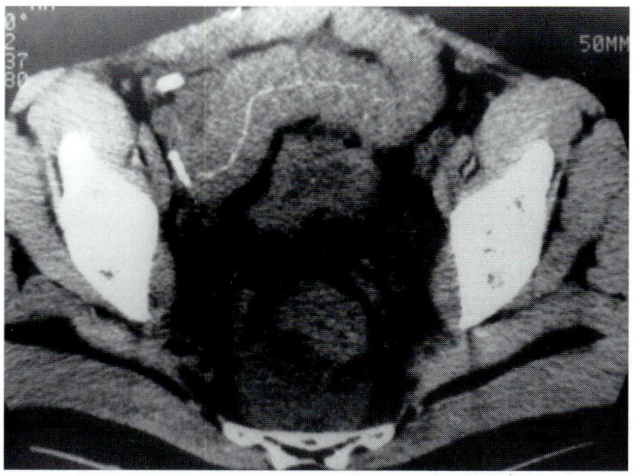

Fig. 13.6. Normal segmental pancreatic graft on plain computed tomography. The graft is positioned extraperitoneally over the bladder. The graft section and the pancreatic duct are occluded by neoprene

al. 1989). Multiple phased-array coils provide better signal-to-noise ratios than body coils. The protocol usually includes axial and coronal spin-echo T1-weighted and fast spin-echo T2-weighted sequences. The coronal view is very useful for imaging the entire gland (Fig. 13.8). The normal pancreatic parenchyma shows the same intermediate signal intensity as the renal cortex on T1-weighted images and approximately the same signal intensity as that of muscle on T2-weighted images (Fig. 13.9a,b). Pancreatic vessels can be imaged selectively with MR angiography techniques (Brichaux et al. 1991) (Fig. 13.9c). Intravenous infusion of gadolinium chelates has also been proposed by some investigators (Fernandez et al.

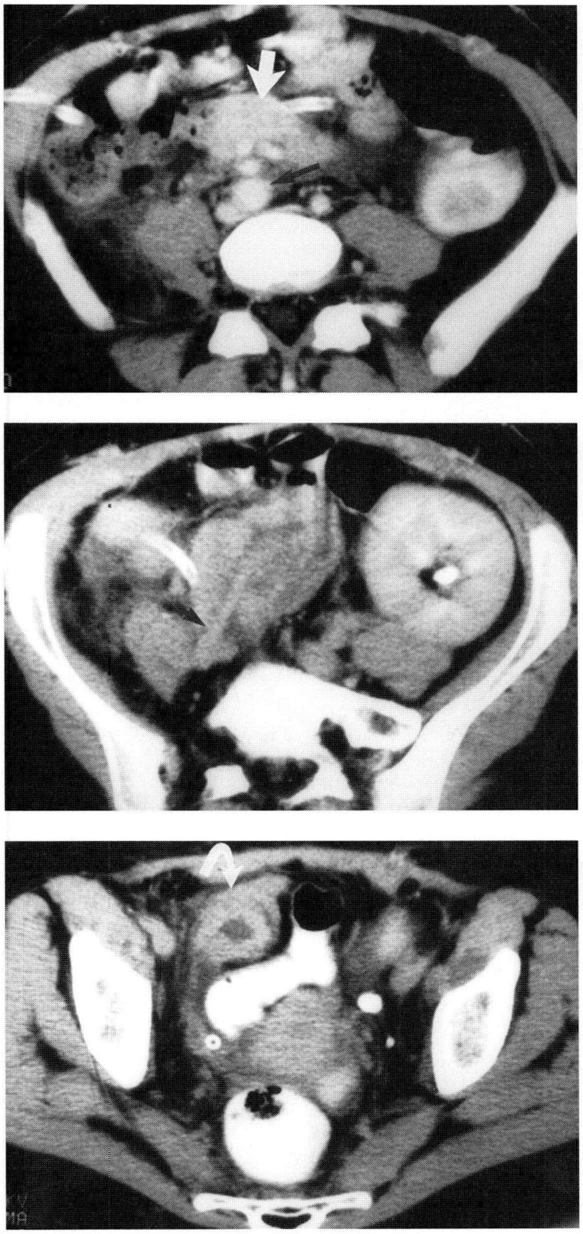

Fig. 13.7a–c. Normal total pancreatic graft on enhanced computed tomography. **a** Section of the pancreatic isthmus (*white arrow*). Splenic vessels and the superior mesenteric artery are visible at its posterior aspect in front of the right iliac artery (*black arrow*), which is enlarged by the patch. **b** Lower section on the pancreatic head. Visualization of the venous anastomosis (*arrow*). **c** Lower section on the duodenal stump (*arrow*)

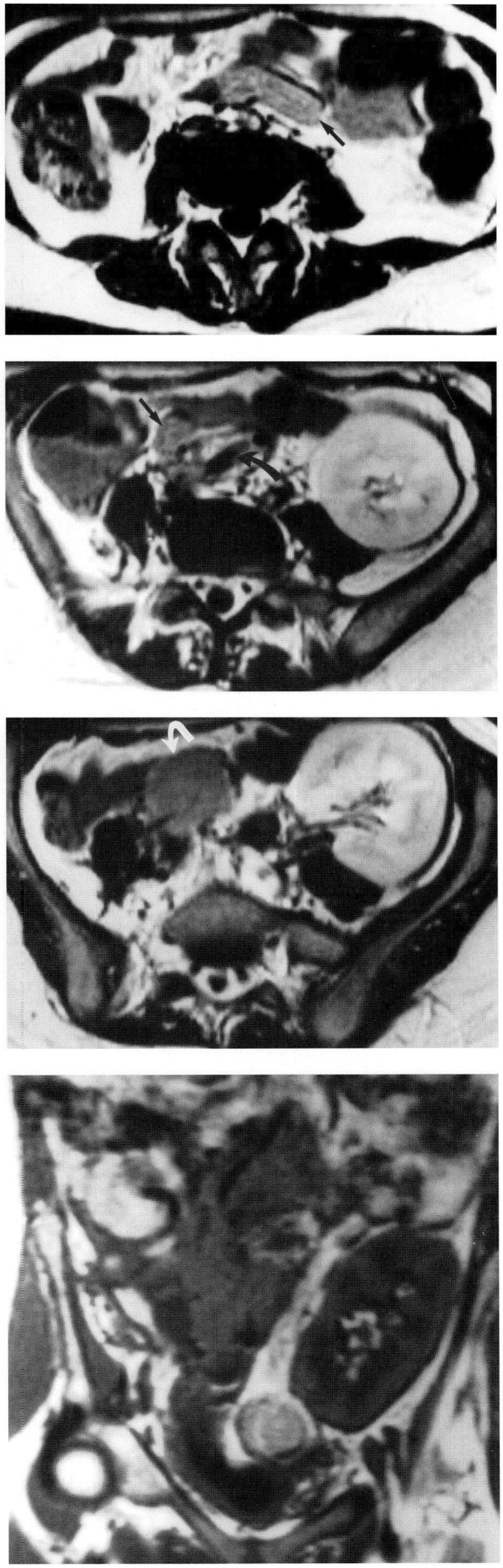

Fig. 13.8a–d. Normal total pancreatic graft on T1-weighted magnetic resonance (MR) imaging. **a** Axial section of the pancreatic tail (*black arrow*). **b** Axial section of the pancreatic isthmus (*black arrow*) with pancreatic vessels at their posterior aspect (*black curved arrow*). **c** Lower section on the pancreatic head (*white arrow*). **d** Coronal Tl-weighted MR image of both grafts, the pancreatic graft in the right flank and the concomitant renal graft in the left iliac fossa

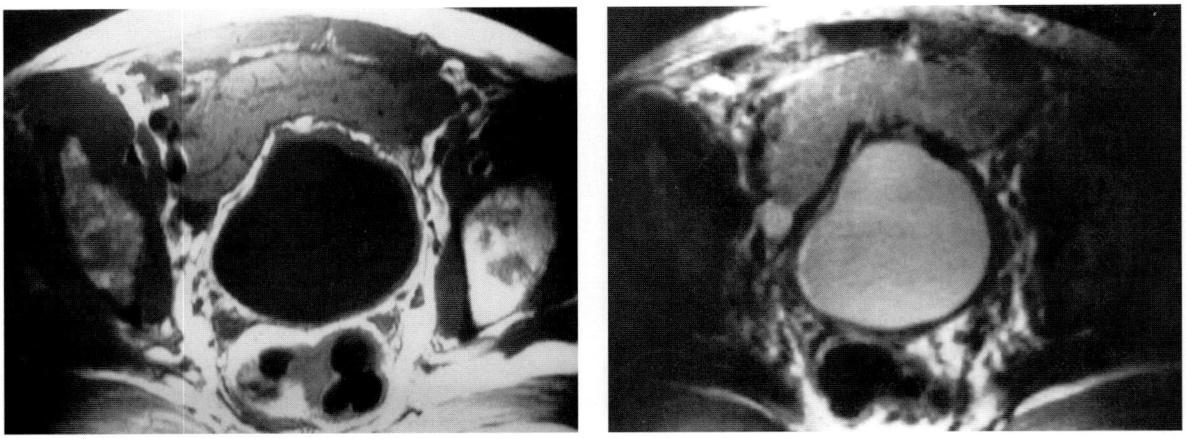

a b

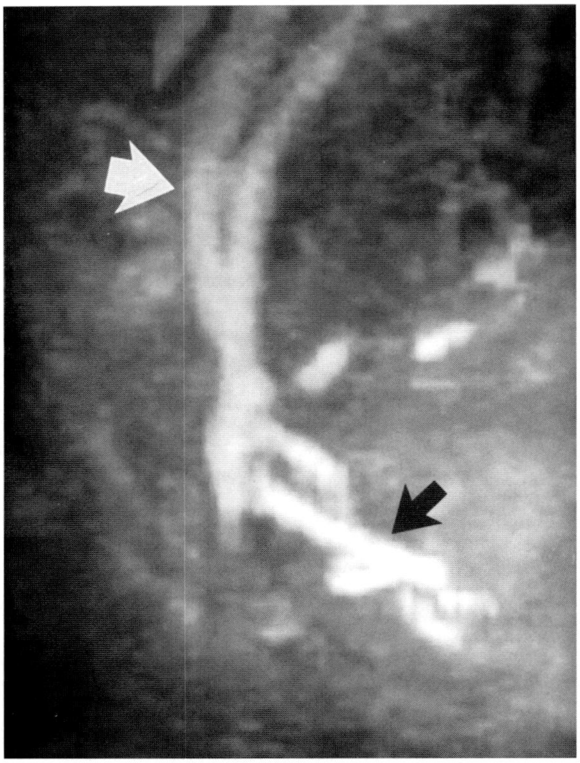

c

Fig. 13.9a–c. Normal segmental pancreatic graft with magnetic resonance imaging (MRI) (Helmholtz coil). **a** On a Tl-weighted image, the pancreas is homogeneous with intermediate signal intensity. The pancreatic duct displays low signal intensity since it is occluded with neoprene. **b** On the T2-weighted image, the signal intensity is lower than that of urine and approximately equal to that of fat. **c** The time-of-flight MR angiographic technique allows visualization of the pancreatic vessels (*black arrow*) and iliac vessels (*white arrow*) of this segmental graft (coronal vein)

1991) to study the dynamic enhancement of the pancreas: 98% enhancement was observed in normal glands during the first minute. Given that gadolinium chelates have no nephrotoxicity, the use of MRI in pancreas transplant monitoring will probably increase in the future, as it has for kidney transplants.

Retrograde cystography may be helpful when a complication of pancreaticoduodenocystostomy is suspected (Woolsey et al. 1987). An iodine contrast agent is infused into the bladder and then refluxes into the duodenal segment. Overdistension of the bladder must be avoided in the postoperative period.

Angiography is currently used only when a vascular complication is suspected. Conventional or digital intra-arterial angiography can be performed through a contralateral femoral approach (Fig. 13.10) or through an ipsilateral approach using a balloon occlusion catheter.

13.4.2 Imaging of Complications

Complications of pancreatic transplantation are extremely frequent. Almost 20% of early graft losses are related to a postoperative technical failure. Clin-

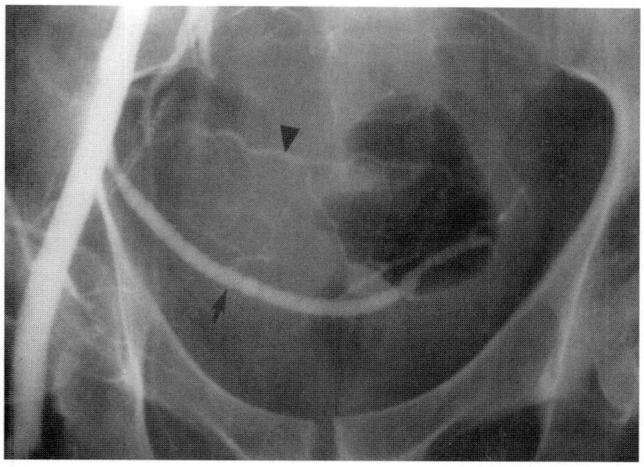

Fig. 13.10. Conventional arteriography of a segmental allograft, showing the splenic artery (*arrow*) and the dorsal pancreatic artery (*arrowhead*) communicating by several arcades

ical laboratory follow-up during the early post-transplantation period includes serum and urine levels of glucose, amylase, and C-peptide. Hyperglycemia during the first 2 weeks after transplantation suggests a surgical complication because rejection occurs only rarely that soon. After the first 2 weeks, rejection should be considered among the differential diagnoses if serum glucose rises.

13.4.2.1 Rejection

Rejection is frequent in pancreatic transplantation, occurring in approximately 35% of cases. It remains the major cause of graft loss (Gruessner and Sutherland 1996). Acute rejection is characterized by inflammation with accumulation of mononuclear phagocytes and usually responds to immunotherapy. Conversely, chronic rejection consists of fibrosis and pronounced vascular changes usually not amenable to therapy (Nelson et al. 1996). Clinical diagnosis of rejection is subtle because its symptoms, which include abdominal pain, fever, ileus, and graft tenderness, are very infrequent. When rejection occurs, endocrine function is altered several days after deterioration of exocrine function. Consequently, hyperglycemia occurs late. Moreover, a decrease in urinary amylase levels is neither a sensitive nor specific means of diagnosing rejection. In combined pancreas-kidney transplantations, renal rejection is associated with pancreatic rejection in almost 50% of cases, giving some diagnostic value for pancreatic rejection to the increase of creatinine levels.

Imaging studies show subtle changes suggesting the diagnosis of rejection. Their principal role is to rule out other surgical complications.

In acute rejection, the size of the graft increases. This finding, which is displayed by all of the various imaging techniques, is unfortunately not specific. Sonography of the pancreatic parenchyma shows inhomogeneous echo texture or decreased echogenicity with graft swelling, loss of marginal definition, and, rarely, dilatation of the pancreatic duct. On CT, areas of spontaneous increased density may be observed with infiltration of the peripancreatic fat. These CT findings are not specific because they are also observed with pancreatitis (Moulton et al. 1989). A rise in the resistive index above 0.7 was reported to be strongly correlated with the diagnosis of rejection (Patel et al. 1989). However, more recent studies have failed to confirm this correlation (Aideyan et al. 1997; Nelson et al. 1996; Wong et al. 1996). With MRI, the signal intensity of the pancreatic parenchyma decreases on T1-weighted images (normally identical to renal cortex intensity) and increases on T2-weighted images (normally identical to muscle intensity) (Yuh et al. 1989). These changes are diffuse within the gland and sometimes multifocal. In the diagnosis of rejection, MRI was initially reported to have 100% sensitivity, 76% specificity, and 100% negative predictive value (Yuh et al. 1989). Valhey et al. (1988) also found a significant difference between the calculated T2 of normal and that of rejecting allografts. However, these studies lacked histopathologic correlations and the results have not been confirmed by others (Fernandez et al. 1991; Kelcz et al. 1991). During dynamic MRI, enhancement of signal intensity after infusion of gadolinium is delayed in patients undergoing rejection (42% during the first minute), but such a delay is also observed with pancreatic infarction (Fernandez et al. 1991).

In chronic rejection, the size of the gland is decreased and the pancreatic duct may be dilated on all imaging techniques (Fig. 13.11). However, such changes are also compatible with a normally functioning gland (Fig. 13.12). Echogenicity is increased on sonograms (Low et al. 1990). To our knowledge, Doppler resistive indices have not been evaluated in chronic rejection. On CT, the density of the gland may appear slightly inhomogeneous or normal (Moulton et al. 1989) and on MRI, preliminary results have shown a decreased signal intensity on both T1- and T2-weighted images (Yuh et al. 1989).

Because of the poor sensitivity and specificity of these imaging features, diagnosis of rejection often

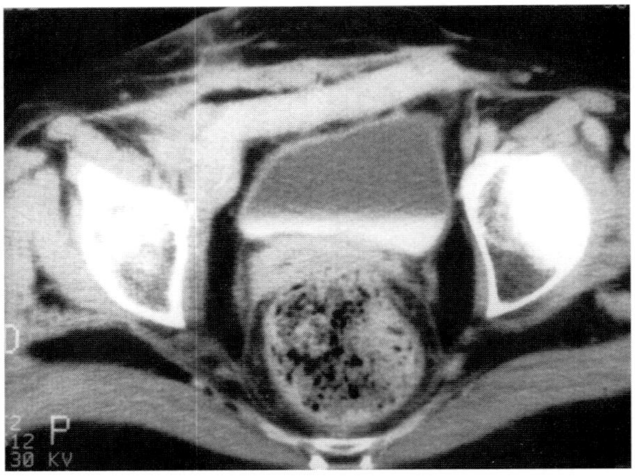

Fig. 13.11. Chronic rejection. The size of the graft is decreased but the parenchyma is still homogeneous

a

b

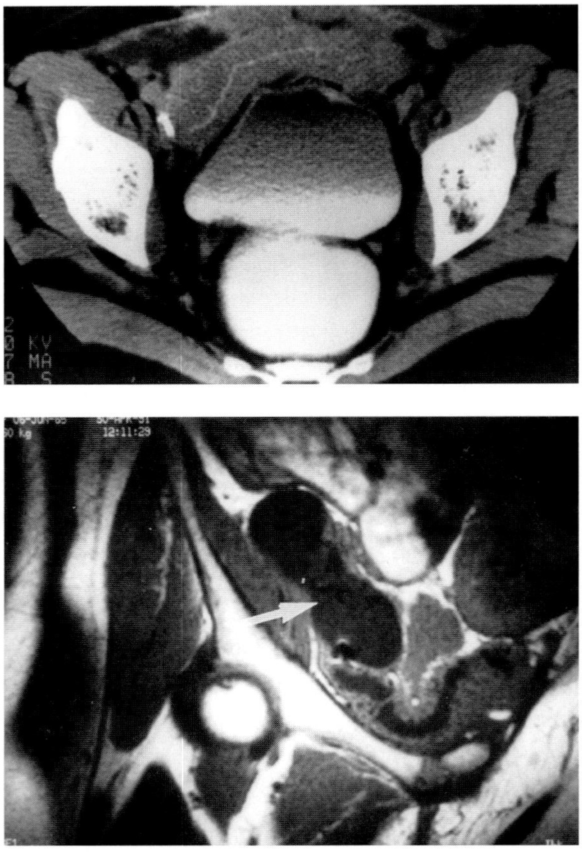

Fig. 13.12. a Normally functioning segmental graft imaged with computed tomography 1 week after transplantation. Note the presence of a small fluid collection anterior to the right external iliac vessels. b The T1-weighted coronal image 6 months later shows a gland decreased in size, enlargement of the pancreatic duct, and enlargement of the iliac collection (lymphocele) (*arrow*). Endocrine secretion was still present

requires histopathologic sampling obtained by percutaneous biopsy. Biopsy of the pancreatic gland is now performed with good safety, either percutaneously under guidance by US (Wong et al. 1996) or CT (Aideyan et al. 1996), or transduodenally during cystoscopy with US guidance (Nelson et al. 1994), with a 90%–95% success rate. Bleeding is observed in 2%–8% of cases.

13.4.2.2
Graft Pancreatitis

In graft pancreatitis, pancreatic fluid and enzymes accumulate around the graft, infiltrating the peripancreatic fat or producing ascites and collections. Some of these inflammatory changes are common after surgery, being favored by ischemia and physical manipulation. Simple bladder drainage allows regression of graft pancreatitis. After the early postoperative period, this complication can be caused by urinary reflux (the most frequent) or by an ampullary mucous plug. Diagnosis of reflux pancreatitis is based on the association of right flank pain, elevation of serum amylase, absence of pancreatic leak, edema of the pancreas without collection or abscess on CT, and resolution of symptoms within 24 h of urinary catheter drainage. Its incidence ranges from 11% to 17%. On imaging, the size of the gland is generally increased and the pancreatic duct dilated. Pancreatic parenchyma shows inhomogeneous echogenicity on sonogram and increased and inhomogeneous density on CT with infiltration of the peripancreatic fat (Moulton et al. 1989) (Fig. 13.13). Although these US and CT changes are not specific (they are also observed in acute rejection, peripancreatic infection, vascular complications, and exocrine leaks), the latter technique is the examination of choice for evaluating complications of pancreatitis. Just as in native gland pancreatitis, CT delineates parenchymal necrosis, phlegmon or abscess formation, peripancreatic collections, pseudocysts, and vascular erosion with pseudoaneurysm.

13.4.2.3
Fluid Collections

A small amount of fluid is very commonly encountered around the pancreatic allograft (Fig. 13.14) with little clinical consequence and requiring no treatment. However, actual collections may develop, necessitating characterization, if possible, for appropriate treatment. Such fluid collections may involve

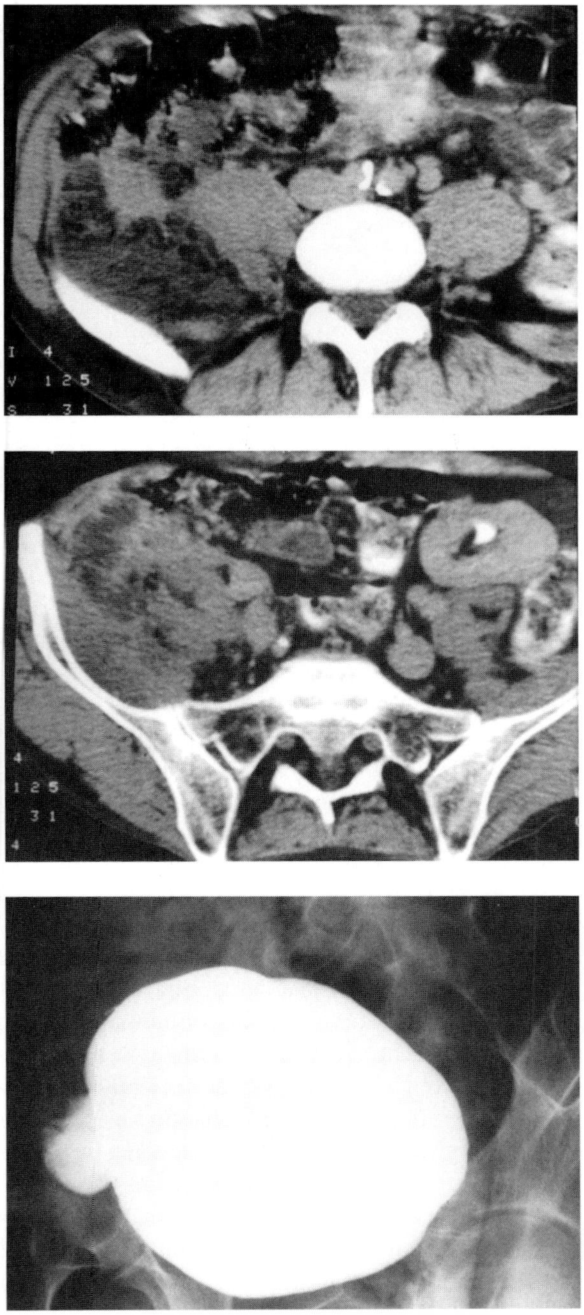

Fig. 13.13a–c. Acute pancreatitis. **a,b** On both axial computed tomography sections, the pancreas (*arrows*) shows irregular borders and the surrounding fat is infiltrated. **c** Retrograde cystography shows reflux into the duodenal stump

pancreatic fluid (Fig. 13.14), blood, lymph (Fig. 13.12b), urine, or pus. Pancreatitis, infection, and vascular complications all predispose to bleeding. Urinomas are due to an anastomotic leak or necrosis of the allograft. Infections with the formation of an abscess can be favored by the presence of a collection (urinoma or hematoma), by a urinary tract infection, or by pancreatitis. Furthermore, abscess can induce the onset of pancreatitis. Any infection of a collection must be considered as severe because it may lead to loss of the graft.

Sonography allows detection of most retroperitoneal collections, but analysis of their content and extent is easier with CT (Patel et al. 1991). However, CT usually calls for intravenous infusion of iodine contrast medium which may be contraindicated in patients with impaired renal function. In such cases, MRI is preferable. Except for hematomas, which show a high spontaneous density on CT and characteristic signal intensity changes on MRI, determining the nature of the fluid is difficult. Gas bubbles within the collection are suggestive of infection, but may also be observed with bowel fistula, pancreatic necrosis after vascular thrombosis and in noninfected hematomas (Vas et al. 1989), as described in liver traumas. Identification of urinomas secondary to urinary leaks requires bladder scintigraphy or cystography (see Sect. 13.4.2.5).

Characterization of collections is reliant upon percutaneous sonographically guided or CT-guided aspiration of the fluid for measurement of creatinine and amylase levels, and for microbial analysis. Percutaneous drainage of these collections is important for treatment, obtaining either definitive remission or the postponement of surgical intervention until local conditions are more propitious (Gissel-Letourneau et al. 1988). The choice of guiding percutaneous drainage by sonography or CT depends on bowel or vessel proximity. When a pancreatic or duodenal fistula is present, drainage must be maintained for a longer period. The complication rate of drainage is around 3%.

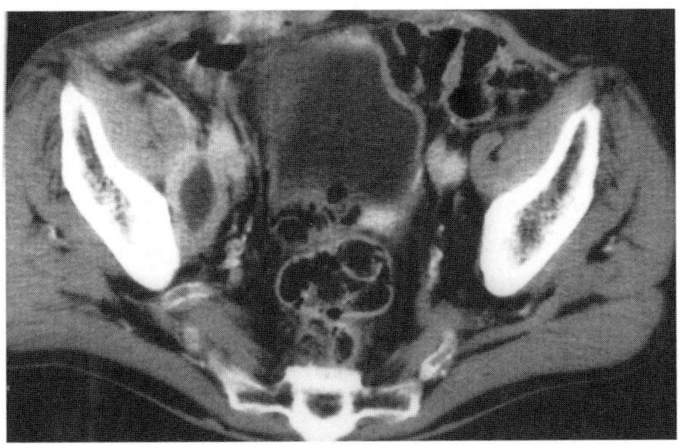

Fig. 13.14. Pelvic collection of pancreatic fluid with a thick capsule behind the external iliac vessels. This collection was treated using computed tomography-guided percutaneous drainage

13.4.2.4
Vascular Complications

Vascular complications are also very frequent, comprising predominantly venous thrombosis which occurs in 10%–15% of cases, usually during the first week after transplantation (Dunn and Sutherland 1991). Clinically, venous thrombosis of the graft results in a pattern of abdominal or back pain, hyperglycemia, decreased urine amylase, and, in some cases, hematuria secondary to necrosis of the graft. Usually, vascular thrombosis leads to graft loss. Many factors are involved in this process, including intraoperative trauma, prolonged cold ischemia, intrapancreatic microthrombi, vascular kinking, compression of the venous anastomosis, excessively slow venous flow due to oversized venous conduits, and, possibly, to thrombogenic properties of cyclosporine. Arterial stenoses are also frequent and multifactorial, analogous to their pathogenesis in renal transplantation (rejection, surgery, kinking, peripancreatic inflammation).

Arterial and venous thrombosis can be detected by Doppler sonography (Snider et al. 1991). Venous pancreatic flow is very slow and the operator should verify that the maximum sensitivity has been set to slow flow before advancing a diagnosis of venous thrombosis. Perfusion scintigraphic study confirms the diagnosis by the absence of tracer fixation within the gland (Boiskin et al. 1990; Snider et al. 1991). In venous thrombosis, a very high resistive index with a holodiastolic reflux may be noted in the pancreatic arteries (Boiskin et al. 1990; Foshager et al. 1997). MR angiography may prove useful in the future. Segmental venous thrombosis may also be encountered with subsequent development of a cavernoma (Fig. 13.15).

Color Doppler flow imaging helps to detect arterial stenoses, pseudoaneurysms (postoperative or favored by graft pancreatitis), and post-biopsy arteriovenous fistulas (Snider et al. 1991). Diagnosis of stenosis is based on a turbulent flow with high peak systolic velocities. Angiography makes it possible to confirm this diagnosis and to treat the lesion by percutaneous angioplasty during the same procedure.

13.4.2.5
Urological Complications

With the change from enteric to bladder drainage, the formerly general surgical complication profile of pancreatic transplantation has shifted towards a urological complication profile. Urological complications include duodenocystostomy fistula, hematuria, urinary tract infections, dysuria syndrome, urethral disruption, urethral stricture, and, rarely, autodigestion of the glans penis (Hickey et al. 1997). Most of these complications are related to activation of pancreatic enzymes, favored by the presence of the duodenum, and urinary infections, favored by the change in urinary pH.

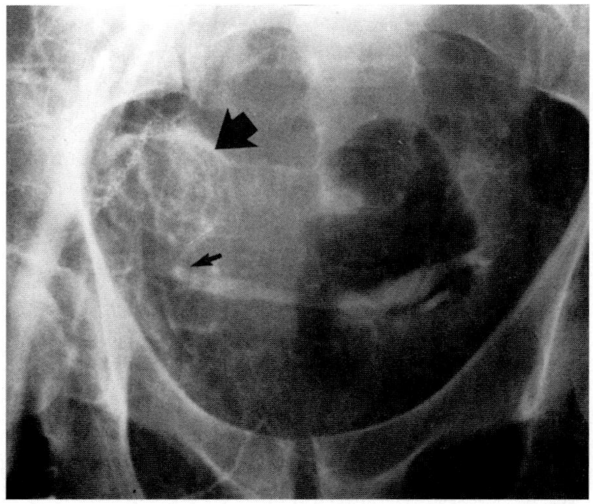

Fig. 13.15. Venous phase of a conventional arteriography. Segmental thrombosis of the splenic vein (*arrow*), with development of a cavernoma (*large arrow*)

Duodenocystostomy fistulas occur in 7%–14% of transplantations with bladder drainage. Those that occur early after surgery are predominantly related to duodenal ischemia, and those that occur later are often triggered by cytomegalovirus infection or duodenal ulceration. Associated infection is frequent with a high risk of graft loss. Imaging methods include conventional, scintigraphic, and CT cystography. Longley et al. (1990) showed that CT cystography can visualize leaks that are not demonstrated by conventional cystography. Eckhoff et al. (1994) have reported 99m-Tc voiding cystography to be superior to conventional voiding cystography. CT cystography, with full bladder and post-voiding acquisitions, is reportedly very accurate (96%) (Bischof et al. 1995). Aside from leaks, CT shows intraperitoneal collections and inflammatory changes in the area of the duodenocystostomy. Most early leaks may be treated conservatively by means of in-dwelling Foley catheter drainage of the bladder. Large and late leaks typically require surgical correction with, in some cases, enteric conversion.

Chemical urethritis occurs essentially in males, but has also been described in females (Sollinger et al. 1993; ELKHAMMAS et al. 1994; LECOUVET et al. 1994). This can lead to urethral stricture and disruption. Disruption most often involves the bulbar urethra or bulbomembranous junction and appears to be favored by recent urinary instrumentation (DUMAS et al. 1996). This diagnosis should be considered when patients present with dysuria, and verified with the aid of retrograde urethrography (Fig. 13.16).

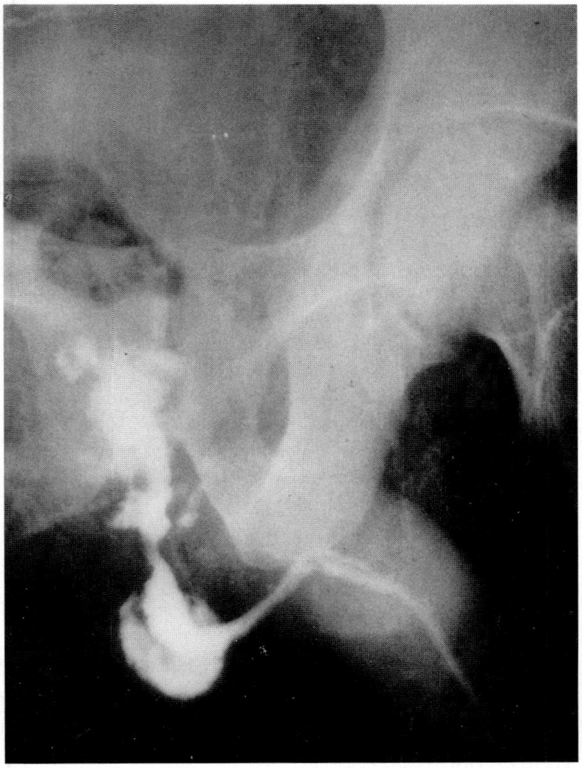
a

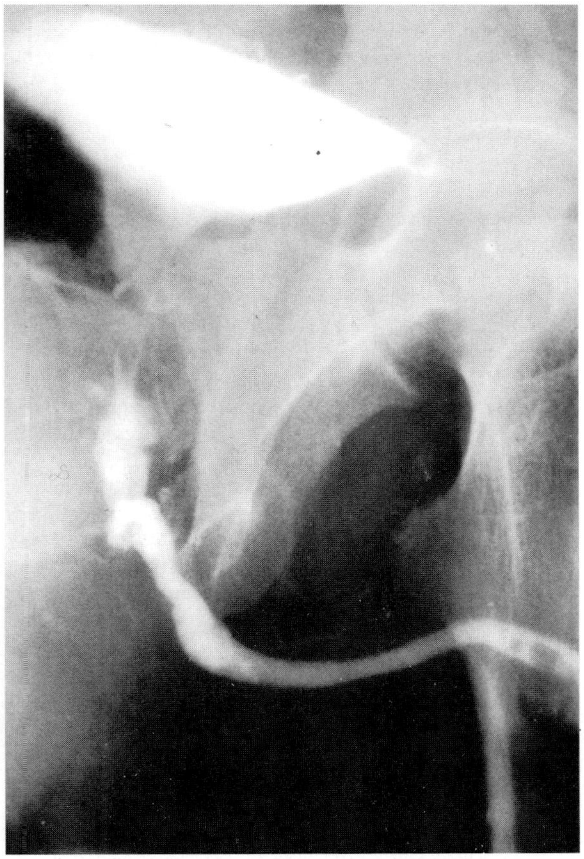
b

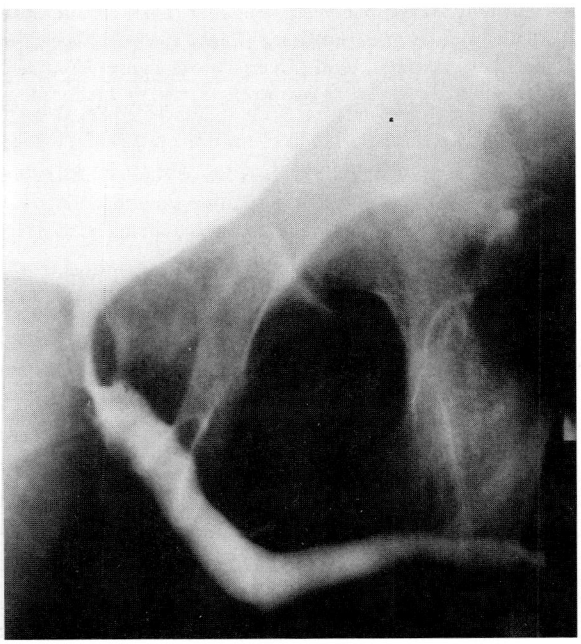
c

Fig. 13.16a–c. Chemical urethritis in a male recipient presenting with retention. **a** Voiding cystourethrogram shows an irregular urethral lumen and fistulas. **b** Reexamination after 6 weeks of bladder drainage shows regression of fistulas and stenosis of the proximal urethra. **c** Last assessment 3 weeks after urethrotomy. [With permission from LECOUVET et al. (1994)]

References

Abouna GM, Kremer GD, Daddah SK, et al. (1983) Fate of transplanted kidneys with diabetic nephropathy. Lancet II:1274–1276

Aideyan OA, Schmidt AJ, Trenkner SW, Hakim NS, Gruessner RWG, Walsh JW (1996) CT-guided percutaneous biopsy of pancreas transplants. Radiology 201:825–828

Aideyan OA, Foshager MC, Benedetti E, Troppmann C, Gruessner RWG (1997) Correlation of the arterial resistive index in pancreas transplants of patients with transplant rejection. AJR 168:1445–1447

Bischof TP, Thoeni RF, Melzer JS (1995) Diagnosis of duodenal leaks from kidney-pancreas transplant in patients with duodenovesical anastomoses: value of CT cystography. AJR 165:349–354

Boiskin I, Sandler MP, Fleischer AC, Nylander WA (1990) Acute venous thrombosis after pancreas transplantation: diagnosis with duplex Doppler sonography and scintigraphy. AJR 154:529–531

Brichaux JC, Grenier N, Douws C, Revel P, Potaux L, Franconi JM (1991) MR angiography of renal and pancreatic transplant arteries (abstract). Society of Magnetic Resonance in Medicine, San Francisco, Book of abstracts, p 140

Dumas MD, Bude RO, Sonda PL, Cohan RH, Merion RM (1996) Urethral disruption with urinary extravasation: a delayed complication of pancreatic transplantation. Radiology 201:761–765

Dunn DL, Sutherland DER (1991) Pancreatic transplantation. In: Gissel-Letourneau J, Day DL, Ascher NL (eds) Radiology of organ transplantation. Mosby Year Book, St. Louis, p 237

Eckhoff DE, Ploeg RJ, D'Allessandro AM et al (1994) Efficacy of 99m-Tc voiding cysto-urethrogram for detection of duodenal leaks after pancreas transplantation. Transplant Proc 26:462–463

Elkhammas EA, Henry ML, York JP et al (1994) Pancreas transplantation and dysuria. J Urol 152:881–883

Fernandez M, Bernardino ME, Neylan JF, Olson RA (1991) Diagnosis of pancreatic transplant dysfunction: value of gadopentetate dimeglumine-enhanced MR imaging. AJR 156:1171–1176

Foshager MC, Hedlund LJ, Troppman C, Benedetti E, Gruessner RW (1997) Venous thrombosis of pancreatic transplants: diagnosis by duplex sonography. AJR 169:1269–1273

Gaber AO, el-Gebely S, Sugathan P et al (1995) Early improvement in cardiac function occurs for pancreas-kidney but not diabetic kidney-alone transplant recipients. Transplantation 57:816

Gissel-Letourneau J, Junter DW, Crass JR, Thompson WM, Sutherland DER (1988) Percutaneous aspiration and drainage of abdominal fluid collections after pancreatic transplantation. AJR 150:805–809

Gruessner RWG, Sutherland DER (1996) Clinical diagnosis in pancreatic allograft rejection. In: Solez K, Racusen LC, Billingham ME (eds) Solid organ transplant rejection mechanisms, pathology and diagnosis. Dekker, New York, pp 455–499

Hathaway DK, Hartwig MS, Milstead J, Elmer D, Evans S, Gaber AO (1994) Improvement of quality of life reported by diabetic recipients of kidney-only and pancreas-kidney allografts. Transplant Proc 26:512

Hickey DP, Bakthavatsalam R, Bannon A, O'Malley K, Corr J, Little DM (1997) Urological complications of pancreatic transplantation. J Urol 157:2042–2048

International Pancreas Transplant Registry (1995) Pancreas transplant results in the USA with comparison to non-USA data in the international registry. Presented at the 5th congress of the International Pancreas and Islet Transplant Association, Miami Beach, Florida, 18–22 June

Kelcz F, Sollinger HW, Pirsch JD (1991) MRI of the pancreas transplant: lack of correlation between imaging and clinical status. Magn Reson Med 21:20–38

Kennedy WR, Navarro X, Goetz FC, Sutherland DE, Najarian JS (1990) Effects of pancreatic transplantation on on diabetic neuropathy. N Engl J Med 322:1031

Kuni CC, Du Cret RP, Boudreau RJ (1989) Pancreas transplants: evaluation using perfusion scintigraphy. AJR 153:57–61

Lecouvet F, Mourad M, Wese FX, Abi-Aad A, Dardenne An, Squifflet JP (1994) Urétrite chimique sévère au décours d'une greffe combinée rein-pancréas. Rev Im Med 6:239–243

Longley DG, Dunn DL, Gruessner R, Halvorsen RA, Sutherland DER, Gissel-Letourneau J (1990) Detection of pancreatic fluid and urine leakage after pancreas transplantation: value of CT and cystography. AJR 155:997–1000

Low R, Kuni CC, Gissel-Letourneau J (1990) Pancreas transplant imaging: an overview. AJR 155:13–21

Moulton JS, Munda R, Weiss MA, Lubbers DJ (1989) Pancreatic transplants: CT with clinical and pathologic correlation. Radiology 172:21–26

Nelson NL, Lowell JA, Taylor RJ, Stratta RJ (1994) Pancreas transplants: efficacy of US-guided cystoscopic biopsy. Radiology 191:283–284

Nelson NL, Largen PS, Stratt RJ et al (1996) Pancreas allograft rejection: correlation of transduodenal core biopsy with Doppler resistive index. Radiology 200:91–94

Patel B, Wolverson MK, Mahanta B (1989) Pancreatic transplant rejection: assessement with duplex US. Radiology 173:131–135

Robertson RP (1992) Seminars in medicine of the Beth Israel Hospital, Boston: pancreatic and islet transplantation for diabetes-cures or curiosities? N Engl J Med 327:1861

Snider JF, Hunter DW, Kuni CC, Castaneda-Zuniga WR, Gissel-Letourneau J (1991) Pancreatic transplantation: radiologic evaluation of vascular complications. Radiology 179:749–753

Sollinger HW, Messing EM, Eckhoff DE et al (1993) Urological complications in 210 consecutive simultaneous pancreas/kidney transplants with bladder drainage. Ann Surg 218:561–570

Sutherland DER, Goetz FC, Najarian JS (1987) Pancreas transplantation at the University of Minnesota: donor and recipient selection, operative and postoperative management, and outcome. Transplant Proc 19:63–74

The Diabetes Control and Complications Trial Research Group (1993) The effect of intensive treatment of diabetes on the development and progression of long term complications in insulin-dependent diabetes mellitus. N Engl J Med 329:977

Valhey TN, Glazer GM, Francis IR, Li K, Dafoe DC, Aisen AM, Smid DM (1988) MR diagnosis of pancreatic transplant rejection. AJR 150:557–560

Vas W, Patel B, Mahanta B, et al. (1989) Innocuous gas collections in pancreatic allografts demonstrated by computed tomography. Gastrointest Radiol 14:118–122

West KM, Erdreich LJ, Stober JA (1980) A detailed study of risk factors for retinopathy in diabetes. Diabetes 29:501–508

Wong JJ, Krebs TL, Klassen DK et al (1996) Sonographic evaluation of acute pancreatic transplant rejection: morphology-Doppler analysis versus guided percutaneous biopsy. AJR 166:803–807

Woosley EJ, Tauscher JR, Dafoe DC (1987) Pancreas transplantation with pancreatico-duodeno-cystostomy for exocrine drainage: cystographic findings. AJR 149:507–509

Yang HC, Neumyer MM, Thiele BL, Gifford RRM (1990) Evaluation of pancreatic allograft circulation using color Doppler ultrasonography. Transplant Proc 22:609–611

Yuh WTC, Hunsicker LG, Nghiem DD, Sato Yutaka, Smith JL, Wright FH, Corry RJ (1989) Pancreatic transplants: evaluation with MR imaging. Radiology 170:171–17

14 The Postoperative Pancreas

F. Grabenwöger, A.M. Herneth, R. Függer, G. Lechner

CONTENTS

14.1 Introduction

The incidence of pancreatic cancer, periampullary malignancies, and intractable pancreatitis is rising worldwide (DiMagno 1991). The group of periampullary carcinomas includes adenocarcinoma of Vater's papilla and carcinomas of the distal choledochal and pancreatic ducts. In Europe, an incidence of pancreatic adenocarcinoma of approximately 10/100 000 is reported (Büchler et al. 1996) and, untreated, has an expected survival of 3–6 months (Schenk et al. 1998). Surgery remains the only curative therapy in patients with pancreatic malignancies. Over the last two decades, perioperative mortality dropped precipitously from 45% to less than 5%, and 5-year survival rates improved for both pancreatic cancer and periampullary malignancies, rising to 20% and 40%, respectively (Grace et al. 1986; Yeo and Cameron 1991; Cameron et al. 1993; Gordon et al. 1995).

The most frequent malignancy of the pancreas is adenocarcinoma, which accounts for more than 85% of all pancreatic neoplasias and is found in about 80% of cases in the pancreatic head (Büchler et al. 1996). Less common are periampullary carcinomas and endocrine neoplasias (apudomas) such as insulinoma and gastrinoma. Benign tumors such as lipoma, fibroma, or lipofibroma are exceedingly rare.

At the time of diagnosis, only 20% of pancreatic adenocarcinomas are resectable, due to tumor size, tumor invasion, and nodal or distant metastases (Bakkevold et al. 1992; Strasberg et al. 1997).

According to the location, extent, and malignant or benign nature of the pancreatic disease, four different surgical strategies are currently performed: pancreaticoduodenectomy and its modifications, duodenum-preserving pancreatic head resection, distal pancreatectomy, and tumor enucleation.

Knowledge of the various surgical procedures performed is essential for the radiologist to differentiate a regular postoperative anatomy from a pathologic situation. Therefore, the objectives of this chapter are to give an overview of the currently performed procedures in pancreatic surgery and their typical complications, and to review the role of modern imaging modalities in the management of the postoperative patient.

F. Grabenwöger, MD, Department of Radiology (7F), Allgemeines Krankenhaus, University of Vienna, Währinger Gürtel 18—20, A-1090 Vienna, Austria
A.M. Herneth, MD, Department of Radiology (7F), Allgemeines Krankenhaus, University of Vienna, Währinger Gürtel 18-20, A-1090 Vienna, Austria
R. Függer, MD, Department of General Surgery, Allgemeines Krankenhaus, University of Vienna, Währinger Gürtel 18-20, A-1090 Vienna, Austria
G. Lechner, MD, Department of Radiology (7F), Allgemeines Krankenhaus, University of Vienna, Währinger Gürtel 18-20, A-1090 Vienna, Austria

14.2 Surgical Procedures

14.2.1 Pancreaticoduodenectomy

14.2.1.1 Standard Whipple Procedure

A.O. WHIPPLE introduced pancreaticoduodenectomy as a single-stage procedure (WHIPPLE et al. 1935). This operation includes en bloc resection of the pancreatic head to the level of the superior mesenteric vein, the distal common bile duct, the gallbladder, the entire duodenum, the pylorus, and the distal stomach. Reconstruction of the gastrointestinal tract continuity utilizes the proximal jejunum for pancreaticojejunostomy, choledochojejunostomy, and gastrojejunostomy (Fig. 14.1a). The retrocolic or antecolic placement of the anastomotic loop depends on the anatomic situation and the surgeon's preference.

This procedure is associated with serious complications. The most feared postoperative complication is leakage of pancreaticojejunostomy (15%–20%) with possible consecutive biliary peritonitis (YEO et al. 1997). To avoid biliary reflux and blind loop syndrome with ascending cholangitis, an additional enteroenteric anastomosis is performed (Braun's anastomosis) (Fig. 14.1b).

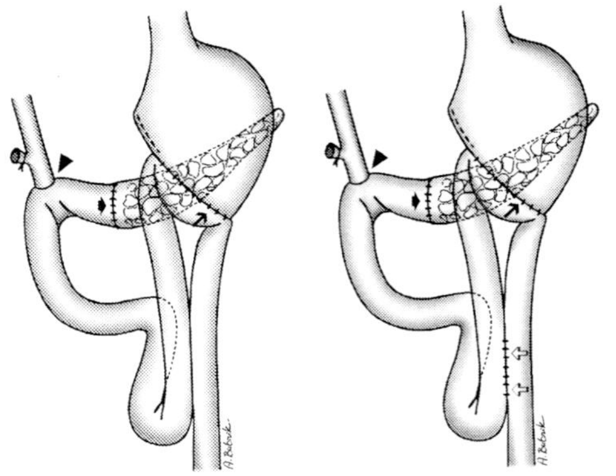

Fig. 14.1a,b. Standard Whipple procedure (pancreaticoduodenectomy). En bloc resection of the head of the pancreas, the distal common bile duct, the gallbladder, the entire duodenum, the pylorus, and the distal stomach. The gastrointestinal tract is reconstructed with an end-to-end pancreaticojejunostomy (*short arrow*), an end-to-side choledochojejunostomy (*arrowhead*), and a side-to-side gastrojejunostomy (*long arrow*). **b** In addition to the standard Whipple procedure, an enteroenterostomy (Braun's anastomosis) (*open arrows*) is performed to avoid biliogastric reflux and blind loop syndrome. *Short arrow*, pancreaticojejunostomy; *arrowhead*, choledochojejunostomy; *long arrow*, gastrojejunostomy

14.2.1.2 Modified Whipple Procedure

In most centers, the standard Whipple procedure is still performed. However, some technical modifications have been introduced mainly to reduce surgical postoperative complications.

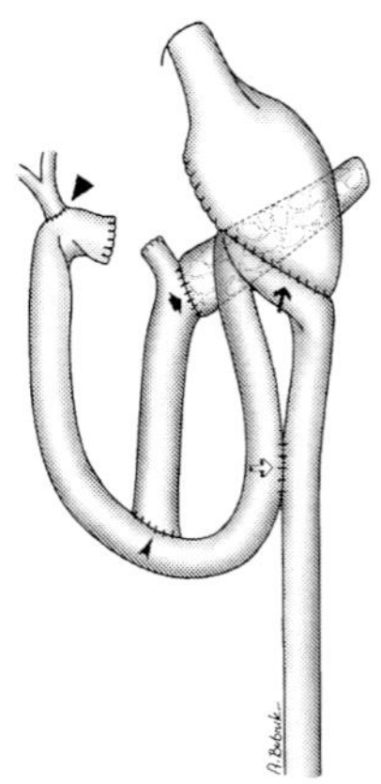

Fig. 14.2. Modified Whipple procedure. After standard pancreaticoduodenectomy, an end-to-side anastomosis of the pancreatic remnant with a separated jejunal loop is performed (*short arrow*, pancreaticojejunostomy; *small arrowhead*, jejunojejunostomy). *Large arrowhead*, end-to-side choledochojejunostomy; *long arrow*, side-to-side gastrojejunostomy; *open arrow*, side-to-side enteroenterostomy

14.2.1.2.1 MODIFIED WHIPPLE PROCEDURE WITH A SEPARATED ENTERIC LOOP

Performing pancreaticojejunostomy and choledochojejunostomy by separated enteric loops avoids biliary peritonitis in the case of insufficiency of the pancreaticojejunostomy and, therefore, markedly reduces perioperative mortality (Fig. 14.2).

A further modification to the Whipple procedure was to occlude the residual pancreatic duct with fibrin glue, histoacryl, or neoprene (CAVALLINI et al. 1991). This technique was thought to reduce both the incidence of ascending pancreatitis and the incidence of leakage of the pancreaticojejunostomy due to aggressive exocrine pancreatic juice. This modification, however, did not change the incidence of anastomotic dehiscence or pancreatitis significantly and has therefore been abandoned.

14.2.1.2.2
PYLORUS-PRESERVING
PANCREATICODUODENECTOMY

The pylorus-preserving pancreaticoduodenectomy (Fig. 14.3) has been proposed to reduce perioperative morbidity and mortality due to shortened operative time and reduced postgastrectomy complications (TRAVERSO and LONGMIRE 1978). This procedure eliminates gastric resection and leaves a 2-cm cuff of duodenum for enteric reconstruction as a pylorojejunostomy. Pancreaticojejunostomy and choledochojejunostomy are performed in a similar way to the standard Whipple procedure. This technique is used rather as a treatment of benign pancreatic diseases and periampullary cancer than as therapy of pancreatic adenocarcinoma (TAKADA et al. 1997; BÜCHLER et al. 1997).

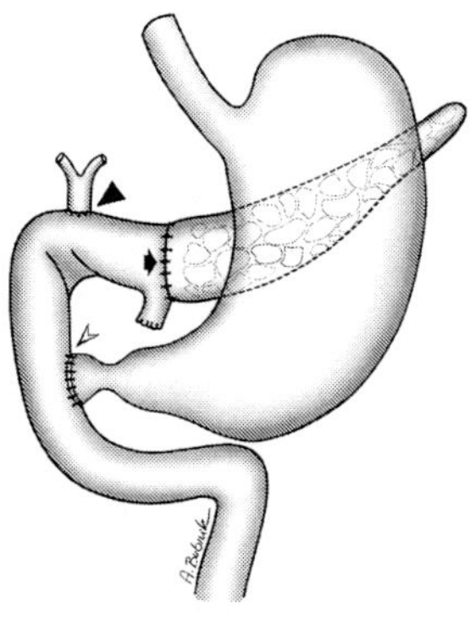

Fig. 14.3. Pylorus-preserving pancreaticoduodenectomy. Resection of the pancreatic head, the entire duodenum, the distal common bile duct, and the gallbladder. Reconstruction with end-to-side (end-to-end) pancreaticojejunostomy (*short arrow*), end-to-side choledochojejunostomy (*closed arrowhead*), and an end-to-side pylorojejunostomy (*open arrowhead*)

14.2.1.3 Total Pancreaticoduodenectomy

It has been hypothesized that pancreatic adenocarcinoma is a multicentric disease with early tumorseeding and, therefore, tumor recurrence can only be decreased by total resection of the pancreas (CONNOLLY 1987). Another indication for this technique was pan-pancreatitis resistant to therapy. This operation has not gained much acceptance because of the elimination of all exocrine and endocrine pancreatic function, requiring lifelong exogenous pancreatic enzyme and insulin supplementation (BÜCHLER and FRIESS 1993). Furthermore, there was no significant difference in the 5-year survival rate of patients with total pancreaticoduodenectomy compared to those who underwent the Whipple procedure.

With this operative technique, the entire pancreas, the duodenum, as well as the distal stomach, get resected en bloc. The enteric continuity is reconstructed with a gastrojejunostomy and a Roux-en-Y choledochojejunostomy (Fig. 14.4).

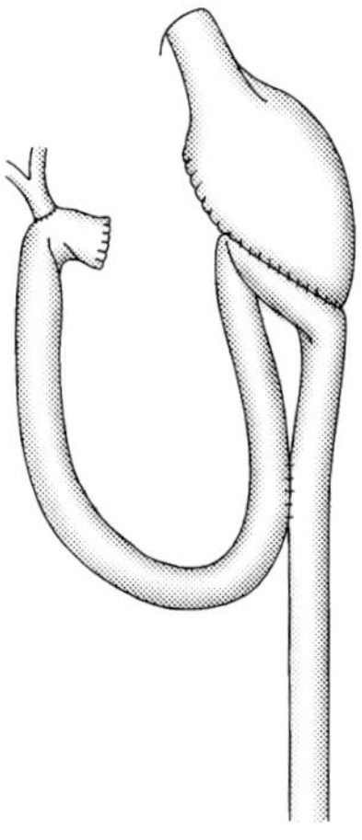

Fig. 14.4. Total pancreaticoduodenectomy. En bloc resection of the pancreas, the distal common bile duct, the gallbladder, the entire duodenum, the pylorus, and the distal stomach. Reconstruction with end-to-side choledochojejunostomy (*arrowhead*), side-to-side gastrojejunostomy (*closed arrow*), and side-to-side enteroenterostomy (*open arrow*) (Braun's anastomosis)

14.2.2 Duodenum-Preserving Pancreatic Head Resection

This operation is not a generally used procedure, but is performed by some centers for the treatment of non-malignant pancreatic pseudotumors of the pancreatic head, and in cases of chronic pancreatitis due to pancreas divisum (BÜCHLER et al. 1997; WIDMAIER et al. 1997). The advantage of this method is the preservation of the biliary and the gastroduodenal tracts (Fig. 14.5).

14.2.3 Distal Pancreatectomy

Indications for distal pancreatectomy are tumors of the left-sided pancreas. The pancreatic tail and parts of the pancreatic body are resected. Usually, splenectomy has to be performed for anatomical or techni-

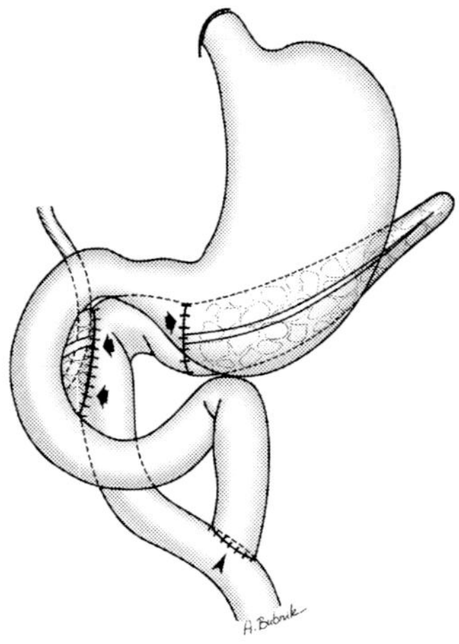

Fig. 14.5. Duodenum-preserving pancreatic head resection. Subtotal resection of the pancreatic head leaving the periampullary pancreatic tissue and the choledochal duct in situ. The pancreatic remnants are sutured end-to-end and end-to-side to a separated jejunal loop (*short arrows*). *Arrowhead*, enteroenterostomy

cal reasons. This operation has a lower complication rate than pancreaticoduodenectomy (Fig. 14.6a,b).

14.2.4 Tumor Enucleation

Tumor enucleation is restricted to well-defined or encapsulated benign pancreatic lesions such as benign apudomas (e.g., insulinoma), lipoma, fibroma, and postpancreatic pseudotumorous lesions.

14.2.5 Palliative Treatment

Palliative hepatojejunostomy in the case of biliary obstruction has been replaced by interventional radiology and endoscopy, with or without stenting in most cases (Beger et al. 1994; Laugier and Renou 1998). In patients with gastroduodenal obstruction, stenting is rarely performed and a gastrojejunostomy is still used as a palliative operation (Fig. 14.7a,b).

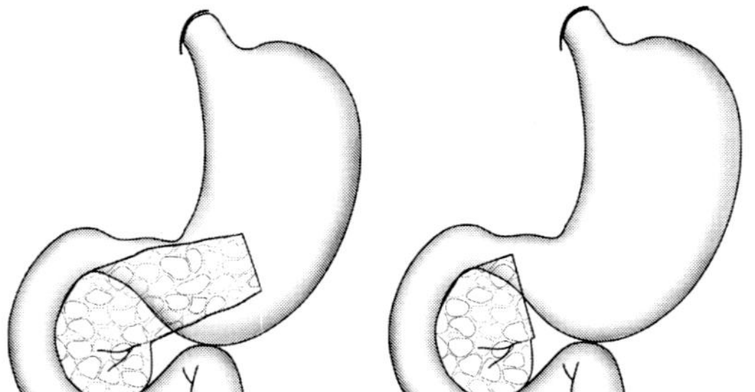

a b

Fig. 14.6a,b. Distal pancreatectomy. In the case of a left-sided pancreatic tumor, distal (**a**) or extended distal pancreatectomy (**b**) is performed

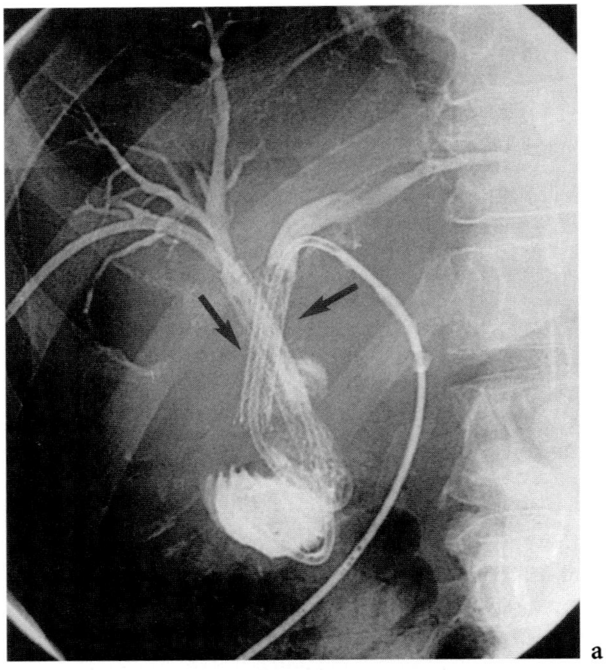

a

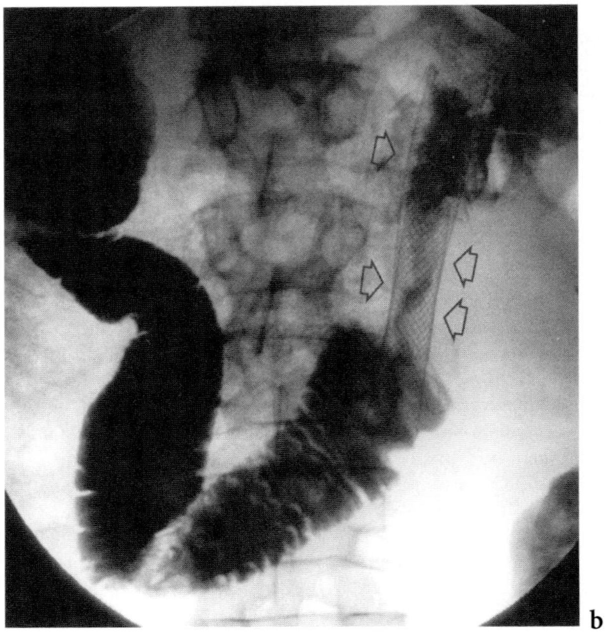

b

Fig. 14.7a,b. Tumor stenosis of the biliodigestive anastomosis and the afferent loop in a patient 3 months after the Whipple procedure for carcinoma of the distal common bile duct. Percutaneous transhepatic cholangiography and stenting of the biliodigestive anastomosis (*arrows*) (**a**), as well as stenting of the afferent loop (*open arrows*) (**b**)

14.3 Postoperative Imaging

Plain film, upper GI series, sonography, computed tomography (CT), and magnetic resonance imaging (MRI) are used to evaluate the postoperative pancreas.

14.3.1 Perioperative and Postoperative Period

The use of abdominal plain films are confined to the peri- and postoperative period in the case of suspected ileus or free air due to anastomotic dehiscence.

Upper GI series with non-ionic, water-soluble contrast medium given orally or administered via nasogastric tube is performed in the case of suspected dehiscence of enteroenteric anastomosis or possible obstruction of the gastrojejunostomy.

In the perioperative period, the efficacy of sonography is impaired by postoperative free abdominal air and/or increased bowel gas due to paralysis.

Spiral CT is superior to all other imaging modalities to demonstrate the normal postoperative anatomy (Fig. 14.8a,b) and complications such as abscesses, bilomas, and hematomas. For this purpose, the entire abdomen needs to be investigated.

14.3.2 Follow-up Period

Upper GI series are used to demonstrate the regular postoperative situation at the gastroenteric and enteroenteric anastomosis (Fig. 14.9). Normally, the afferent loops (e.g., choledochojejunostomy and separated pancreaticojejunostomy) and the enteroenteric anastomosis (Braun's anastomosis) are not visualized. Furthermore, upper GI series can demonstrate inflammatory or ulcerative disease of the gastric remnant or at the gastrojejunostomy.

Sonography is frequently used in late follow-up for the detection of local tumor recurrence or liver metastases. However, contrast-enhanced spiral CT is far superior to other techniques and should be used as the primary imaging modality (Fig. 14.10). Several modifications such as tri-phasic, bolus-guided, spiral hydro-CT may increase accuracy in the detection of tumor recurrence (Lentschig et al. 1996; Richter et al. 1996; Dux et al. 1996).

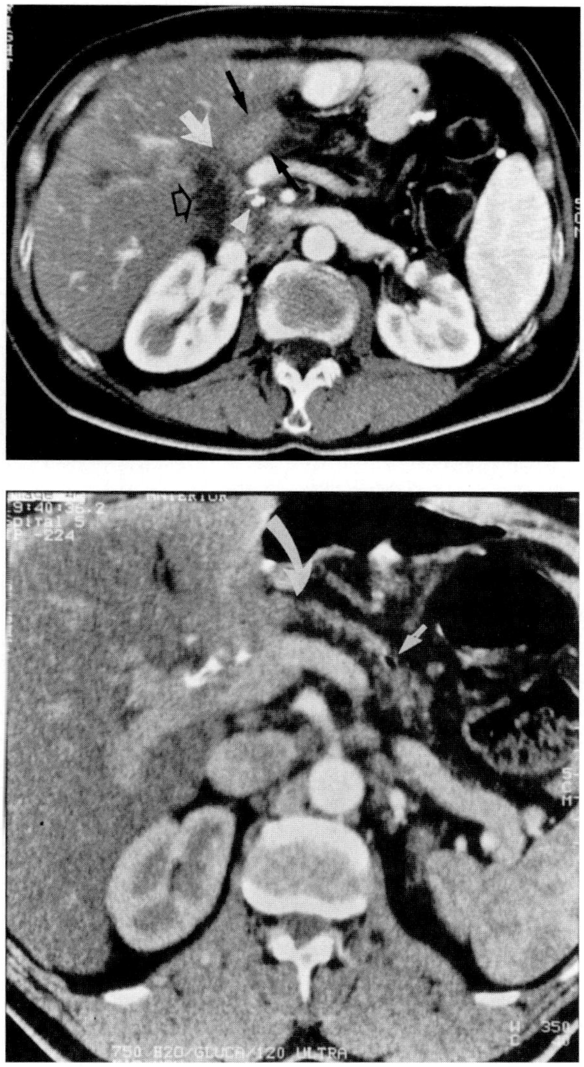

a

b

Fig. 14.8a,b. Regular postoperative anatomy after a standard Whipple procedure for adenocarcinoma of the pancreatic head, demonstrated with contrast-enhanced spiral computed tomography of the upper abdomen. Both the pancreatic remnant (*black arrows*) and the choledochojejunostomy (*white arrow*) are of regular appearance. Metallic clips (*arrowhead*) are seen within the pancreatic bed. Note the well-distended blind jejunal loop (*open arrow*). **b** Regular postoperative anatomy after a modified Whipple procedure for mucous cystadenoma in the pancreatic head. Regular appearance of the atrophic pancreatic remnant and the pancreaticojejunostomy (*curved arrow*). Note the small air bubble within the pancreatic duct (*straight arrow*), which can frequently be seen after pancreaticojejunostomy

In comparison to CT, MRI plays a minor role in the evaluation of tumor recurrence (Fig. 14.11). However, for investigation of the biliary tract, biliodigestive anastomosis, and the pancreatic duct, MRI is superior to other techniques and has replaced percutaneous transhepatic cholangiography in many

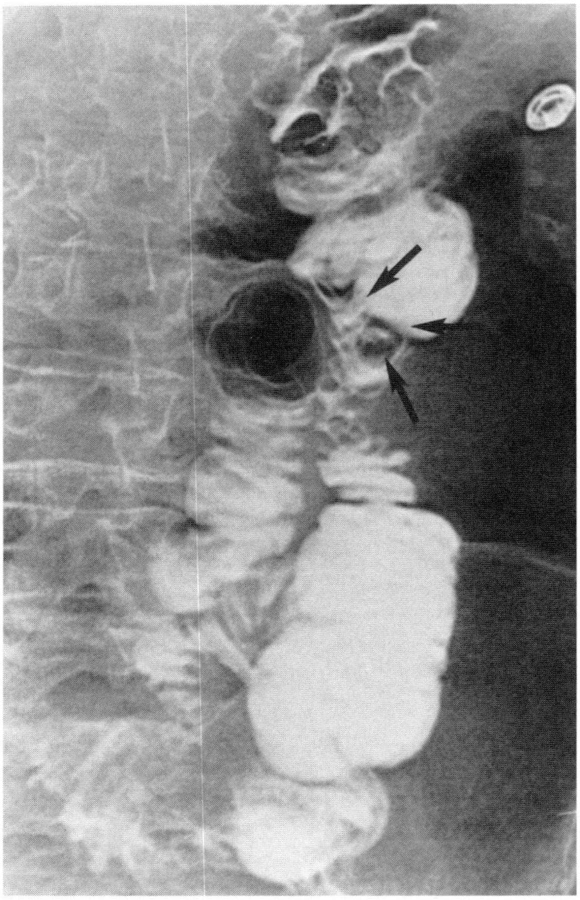

Fig. 14.9. Upper abdominal series with water-soluble non-ionic contrast material 14 months after total pancreatectomy for carcinoma of the pancreatic duct. Normal anatomy of the gastrojejunostomy (*arrows*)

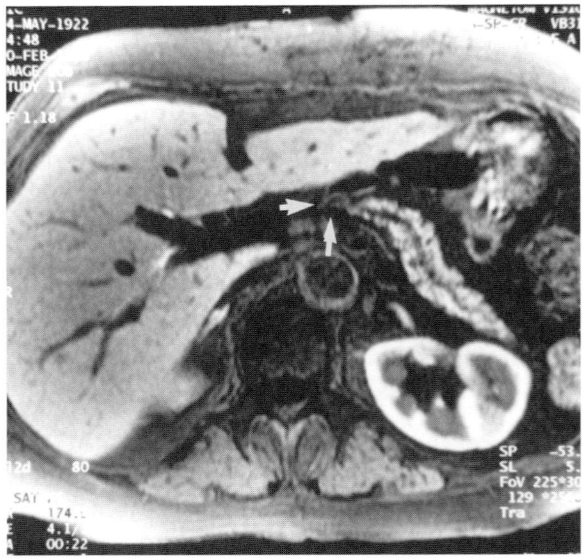

Fig. 14.11. Modified Whipple procedure for carcinoma of the pancreatic head. Contrast-enhanced magnetic resonance imaging (T1-weighted gradient-echo sequence, fat saturation) shows a normal postoperative anatomy. The pancreatic remnant is unremarkable with a slightly pronounced pancreatic duct. Regular appearance of the pancreaticojejunostomy (*arrows*)

a

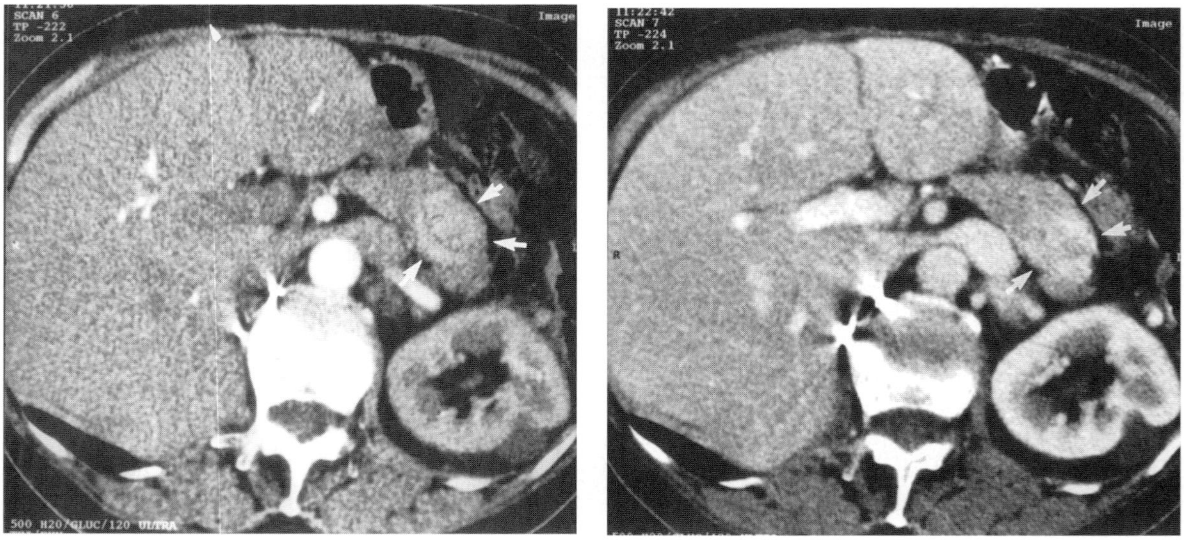

b

Fig. 14.10a,b. Tri-phasic computed tomography of the pancreas 17 months after distal pancreatectomy for metastases of hypernephroma in the pancreatic tail. Both in the arterial phase (**a**) and the portal phase (**b**), a hyperdense lesion of 3 cm in diameter is visible in the pancreatic remnant, indicating tumor recurrence (*arrows*) cases. These structures are best visualized with half-Fourier single-shot turbo spin-echo (HASTE), fat-suppressed T2-weighted and three-dimensional turbo spin-echo sequences (PAVONE et al. 1997; LOMANTO et al. 1997).

14.4 Postoperative Complications

Perioperative mortality in patients who have undergone the Whipple procedure has been reduced during recent years due to the improvement of the surgical technique, anesthesia, and intensive care support (DEL FERNANDEZ et al. 1995). In centers specified in pancreatic surgery, a perioperative mortality of less than 5 % is achieved (CAMERON et al. 1993).

14.4.1 Anastomotic Dehiscence and Abscess Formation

The most frequent postoperative complication is pancreatic fistulas due to leakage of the pancreaticojejunostomy (15%–20%) (BÜCHLER et al. 1996; YEO et al. 1997). Abscess formation is rare and is avoided by drainage of the anastomotic site (SIKORA and POSNER 1995). In the case of suboptimal drainage and/or infection, the fistulas will persist and lead to abscess formation. Less frequently, an abscess may develop at other sites of the abdomen (e.g., subphrenic) with or without radiologic demonstration of a leakage. With contrast-enhanced spiral CT, abscesses are best differentiated from other fluid collections such as biloma or hematoma (Fig. 14.12a,b).

Much less frequent dehiscence of the biliodigestive anastomosis may occur (5%), which is eventually followed by biloma (Fig. 14.13a) (STRASBERG et al. 1997). With proper drainage, spontaneous healing usually occurs (Fig. 14.13b).

Dehiscence of the gastrojejunostomy is rare due to technical advances, absorbable suture materials, and the introduction of stapling devices.

14.4.2 Acute Postoperative Pancreatitis

Postoperative edema of the pancreatic remnant occurs frequently, caused by surgical manipulation, and usually resolves without specific treatment. In a few cases, pancreatic necrosis develops and may be complicated by anastomotic leakage, abscess formation, and peritonitis (Fig. 14.14). Necrotic pancreatitis may be complicated by infection in 10% of cases, which is associated with a high mortality rate and has to be treated either by CT-guided percutaneous drainage or by necrosectomy (BEGER et al. 1997; RAU et al. 1997; FREENY et al. 1998).

14.4.3 Pancreatic Pseudocysts

Pancreatic pseudocyst is a late complication and is usually found several weeks after surgery. These

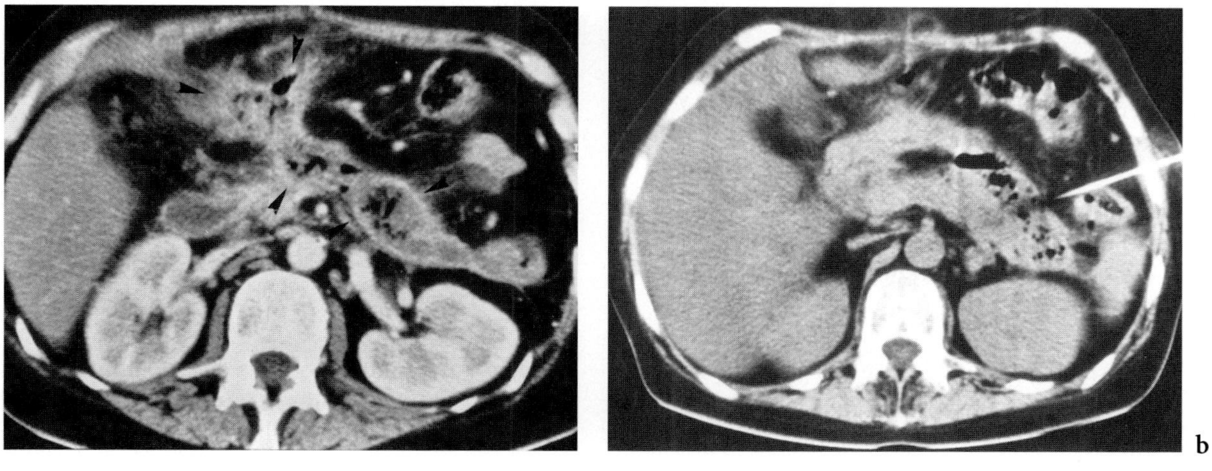

a b

Fig. 14.12. a Abscess formation 3 weeks after a modified Whipple procedure for chronic pancreatitis of the pancreatic head and biliary obstruction. Contrast-enhanced spiral computed tomography (CT) shows an ill-defined pancreatic remnant. An inhomogeneously structured, encapsulated liquid collection with marginal contrast enhancement and multiple gas bubbles indicating abscess formation can be observed (*arrowheads*). **b** Interventional CT-guided drainage of the abscess was successfully performed

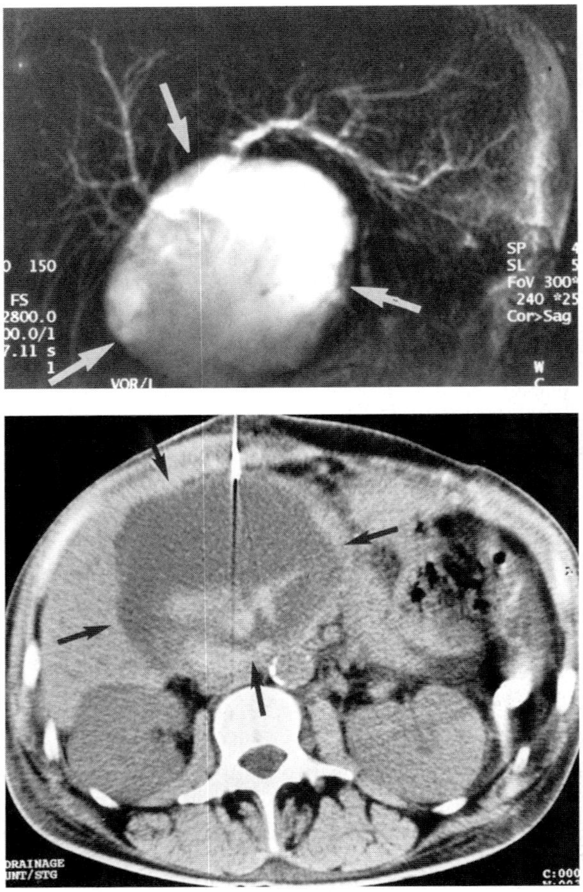

Fig. 14.13a,b. Biloma 3 weeks after a modified Whipple procedure for chronic pancreatitis. **a** Cholangio-magnetic resonance imaging (half-Fourier single-shot turbo spin echo) shows dilated biliary tree and a 10-cm biloma at the liver hilus following leakage of the biliodigestive anastomosis. **b** Computed tomography-guided drainage of the biloma was successfully performed

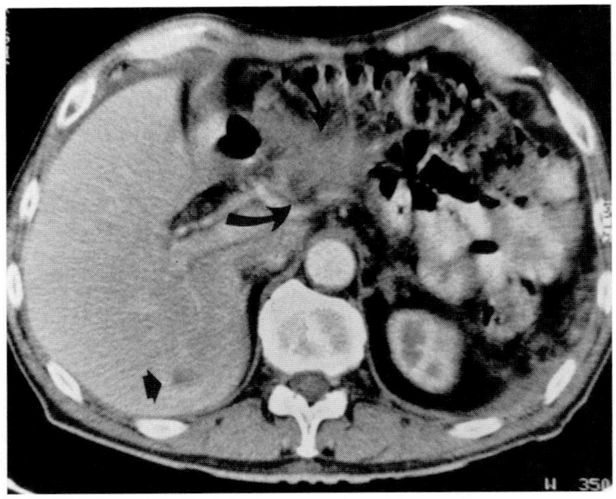

Fig. 14.14. Contrast-enhanced spiral computed tomography of the upper abdomen 3 weeks after a Whipple procedure for carcinoma of the pancreatic head. An ill-defined and inhomogeneously structured pancreatic remnant indicating pancreatitis is observed (*curved arrow*), which resolved spontaneously under conservative treatment. Metastatic lesion in the

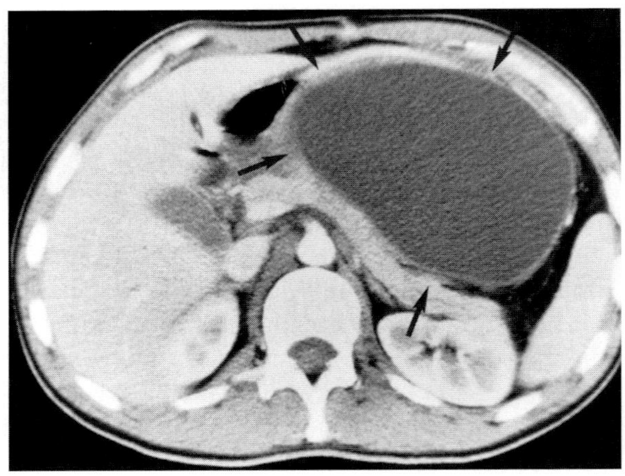

Fig. 14.15. Large pancreatic pseudocyst in the left upper abdomen 2 weeks after enucleation of a benign insulinoma of the pancreatic body. Contrast-enhanced spiral computed tomography (CT) of the upper abdomen shows a homogeneous, hypodense lesion, which was successfully treated with CT-guided percutaneous drainage

pseudocysts are often asymptomatic; however, they may increase in size and cause clinical symptoms. Interventional radiology is the treatment of choice (Fig. 14.15).

14.4.4 Stenosis of the Biliodigestive and Gastroenteric Anastomosis

Stenosis of the biliodigestive and gastroenteric anastomosis may be caused by inflammation, fibrosis, or by compression and infiltration due to tumor growth. In the case of jaundice or bowel obstruction, interventional procedures such as balloon dilatation or stenting may be used for treatment (see Fig. 14.7a,b).

14.4.5 Tumor Recurrence

A major determinant of survival is tumor recurrence, which is closely related to operative and histopathological staging of the tumor. After curative resection, the 5-year survival rate ranges between 5%–40%, the best prognosis shown among patients with UICC stage I (T_1 or T_2, N_0, M_0) (Crist and Cameron 1992; Geer and Brennan 1993).

14.4.5.1
Local Recurrence

Local recurrence results from residual tumor in lymph nodes, pancreatic remnants, fatty tissue, and perineural invasion. Typically, clinical and radiological signs of tumor recurrence appear 12–18 months after radical tumor resection (Strasberg et al. 1997; Yeo et al. 1997). Contrast-enhanced spiral CT is the imaging modality of choice in the case of suspected tumor recurrence or liver metastases (Fig. 14.16a,b).

14.4.5.2
Distant Metastases

At the time of primary diagnosis, 50%–80% of patients already present with distant metastases and these patients are not eligible for curative surgery (Auerbach et al. 1997; Büchler et al. 1996). Also, in patients where curative resection was possible, the liver is the most common site of occurrence of distant metastases with or without local tumor recurrence. In almost all patients who die from pancreatic cancer, liver metastases have developed (Fig. 14.17a,b). Other sites of distant metastases are the lung and the skeleton.

There is no generally accepted regimen for the follow-up of patients after radical resected pancreatic cancer. At our institution, contrast-enhanced spiral CT and laboratory tests are performed alternately every 3 months for the first 2 postoperative years.

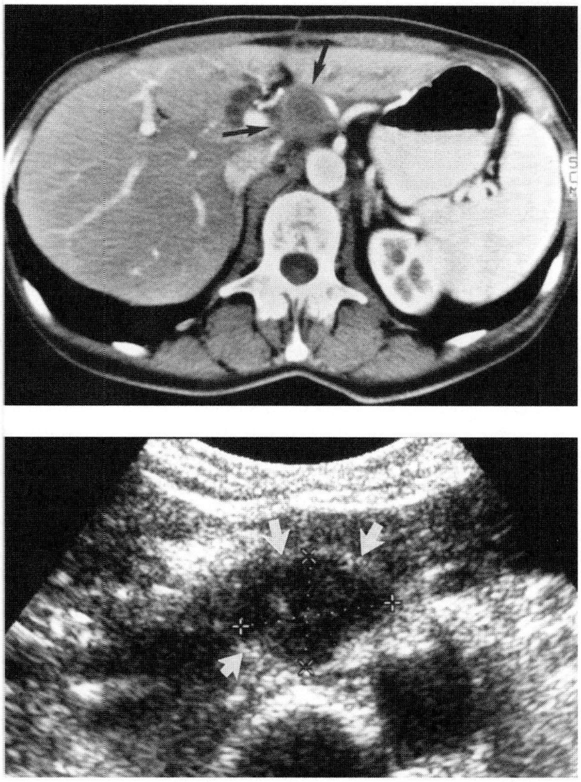

Fig. 14.16. Contrast-enhanced spiral computed tomography (**a**) and sonography of the upper abdomen (**b**) 6 months after a Whipple procedure for carcinoma of the choledochal duct. Lymph node metastasis of 3 cm in diameter was detected between the celiac artery and the portal vein

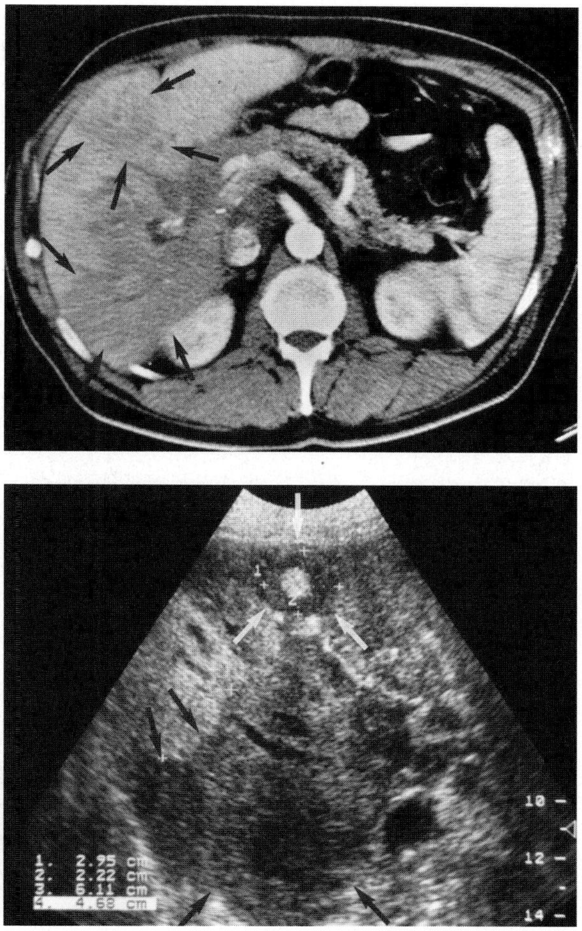

Fig. 14.17a,b. Liver metastases 19 months after a modified Whipple procedure for carcinoma of the choledochal duct. Contrast-enhanced spiral computed tomography of the upper abdomen (**a**) and sonography of the liver (**b**). Diffuse inhomogeneously structured liver parenchyma indicating diffuse metastases (*arrows*). There is no sign of local recurrence. The pancreaticojejunostomy is well seen

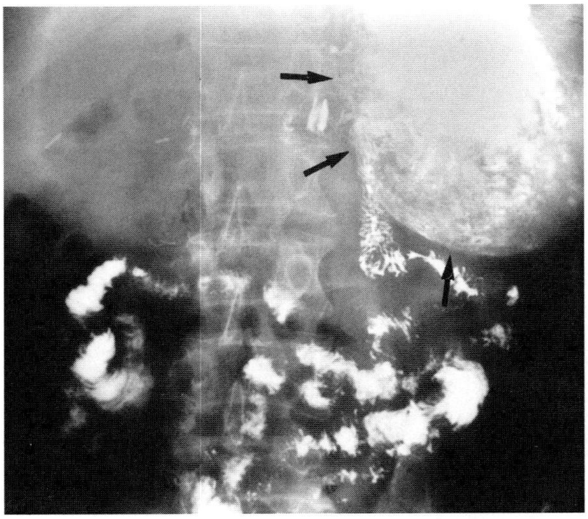

Fig. 14.18. Upper abdominal series 10 days after a Whipple procedure for chronic pancreatitis. Distended gastric remnant with large amounts of fasting stomach contents (*arrows*) and prolonged gastric emptying due to stenosis following inflammation and mucosal swelling of the gastroenteric anastomosis

14.4.6 Digestive Sequelae

Among the morbidities of pancreaticoduodenectomy are those that may be seen in any patient undergoing hemigastrectomy, such as dumping, bile-reflux gastritis, and marginal ulceration. The latter has been caused by the advent of H_2-blocker therapy. Delayed gastric emptying can occur after both the pancreaticoduodenectomy and pylorus-preserving procedures and may affect 25%–40% of patients. This sequela, however, is self-limiting and rarely extends beyond 6 weeks (Fig. 14.18) (Strasberg et al. 1997). Greasy stools and diabetes may also occur and are often long-lasting and may require lifelong therapy (McLeod et al. 1995; Müller et al. 1997).

References

Auerbach M, Wampler GL, Lokich JJ, Fryer D, Ahlgren JD (1997) Treatment of advanced pancreatic carcinoma with a combination of protracted infusional 5-fluorouracil and weekly carboplatin: a Mid-Atlantic Oncology Program Study. Ann Oncol 8:439–444

Bakkevold KE, Arnesjo B, Kambestad B (1992) Carcinoma of the pancreas and papilla of Vater-assessment of resectability and factors influencing resectability in stage I carcinomas. A prospective multicentre trial in 472 patients. Eur J Surg Oncol 18:494–507

Beger HG, Buchler MW, Friess H (1994) Surgical results and indications for adjuvant measures in pancreatic cancer. Chirurg 65:246–252

Beger HG, Schoenberg MH, Link KH, Safi F, Berger D (1997) Duodenum-preserving pancreatic head resection – a standard method in chronic pancreatitis. Chirurg 68:874–880

Büchler M, Friess H (1993) Inhibition of pancreatic secretion to prevent postoperative complications following pancreatic resection. Acta Gastroenterol Belg 56:271–278

Büchler MW, Uhl W, Malfertheiner P (1996) Pankreaserkrankungen: Akute Pankreatitis, chronische Pankreatitis, Tumore. Karger, Basel

Büchler MW, Baer HU, Seiler C, Reber-Pum Sadowski C, Friess H (1997) Duodenum preserving resection of the head of the pancreas: a standard procedure in chronic pancreatitis. Chirurg 68:364–368

Cameron JL, Pitt HA, Yeo CJ, Lillemoe KD, Kaufman HS, Coleman J (1993) One hundred and fifty-five consecutive pancreaticoduodenectomies without mortality. Ann Surg 217:430–438

Cavallini M, Tallerini A, Stipa F (1991) Occlusion of the duct with a fibrin glue and preservation of the pylorus after resection of the duodenum and head of the pancreas for periampullary carcinoma. Minerva Chir 46:733–739

Connolly MM (1987) Survival in 1001 patients with carcinoma of the pancreas. Ann Surg 206:358

Crist DW, Cameron JL (1992) The current status of the Whipple operation for periampullary carcinoma. Adv Surg 25:21–49

del Fernandez C, Rattner DW, Warshaw AL (1995) Standards for pancreatic resection in the 1990 s. Arch Surg 130:295–300

DiMagno EP (1991) Pancreatic adenocarcinoma (1893–1991). In: Textbook of gastroenterology, vol 2. Yamada

Dux M, Richter GM, Roeren T, Heuschen U, Kauffmann GW (1996) Gastrointestinal imaging with hydrosonography and hydro-CT. Rofo Fortschr Geb Rontgenstr Neuen Bildgeb Verfahr 164:359–367

Freeny PC, Hauptmann E, Althaus SJ, Traverso LW, Sinanan M (1998) Percutaneous CT-guided catheter drainage of infected acute necrotizing pancreatitis: techniques and results. AJR Am J Roentgenol 170:969–975

Geer RJ, Brennan MF (1993) Prognostic indicators for survival after resection of pancreatic adenocarcinoma. Am J Surg 165:68–73

Gordon TA, Burleyson GP, Tielsch JM, Cameron JL (1995) The effects of regionalization on cost and outcome for one general high-risk surgical procedure. Ann Surg 221:43–49

Grace PA, Pitt HA, Tomkins RK (1986) Decreased morbidity and mortality after pancreatoduodenectomy. Am J Surg 151:141

Laugier R, Renou C (1998) Endoscopic ductal drainage may avoid resective surgery in painful chronic pancreatitis without large ductal dilatation. Int J Pancreatol 23:145–152

Lentschig MG, Reimer P, Rummeny E, Grenzheuser C, Daldrup HE, Berns T, Dinse P, Sulkowski U, Peters PE (1996) The value of 3-phase spiral CT and magnetic resonance tomography in preoperative diagnosis of pancreatic carcinoma. Radiologe 36:406–412

Lomanto D, Pavone P, Laghi A Panebianco V, Mazzocchi P, Fiocca F, Lezoche E Passariello R, Speranza V (1997) Magnetic resonance-cholangiopancreaticography in the diagnosis of biliopancreatic diseases. Am J Surg 174:33–38

McLeod RS, Taylor BR, O'Connor BI, Greenberg GR, Jeejeebhoy KN, Royall D, Langer B (1995) Quality of life, nutritional status and gastrointestinal hormone profile following the Whipple procedure. Am J Surg 169:179–185

Muller MW, Friess H, Beger HG, Kleeff J, Lauterburg B, Glasbrenner B, Riepl RL, Buchler MW (1997) Gastric emptying following pylorus-preserving Whipple and duodenum-preserving pancreatic head resection in patients with chronic pancreatitis. Am J Surg 173:257–263

Pavone P, Laghi A, Catalano C, Broglia L, Panebianco V, Messina Am, Salvatori FM, Passariello R (1997) MR cholangiography in the examination of patients with biliary-enteric anastomosis. AJR Am J Roentgenol 169:807–811

Rau B, Uhl W, Buchler MW, Beger HG (1997) Surgical treatment of infected necrosis. World J Surg 21:155–161

Richter GM, Simon C, Hoffmann V, DeBernardinis M, Seelos R, Senninger N, Kauffmann GW (1996) Spiral hydro-CT of the pancreas in the thin-slice method. Radiologe 36:379–405

Schenk M, Severson RK, Pawlish KS (1998) The risk of subsequent primary carcinoma of the pancreas in patients with cutaneous malignant melanoma. Cancer 82:1672–1676

Sikora SS, Posner MC (1995) Management of the pancreatic stump following pancreaticoduodenectomy. Br J Surg 82:1590–1597

Strasberg SM, Drebin JA, Soper NJ (1997) Evolution and current status of the Whipple procedure: an update for gastroenterologists. Gastroenterology 113:983–994

Takada T, Yasuda H, Amano H, Yoshida M, Ando H (1997) Results of a pylorus-preserving pancreatoduodenectomy for pancreatic cancer: a comparison with results of the Whipple procedure. Hepatogastroenterology 44:1536–1540

Traverso LW, Longmire WPJ (1978) Preservation of the pylorus in pancreaticoduodenectomy. Surg Gynecol Obstet 146:959

Widmaier U, Schmidt A, Schlosser W, Beger HG (1997) Duodenum preserving resection of the head of the pancrease in therapy of pancreas divisum. Chirurg 68:180–186

Whipple AO, Parsons WB, Mullins CR (1935) Treatment of carcinoma of the ampulla of Vater. Ann Surg 102:763

Yeo CJ, Cameron JL (1991) The pancreas. Textbook of surgery. Sabiston DC Jr (ed) Durham, NC pp 1076–1107

Yeo CJ, Cameron JL, Sohn TA, Lillemoe KD, Pitt HA, Talamini MA, Hruban RH, Ord SE, Sauter PK, Coleman J, Zahurak ML, Grochow LB, Abrams RA (1997) Six hundred fifty consecutive pancreaticoduodenectomies in the 1990s: pathology, complications and outcomes. Ann Surg 226:248–257; discussion 257–260

Subject Index

List of Contributors

Albert L. Baert, MD
Professor
Department of Radiology
University Hospital K.U.L.
Herestraat 49
B-3000 Leuven
Belgium

P. H. Bernard, MD
Practicien Hospitalier, Service des Maladies de l'Appareil Digestif (Pr Quinton)
Centre Hôpitalier et Universitaire
Hôpital Saint-André
1, Rue Jean Borguet
F-33075 Bordeaux Cédex
France

J.C. Brichaux, MD
Service de Radiologie
Groupe Hospitalier Pellegrin
Place Amélie-Raba-Léon
F-33076 Bordeaux Cédex
France

Jean-Michel Bruel, MD
Professor of Radiology
Hôpital Saint-Eloi
Avenue Bertin Sans
F-34059 Montpellier Cédex
France

M. Brun, MD
Service de Radiologie A
Hôpital Pellegrin
Place A Raba Léon
F-33076 Bordeaux
France

P. Brys, MD
Resident
Department of Radiology
University Hospital K.U.L.
Herestraat 49
B-3000 Leuven
Belgium

J. F. Chateil, MD
Service de Radiologie A
Hôpital Pellegrin
Place Amélie-Raba-Léon
F-33076 Bordeaux Cédex
France

B. Claikens, MD
Department of Radiology
University Hospital K.U.L.
Herestraat 49
B-3000 Leuven
Belgium

F. Diard, MD
Professeur de Radiologie
Service de Radiologie A
Hôpital Pellegrin
Place Amélie-Raba-Léon
F-33076 Bordeaux Cédex
France

B. Dousset, MD
Hôpital Cochin
Service de Chirurgie Digestive
Assistance Publique
Hôpitaux de Paris
27 rue du Faubourg Saint-Jacques
F-75679 Paris Cédex 14
France

C. Douws, MD
Service de Radiologie
Groupe Hospitalier Pellegrin
Place Amélie-Raba-Léon
F-33076 Bordeaux Cédex
France

Jacques Drouillard, MD
Professeur de Radiologie
Université de Bordeaux II
Hôpital Haut Lévêque - U.S.N. - C.H.U. Bordeaux
Avenue de Magellan
F-33604 Pessac
France

P. M. Dubois
Professeur
CNRS-URA 1454, Université Claude Bernard
Faculté de Médicine Lyon Sud
Laboratoire d'Histologie et d'Embryologie, BP 12
F-96900 Oullins
France

Jean-Francois Flejou, MD
Associate Professor
Department of Pathology, Hôpital Beaujon
100, Bd du Général Leclerc
F-92118 Clichy
France

R. Függer, MD
Department of General Surgery
Allgemeines Krankenhaus
University of Vienna
Währinger Gürtel 18–20
A-1090 Vienna
Austria

F. Grabenwöger, MD
Department of Radiology (7F)
Allgemeines Krankenhaus
University of Vienna
Währinger Gürtel 18–20
A-1090 Vienna
Austria

P. Grelet, MD
Service de Radiologie
Hôpital Saint-André
1, Rue Jean Burguet
F-33075 Bordeaux Cédex
France

J. Grellet, MD
Groupe Hospitalier Pitié – La Salpétrière
Service Central de Radiologie
Assistance Publique
Hôpitaux de Paris
47–83 Boulevard de l'Hôpital
F-75651 Paris Cédex 13
France

N. Grenier, MD
Service de Radiologie
Groupe Hospitalier Pellegrin
Place Amélie-Raba-Léon
F-33076 Bordeaux Cédex
France

A.M. Herneth, MD
Department of Radiology (7F)
Allgemeines Krankenhaus
University of Vienna
Währinger Gürtel 18–20
A-1090 Vienna
Austria

Günter Klöppel, MD, PhD
Professor and Chairman
Klinikum der Christian-Albrechts-Universität zu Kiel
Department of Pathology
University of Kiel
Michaelisstraße 11
D-24105 Kiel
Germany

Francois Laurent, MD
Professeur de Radiologie
Université de Bordeaux II
Hôpital Haut Lévêque - U.S.N.-
C.H.U. Bordeaux
Avenue de Magellan
F-33604 Pessac
France

R. Lecesne, MD
Service d'Imagerie Médicale
Radiologie Diagnostique et Thérapeutique
Université de Bordeaux II
Hôpital Haut Lévêque, USN
C.H.U. Bordeaux
Avenue de Magellan
F-33604 Pessac
France

G. Lechner, MD
Department of Radiology (7F)
Allgemeines Krankenhaus
University of Vienna
Währinger Gürtel 18--20
A-1090 Vienna
Austria

Paul Legmann, MD
Professor
Hôpital Cochin, Service de Radiologie
Assistance Publique, Hôpitaux de Paris
27 rue du Faubourg Saint-Jacques
F-75679 Paris Cédex 14
France

Guy Marchal, MD
Professor
Department of Radiology
University Hospital K.U.L.
Herestraat 49
B-3000 Leuven
Belgium

Didier Mathieu, MD
Professor of Radiology
Hôpital Henri Mondor
51, Avenue du Maréchal de Lattre
de Tassigny
F-94010 Créteil Cédex
France

E. Ponette, MD
Professor
Department of Radiology
University Hospital K.U.L.
Herestraat 49
B-3000 Leuven
Belgium

Alain Rahmouni, MD
Assistant Professor
Department of Radiology
Hôpital Henri Mondor
51, Avenue du Maréchal de Lattre
de Tassigny
F-94010 Créteil Cédex
France

J.W.A.J Reeders, MD
Department of Diagnostic Radiology
Academic Medical Center
Meibergdreef 9
1105 AZ Amsterdam Zuidoost
The Netherlands

Hans Rigauts, MD
Resident
Department of Radiology
University Hospital K.U.L.
Herestraat 49
B-3000 Leuven
Belgium

A. Roche, MD
Service de Radiodiagnostic
Unité de Radiologie Interventionnelle
et Vasculaire
Institut Gustave Roussy
Rue Camille Desmoulins
F-94805 Villejuif Cédex
France

E. Schlüter, MD, PhD
Department of Pathology
Academic Hospital Jette
Free University of Brussels
Laarbeeklaan 101
B-1090 Brussels
Belgium

N.J. Smits, MD
Department of Gastrointestinal Radiology
and Hepato-Pancreato-Biliary Imaging
Academic Medical Center
Amsterdam
The Netherlands

Patrice Taourel, MD
Assistant Professor
Hôpital Saint-Eloi
Avenue Bertin Sans
F-34059 Montpellier Cédex
France

E. Thérasse, MD
Service de Radiodiagnostic
Unité de Radiologie Interventionnelle
et Vasculaire
Institut Gustave Roussy
Rue Camille Desmoulins
F-94805 Villejuif Cédex
France

H. Trillaud, MD
Fellow in Radiology
Service de Radiologie
Groupe Hôspitalier Pellegrin
Place Amélie-Raba-Léon
F-33076 Bordeaux Cédex
France

O.M. Van Delden, MD
Department of Gastrointestinal Radiology
and Hepato-Pancreato-Biliary Imaging
Academic Medical Center
Amsterdam
The Netherlands

Lieven Van Hoe, MD, PhD
Assistant Professor
Department of Radiology
University Hospital K.U.L.
Herestraat 49
B-3000 Leuven
Belgium

W. Van Steenbergen, MD
Professor
Department of Internal Medicine
Liver Unit
University Hospital K.U.L.
Herestraat 49
B-3000 Leuven
Belgium

O. Vignaux, MD
Hôpital Cochin
Service de Radiologie
Assistance Publique
Hôpitaux de Paris
27 rue du Faubourg Saint-Jacques
F-75679 Paris Cédex 14
France

Valérie Vilgrain, MD
Professor
Department of Radiology
Hopital Beaujon
100, Boulevard du Général Leclerc
F-92118 Clichy
France

Medical Radiology
Diagnostic Imaging and Radiation Oncology

Titles in the series already published

Diagnostic Imaging

Innovations in Diagnostic Imaging
Edited by J.H. Anderson

Radiology of the Upper Urinary Tract
Edited by E.K. Lang

The Thymus - Diagnostic Imaging, Functions, and Pathologic Anatomy
Edited by E. Walter, E. Willich, and W.R. Webb

Interventional Neuroradiology
Edited by A. Valavanis

Radiology of the Pancreas
Edited by A.L. Baert, co-edited by G. Delorme

Radiology of the Lower Urinary Tract
Edited by E.K. Lang

Magnetic Resonance Angiography
Edited by I.P. Arlart, G.M. Bongartz, and G. Marchal

Contrast-Enhanced MRI of the Breast
S. Heywang-Köbrunner and R. Beck

Spiral CT of the Chest
Edited by M. Rémy-Jardin and J. Rémy

Radiological Diagnosis of Breast Diseases
Edited by M. Friedrich and E.A. Sickles

Radiology of the Trauma
Edited by M. Heller and A. Fink

Biliary Tract Radiology
Edited by P. Rossi

Radiological Imaging of Sports Injuries
Edited by C. Masciocchi

Modern Imaging of the Alimentary Tube
Edited by A. R. Margulis

Diagnosis and Therapy of Spinal Tumors
Edited by P. R. Algra, J. Valk, and J. J. Heimans

Interventional Magnetic Resonance Imaging
Edited by J. F. Debatin and G. Adam

Abdominal and Pelvic MRI
Edited by A. Heuck and M. Reiser

Orthopedic Imaging
Techniques and Applications
Edited by A.M. Davies and H. Pettersson

Radiology of the Female Pelvic Organs
Edited by E.K.Lang

Magnetic Resonance of the Heart and Great Vessels
Clinical Applications
Edited by J. Bogaert, A. J. Duerinckx, and F. E. Rademakers

Modern Head and Neck Imaging
Edited by S. K. Mukherji and J. A. Castelijns

Radiological Imaging of Endocrine Diseases
Edited by J. N. Bruneton in collaboration with B. Padovani and M.-Y. Mourou

Trends in Contrast Media
Edited by H. S. Thomsen, R. N. Muller, and R. F. Mattrey

Functional MRI
Edited by C. T. W. Moonen and P. A. Bandettini

Radiology of the Pancreas
2nd Revised Edition
Edited by A. L. Baert
Co-edited by G. Delorme and L. Van Hoe

Radiation Oncology

Lung Cancer
Edited by C.W. Scarantino

Innovations in Radiation Oncology
Edited by H.R. Withers and L.J. Peters

Radiation Therapy of Head and Neck Cancer
Edited by G.E. Laramore

Gastrointestinal Cancer – Radiation Therapy
Edited by R.R. Dobelbower, Jr.

Radiation Exposure and Occupational Risks
Edited by E. Scherer, C. Streffer, and K.-R. Trott

Radiation Therapy of Benign Diseases - A Clinical Guide
S.E. Order and S.S. Donaldson

Medical Radiology
Diagnostic Imaging and Radiation Oncology

Titles in the series already published

Radiation Oncology

Interventional Radiation Therapy Techniques - Brachytherapy
Edited by R. Sauer

Radiopathology of Organs and Tissues
Edited by E. Scherer, C. Streffer, and K.-R. Trott

Concomitant Continuous Infusion Chemotherapy and Radiation
Edited by M. Rotman and C.J. Rosenthal

Intraoperative Radiotherapy – Clinical Experiences and Results
Edited by F.A. Calvo, M. Santos, and L.W. Brady

Radiotherapy of Intraocular and Orbital Tumors
Edited by W.E. Alberti and R.H. Sagerman

Interstitial and Intracavitary Thermoradiotherapy
Edited by M.H. Seegenschmiedt and R. Sauer

Non-Disseminated Breast Cancer
Controversial Issues in Management
Edited by G.H. Fletcher and S.H. Levitt

Current Topics in Clinical Radiobiology of Tumors
Edited by H.-P. Beck-Bornholdt

Practical Approaches to Cancer Invasion and Metastases
A Compendium of Radiation Oncologists' Responses to 40 Histories
Edited by A.R. Kagan with the Assistance of R.J. Steckel

Radiation Therapy in Pediatric Oncology
Edited by J.R. Cassady

Radiation Therapy Physics
Edited by A.R. Smith

Late Sequelae in Oncology
Edited by J. Dunst and R. Sauer

Mediastinal Tumors. Update 1995
Edited by D.E. Wood and C.R. Thomas, Jr.

Thermoradiotherapy and Thermochemotherapy
Volume 1:
Biology, Physiology, and Physics
Volume 2:
Clinical Applications
Edited by M.H. Seegenschmiedt, P. Fessenden, and C.C. Vernon

Carcinoma of the Prostate
Innovations in Management
Edited by Z. Petrovich, L. Baert, and L.W. Brady

Radiation Oncology of Gynecological Cancers
Edited by H.W. Vahrson

Carcinoma of the Bladder
Innovations in Management
Edited by Z. Petrovich, L. Baert, and L.W. Brady

Blood Perfusion and Microenvironment of Human Tumors
Implications for Clinical Radiooncology
Edited by M. Molls and P. Vaupel

Radiation Therapy of Benign Diseases. A Clinical Guide
2nd Revised Edition
S.E. Order and S.S. Donaldson

Carcinoma of the Kidney and Testis, and Rare Urologic Malignancies
Innovations in Management
Edited by Z. Petrovich, L. Baert, and L.W. Brady

Progress and Perspectives in the Treatment of Lung Cancer
Edited by P. Van Houtte, J. Klastersky, and P. Rocmans

Springer and the environment

At Springer we firmly believe that an international science publisher has a special obligation to the environment, and our corporate policies consistently reflect this conviction.
We also expect our business partners – paper mills, printers, packaging manufacturers, etc. – to commit themselves to using materials and production processes that do not harm the environment. The paper in this book is made from low- or no-chlorine pulp and is acid free, in conformance with international standards for paper permanency.